# Sterile Compounding and Aseptic Technique

## Concepts, Training, and Assessment for Pharmacy Technicians

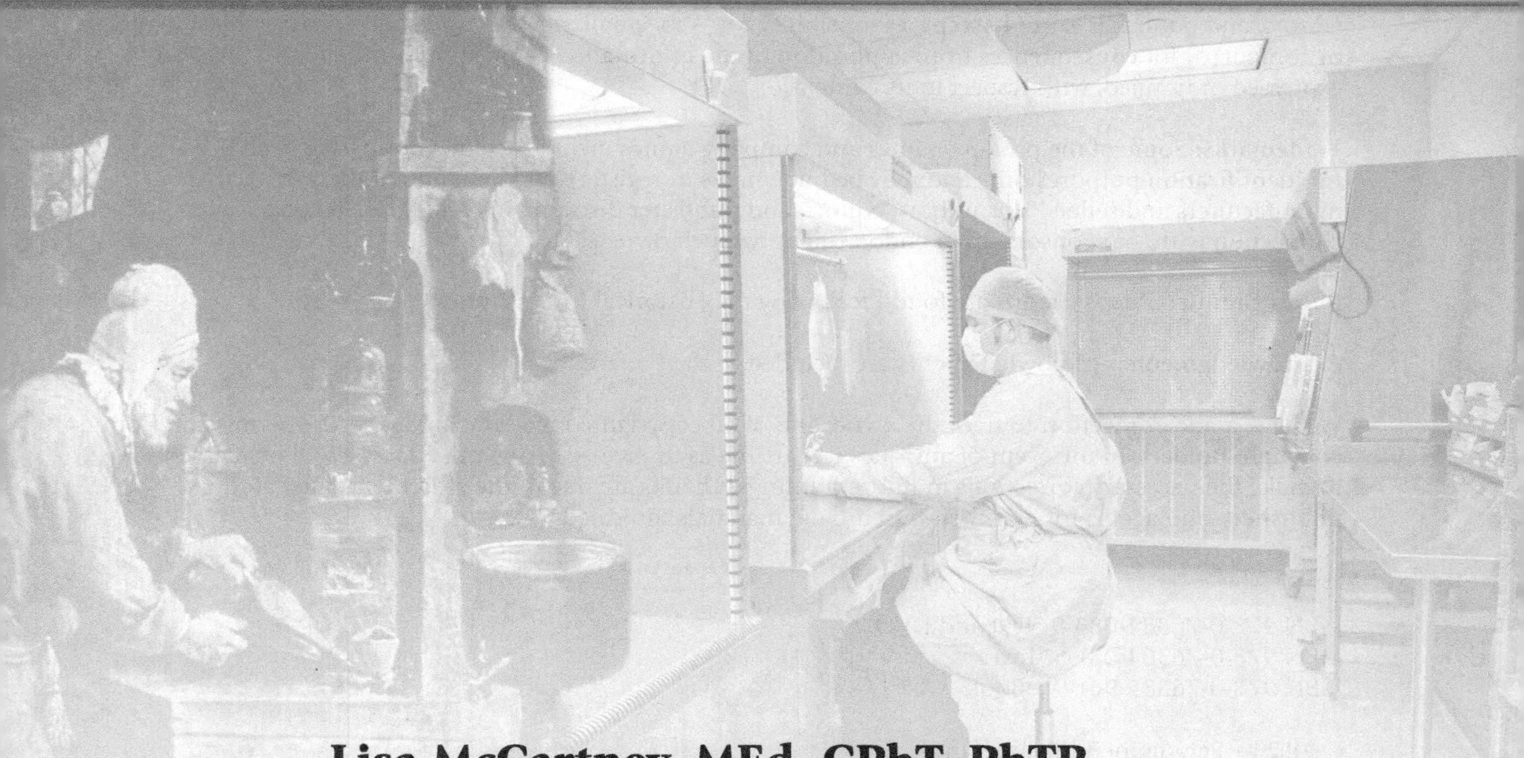

Lisa McCartney, MEd, CPhT, PhTR

PARADIGM
EDUCATION SOLUTIONS
St. Paul

| | |
|---|---|
| **Managing Editor:** | Brenda M. Palo |
| **Editor and Writer:** | Nancy Papsin |
| **Production Editor:** | Bob Dreas |
| **Senior Graphic Designer:** | Leslie Anderson |
| **Senior Design and Production Specialist:** | Jaana Bykonich |
| **Photo Researchers:** | Nancy Papsin, Stefan Johansson, Stephanie Schempp, Cassie Kunshier |
| **Copy Editor:** | Melanie P. Hagge |
| **Proofreaders:** | Sarah Kearin, Stefan Johansson, Melanie P. Hagge |
| **Indexer:** | Schroeder Indexing Services |
| **Permissions Coordinator:** | Lindsay Ryan |
| **Cover Images:** | Courtesy of the National Library of Medicine (left); George Brainard (right) |
| **Illustrators:** | Cohographics, Rolin Graphics, Inc. |



**Photo Credits:** Photo Credits are found following the Historical Images Index.

**Acknowledgments:** Acknowledgments are included in the Preface.



ISBN 978-0-76384-083-9 Text and DVD
ISBN 978-0-76384-081-5 Text
ISBN 978-0-76385-961-9 eBook


875 Montreal Way
St. Paul, MN 55102
Email: educate@emcp.com
Website: www.emcp.com



Printed in the United States of America

28 27 26 25 24 23 22 21 4 5 6 7 8 9 10 11

# Brief Contents

# Table of Contents

# Preface

*Sterile Compounding and Aseptic Technique: Concepts, Training, and Assessment for Pharmacy Technicians* provides technician-focused instruction and training for the successful production of sterile parenteral preparations, a major responsibility of the pharmacy technician in hospitals, long-term care facilities, and home healthcare. This important work requires mastery of aseptic technique: the procedures that ensure patient safety and consistent, pathogen-free products.

This book is both a textbook and a training manual, first introducing the student to the history, methods, and regulation of sterile compounding and aseptic technique, and then leading students through multiple layers of procedural instruction that help to ensure learning. Various activities and exercises challenge students to demonstrate knowledge and effective technique through independent, small-group, and large-group options. Written in compliance to the most recent USP Chapter <797> pharmacy practice standards, *Sterile Compounding and Aseptic Technique* provides a working knowledge of the essential aspects of this subject, including:

- The history and context of current standards, prior legislation, and the origins of the need for pharmacy and sterile compounding
- The tools, materials, and environments involved, and the methods of handling and cleaning them as required by industry standards
- Pertinent terminology and abbreviations
- Interpreting medication orders and interpreting and creating labels
- Personal garbing and cleanliness procedures
- Methods for preparing common types of parenteral products, such as large- and small-volume preparations using drugs provided in vials and ampules, as well as specialized products for pediatrics, narcotics, TPN, and chemotherapy

## Alignment with Current Standards and Certifications

This book helps students master aseptic technique and, importantly:

- Aligns with USP Chapter <797> Revised Standards
- Prepares students for passing process validation checklists given by instructors during course training and by pharmacy supervisors during on-the-job initial and annual aseptic technique validation
- Aligns with ASHP's Model Curriculum for Pharmacy Technician Training
- Provides comprehensive coverage of all procedures and techniques related to the ACPE skill set for IV admixtures
- Prepares students to earn ACPE certification in sterile compounding and aseptic technique as granted by an ACPE-accredited CPE provider
- Helps students to prepare for the Pharmacy Technician Certification Exam (PTCE)

# Organization of the Text

*Sterile Compounding and Aseptic Technique* contains fourteen chapters divided into two units. Unit 1, "Exploring the Basics of Sterile Compounding," introduces students to the field, describing the tools, materials, and environments required, the standards and legislation involved, and the methods for creating and interpreting the documentation associated with sterile compounding work. The exploratory labs in the Unit 1 chapters offer the step-by-step instruction and thorough training that students need to understand the skills necessary for professional laboratory compounding procedures.

Unit 2, "Compounding Sterile Preparations," begins the more traditional laboratory section of the textbook, first teaching garbing and cleaning techniques and then guiding students as they prepare sterile products in the laboratory environment. The second unit progresses from the most simple procedures—such as performing a correct hand washing—to increasingly complex procedures that cover the preparation of parenteral products, ending with the final, in-depth chapter on preparing chemotherapy products.

# Appendices

Four appendices are included in the book. Appendix A, Student Answer Key for Concepts Self-Check, provides answers to the Concepts Self-Check questions. Appendix B, Useful Reference Tables, offers supplemental information for the Chapter 4 content. Appendix C, Resources for Chemotherapy Compounding, contains essential guidelines for the Chapter 14 content. Lastly, Appendix D, the Process Validation Checklists, provides the process validation forms that correspond with the Procedural Labs of Chapters 6–14.

> *SPECIAL NOTE ON APPENDIX D:* The Appendix D checklists are appropriate for use during pharmacy "in-house" initial and annual training evaluations, provided that only those personnel who achieve 100% compliance be validated as having the necessary skills, technique, and ability to perform sterile compounding and aseptic technique procedures.
>
> It is considered best practice that all personnel who prepare compounded sterile preparations complete an ACPE-accredited certification course in sterile compounding and aseptic technique (i.e., IV certification). Instruction may be provided through classroom lecture, online distance learning, self-study modules, or a combination of these methods. Experiential training should be provided by a skilled and experienced ACPE-certified instructor in a hospital pharmacy or laboratory facility that utilizes state-of-the-art equipment and supplies. Instruction and training for sterile compounding personnel should follow current USP <797> standards, and be in alignment with ASHP's Model Curriculum for Pharmacy Technician Training.
>
> For more information on ACPE certification in sterile compounding and aseptic technique (also know as IV certification), please refer to the Internet Resource Center at www.paradigmcollege.net/sterilecomp or contact the author directly at lmccartney@emcp.com.

# Chapter Features

Each chapter includes learning objectives, a topic-related historical introduction, a Concepts section that discusses the central ideas and techniques and concludes with an independent student assessment, a Training section that studies important supplies and procedures in depth, an exploratory or procedural lab that provides step-by-step technique, and an Assessment section that contains a chapter summary, a listing of key terms, ten multiple-choice questions, three critical thinking questions (one requiring Internet research), one higher-level challenge activity, and a listing of additional topics for students to explore.

A key feature of this text is the step-by-step instruction for every lab, fine-tuned over the author's extensive career and teaching experience. These steps provide clear details on locating important topical information, preparing to enter the work environment, and compounding sterile preparations while ensuring total aseptic conditions. Many steps are illustrated with full-color photographs of the described technique, and the Chapters 6–14 videos offer brief but clear demonstrations of every skill and task.

Other chapter features include:

- Three distinct marginalia tips:
  - POINTER A Pointer that offers tips grounded in best practice knowledge
  - BE AWARE A Safety Alert that calls attention to possible safety concerns
  - A USP Chapter <797> tip that highlights important regulations from Chapter <797> of the *USP Pharmacists' Pharmacopeia*
- Beautiful and varied educational images in the chapter opener, including vintage and historical photos and drawings (catalogued in the Historical Images Index) that inspire further interest and study
- Photos and photo sequences that accompany lab steps, and photos, figures, and tables in Parts 1 and 2 that enhance student understanding of concepts and techniques
- A training video DVD icon that alerts students to watch the associated chapter video demonstration
- A layered chapter structure that reinforces the subject matter that students must later demonstrate with 100% accuracy in order to pass rigorous competency requirements

# Additional Resources for the Student

In addition to the student textbook, the following tools and resources are available to students.

## Student Resources DVD

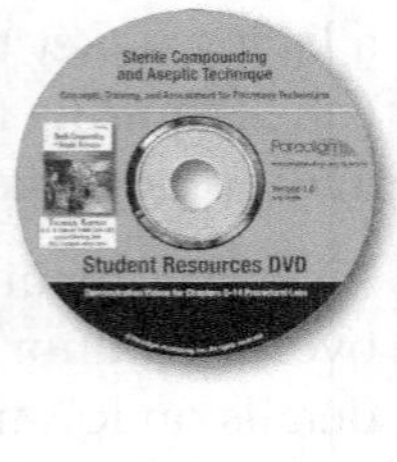


The Student Resources DVD included with each textbook contains video demonstrations of the nine procedural labs of Unit 2 (Chapters 6–14). The author introduces and narrates each video and performs each lab procedure. These videos are intended to supplement your learning process, and the author recommends your viewing them several times as you practice and perfect your aseptic technique.

## Internet Resource Center

The Internet Resource Center for this title is located at www.paradigmcollege.net/sterilecomp. This website provides additional resources, such as Spanish for Pharmacy Technicians, guidelines for dispensing medications, links to professional resources, and much more. Access to the site is free.

## eBook

For students who prefer studying with an eBook, this text is available in an electronic form. The Web-based, password-protected eBook features dynamic navigation tools, including bookmarking, a linked table of contents, and the ability to jump to a specific page. The eBook format also supports helpful study tools, such as highlighting and note taking.

# Resources for the Instructor

## *Instructor's Guide* and DVD with EXAMVIEW

The print *Instructor's Guide* offers course planning tools, syllabus suggestions, chapter-specific teaching hints, and answers for all end-of-chapter exercises.

All of the resources from the print *Instructor's Guide* are also provided on the Instructor Resources DVD. In addition, the DVD includes PowerPoint presentations and the EXAMVIEW Assessment Suite, a full-featured computerized test generator offering instructors a wide variety of options for generating both print and online tests. The test banks provide 35 multiple-choice questions for each chapter. Instructors can create custom tests using the chapter item banks and edit questions or add new items of their own design.

## Internet Resource Center

Many of the features that appear in the print *Instructor's Guide* and on the Instructor Resources DVD are also available on the password-protected section of the Internet Resource Center for this title at www.paradigmcollege.net/sterilecomp.

# Additional Pharmacy Technician Textbooks from Paradigm

In addition to *Sterile Compounding and Aseptic Technique*, Paradigm Publishing, Inc. offers other titles designed specifically for the pharmacy technician curriculum:

- *Pharmacy Labs for Technicians, Second Edition*
- *Pharmacology Essentials for Technicians*
- *Pharmacology for Technicians, Fifth Edition*
- *Pharmacology for Technicians Workbook, Fifth Edition*
- *Pharmacy Practice for Technicians, Fifth Edition*
- *Pharmacy Calculations for Technicians, Fifth Edition*
- *Certification Exam Review for Pharmacy Technicians, Third Edition*

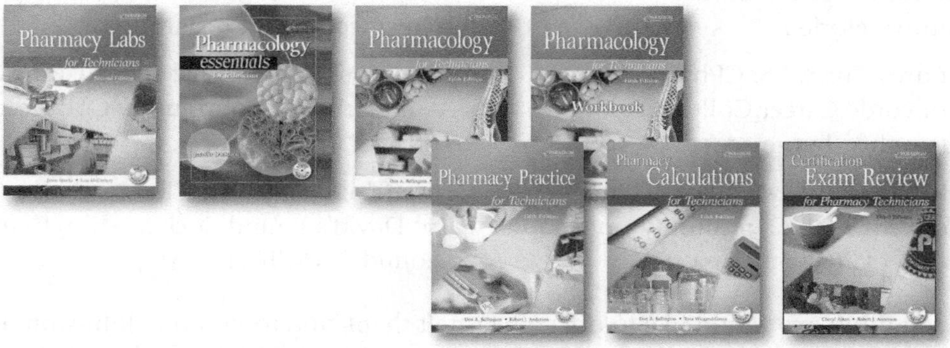


# About the Author

**Lisa McCartney**, MEd, CPhT, PhTR, has been an ACPE-certified instructor in sterile product preparation and aseptic technique since 1997. She is the department chair for the ASHP-accredited pharmacy technology program at Austin Community College, where she specializes in teaching hospital pharmacy courses, including sterile product preparation. She has been educating pharmacy technicians since 1999. Lisa has worked as a pharmacy technician for more than 30 years and spent 15 years as a lead IV trainer and supervisor in the busy hospital pharmacy of a Level I trauma center. She has also worked in the community, pediatric, and oncology pharmacy settings. She became a PTCB-certified pharmacy technician in 1995 and has been registered with the State of Texas since 2005. She received her AAS degree in Pharmacy Technology from Weatherford College, Weatherford, Texas in 2008. In 2011, she received her BAAS degree with an emphasis in Occupational Education from Texas State University in San Marcos. In 2013, she received her master's degree in Education from Texas State University. Lisa is a 2011 International NISOD Award winner for *Teaching and Leadership Excellence*. In 2012, she received the Roy Kemp award from the Pharmacy Technician Educator's Council, and in 2013, the Mike Knapp award from the Texas Society of Health-System Pharmacists. Lisa is the co-author of the Paradigm Publishing book, *Pharmacy Labs for Technicians*. Lisa currently serves on the board of the Pharmacy Technician Educator's Council and is the chair-elect for the technician executive committee for the Texas Society of Health-System Pharmacists and serves on the USP Chapter <797> Expert Panel for the United States Pharmacopeia.

# Acknowledgments

The author and editors are grateful to the many professionals who provided constructive feedback by reviewing project proposals, drafts of manuscript, or early versions of the text. The following individuals participated in the development of *Sterile Compounding and Aseptic Technique*:

Larry M. Allen, MBA, PhD, RPh
Arapahoe Community College
Littleton, Colorado

Linda Calvert, BS, MS
Front Range Community College
Westminster, Colorado

April B. Cortright, CPhT
Sanford Brown Institute
Tampa, Florida

Andrea Curry, BS, CPhT
Concorde Career College
Memphis, Tennessee

Michelle "Shelly" Dillon, CPhT
Bossier Parish Community College
Bossier City, Louisiana

Candice Geiger, BS, CPhT
Midlands Technical College
Columbia, South Carolina

Richard Nunez, RPhT, CPhT
Everest College
San Francisco, California

Tonya Phillips, BS, CPhT
Piedmont Technical College
Greenwood, South Carolina

Stephanie E. Smith-Baker, BS, CPhT, CAHI
Anne Arundel Community College
Arnold, Maryland

Lisa Thibodeaux, CPhT
St. David's Round Rock Medical Center
Round Rock, Texas

In addition, we would like to offer a heartfelt thank-you to Philip E. Johnston, RPh, and Margaret Wallace, PharmD, for their thorough and careful review of early pages of the textbook content and end-of-chapter materials, and beta versions of the procedural videos. The editorial team also thanks George Brainard of George Brainard Photography, for his excellent in-laboratory photographs of supplies, equipment, and technique; and Alex Valkema, owner and director of O'Blivion Pictures, for his production of the procedural videos on the Student Resources DVD.

Finally, Jeff Johnson of Minneapolis, Minnesota, prepared the test bank materials and Janet Blum of Ontario, Canada, prepared the PowerPoint slides for the Instructor's DVD; and Judy Peterson of Two Harbors, Minnesota, created the supplemental test materials. We thank them for their contributions.

The author and editorial staff invite your comments on the text and its supplements. Please reach us by clicking the Contact Us link at www.paradigmcollege.net/sterilecomp.

# Author's Acknowledgments

I have so many people to thank for their support, love, and encouragement throughout the writing and production of this book. I would like to dedicate this book to them. To my family—for your wry and twisted sense of humor, thanks and love to each of you; remember that there's plenty of room for everyone at the Rattlesnake Ranch. To the Robinsons, and the rest of my Austin family—thank you for your understanding and support; I love you. To my dear friend and fellow author Susan Guthrie—my door is always open; I love you. To my JUMP team and everyone at USM—without your support and encouragement, I would have never jumped out of a perfectly good airplane, nor written a book. Thank you to all of the educators—who continue to inspire me to be the best teacher that I can be; especially Phil Sheldon, who encouraged me in the 12th grade to pursue my dream of becoming an author. To everyone at ACC—in appreciation of your dedication to providing an exceptional learning environment for our students; I am blessed to work with such amazing people. To George Brainard—your wonderful photos have enhanced the book immeasurably. To Alex Valkema and Nick Myers—for your creativity and humor during the photo and video sessions; I look forward to seeing the blooper reel. To Jason Sparks—for asking me to co-author the *Pharmacy Labs for Technicians* book, setting this all in motion. To Brenda Palo and Nancy Papsin—the editorial dream team—when we take *BNH's and the Zone of Turbulence* on tour, I will be more than honored to share the stage with you! To Rebecca LaBrum—for your "pharmacy eyes" and last-minute editing support. To the pharmacy technicians that I have been fortunate enough to work with over the years—know that what you do, and the dedication with which you provide quality pharmacy services, does make a difference in the lives of those you serve. To my mentors John-Roger, John Morton, and doctors Ron and Mary Hulnick—you have inspired me to create the life of my dreams and then go out and live it; I appreciate you more than words can say. Most important, to my partner Liz LaRue—without your tremendous patience and encouragement, this book simply would not have been written. For you, my most heartfelt acknowledgment. I am so grateful for the light and joy you bring to my life. I am humbled and blessed by your loving, kindness, and support, and I am so very thankful that we are on this journey together. Finally, thank you, Spirit, for this life and all its many blessings!

Namaste
~Lisa

# Oath of a Pharmacy Technician

I dedicate myself to providing pharmacy technician services of the highest quality to all patients, regardless of situation or circumstance, and I will consider the health and safety of my patients my primary concern.

I will uphold the highest principles of moral, ethical, and legal conduct, and will perform my duties with honesty and integrity.

I will use my knowledge, skills, and abilities to ensure optimal patient treatment outcomes, while always operating within the pharmacy technician's scope of practice.

I will maintain patient confidentiality, promote individual dignity, and treat all patients with respect, compassion, and appreciation for diversity.

I will work closely with pharmacists and other healthcare professionals to ensure that quality pharmaceutical care is dispensed without error.

I will strive to provide excellent customer service and effective communication, supported by an exceptional work ethic, while maintaining absolute accuracy and ensuring patient health and safety.

I will stay informed regarding developments in the field of pharmacy and will maintain professional competency, striving to continually enhance my knowledge, skills, and expertise.

I will participate in the evolution of a pharmaceutical practice that improves patient care, and will actively support organizations that further the profession and support the advancement of pharmacy technicians.

I will respect, value, and support my colleagues; foster a sense of loyalty and duty to the profession of pharmacy; and actively participate as a member of the healthcare team.

I will strive to conduct myself with professionalism and integrity and maintain a full appreciation of the responsibility that the public entrusts to me.

# Unit 1

# Exploring the Basics of Sterile Compounding

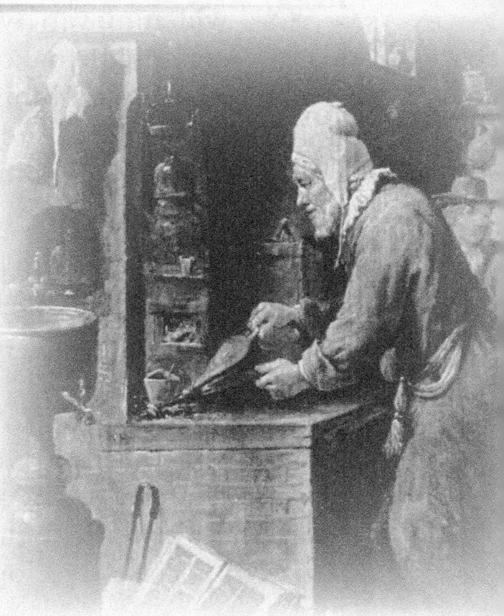



## Early Pharmacy as Art

We can trace the origins of pharmacy back to the earliest civilizations, when the women and men who were healers in their communities used local flowers, herbs, and other natural substances to treat illness and disease. Varied cultures from every continent have long demonstrated an understanding of the healing properties of such materials, as supported by the numerous archaeological digs that have uncovered ancient writings, tools, and instruments related to healing work.

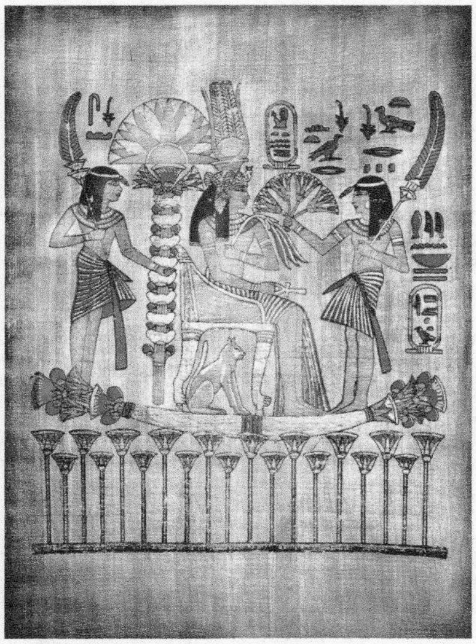

Evidence of pharmaceutical compounding can also be found in the stories of several religious traditions. Ancient Islamic texts tell of the medicinal properties of plants and the use of various chemical compounds to promote healing. The excavation of numerous Egyptian tombs provides evidence that religious ceremonies, such as burials, used compounded ointments, salves, and perfumes. The Christian Nativity story is another example of the link between religion and the origin of pharmacy. This story includes a wise man who gifts the healing substance myrrh to the newborn baby Jesus. Myrrh is still used today as a homeopathic treatment for inflammatory conditions of the mouth and gums, and to treat chronic cough.

As world cultures developed due to expanding opportunities for travel, information gleaned from focused study, and increased cross-cultural

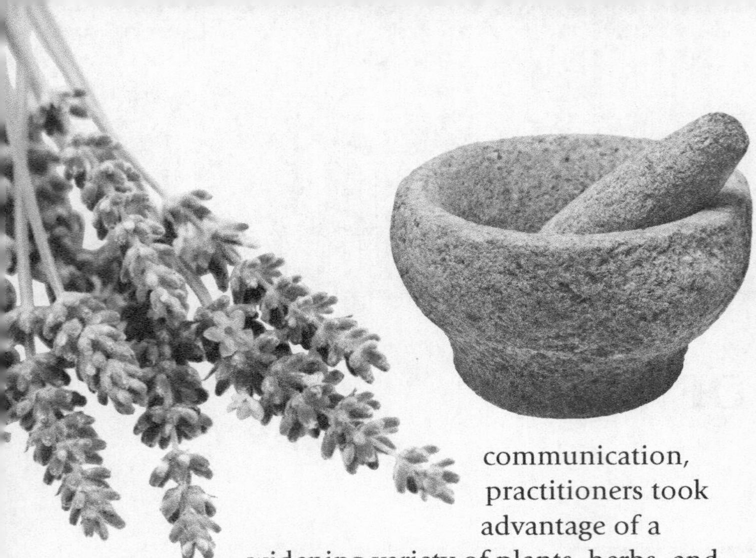

communication, practitioners took advantage of a widening variety of plants, herbs, and other medicinal compounds. Their careful work, artfully combining the products of the natural world into helpful compounds, gradually developed into the healing art known today as pharmacy.

Some notable people who have been instrumental in the creation and development of pharmacy include the Greek physicians Hippocrates (ca. 460 BCE – ca. 370 BCE) and Galen (129 CE – 216 CE). Hippocrates is often referred to as "The Father of Medicine" and is credited with encouraging a scientific approach to medicine and pharmacy, helping to debunk early myths that illness was caused by evil spirits. Hippocrates developed the concept of the body's four **humors**: blood, phlegm, black bile and yellow bile. Each was associated with a particular organ: blood with the heart; phlegm, the lungs; black bile, the spleen; and yellow bile, the gallbladder. When the humors were harmonious and in balance an individual maintained a healthful state, or **eucrasia** (meaning "good mixture"). If one humor became excessive and upset the body's equilibrium, the diagnosis was **dyscrasia** (meaning "bad mixture"), and illness or disease ensued. Galen is commonly known as "The Father of Pharmacy" for his efforts to systematically classify the pharmaceuticals used to treat illness and disease. Works of historic Greek literature, such as *The Iliad* and *The Odyssey*, tell the tales of some of the women who were instrumental in the development of ancient pharmacy. For example, Agamede, Princess of Elis, was a well-known healer who used herbal compounds and medicinal tinctures to treat soldiers wounded in the Trojan War.

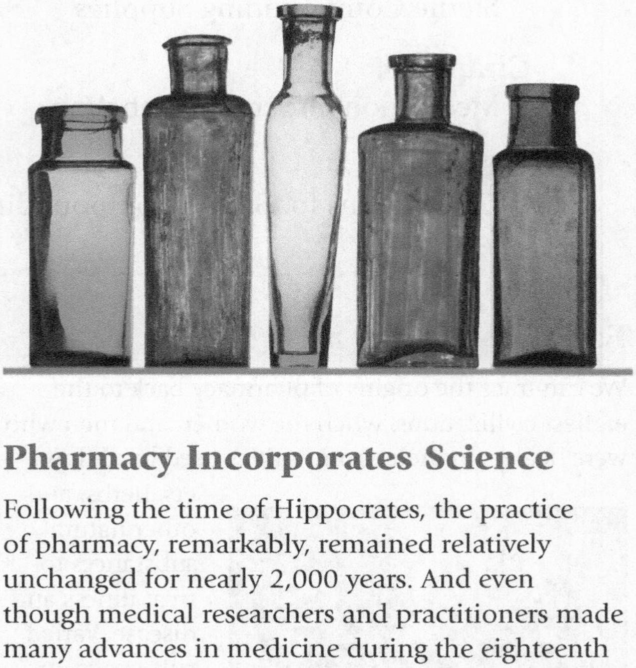

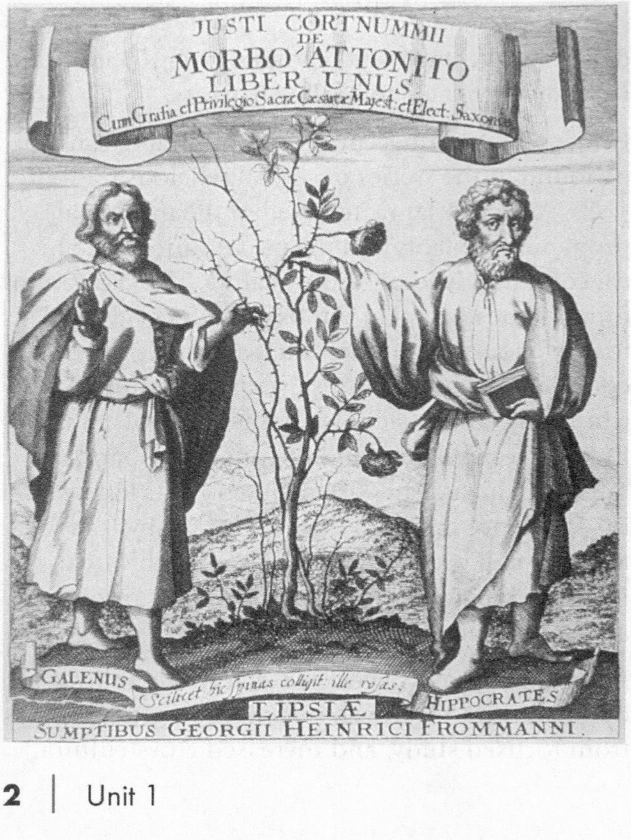
JUSTI CORTNUMMII
DE
MORBO ATTONITO
LIBER UNUS
Cum Gratia et Privilegio Sacræ Cæsareæ Majest: et Elect: Saxon:
GALENUS
HIPPOCRATES
LIPSIÆ
SUMPTIBUS GEORGII HEINRICI FROMMANNI

## Pharmacy Incorporates Science

Following the time of Hippocrates, the practice of pharmacy, remarkably, remained relatively unchanged for nearly 2,000 years. And even though medical researchers and practitioners made many advances in medicine during the eighteenth century, these advances did not significantly affect pharmacy until the mid-nineteenth century when Dr. Joseph Lister and Louis Pasteur made some important discoveries. In 1867, Lister determined that hospital deaths would decrease significantly if personnel thoroughly cleaned surgical instruments and environments before using them. In the 1870s, Louis Pasteur's work with germ theory led doctors to realize the importance of hand washing and proper sanitization in preventing the transmission

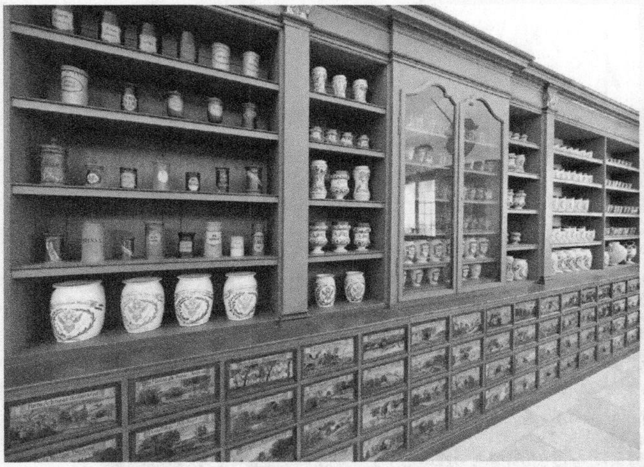

of disease. In fact, Lister's and Pasteur's work led to the development of pharmacy procedures and techniques that eventually expanded to become the sterile compounding and aseptic technique practices of today.

Modern pharmaceutical science uses a combined understanding of chemistry, botany, and herbology to discover and synthesize the medications used to treat a wide variety of conditions. Pharmacists and pharmacy technicians work with physicians, nurses, and other healthcare practitioners to dispense medications that treat illness, injury, and disease. Compounding practices have evolved from the creative, but slower, trial-and-error process of mixing tinctures, balms, and liniments in the small chemists' hutches of drugstores to the precise sterile compounding procedures performed in today's sleek, modern pharmacy facilities.

Although pharmacy has gained a scientific and technical framework over the last 150 years, its association as an art remains. In fact, the current edition of *Merriam-Webster's Collegiate Dictionary* defines pharmacy firstly as "the art, practice, or profession of preparing, preserving, compounding, and dispensing medical drugs."

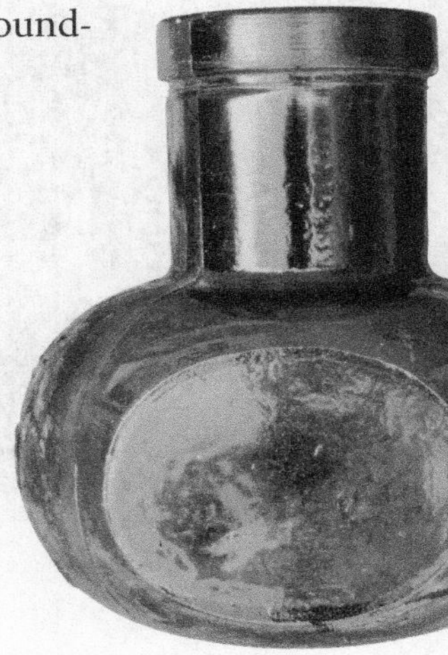

## Unit 1 Overview: Five Exploratory Labs

Unit 1 of this textbook offers a basic overview of the origins of sterile compounding and introduces the regulations outlined in the *USP Pharmacists' Pharmacopeia*. (Additional details and specific procedures are provided in Unit 2.) This unit discusses the proper environment, equipment, and supplies necessary for sterile compounding. It also highlights pertinent terminology and abbreviations related to pharmacy practice as well as explains how to interpret medication orders and prescriptions, verify medication labeling, and perform pharmaceutical calculations. The chapters in Unit 1 are ordered to provide a firm foundation of knowledge about sterile compounding basics, and each chapter builds on those that precede it.

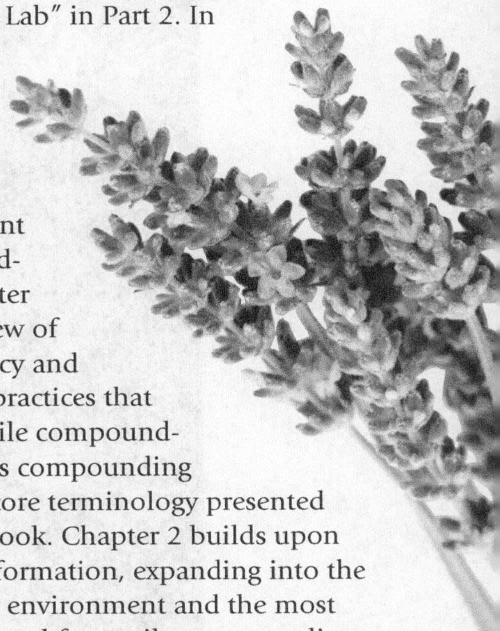

Each chapter in Unit 1 contains three parts, with an "Exploratory Lab" in Part 2. In the exploratory labs, you begin to learn about, understand, and investigate your role, responsibilities, and work environment as a sterile compounding technician. Chapter 1 provides an overview of the origin of pharmacy and the development of practices that eventually led to sterile compounding. It also introduces compounding regulations and the core terminology presented throughout the textbook. Chapter 2 builds upon that foundational information, expanding into the sterile compounding environment and the most important and basic tool for sterile compounding, the hood. Chapter 3 introduces the additional tools and equipment you will use for sterile compounding. Once you are aware of the tools of the trade, Chapter 4 brings you to the next step: interpreting medication orders and reading pharmacy labels. In Chapter 5, you work from medication orders and pharmacy labels to determine and perform the pharmacy calculations central to mixing compounded sterile preparations (CSPs). Once you have mastered the pharmacy calculations of Chapter 5, you will have completed the "basics" section of the textbook and will be ready to learn about and practice the pharmacy sterile compounding procedures of Unit 2.

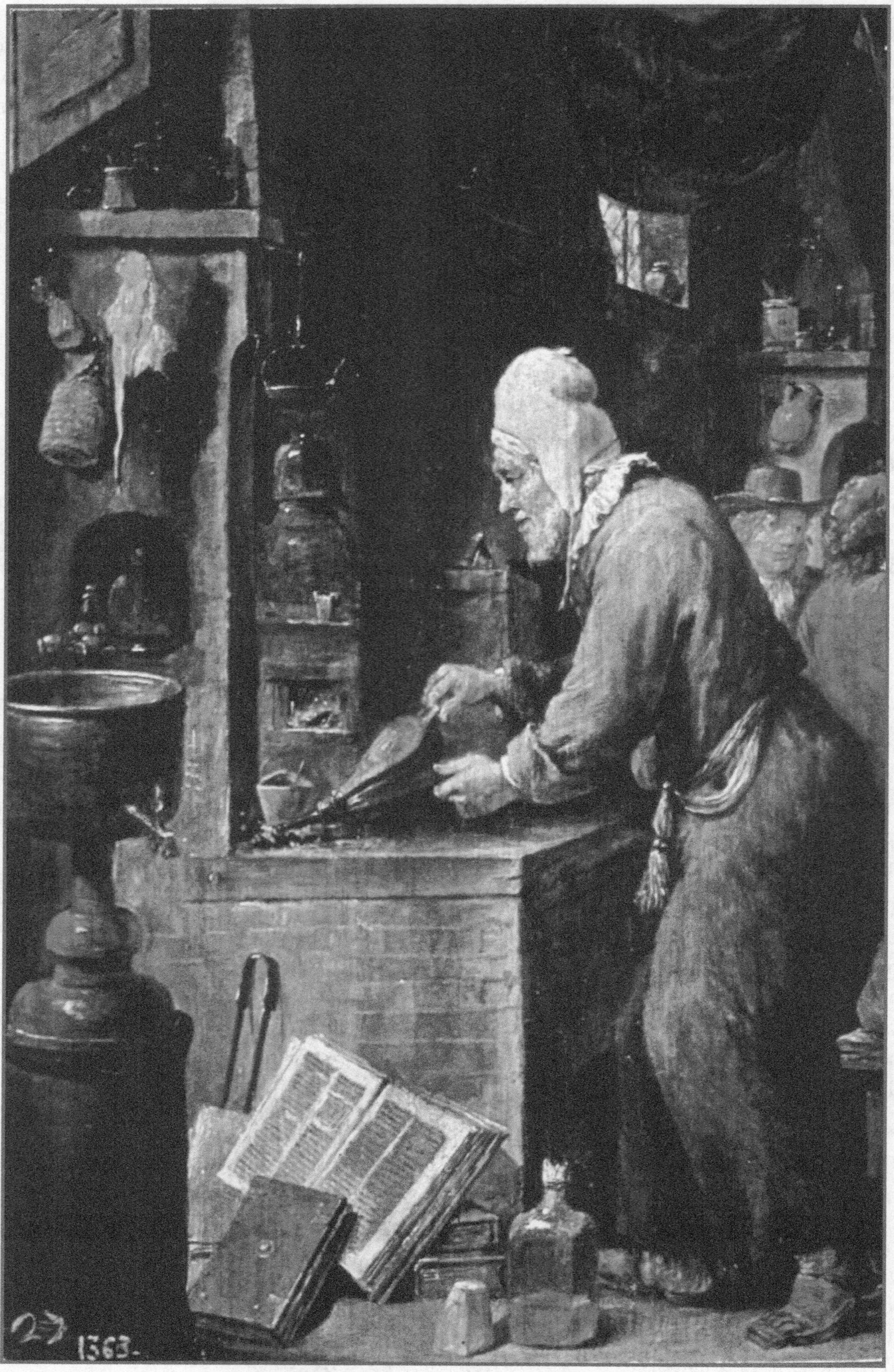
1363-

# Chapter 1

# Sterile Compounding as a Pharmacy Technician

## Learning Objectives

- Gain an awareness of the historical roots of pharmacy and sterile compounding.
- Define sterile compounding and aseptic technique.
- Describe the ways in which sterile compounding and aseptic technique processes may affect patient health and safety.
- Define the objectives of USP Chapter <797>.
- Understand the training requirements for pharmacy technicians who prepare sterile products, and describe the process validation tool used for technique evaluation.
- Recognize various quality assurance and end-product testing procedures.
- Determine appropriate responses to medication safety questions.
- Demonstrate an awareness of the ethical issues in pharmacy.

The art of compounding, or the mixing of several different agents, can be traced back to the ninth century in Mesopotamia and the Middle East. At that time, doctors, midwives, mystics, and learned members of religious orders experimented with chemical processes to create luxury products for religious leaders and royalty. By the Middle Ages, compounding practices had spread to Europe, where craftspeople, or artisans, began combining flowers, herbs, and other natural substances to create medicinal elixirs, powders, and ointments with the power to cure the sick and injured and—many believed—to prolong life.

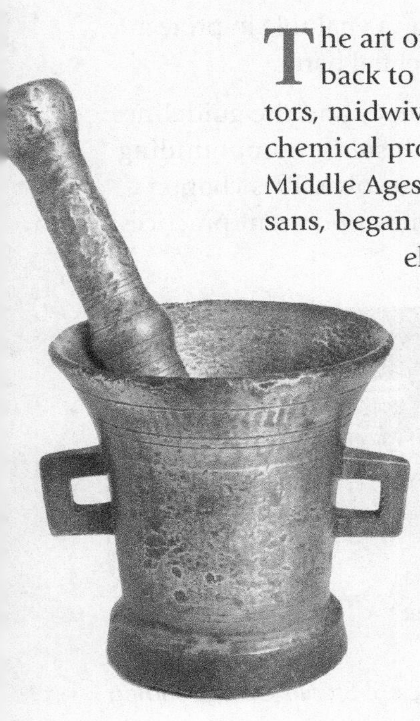

These skilled compounding artisans were known as **alchemists** and were revered by people from all segments of society. These artisans and their compounding pharmacies, or **apothecaries**, sprang up all across the European continent. Their work was frequently rooted in the spiritual beliefs of the time and was often shrouded in mysticism. In fact, many of the compounds that alchemists prepared were thought to have magical properties. Early pharmacy practitioners quickly became associated with their main tool for grinding and mixing the ingredients by hand: the mortar and pestle.

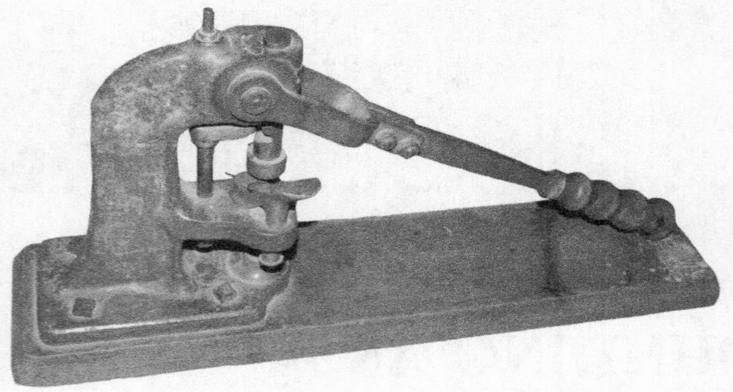

## Evolution of Compounding

In the late 1800s, the influence of the Industrial Revolution, which began in Great Britain but quickly spread to the United States, changed the practice of compounding from a hands-on art to a scientific process. Automated machinery produced higher volumes of syrups, elixirs, powders, and other drug forms with increased speed. Yet despite the advent of pharmaceutical manufacturing, pharmacists continued to use their knowledge of compounding for 80% of the prescriptions they filled. Although they incorporated mass-manufactured ingredients, they still needed to perform compounding tasks to fill the prescriptions written by physicians. Many pharmacists continued to roll their own pills and formulate their own liquids and powders and, like their artisanal predecessors, they turned to the healing powers of nature. They used plants such as belladonna (for headaches), foxglove (for heart ailments), bloodroot (for throat infections), and St. John's Wort (for burns) in their compounding preparations. Thus, apothecaries thrived well into the nineteenth century as people continued to rely on the potions and cures of these mystical chemists.

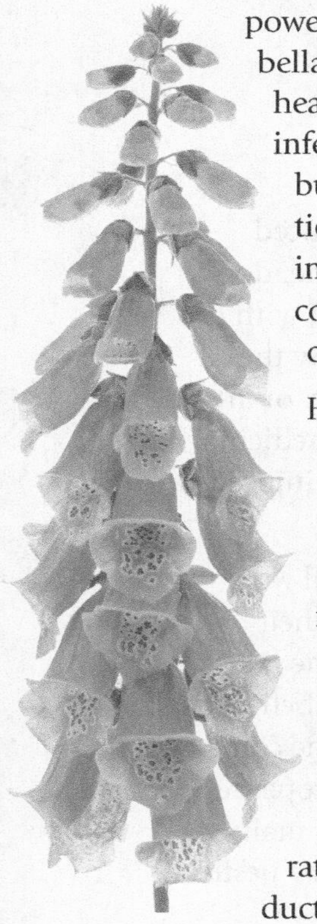

However, by the mid-twentieth century, in most areas of the world, pharmaceutical compounding became less and less common in a pharmacist's daily practice. Relying on large manufacturing plants, pharmaceutical manufacturers synthesized drugs into stable, uniform, high-quality medications in various dosage forms—primarily oral solids, oral liquids, and topical preparations. In the United States, the production capacity of such plants enabled more drugs that met federal standards for purity and quality to be available to more patients. As a result, pharmacists were compounding only about one-fourth of the total prescriptions that they filled, and their role shifted from both creating and dispensing medications to primarily dispensing them.

## Sterile Product Preparation

Toward the end of the twentieth century, an increased need for intravenous admixture services, injectable dosage forms, and individualized medications led to a dramatic rise in the number of practitioners and environments involved worldwide in sterile product preparation. These increases came about as physicians recognized the advantages of personalized medication dosing. Such dosing allowed physicians to provide more exact and specialized treatment for each patient. Increased allergic reactions to various inactive ingredients in manufactured drugs, as well as a need to provide medications to patients who were unable to tolerate the oral dosage form, also increased the use of sterile compounding.

Still, it wasn't until the early 1990s that pharmacy practitioners realized the need to implement safer practices related to sterile compounding and aseptic technique. Independent scientific research had determined that **compounded sterile preparations (CSPs)** at times provided both a fertile breeding ground for bacteria and a perfect vehicle for transmitting bacteria to the patient recipient. Fortunately, multiple studies recognized that correct sterile compounding practices could play a vital role in protecting the patient from this potential harm.

Today, the practice of pharmacy and the guidelines and regulations under which sterile compounding personnel work continue to evolve. This chapter provides you with an overview of current practices and regulations.

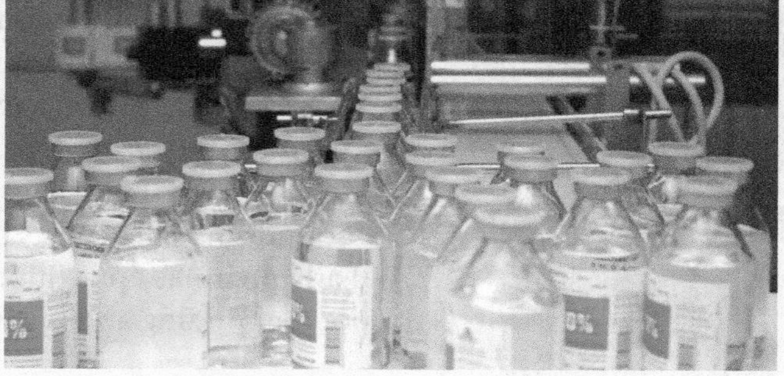

# Part 1: Concepts

The pharmacy practice of **sterile compounding** involves the dilution, mixing, and injection of various medication products using aseptic technique. **Aseptic technique** is performed by **sterile compounding personnel** or *sterile products personnel*. Aseptic technique is vital to the compounding process to avoid the introduction of pathogenic organisms or other contaminants into a sterile environment or preparation. Failure of pharmacy personnel to follow the protocol of aseptic technique may lead to **microbial contamination** of the medication, resulting in serious illness or, possibly, death for patient recipients due to infection. Therefore, it is critical for patient health and safety that you, as a pharmacy technician, become well-versed in aseptic technique and the procedures for sterile compounding.

**POINTER**

The word *aseptic* comes from the Latin prefix *a*, meaning "not or without" and *sepsis*, meaning "characterized by putrefaction or decay." Therefore, *aseptic* describes something that is without pathogens or is free from infection.

## Roles and Responsibilities of IV Technicians

Pharmacy technicians play a major role in preparing compounded sterile preparations (CSPs) in pharmacies. These specialized technicians—often referred to as sterile compounding technicians, intravenous (IV) admixture technicians, or simply IV technicians—are largely responsible for preparing injectable medications for patients in hospital and home healthcare settings who are unable to swallow oral medications, whose digestive systems preclude the use of oral medications, or whose conditions necessitate a more rapid delivery of medication into the blood supply. Injectable medications may be delivered to the patient via **parenteral routes of administration**.

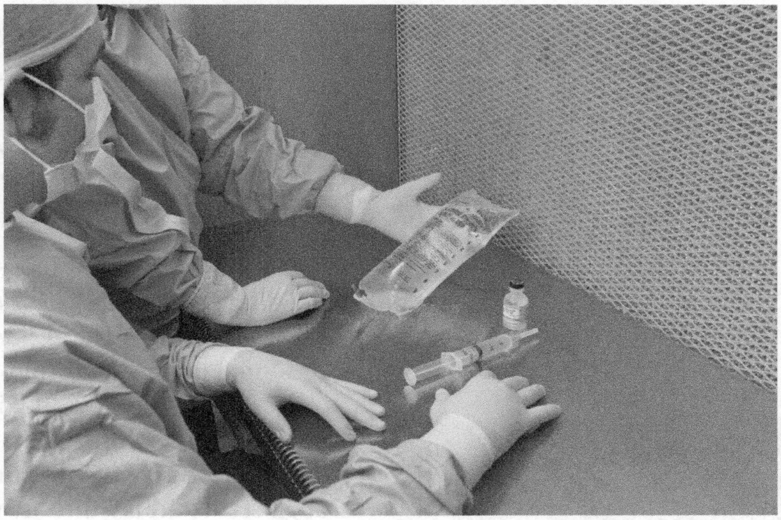

Pharmacist checking the IV technician's work.

The term *parenteral route of administration* refers to the method of medication administration by any route other than through the alimentary canal (the digestive tract). In general, this means every method other than by mouth or rectum, including the **intravenous (IV)**, **intramuscular (IM)**, **subcutaneous (Sub-Q)**, and **intrathecal (IT)** routes. The majority of medications prepared by sterile compounding technicians are administered through an IV.

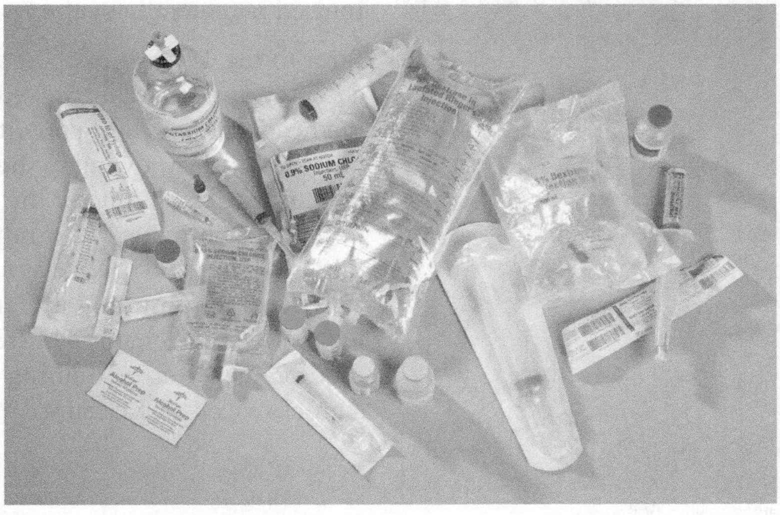

Various sterile compounding supplies.

Parenteral solutions are sterile, injectable solutions that are administered to the patient by one of the parenteral

**POINTER**
Medication can also be administered topically, intranasally, by inhalation, or instilled into the ear or eye. These types of medications are generally provided by the manufacturer ready to administer and will not require preparation by sterile compounding personnel.

routes of administration. CSPs are comprised of small-volume or large-volume parenteral solutions to which a medication or additive has been added during sterile compounding procedures. The typical volumes for these various routes of administration are listed in Table 1.1.

**Table 1.1 Typical Volume for Various Routes of Administration**

The volumes given below may vary according to the age or size of the patient and the dosing guidelines of the drug to be administered. Sterile compounding personnel should consult their facility's P&P manual or the drug's product insert for administration guidelines.

| |
|---|
| Intradermal (ID) ≤ 0.1 mL |
| Subcutaneous (Sub-Q) ≤ 1 mL |
| Intramuscular (IM) ≤ 3 mL |
| Intrathecal (IT) 1 mL–10 mL<br>(larger volumes may be administered via syringe pump or epidural cassette pump) |
| IV Push (IVP) 1 mL–60 mL<br>(volumes ≥ 10 mL are usually administered via syringe pump) |
| IVPB 25 mL–250 mL<br>(infusion rate controlled via tubing's roll clamp or IV pump) |
| IV > 250 mL<br>(infusion rate controlled via IV pump) |

Small-volume CSPs are those of a volume ranging from less than 1 mL to as much as 250 mL, depending on the required route of administration. Some small-volume CSPs are administered by the **intravenous piggyback (IVPB)** route of administration. Often, a drug is diluted in powder form with a solvent such as sterile water or **normal saline (NS)**. The diluted drug is drawn into a syringe and injected into a sterile IVPB base solution such as **dextrose 5% in water ($D_5W$)** or 0.9% sodium chloride (NS). The nurse then injects the final prepared solution through sterile tubing directly into the patient's vein.

Large-volume CSPs are those with a volume of 500 mL or greater and are infused parenterally by the IV route of administration.

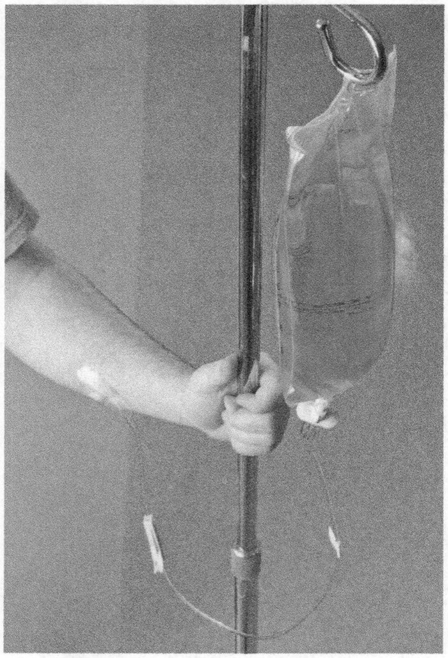
A patient receiving IV therapy.

Prior to the 1980s, most CSPs were prepared at the patient's bedside by a doctor or nurse. This proved problematic due to a high incidence of medication errors and patient infections. Today, most CSPs are prepared in the pharmacy, owing to dramatic improvements in technology and a better understanding of the need for sterile compounding procedures designed to provide uniformly safe CSPs. The use of the **laminar airflow workbench (LAFW)** as a tool for sterile product preparation has also become commonplace. In 2008, revisions to USP Chapter <797> led to sweeping changes in sterile compounding practices and set forth requirements for the training and testing of sterile compounding personnel as well as guidelines for all aspects of aseptic technique.

## The Effect of Aseptic Technique on Patient Health and Safety

Correct sterile compounding and aseptic technique procedures—performed by well-trained personnel in a clean, controlled environment—are essential to patient health and safety. To ensure that these aseptic practices are strictly followed, sterile compounding technicians must undergo frequent and comprehensive evaluations based on such tools as process validation checklists and numerous quality assurance and end-product testing procedures. These safeguards not only prevent medication errors but hold technicians to the highest quality-control standards. The **United States Pharmacopeia (USP)**, a nongovernmental regulatory organization, oversees quality control of pharmacy practices by establishing public standards for the preparation and dispensing of prescription and over-the-counter medications as well as other healthcare products. Guidelines set forth by the USP are used by government agencies, such as Joint Commission or Center for Medicare and Medicaid Services (CMS). These agencies determine whether or not healthcare institutions receive government reimbursement for their products.

### USP

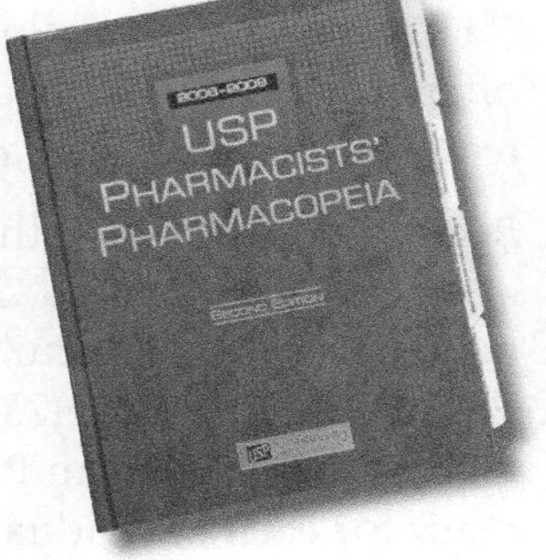


The *USP Pharmacists' Pharmacopeia* is an official publication whose guidelines are a mainstay for both pharmacists and pharmacy technicians. This large, hardcover book currently has a blue cover, as shown at right. You will likely observe pharmacy personnel frequently consulting this book, commonly called the *USP*, in pharmacy practice.

In your own practice as a sterile compounding technician, the most relevant part of this large book is a single chapter titled "Chapter <797> Pharmaceutical Compounding – Sterile Preparations." This important chapter currently falls on pages 779–831 in Section 7 and sets practice standards regarding the preparation of sterile compounds. Referenced in this textbook as USP Chapter <797>, it covers topics such as the training and responsibilities of the personnel who prepare sterile products, quality assurance, environmental quality control, the storage of sterile compounds, and the importance of **beyond-use dating (BUD)**. BUD is the date or time after which a CSP is no longer sterile, stable, or effective and must not be used.

The chapter also identifies four specific risk levels for CSPs: **low-risk**, **medium-risk**, **high-risk**, and **immediate-use**. Each of the risk levels is assigned according to the potential for microbial contamination during sterile compounding. Within each risk level, the *USP* designates the types of preparations that may be compounded and the special training and testing required for sterile compounding personnel. Chapter 2 of this textbook covers additional information on risk levels and suitable sterile compounding environments.

You should also be aware that in order to provide additional guidance with interpreting and following the important regulations of USP Chapter <797>, the *USP* has produced a supplemental guidebook for sterile compounding personnel. The guide-

**POINTER**

The *USP <797> Guidebook* is now available to healthcare providers in a dual publication known as the *USP-NF*, or the *United States Pharmacopeia – National Formulary*. This publication combines the traditional *USP* with a copy of the *National Formulary*, a list of all medications approved for use within the United States.

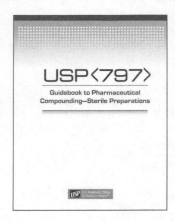


book is smaller than the big blue book, produced with a soft cover, and titled *USP <797> Guidebook to Pharmaceutical Compounding – Sterile Preparations*. You may find this softcover book kept in your pharmacy, consulted regularly, and commonly referred to as the *USP <797> Guidebook*.

## Training and Testing Requirements

To work in a sterile compounding facility in most states, personnel must be certified pharmacy technicians and must undergo additional training and testing on the compounding of sterile products. Every state has its own regulations regarding the training and testing of pharmacy technicians. After years of advocacy by pharmacy technician organizations and educators, laws are slowly being enacted to provide more standardization in the requirements for pharmacy technician education and training. At a minimum, most states now require that pharmacy technicians pass a national certification exam. Two pharmacy technician certification exams are offered in the United States. The most widely used exam is the **Pharmacy Technician Certification Exam (PTCE)**, offered by the Pharmacy Technician Certification Board (PTCB) and accepted by all of the U.S. **Boards of Pharmacy**. The **Exam for the Certification of Pharmacy Technicians (ExCPT)**, offered by the Institute for the Certification of Pharmacy Technicians (ICPT), is currently accepted by only a portion of the State Boards of Pharmacy.

Regulations regarding the training and testing of sterile compounding technicians are not as well defined. Some agencies that develop guidelines for the training of personnel who perform sterile compounding include the Accreditation Council for Pharmacy Education (ACPE), the American Society of Health-Systems Pharmacists (ASHP), the American Pharmacists Association (APhA), and the Board of Pharmacy for each individual state. Many of these organizations refer to USP Chapter <797> as a guideline for developing policies related to sterile compounding and personnel training. Another tool widely used in the development of comprehensive training programs for pharmacy technicians is the ASHP's ***Model Curriculum for Pharmacy Technician Training***.

It is considered **best practice** that all personnel who prepare sterile products complete an ACPE-accredited training program in sterile product preparation and aseptic technique. At a minimum, sterile compounding technicians should either be experienced and knowledgeable pharmacy technicians with strong backgrounds in math and science, or students who have graduated from well-designed pharmacy technician schools or training programs. It is standard practice that sterile compounding students complete a minimum of 40 hours of hands-on training in a laboratory setting, along with classroom instruction, independent study assignments, written exams, and process validation procedures designed to prepare trainees to work in IV rooms.

In addition, sterile compounding employees should receive a minimum of 40 hours of practical on-the-job training in IV rooms and must pass intensive process validation evaluations and quality assurance testing prior to making sterile products for patient administration. USP Chapter <797> requires that sterile compounding personnel undergo annual recertification, which includes a written exam, a process validation evaluation, and the completion of a media-fill kit.

## Process Validation

Sterile compounding personnel must undergo process validation for each aspect of the training process. During **process validation**, instructors observe, critique, and grade students' technique on specialized process validation checklists. These checklists break down each technique into small components that are separately evaluated and graded. These components include sterile garbing and gloving, horizontal laminar airflow hood cleaning, vial preparation, ampule preparation, and large-volume parenteral preparation. Chapters 6–14 discuss the process validation checklists for procedural laboratory techniques, and the checklists themselves are located in Appendix D.

## Quality Assurance

Sterile compounding personnel must also undergo various **quality assurance procedures** as part of the training process. For instance, students confirm their ability to aseptically don sterile garb and gloves by providing evidence of a negative-growth fingertip test. Students must also demonstrate how to properly clean and disinfect a hood, a process evaluated by culturing the hood's surface. As another quality assurance procedure, students must correctly complete an **aseptic technique testing kit**, often referred to as a media-fill kit, process validation kit, Gro-Med kit, or ATTACK kit. Lastly, **end-product testing** evaluates a student's sterile compounding techniques by assessing their prepared products for contamination and also verifying that the products contain the proper type and amount of medication.

Before sterile compounding personnel can make sterile products for patient administration, they must complete this type of testing and demonstrate 100% compliance with aseptic technique requirements. In addition, all personnel who prepare sterile products should successfully complete process validation and an aseptic technique testing kit at least once a year. Sterile compounding personnel who fail to demonstrate correct aseptic technique during the annual recertification process must undergo mandatory retraining. Retraining must also take place any time a pharmacy authority observes a break in technique. The individuals being retrained must then undergo additional process validation and aseptic technique testing in which they must demonstrate 100% compliance before being allowed to return to sterile compounding. Technicians who cannot demonstrate 100% compliance with aseptic technique after thorough retraining will *not* be allowed to compound sterile products.

In sterile compounding pharmacies, process validation and other quality-assurance testing procedures are critical controls to ensure the safety of the compounding process and the integrity of the end product.

## Medication Safety

Quality assurance procedures are critical in every healthcare setting to ensure the safe dispensing and administration of medication to patients. Adherence to medication safety standards is the responsibility of every healthcare professional. Any breach of these established guidelines could lead to a **medication error**, a preventable event in which a patient is harmed by a medication or would have been harmed if the medication had been administered. Although every medication order brings with it the possibility of a medication error, healthcare workers who dispense or administer

> **POINTER**
> Pharmacy technicians should always defer to pharmacists for questions requiring professional judgment, such as those concerning medication prescribing and dosing as well as drug identification and administration.

medications must diligently verify the **five patient "rights" of correct drug administration**: right patient, right drug, right dose, right route, and right time.

Medication errors in sterile compounding pharmacies typically involve incorrect drugs ("right drug" errors) or errors in pharmacy calculations ("right dose" errors). Chapters 4 and 5 provide additional information on how to avoid these types of errors.

## Monitoring of Medication Errors

> **POINTER**
> Self-reporting of medication errors is a valuable learning tool for both healthcare employees and pharmacy regulatory organizations. Because data from self-reported errors can influence positive changes in published patient safety guidelines, self-reporting is encouraged among pharmacy personnel.

Several agencies and organizations track medication errors with the goal of providing evidence-based information and guidelines designed to decrease the incidence of medication errors. The **Institute for Safe Medication Practices (ISMP)** is a nonprofit organization that educates the healthcare community and consumers about safe medication practices. The ISMP publishes a list of abbreviations that most pharmacies and institutions want to eliminate from use. **MedWatch**, a voluntary program of the **Food and Drug Administration (FDA)**, supports healthcare workers in the reporting of medication errors and **adverse drug effects (ADEs)**. The Joint Commission, formerly the Joint Commission on Accreditation of Healthcare Organizations (JCAHO), has several programs designed to decrease medication errors and improve patient safety.

> **POINTER**
> The "system" referred to at right includes all actions and people involved in the process of preparing and delivering medications, both in the pharmacy itself and within the larger system of healthcare. Some components of this complex system include labeling, workflow, communication, interruptions, personnel issues, and technique repetition.

In addition to these regulatory agencies, every pharmacy has its own policies and procedures in place to reduce medication errors and encourage error reporting. To effectively do so, pharmacies must foster a culture of safety. When an error is made, a pharmacy must examine the system that allowed the error to occur, rather than placing blame on the individual responsible for the error. When a pharmacy poses questions that explore the circumstances surrounding the medication error, beneficial changes to pharmacy protocol may result. Some possible questions include: How would you describe the workload in the pharmacy when the medication error was made? What type of distractions might have affected the employee's performance? Considering the type of error made, would better package labeling or bar-coded packaging have prevented the error? By examining the conditions and processes that led to an error, pharmacy personnel can discover ways to change their policies and procedures to reduce the likelihood of repeating the error. Once processes have been changed to reduce the chance of error, individuals are then held responsible for adhering to those improved processes.

## Ethical Issues in Pharmacy Practice

A number of legal and ethical concerns are related to pharmacy practice. Many center on reducing and reporting medication errors. Each state's Board of Pharmacy provides legal guidelines and oversight for pharmacy practice. In addition, most states have regulations defining mandatory error-reporting procedures.

Like other pharmacy personnel, pharmacy technicians are legally and ethically bound to provide safe and effective care for the patients they serve. To assist technicians in fulfilling these responsibilities, the American Association of Pharmacy Technicians (AAPT) publishes the *Code of Ethics for Pharmacy Technicians.* This publication serves as a standard for technicians faced with ethical and legal decisions and is discussed briefly on page 15.

# Concepts Self-Check

## Check Your Understanding

*Write your answers on a separate sheet of paper, as modeled in these examples:* 1d; 2c; 3b; *etc. Check your answers using the Answer Key in Appendix A.*

**1.** Sterile compounding technicians do not generally prepare medications that are delivered by which of the following routes?

a. IM
b. IV
c. Sub-Q
d. PR

**2.** Which of the following organizations sets standards for the purity, quality, strength, and consistency of prescription and over-the-counter medications?

a. ACPE
b. ASHP
c. USP
d. PTCE

**3.** Which of the following exams are required by most states for the certification of pharmacy technicians?

a. either the PTCE or ExCPT
b. either the PTCE or the PTCB
c. either the ExCPT or the PTCB
d. either the ExCPT or the ICPT

**4.** At a minimum, how often must sterile compounding personnel undergo process validation to show 100% compliance with aseptic technique?

a. annually after the completion of initial training
b. at the completion of initial training, annually thereafter, and upon evidence of poor technique
c. semi-annually after completion of initial training
d. at the completion of initial training, and upon evidence of poor technique

**5.** The primary purpose of the AAPT publication *Code of Ethics for Pharmacy Technicians* is to

a. explain the laws that must be followed by pharmacy technicians.
b. define the ethical responsibilities of pharmacy technicians.
c. list the duties of pharmacy technicians.
d. discuss the morals that must be followed by pharmacy technicians.

## Apply Your Knowledge

*On a separate sheet of paper, write your answer to the question posed in the paragraph below. Use complete sentences and take time to create a thorough and thoughtful response. Check your answer against the Answer Key in Appendix A.*

In Part 1 of this chapter, you learned that correct aseptic technique plays a vital role in patient care and safety. With that in mind, what should you do if you accidentally contaminate the sterile product in the course of preparing a medication for IV administration?

# Part 2: Training

## Examine the Resources and Supplies

### USP

Personnel who work in the sterile compounding room must be familiar with the *USP*. As discussed in Part 1 of this chapter, pharmacists and pharmacy technicians use the *USP* as a reference and guide because it offers valuable information on nearly every aspect of pharmacy practice. Pharmacy personnel may refer to the *USP* to ascertain and develop appropriate policies and procedures for pharmacy operations. It is especially important that personnel who prepare sterile products be familiar with the objectives and content of USP Chapter <797>. Sterile products personnel must pay special attention to the training and testing requirements of the sterile compounding technician as defined in USP Chapter <797> and to the information regarding low- and medium-risk levels (the risk level conditions under which most sterile products are prepared). Pharmacy technicians using the *USP* as a resource will build familiarity with its contents and gain a solid understanding of why it is such a valuable resource in pharmacy practice.

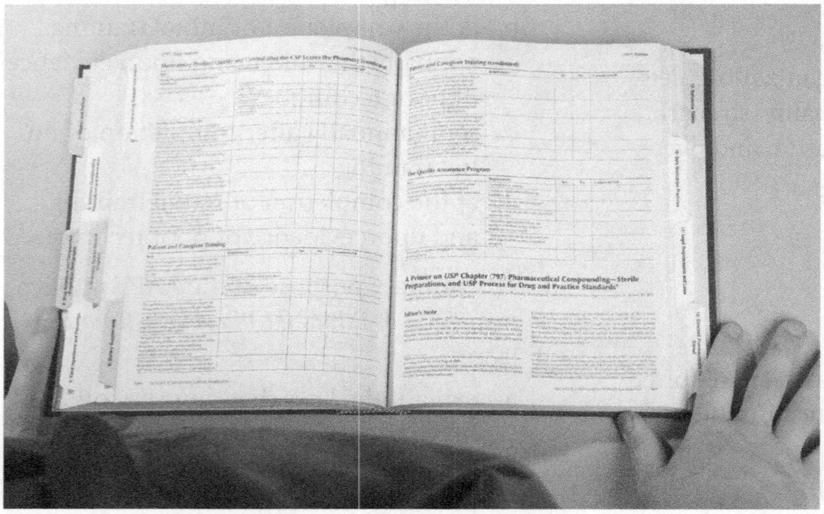

IV technician reviewing *USP* <797> for sterile compounding.

**POINTER**

In your career as a sterile compounding technician, you will undergo two separate types of process validation. The first validation is specific to your training period, prior to certification or course completion, and involves the instructor checklists. The second validation is specific to your role as an employee on the job site and is required prior to your preparation of "live" IVs.

### Process Validation Checklists

Process validation checklists are an important part of aseptic technique training. Each checklist corresponds to a particular aspect of aseptic technique and serves as an evaluative tool for instructors to test students' competency. Once you become a sterile compounding technician, process validation checklists serve as study aids to help you prepare for your initial and annual competency tests. Chapters 6–14 contain procedural labs that require your instructor to complete a process validation checklist as you perform the lab. It is considered best practice for you, as a sterile compounding technician, to read the corresponding checklist before you begin the procedural lab and after you complete it. You are also encouraged to practice the steps in the procedural lab *several times* prior to instructor observation for competency evaluation.

## Aseptic Technique Testing Kit

Several different types of aseptic technique testing kits are available. These kits are used to confirm sterile compounding and aseptic technique competency, to assess technique failures, and to design corrective actions. The **media-fill kit** is one of the most commonly used aseptic technique testing kits for initial training and annual validation and usually includes one or more vials or ampules and a small-volume PVC bag (typically 50 mL or 100 mL) containing a soy-broth testing solution. Most testing kits require the technician to make multiple withdrawals from a vial or an ampule and then make multiple injections into the bag. The technician then incubates the bag for the period of days specified by the product's manufacturer. The soy-broth medium is designed to test the compounder's aseptic technique. If the person being tested has a **break in technique**, visible particles will develop in the bag. These particles simulate bacterial growth.

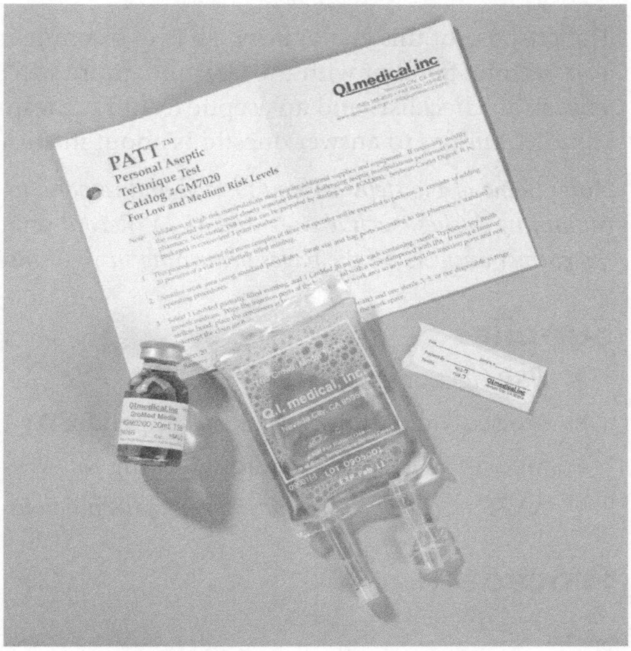

The contents of an aseptic technique testing kit.

## Code of Ethics

Many pharmacy technician training programs develop a code of ethics for pharmacy technicians. This code of ethics is frequently part of a training program's student handbook and is sometimes recited by students during the program's graduation ceremony. The code outlines and defines the ethical responsibilities of the pharmacy technician, often including guidelines that promote patient health and safety and encourage honest and dependable actions by the pharmacy technician. Although a pharmacy technician program may develop its own code of ethics, the most widely used and recognizable one is the AAPT's *Code of Ethics for Pharmacy Technicians*. This code defines specific ethical responsibilities of every pharmacy technician. Some tenets of the code include integrity, safety, respect, competency, confidentiality, and a duty to uphold the legal regulations under which the pharmacy technician practices.

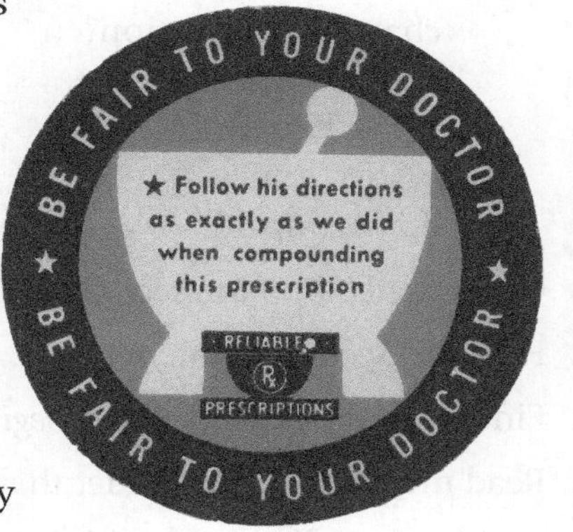
BE FAIR TO YOUR DOCTOR
★ Follow his directions as exactly as we did when compounding this prescription
RELIABLE
℞
PRESCRIPTIONS
BE FAIR TO YOUR DOCTOR

# Exploratory Lab

The purpose of this exploratory lab is to examine important resources and tools used in pharmacy practice. You become familiar with the *USP* and, more specifically, USP Chapter <797>. You also investigate process validation checklists and an aseptic technique testing kit. In addition, you use the *Code of Ethics for Pharmacy Technicians* to answer questions about medication safety and ethics in pharmacy practice.

***Note:*** *Some of the steps ask you to read and respond to one or more multiple-choice questions (marked by numbers containing dashes, such as* **1–1** *and* **1–2***). Record your answers to these multiple-choice questions by either circling the correct answers on the pages or turning in your answers as directed by your instructor.*

## Supplies

- *USP* (text or website)
- Process Validation Checklists (Appendix D)
- Media-Fill Aseptic Technique Testing Kit
- AAPT's *Code of Ethics for Pharmacy Technicians*

## Procedure

### *Using the USP*

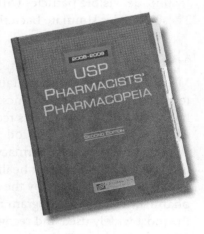


1. Open the *USP* to the Contents page.
2. Answer the following multiple-choice question, recording your answer as directed by your instructor.

   **2–1.** Which section of the *USP* provides pharmacy-related general chapter information?
   a. Section 2
   b. Section 6
   c. Section 7
   d. Section 10
3. Open the *USP* to the section on Pharmacy-Related General Chapters.
4. Find the Section Contents page.
5. Find Chapter <797> (*official beginning June 1, 2008*).
6. Read the information under the heading *Organization of this Chapter*.
7. Answer the following multiple-choice question, recording your answer as directed by your instructor.

   **7–1.** Which of the following is *not* listed as a main section of USP Chapter <797>?
   a. Responsibilities of All Compounding Personnel
   b. Verification of Compounding Accuracy and Sterility
   c. Storage and Beyond-Use Dating
   d. Quality Assurance Program for CSPs for Veterinary Use
8. Turn to the Chapter <797> paragraph titled "Responsibility of Compounding Personnel" and read all of the related information.
9. Answer the following multiple-choice question, recording your answer as directed by your instructor.

9–1. According to USP Chapter <797>, which of the following statements is *not* true regarding the Responsibility of the Compounder?
   a. Perform antiseptic hand cleansing and disinfection of nonsterile compounding surfaces.
   b. Use laminar flow clean-air hoods, barrier isolators, and other contamination control devices that are appropriate for the risk level.
   c. Identify, weigh, and measure ingredients.
   d. Reduce solid ingredients to the smallest reasonable particle size.

**10.** Find the Chapter <797> paragraph titled "Verification of Compounding Accuracy and Sterility" and read the first three paragraphs in that section.

**11.** Answer the following multiple-choice question, recording your answer as directed by your instructor.

11–1. According to USP Chapter <797>, which statement regarding the Verification of Compounding Accuracy and Sterilization is true?
   a. Achieving and maintaining sterility and freedom from contamination is not the responsibility of the pharmacy technician.
   b. It is the pharmacist's responsibility to ensure that the sterile compound is free from microbial contamination.
   c. Verification requires planned testing designed to demonstrate effectiveness of all procedures critical to the accuracy and purity of finished CSPs.
   d. Packaged and labeled CSPs do not need to be inspected for physical integrity and expected appearance.

**12.** Temporarily set the *USP* aside; you will need it to answer Questions 22–1 and 22–2 in this procedure section.

### *Understanding Process Validation*

**13.** Open your textbook to Appendix D.

**14.** Read through each of the process validation checklists in Appendix D.

**15.** Use the information in Appendix D to answer the following multiple-choice questions, recording your answers as directed by your instructor.

15–1. According to Appendix D of this textbook, how many separate process validations must be completed?
   a. 7
   b. 8
   c. 9
   d. 10

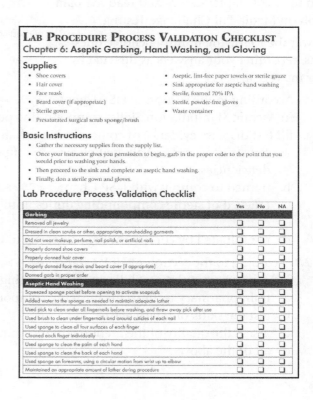

**LAB PROCEDURE PROCESS VALIDATION CHECKLIST**

**Chapter 6: Aseptic Garbing, Hand Washing, and Gloving**

**Supplies**

- Shoe covers
- Hair cover
- Face mask
- Beard cover (if appropriate)
- Sterile gown
- Presaturated surgical scrub sponge/brush
- Aseptic, lint-free paper towels or sterile gauze
- Sink appropriate for aseptic hand washing
- Sterile, foamed 70% IPA
- Sterile, powder-free gloves
- Waste container

**Basic Instructions**

- Gather the necessary supplies from the supply list.
- Once your instructor gives you permission to begin, garb in the proper order to the point that you would prior to washing your hands.
- Then proceed to the sink and complete an aseptic hand washing.
- Finally, don a sterile gown and gloves.

**Lab Procedure Process Validation Checklist**

| | Yes | No | NA |
|---|---|---|---|
| **Garbing** | | | |
| Removed all jewelry | ❑ | ❑ | ❑ |
| Dressed in clean scrubs or other, appropriate, nonshedding garments | ❑ | ❑ | ❑ |
| Did not wear makeup, perfume, nail polish, or artificial nails | ❑ | ❑ | ❑ |
| Properly donned shoe covers | ❑ | ❑ | ❑ |
| Properly donned hair cover | ❑ | ❑ | ❑ |
| Properly donned face mask and beard cover (if appropriate) | ❑ | ❑ | ❑ |
| Donned garb in proper order | ❑ | ❑ | ❑ |
| **Aseptic Hand Washing** | | | |
| Squeezed sponge packet before opening to activate soapsuds | ❑ | ❑ | ❑ |
| Added water to the sponge as needed to maintain adequate lather | ❑ | ❑ | ❑ |
| Used pick to clean under all fingernails before washing, and threw away pick after use | ❑ | ❑ | ❑ |
| Used brush to clean under fingernails and around cuticles of each nail | ❑ | ❑ | ❑ |
| Used sponge to clean all four surfaces of each finger | ❑ | ❑ | ❑ |
| Cleaned each finger individually | ❑ | ❑ | ❑ |
| Used sponge to clean the palm of each hand | ❑ | ❑ | ❑ |
| Used sponge to clean the back of each hand | ❑ | ❑ | ❑ |
| Used sponge on forearms, using a circular motion from wrist up to elbow | ❑ | ❑ | ❑ |
| Maintained an appropriate amount of lather during procedure | ❑ | ❑ | ❑ |

15–2. According to Appendix D of this textbook, what final score do you need to achieve in order to successfully pass process validation consistent with ACPE standards?

a. 75%
b. 90%
c. 95%
d. 100%

### *Examining the Media-Fill Aseptic Technique Testing Kit*

**16.** Open the media-fill aseptic technique testing kit.

**17.** Explore the contents of the kit.

**18.** Read the manufacturer's instruction sheet included in the kit.

**19.** Notice the details of the procedures that will be performed during the preparation of the media-fill aseptic technique testing kit. Note that these procedures must be successfully completed to verify initial and annual competency in aseptic technique and sterile product preparation.

**20.** Turn to USP Chapter <797> and read the paragraph on Personnel Training and Evaluation in Aseptic Manipulation Skills.

**21.** Turn to USP Chapter <797> and read the paragraph on Media-Fill Challenge Testing.

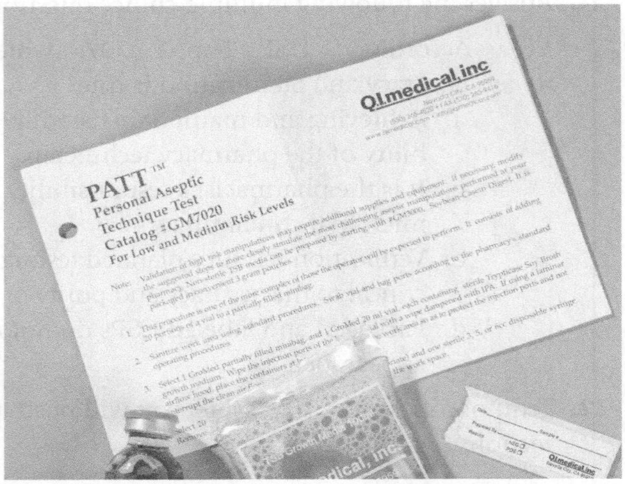


Manufacturer's instruction sheet included in an aseptic technique testing kit.

**22.** Answer the following multiple-choice questions, recording your answers as directed by your instructor.

22–1. According to the section of USP Chapter <797> regarding Personnel Training and Evaluation in Aseptic Manipulation Skills, compounding personnel who fail written tests or whose media-fill test displays evidence of contamination shall be immediately

a. reinstructed and reevaluated by expert compounding personnel to ensure correction of all deficiencies.
b. trained to comply with USP Chapter <797> standards.
c. relieved of sterile compounding duties until she or he passes the pharmacy certification exam.
d. re-evaluated by compounding personnel to ensure correction of deficiencies.

22–2. According to the section of USP Chapter <797> regarding Personnel Training and Evaluation in Aseptic Manipulation Skills, media-fill testing is used to

a. train pharmacy technicians in sterile compounding.
b. test the skills of pharmacists.
c. assess the quality of the aseptic skill of compounding personnel.
d. all of the above

### *Making Ethical Decisions*

**23.** Read the *Code of Ethics for Pharmacy Technicians.* (Your instructor will either direct you to the AAPT website to read this document or provide a handout.)

**24.** Answer the following multiple-choice questions, recording your answers as directed by your instructor.

**24–1.** While processing an outpatient prescription, you notice that a patient who has refused counseling seems confused about his prescription and asks you questions about the medication dosage. Bearing in mind the responsibilities outlined in the *Code of Ethics for Pharmacy Technicians*, what is the best course of action?

a. Answer the patient's question regarding his medication.
b. Refer the patient to the patient information leaflet accompanying the prescription.
c. Refer the patient to the *USP*.
d. Ask the pharmacist to speak with the patient regarding his medication.

**24–2.** While delivering drugs to the nursing unit, you notice that an unauthorized employee has gained access to the narcotic cabinet. You witness the employee placing several narcotic tablets into his pocket and walking away. Bearing in mind the responsibilities outlined in the *Code of Ethics for Pharmacy Technicians*, what is the best course of action?

a. Do nothing. This incident did not happen in the pharmacy and therefore is not your problem.
b. Confront the employee and try to wrestle the narcotics away from him.
c. Return to the pharmacy and notify your supervisor prior to the end of your shift.
d. Immediately notify the unit supervisor and the pharmacy manager, who will contact the police. Write down any details of what you witnessed so that you may give a detailed account of the event.

# Part 3: Assessment

## Chapter Summary

- Pharmacy technicians play an important role in all aspects of medication preparation and delivery and are vital members of the healthcare team.
- Most CSPs are administered by the parenteral route.
- Sterile compounding technicians, or IV technicians, use aseptic technique to assemble CSPs for administration to patients.
- The *USP* provides standards and regulations for the preparation and dispensing of medications and healthcare products.
- Technicians must follow USP Chapter <797> guidelines for the compounding of sterile preparations and strictly adhere to proper aseptic technique to reduce potential contamination of the CSP by pathogenic organisms.
- Failure to follow aseptic technique procedures may cause harm to the patient, which may result in serious injury or death.
- State requirements vary regarding the education, training, certification, and licensure of pharmacy technicians.
- Most states require pharmacy technicians to pass a national pharmacy technician certification exam such as the PTCE.
- Pharmacy technicians should complete an ASHP-accredited pharmacy technician training program prior to taking the PTCE.
- Best practice is that pharmacy technicians who prepare CSPs should complete an ACPE-accredited training program in aseptic technique and sterile product preparation prior to making sterile compounds for patient administration.
- Many federal and state agencies oversee the practice of pharmacy, including the FDA and the State Boards of Pharmacy.
- Numerous professional organizations, including ASHP, APhA, PTCB, and ICPT, strive to improve knowledge of medication and pharmacy practice and support pharmacists and pharmacy technicians by advocating for the pharmacy profession.
- Prior to creating CSPs, pharmacy technicians must undergo rigorous training that should include classroom instruction, independent study, written exams, and multiple process validation evaluations.
- Sterile compounding personnel and the CSPs they prepare must undergo various quality assurance and quality control testing procedures such as the media-fill kit, end-product testing, and gloved-fingertip sampling.
- Pharmacy technician training, testing, evaluation, and quality control procedures help to ensure quality patient care by decreasing the potential for CSP contamination.
- Medication safety is the responsibility of every healthcare worker.
- Verifying the five patient "rights" of correct drug administration can help to prevent medication errors.
- In the sterile compounding environment, most medication errors involve incorrect drugs or pharmacy calculations.
- Many organizations, including the ISMP, FDA, and Joint Commission, work to decrease medication errors and improve medication safety. These organizations also encourage medication error reporting as a vital educational process toward the goal of decreasing medication errors.
- Pharmacy technicians must always act in a legal and ethical manner and may consult the *Code of Ethics for Pharmacy Technicians* when facing an ethical dilemma.

# Key Terms

**adverse drug effect (ADE)** any negative, unintended, or unexpected consequence of a drug, which may or may not result in harmful consequences to the patient; also known as adverse drug reaction (ADR) or adverse event (AE)

**alchemist** a skilled compounding artisan

**apothecary** a shop in which medicines were compounded by skilled artisans using herbs and other natural ingredients; these artisans were themselves often called apothecaries

**aseptic technique** processes and physical preparation methods used by personnel who prepare sterile compounds; meant to prevent the introduction of pathogenic organisms or other contaminants into a sterile environment or preparation

**aseptic technique testing kit** a kit that uses a soy-broth medium to test a student's aseptic technique during multiple withdrawals and injections; the completed kit is incubated for a period of time specified by the product's manufacturer; visible particle growth indicates that aseptic technique was compromised at some point during the completion of the testing kit

**best practice** a requirement, practice, procedure, or guideline that meets or exceeds the highest standards, usually those set by ASHP, that are recognized in pharmacy practice

**beyond-use dating (BUD)** date or time after which a CSP is no longer sterile, stable, or effective and must not be used; also called the expiration date

**Boards of Pharmacy** a state entity that creates, oversees, and enforces state and federal laws and regulations governing the practice of pharmacy within that state; provides licensure and registration for pharmacies, pharmacists, and pharmacy technicians

**break in technique** any incidence of failure to follow aseptic technique procedures and protocols; may be observed, or indicated through media-fill, end-product, process validation, or other testing

**compounded sterile preparations (CSPs)** the mixing of one or more sterile products using aseptic technique; USP Chapter <797> contains extensive information on the risk levels and appropriate procedures related to their preparation. Risk levels are:

- **low-risk CSP** a risk level that refers to sterile compounding situations that meet all of the following conditions: compounded entirely within an ISO Class 5 environment using aseptic technique, mixing no more than three commercially manufactured sterile ingredients, and using no more than two injections into any single container
- **medium-risk CSP** a risk level that refers to sterile compounding situations that meet all of the following conditions: compounded entirely within an ISO Class 5 environment using aseptic technique, and involves the mixing of multiple sterile products using complex aseptic manipulations
- **high-risk CSP** a risk level that refers to sterile compounding situations that meet the following conditions: compounded in an environment worse than ISO Class 5, compounded by incorrectly garbed or gloved personnel, and/or compounded with one or more nonsterile ingredients
- **immediate-use CSP** a risk level intended only for CSPs prepared outside of the pharmacy in emergency situations; administration must begin within one hour of preparation; may not be stored for any length of time

**dextrose 5% in water ($D_5W$)** a sterile solution that contains a concentration of 5% dextrose in water

**dyscrasia** a Greek word meaning "bad mixture"; an abnormal blood chemistry

**end-product testing** a type of quality assurance testing in which a CSP is assayed to verify the strength or concentration of its ingredients as well as to determine its sterility; guidelines for end-product testing are provided in USP Chapter <797>

**eucrasia** a Greek word meaning "good mixture," a state of homeostasis reflecting good health

**Exam for the Certification of Pharmacy Technicians (ExCPT)** an exam offered by the Institute for the Certification of Pharmacy Technicians, a division of Assessment Technologies Institute (ATI); not yet widely accepted as a national certification exam; verify state-based acceptance through your state's Board of Pharmacy

**five patient "rights" of correct drug administration** right patient, right drug, right dose, right time, and right route; designed to reduce the chance of medication error; every healthcare worker who administers or prepares medications should verify these five rights prior to administering a drug to a patient

**Food and Drug Administration (FDA)** U.S. government agency responsible for laws and oversight of all regulations related to the development, manufacture, and labeling of medications within the United States; protects public health and safety by ensuring that food, drugs, and cosmetics are safe, effective, and truthfully labeled

**humor** a component of a medieval medical theory often credited to Hippocrates that believed optimal health may be attained only when the four elemental body fluids, or humors (blood, phlegm, black bile, and yellow bile), were in perfect balance

**Institute for Safe Medication Practices (ISMP)** a nonprofit organization that educates the healthcare community and consumers about safe medication practices

**intramuscular (IM) route** the injection of a sterile medication into a large muscle such as the gluteus maximus or the deltoid muscles

**intrathecal (IT) route** the injection of a sterile medication into the spinal column (between vertebrae)

**intravenous piggyback** an IV solution attached to the main IV bag that provides additional medication to a patient receiving an infusion

**intravenous (IV) route** the injection of a sterile medication into a vein

**laminar airflow workbench** a type of hood, usually with a horizontal airflow, in which sterile products are prepared

**media-fill kit** a testing kit used to evaluate the aseptic technique of sterile compounding personnel; also known as an aseptic technique testing kit (ATTACK)

**medication error** a type of error defined by the National Coordinating Council for Medication Error Prevention and Reporting as "any preventable event that may cause or lead to inappropriate medication use or patient harm while the medication is in the control of the health care professional, patient, or consumer;" may include errors in "prescribing; order communication; product labeling, packaging, and nomenclature; compounding; dispensing; distribution; administration; education; monitoring; and use"

**MedWatch** the FDA's voluntary system for reporting medication errors

**microbial contamination** contamination of a CSP by any microbial organism, bacteria, virus, fungi, or other pathogen; may result in infection or other harm to patients receiving the CSP

**Model Curriculum for Pharmacy Technician Training** a set of standards for the training of pharmacy technicians; ASHP's guide for accredited pharmacy technician training programs

**normal saline (NS)** a sterile solution containing a concentration of 0.9% sodium chloride in water

**parenteral route of administration** a route of supplying medication to a patient other than through the digestive tract; includes the intravenous, intramuscular, subcutaneous, and intrathecal routes

**Pharmacy Technician Certification Exam (PTCE)** a nationally accepted certification exam offered by the PTCB; PTCB-certified pharmacy technicians are designated by the acronym CPhT (Certified Pharmacy Technician)

**process validation** an evaluation checklist that an instructor uses to observe, critique, and grade a student's aseptic technique during the training period; also used as part of the annual recertification process for sterile compounding personnel as regulated by USP Chapter <797>

**quality assurance procedures** methods and tests for ensuring use of proper aseptic technique

**sterile compounding** the process of diluting, mixing, injecting, or otherwise preparing sterile solutions using aseptic technique

**sterile compounding personnel** pharmacy personnel who prepare CSPs

**subcutaneous (Sub-Q) route** injection of a sterile medication into the area just beneath the skin; the formerly accepted abbreviations *SC* and *SQ* are now discouraged

**United States Pharmacopeia (USP)** a nongovernmental regulatory organization that sets public standards for the preparation and dispensing of prescription and over-the-counter medications as well as other healthcare products

**USP Chapter <797>** Chapter <797> of the *United States Pharmacists' Pharmacopeia,* which sets practice standards regarding the preparation of sterile compounds

# Make Connections

*On a separate sheet of paper, write your answers to the following three questions, using complete sentences and making sure your answers are thorough and thoughtful. Note that the third question requires Internet access.*

1. Considering what you've learned so far about sterile compounding and the effects of aseptic technique on patient health and safety, what are the potential consequences of incorrect technique?
2. USP Chapter <797> guidelines require initial and annual competency assessments, which include a written exam, process validation, and media-fill aseptic technique testing. Why is it important for the technician to undergo such rigorous testing? Why is it important to be retested annually?
3. Find and then explore the ".org" website for the *USP*. What is one advantage of having a hard copy of the *USP* on hand in the pharmacy? What is one advantage of accessing the website versus using the hard copy of the *USP*?

# Meet the Challenge

***Scenario*** This "puzzling" activity helps you to become more familiar with some of the key terminology and abbreviations identified in this chapter.

***Challenge*** On your own, read the numbered key-term hints and fill in the associated numbered crossword squares with a key term or related concept from this chapter. The term should both suit the hint and fit within the available number of squares. (Once you have completed this challenge, you might want to create additional crossword puzzles on your own, using the remaining chapter key terms and exchanging your blank puzzles and hints with classmates.)

ACROSS

1 A process validation tool
4 A skilled compounding artisan
6 The number of risk levels associated with sterile compounding
7 An organization that oversees pharmacy continuing education
10 An organization that supports health-system pharmacists
11 The number of procedural labs requiring process validation
12 An organization that sets commercial and industrial standards that often become law
14 Free from pathogenic contaminants
15 A practice that meets or exceeds the highest pharmacy standards
17 A type of certification exam for pharmacy technicians
18 Exploratory and procedural modules tested by process validation
19 The dilution, mixing, and injection of drugs using aseptic technique

DOWN

2 The topic of an AAPT publication for pharmacy technicians
3 The person who prepares sterile compounds
5 Under the skin
8 A sterile injectable medication that may be administered by the IV, IM, or Sub-Q routes
9 Injected into the space around the spine and brain
13 Injected into the vein
14 A type of aseptic technique testing kit
16 The art and science of preparing and dispensing medications

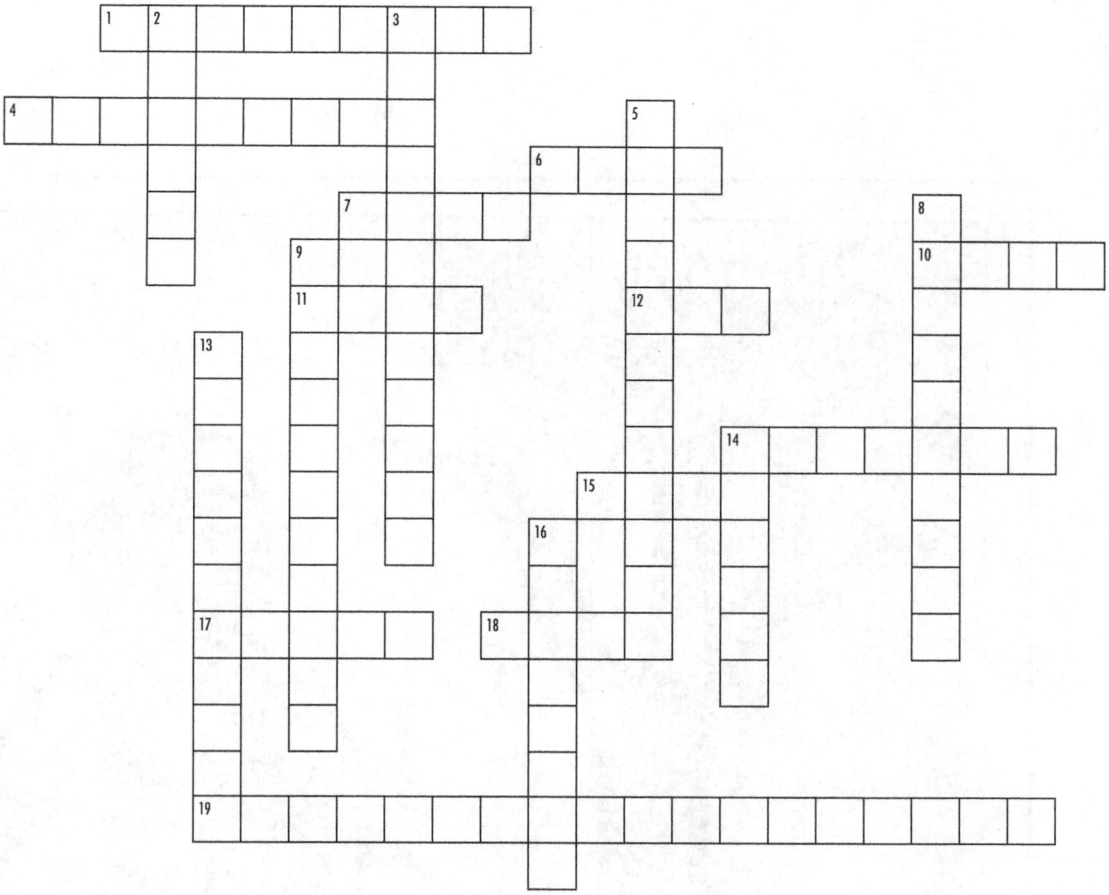


## ADDITIONAL RESOURCES

*Go to the Paradigm Internet Resources Center at* www.paradigmcollege.net/sterilecomp *to access live links related to these Chapter 1 topics:*

- ASHP guidelines
- Process for testing and national certification of pharmacy technicians
- Pharmacy careers, advocacy, and professional support for hospital and health-system pharmacy personnel
- Pharmacy careers, advocacy, and professional support for community and retail pharmacy personnel
- Federal laws and regulations on the manufacture and sale of drugs or other medical products
- Prevention and reporting of medication errors

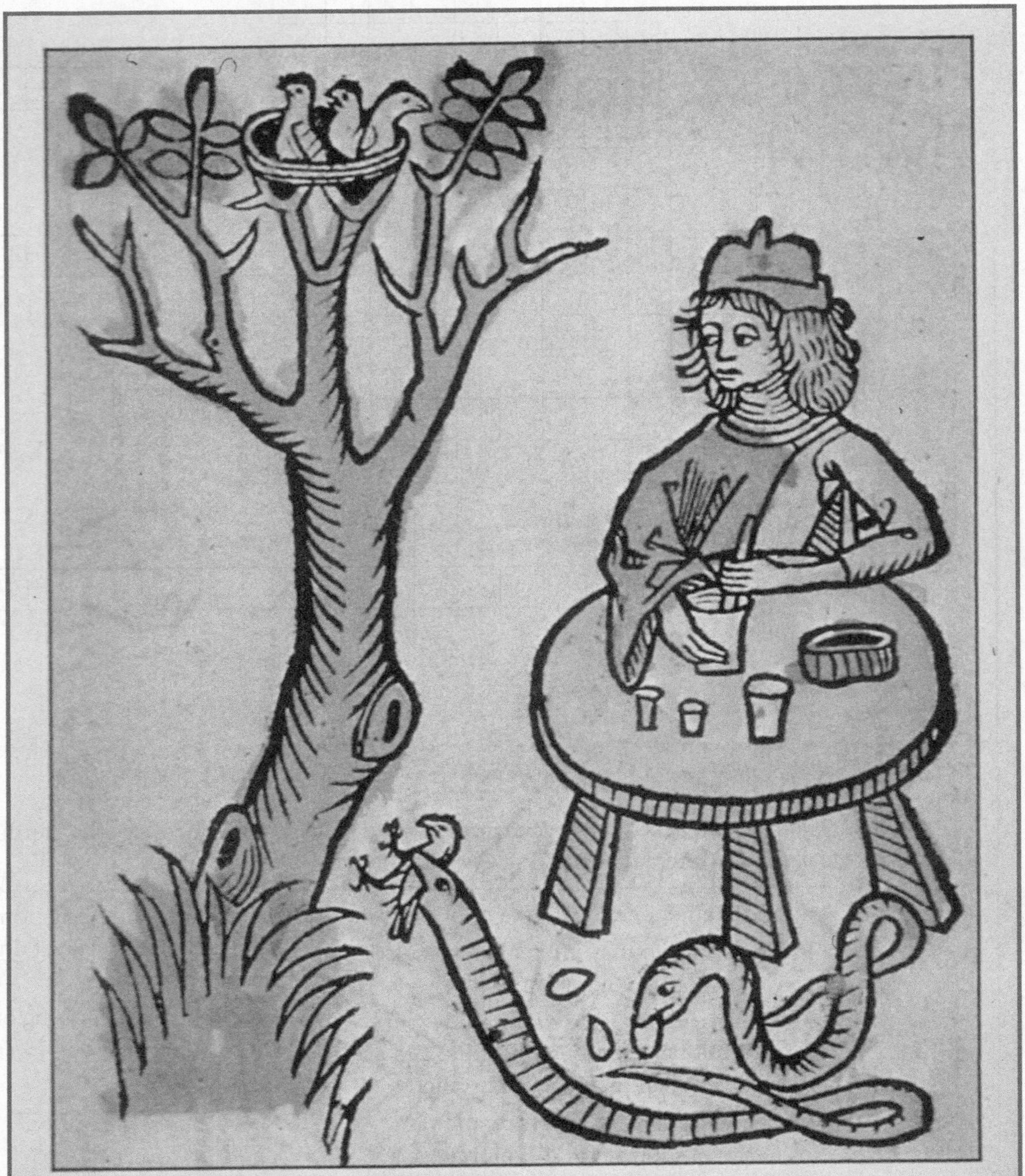

Chapter 2

# The Sterile Compounding Environment

## Learning Objectives

- Identify the origin of the pharmacy clean room and procedures for sterile compounding.
- Describe anteroom and clean room setup and characteristics.
- Understand the various ISO levels that are appropriate for sterile compounding.
- Identify the different types of hoods used for sterile compounding.
- Classify the four sterile compounding risk levels.
- Recognize potential contaminants in the sterile compounding environment.

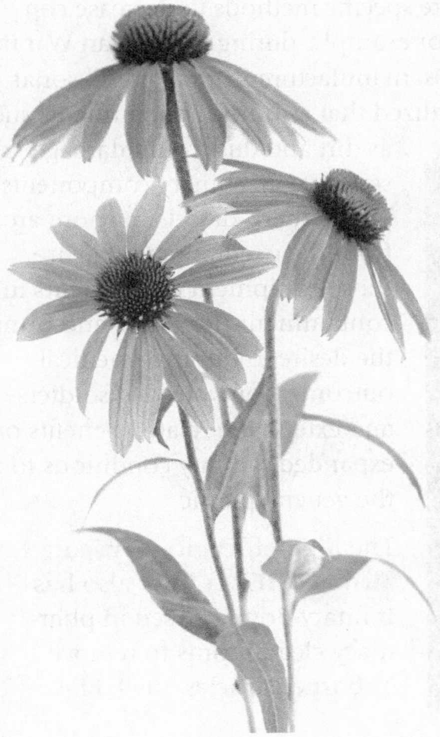

## Early Compounding Environments

During the early history of medicine, healers and alchemists prepared medicinal compounds by grinding plants and herbs with a mortar and pestle. This type of compounding was often done on a wooden table in a back room of the village apothecary shop. Residents of the village received both diagnosis and treatment from the local apothecary. However, royal physicians worked within the walls of the royal palace or in civic buildings and provided their pharmaceutical-compounding services only to ailing and injured members of the ruling elite, including governing officials, the nobility, and members of the ruling class.

Prior to the nineteenth century and the development of parenteral medications, pharmacy compounding was performed in apothecary shops, which were often constructed to provide several small rooms, each serving a very specific purpose. The outermost room served as the display area of the shop. Shelves and counters contained jars filled with prepared medicines and bottles of tinctures and elixirs. The shops often contained at least two inner rooms: one used for the diagnosis and treatment of the patient and the other dedicated to medicinal compounding. Shelves in the inner rooms were stocked with jars of herbs and compounding supplies, along with a myriad of glass bottles and associated copper tubing, which were heated to distill various preparations. In addition, most early apothecary shops maintained a large and varied garden to grow a rich supply of medicinal herbs.

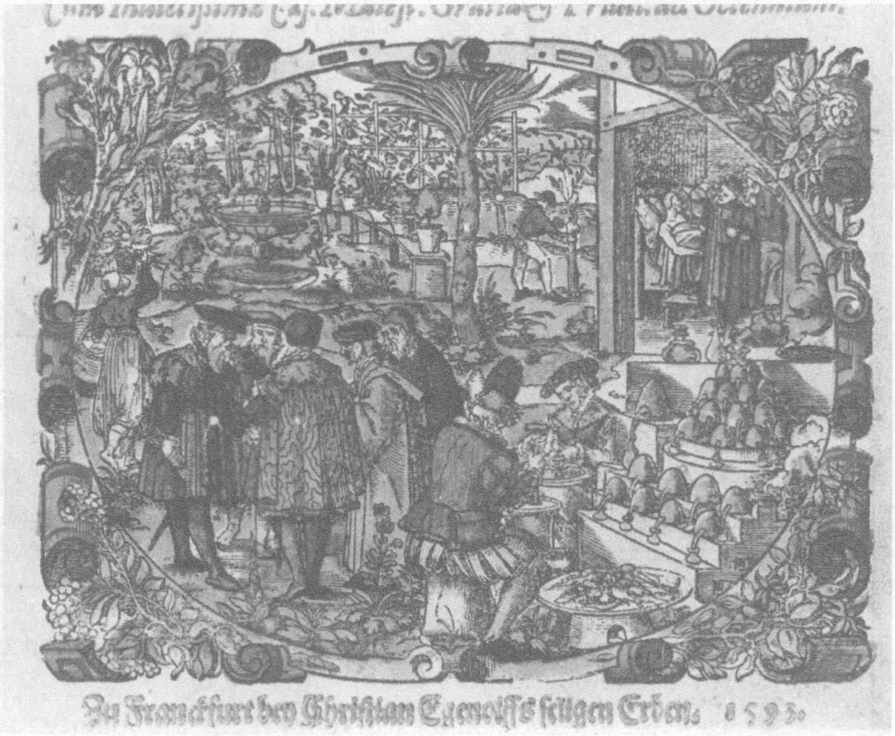

## Clean Room Origins, Types, and Developments

From the mid-1800s until the early 1900s, discoveries and developments in medicine brought about gradual changes in pharmacy and sterile compounding. These changes impacted the areas in which compounds were prepared. Scientific discoveries, including those of Pasteur and Lister, about the transmission of germs led to the use of antiseptics in surgery and medicine and increased awareness of the importance of the compounding environment. Lister's stringent cleanliness practices so significantly decreased patient deaths that he became known as the "Father of Antiseptic Surgery." In fact, hospital surgery rooms were the areas first known as "clean rooms," wherein hospital staff made a concentrated effort to reduce the likelihood of contamination by germs, bacteria, and dust.

In subsequent decades, wartime observations inspired several scientific and medical advances, including more specific methods to decrease contamination. For example, during the Korean War in the early 1950s, manufacturers of radar and sonar equipment realized that airborne contaminants such as dirt and dust could damage sensitive machinery components. The modern-day **clean room** arose from the need to manufacture those equipment components in contaminant-free areas, and from the desire to improve medical outcomes for wounded soldiers and extend the related benefits of expanded sanitary conditions to the general public.

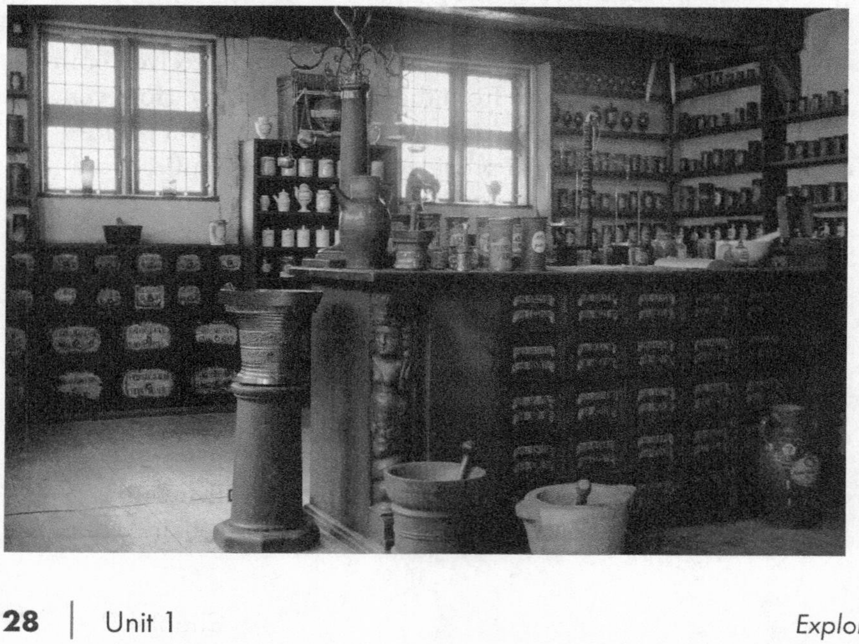

The **high-efficiency particulate airflow (HEPA) filter** also has military origins. Used in pharmacy clean rooms to remove airborne particles, the HEPA

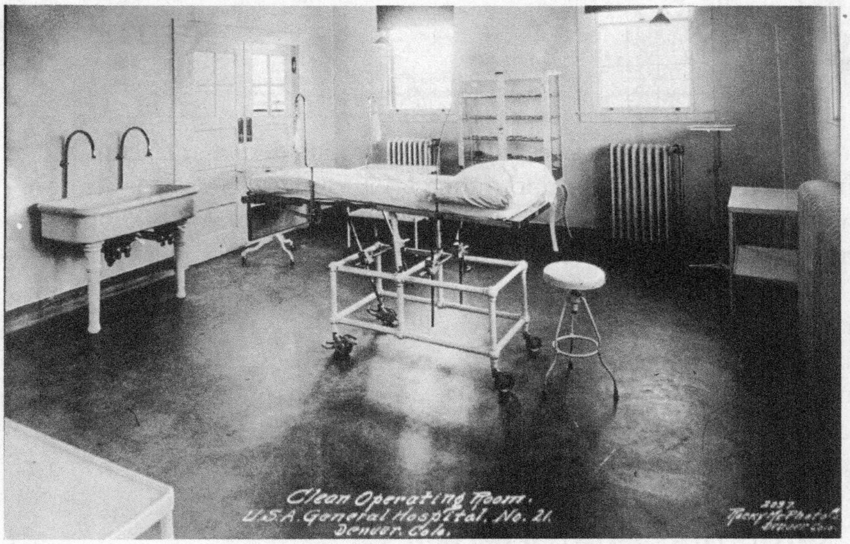


filter was invented during the Manhattan Project to protect scientists working on the atom bomb from exposure to radioactive contaminants in the air. It was declassified in the 1950s, improved in design, and marketed for public use in various technological and medical laboratories.

The U.S. military developed some of the earliest guidelines for the standardized setup and use of clean rooms. In 1960, the first clean room standard was provided by Air Force Technical Order 00-25-203, entitled *Air Force Standard Functional Criteria for the Design and Operation of Clean Rooms*. Today, some of the government agencies that set standards for clean rooms include the U.S. Department of Public Health, the Nuclear Regulatory Commission, the National Aeronautics and Space Administration, and the National Institute of Standards and Technology. These agencies regulate a type of clean room called an **industrial clean room**, which is primarily used for electronic, technology, and military manufacturing. The semiconductor and computer chip manufacturing industries are the primary users of industrial clean rooms. The main goal of the industrial clean room is to create a work area with a reduced quantity of airborne particles.

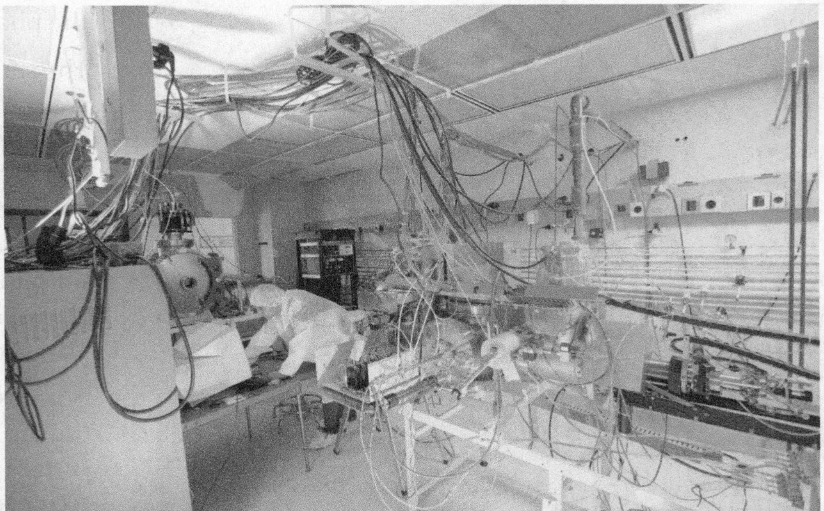

When personnel prepare **biological agents**, **pharmaceuticals**, and sterile compounds, or perform certain kinds of research, they work in another type of clean room known as a hospital, laboratory, or **pharmacy clean room**. This room type is very similar in design to the industrial clean room and shares the general goal of reducing the quantity of airborne particles. However, the primary focus of the pharmacy clean room is to reduce potential contamination by bacteria, viruses, fungi, or other sources of potential infection. Using the pharmacy clean room is one method of decreasing the likelihood of contamination from the work environment during sterile compounding procedures.

Many other tools and strategies can reduce the likelihood of contamination in the compounding environment. The **anteroom** is the room or area located just outside the clean room. The term *anteroom* literally translates as "before room" and is where compounding personnel prepare for entry into the clean room. A horizontal laminar airflow hood or a vertical laminar airflow hood, both of which may also be called a cabinet or workbench, provides the **primary engineering control (PEC)** under which sterile compounds are prepared. In addition, stringent guidelines for the design, setup, maintenance, and cleaning of the anteroom and clean room, as well as standards of conduct for pharmacy personnel, all serve to reduce the risk of contaminating sterile compounds.

# Part 1: Concepts

USP Chapter <797> brought forth sweeping changes to the design and setup of areas in which pharmacy sterile compounding is performed. These changes have caused many pharmacies to completely redesign the layout and function of their sterile compounding areas so that the anteroom and clean room space is separated from the rest of the pharmacy. Some changes necessitated by USP Chapter <797> have required pharmacies to undergo extensive and costly renovations to meet the new standards. Specialized **heating, ventilation, and air conditioning (HVAC)** equipment, clean rooms constructed of **nonporous materials**, and strictly regulated air pressure and humidity control serve to create appropriate anteroom and clean-room environments that are low in particulate matter.

## Anteroom Setup and Characteristics

The anteroom, which may also be called the transition area or ante-area, provides a space where sterile compounding personnel can garb and perform aseptic hand washing. The anteroom is also a place to stage components and supplies prior to entering the clean room. In addition, the anteroom serves as a transition area that helps to maintain required air pressure levels, thereby reducing the need for the **heating, ventilation, and air conditioning (HVAC)** system to manage large disturbances in airflow or changes in temperature or humidity within the clean room. Most sterile compounding pharmacies have an anteroom that is separate from the clean room (see Figure 2.1). However, small facilities that perform only low- or medium-risk sterile compounding may create an ante-area that is separated from the clean room by a simple **line of demarcation**.

Most sterile compounding pharmacies secure a **sticky mat** to the floor at the doorway leading into the clean room. In many cases, that doorway separates the anteroom from the clean room. But in facilities without a separate anteroom, the doorway instead separates the pharmacy from a room that contains both the ante-area (where sterile compounding personnel garb, don shoe covers, and wash) and the clean room itself. In both cases, the sticky mat is placed on the less sterile side of the doorway: either on the anteroom floor or on the pharmacy floor.

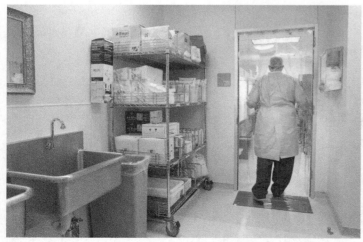

IV technician leaving the anteroom and walking across the sticky mat covering the threshold to the clean room.

The sticky mat is an approximately 18″ × 36″ rectangle intended to help compounders avoid tracking dirt into the sterile compounding area. The back of the mat adheres to the floor and the top of the mat is made up of multiple layers of a sticky substance designed to hold onto the dirt and other loose substances clinging to the bottoms of shoes or shoe covers. These loose particles stick to the mat.

At a designated frequency, you must remove the top layer of the mat to expose a fresh sticky surface and deposit the used layer in a waste receptacle. The frequency varies by facility and compounding volume. Facilities performing a small volume of sterile compounding may have to replace the mat surface daily. Facilities responsible for a large amount of sterile compounding may be required to change out the sticky mat every shift, or even more frequently. Refer to your pharmacy's Policy and Procedure (P&P) manual to determine the requirements for sticky mat replacement.

You may store supplies within the anteroom but should limit items to a small number of materials that are directly required for sterile compound preparation. These items might include syringes, needles, vials, and supplies used in aseptic hand washing or hood cleaning procedures. No horseplay is allowed in the anteroom or clean room. Chewing gum, food, drinks, materials exposed to patients or patient care areas, and nonessential items are also not allowed in the anteroom. Only trained personnel should enter the anteroom. You should avoid storing compounding supplies long-term and should *never* store cardboard or other materials with a high potential for shedding in the anteroom. You must spray or wipe down all supplies with sterile 70% isopropyl alcohol (IPA) or another suitable cleaning agent prior to transporting them from the anteroom into the clean room.

**POINTER**

Consult your facility's P&P manual to determine which additional cleaning agents may be suitable for cleaning within the anteroom and clean room.

**FIGURE 2.1**

**Layout of Hospital Clean Room and Anteroom**

Notice the airflow direction from the high-pressure clean room, through the lower-pressure anteroom, and outward toward the lowest-pressure outer pharmacy area.

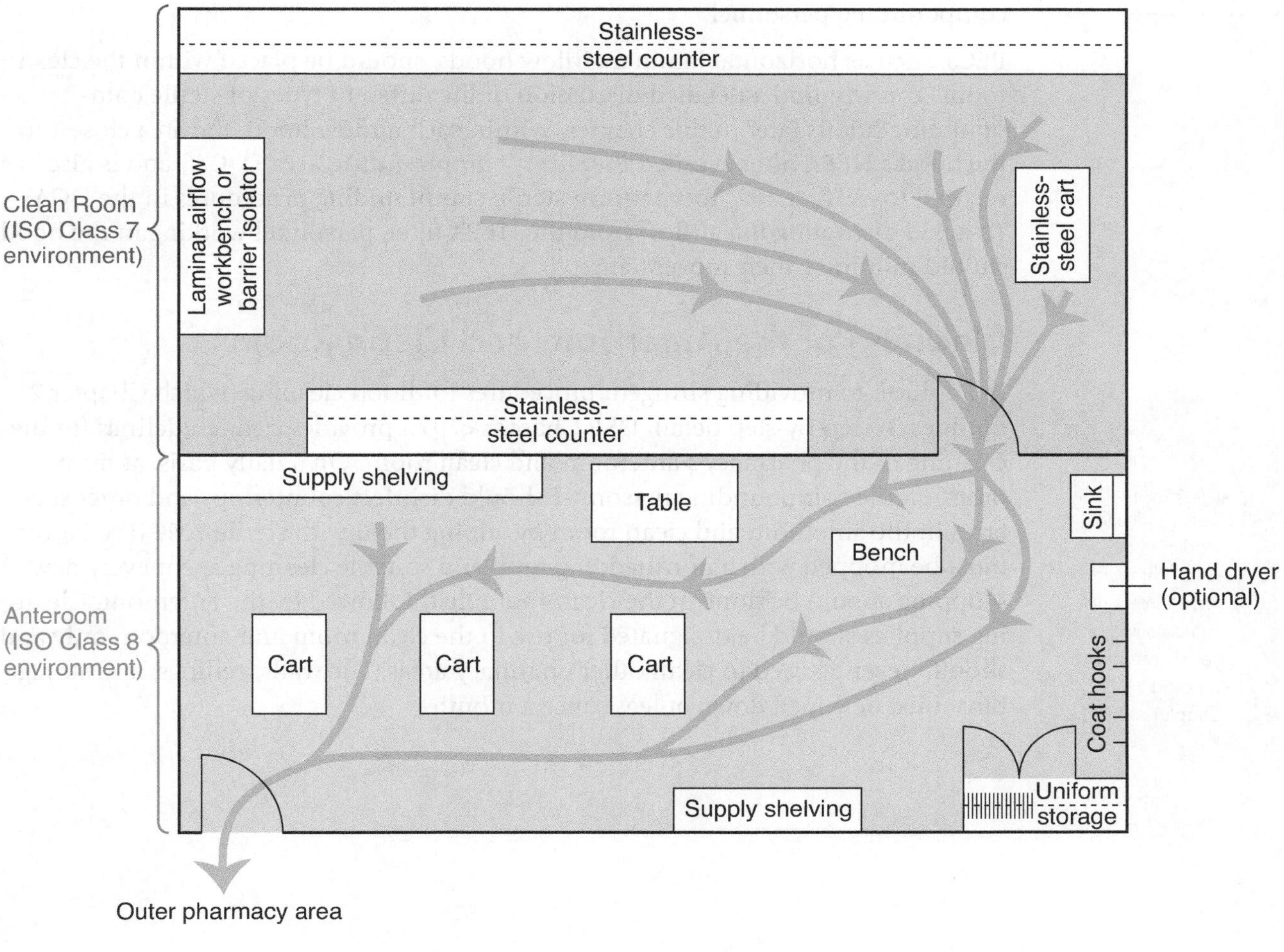

## Clean Room Setup and Characteristics

The clean room is the innermost room within the pharmacy. The laminar airflow hoods are located within the clean room. You may hear the clean room also referred to as the IV room or the buffer area. Access to the clean room is restricted to properly trained and garbed personnel. You must don sterile gloves immediately upon entering the clean room. Bring into the clean room only those supplies needed for the immediate preparation of sterile compounds. Do not locate computers, printers, or other devices that are not essential to the immediate sterile compounding process in the clean room. The floors in the clean room should be coved and heat-sealed to the surrounding walls. Caulk or otherwise seal all joints or cracks in flooring, walls, and ceilings to minimize the buildup of dust and dirt. The surfaces of floors, walls, ceiling tiles, and lighting fixtures must be smooth, nonporous, and easy to clean.

**POINTER**
Plan well and make just one trip into the clean room with all your supplies in order to minimize the airflow disruption created by walking to or from the clean room.

A pharmacy-designated HVAC system should pump HEPA-filtered air into the clean room to create a positive-pressure environment. The positive pressure within the clean room ensures that the airflow moves outward from the clean room, through the anteroom, and continues in the direction of the outer pharmacy area. A positive-pressure environment helps to minimize the travel of dust, spores, and other particles from the outer rooms into the clean room. The humidity and temperature of the clean room should be kept lower than those of the surrounding rooms in order to reduce the potential for bacterial growth and maximize the comfort of sterile compounding personnel.

PECs, such as horizontal laminar airflow hoods, should be placed within the clean room. You will find a detailed discussion of the different types of sterile compounding hoods later in this chapter. Within each airflow hood, the area closest to the hood's HEPA filter is called the **direct compounding area (DCA)** and is also referred to as "first air." You perform sterile compounding procedures in the DCA. To avoid disrupting the airflow from the HEPA filter, personnel working in the hood should minimize their movements.

## Cleaning of the Anteroom and Clean Room

**USP Chapter <797>**
You can find complete guidelines regarding the setup, characteristics, maintenance, and cleaning of the sterile compounding area in USP Chapter <797>.

In addition to providing stringent procedures for hood cleaning, which Chapter 7 outlines in step-by-step detail, USP Chapter <797> provides clear guidelines for the cleaning of the pharmacy's anteroom and clean room. On a daily basis, at minimum, sterile compounding personnel should disinfect countertops and other surfaces in the anteroom and clean room by wiping them with sterile 70% IPA. Floors must be mopped with a nonshedding mop and suitable cleaning agent every day. Mopping should be done in the clean room first, followed by the anteroom. Cleaning supplies should be designated for use in the clean room and anteroom only and should never be used to clean other pharmacy areas. The walls, ceilings, and storage bins must be wiped down at least once a month.

## ISO Environments Appropriate for Sterile Compounding

**Table 2.1 ISO Classifications**

| ISO Class Name | Maximum Particle Count (in particles of 0.5 micron and larger per cubic meter of air) |
|---|---|
| 3 | 35.2 |
| 4 | 352 |
| 5* | 3520 |
| 6 | 35,200 |
| 7 | 352,000 |
| 8 | 3,520,000 |

*The ISO Class 5 rating is synonymous with "Class 100."

The **International Organization for Standardization (ISO)** creates worldwide industrial and commercial standards that often become law. USP Chapter <797> identifies several ISO categories, or classes, that classify the amount of particulate matter in room air. These categories are numbered from Class 3 to Class 8, with a higher number designating a greater allowance for particulate matter. The most restrictive category, therefore, is ISO Class 3 (see Table 2.1).

In general, ISO class stringency within the pharmacy environment increases as you travel from the regular pharmacy areas to the anteroom, to the clean room, and into the hood. In general, the particulate matter contained in regular room air within a pharmacy should be *at or above* the ISO Class 8 range, or approximately 3.52 million particles of 0.5 micron or larger per cubic meter of air. At the next level of stringency, the particulate matter in the pharmacy anteroom must be *no greater than* ISO Class 8. Stricter still, the particulate matter in the clean room should be *no more than* ISO Class 7, or 352,000 particles per cubic meter of air. This ISO Class 7 environment is created through the combined use of HEPA-filtered, positive-pressure air delivered through a designated HVAC system, and nonporous construction components that are not prone to collecting dust. In addition, specially trained personnel sustain the ISO Class 7 environment by performing specific procedures that maintain the cleanliness of the environment.

The air within the DCA of a hood must be ISO Class 5, or no more than 3520 particles per cubic meter of air. In the United States, the ISO Class 5 environment is more commonly known as a Class 100 environment. The ISO Class 5/Class 100 environment within a hood is created by pushing specially filtered air through the various components of the hood or workbench. Chapter 7 of this textbook discusses the components and function of each part of the hood in detail.

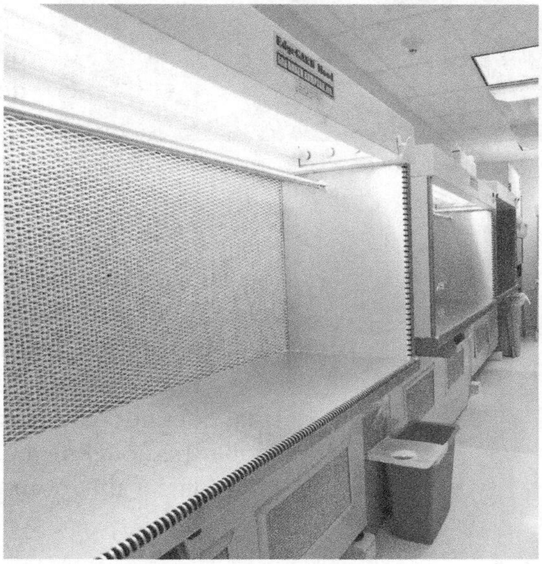

Horizontal LAFW in the clean room.

## Types of Hoods Required for Sterile Compounding

Sterile compounding relies on several types of hoods. Each type has a DCA with HEPA-filtered laminar airflow that provides a Class 100 environment. All of the different hood types may be referred to as primary engineering control (PEC). Sterile compounding personnel perform their work in the following hood types: the **compounding aseptic isolator (CAI)**, the **compounding aseptic containment isolator (CACI)**, the **biological safety cabinet (BSC)**, and the **laminar airflow workbench (LAFW)**. While each hood provides an acceptable DCA, the hoods' design, function, and operation differ in a number of important ways. The most widely used sterile compounding hood in the pharmacy is the horizontal LAFW. Chapter 7 of this textbook discusses in depth this hood type and its function and cleaning. In addition, the lab activities in Chapters 8–13 involve procedures designed to be performed within the horizontal LAFW.

**POINTER**
The LAFW is also commonly referred to as the hood, the horizontal airflow hood, and the horizontal laminar airflow hood. You may hear all of these terms used interchangeably.

***CAI and CACI Hoods*** The CAI is most useful in sterile compounding environments where relatively few compounded preparations are made each day. This type of hood may also be called a **barrier isolator** or an isolator cabinet. The isolator cabinet is a completely enclosed system. Access to the DCA is accomplished by moving supplies through a pass-through window into a small compartment located at the side of the cabinet. The front of the cabinet contains a fixed pair of gloves attached to the inner wall of the cabinet. Sterile compounding personnel place their hands inside the gloves and reach through the inner pass-through window to bring the supplies from the side compartment into the main working space of the isolator cabinet. The IV technician then continues working through the fixed pair of gloves to manipulate the sterile compound within the cabinet. Once the technician has compounded the preparation, she or he returns it to the side compartment, removes the hands from the fixed gloves, and retrieves the sterile compound from the side compartment through the outer pass-through window.

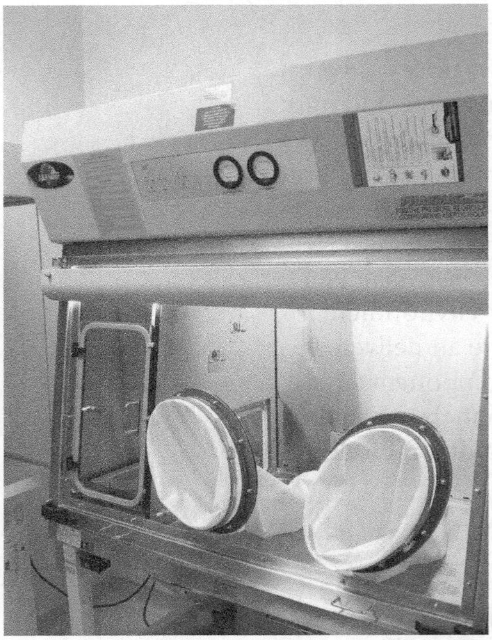
Compounding aseptic containment isolator (CACI).

The CACI is very similar in setup and function to the CAI; however, its design provides greater protection for the worker. According to page 29 of the *USP <797> Guidebook*, the HEPA filter in this type of cabinet is "capable of containing airborne concentrations of the physical size and state of the drug being compounded." If you prepare hazardous drugs in the CACI, you must ensure that the air exhausted from the cabinet is adequately filtered and vented to the outdoors through a specially dedicated pharmacy ventilation system.

***Advantages and Disadvantages of the CAI and CACI Hoods*** The CAI and the CACI hoods have two primary advantages. First, these types of hoods offer a safer environment for the worker because the fully enclosed cabinets limit direct exposure to airborne drugs. Second, because the isolator cabinets are completely enclosed, it is not mandatory to place them in an ISO Class 7 environment, as is always the case with the LAFW- and BSC-type hoods. Instead, facilities may locate CAI and CACI hoods in either an ISO Class 7 or ISO Class 8 environment. This option can be very advantageous to a facility that does not have much space or does not wish to spend hundreds of thousands of dollars remodeling the pharmacy to build an ISO Class 7 clean room in addition to an ISO Class 8 anteroom.

However, the isolator hoods also have some drawbacks. The DCA within the isolator hood is limited in space and can only accommodate a very small number of sterile compounding items at a time. The number of workers who can access the cabinet at any one time is also limited because usually only one or two pairs of fixed gloves are built into the cabinet. Also, the isolator hoods require special operational and cleaning procedures that can be very labor-intensive. Thus, the limited capacity, increased demand on the worker's time, and logistical issues or costs associated with proper venting make the isolator hoods problematic for most of the larger sterile-compounding facilities. In addition, the need for special filtration and correct venting of the CACI may be cost prohibitive.

**USP Chapter <797>**

Cleaning procedures for hoods vary. Consult the isolator manufacturer's handbook for special procedures on the maintenance, use, and cleaning of the CAI and CACI hoods.

***BSC Hood*** The BSC is a special hood for preparing hazardous compounds such as **antineoplastic drugs** and other **chemotherapy** medications. The HEPA-filtered air within a BSC flows downward in a vertical pattern and is then removed from the cabinet through small ventilation holes located at the back and sides of the cabinet. This contaminated air is again HEPA-filtered before being recirculated into the cabinet or ventilated to the outdoors. A Plexiglas shield at the front of the cabinet comes down from the top of the cabinet and stops approximately eight inches above the work surface. The worker stands behind the shield and places the hands into the cabinet to manipulate the sterile compound. This type of cabinet is designed solely to protect the worker from hazardous chemicals. Because of the potential for worker contamination, the BSC should be located in a negative-pressure room that is completely separate from any rooms housing non-BSC hoods. The design of the BSC, as well as the special procedures for its use and cleaning, are detailed in Chapter 14 of this textbook.

**POINTER**

Working with the BSC requires specialized training and testing. Personnel who work in this area must have consistently demonstrated competency in mathematics, excellent aseptic technique, and attention to detail.

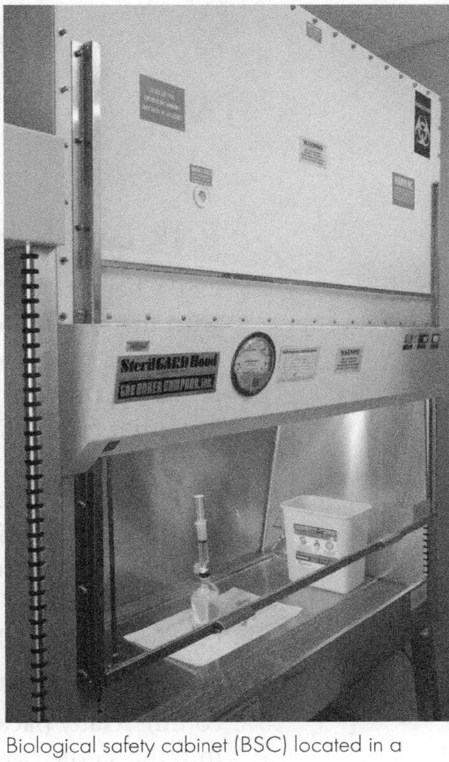

Biological safety cabinet (BSC) located in a negative-pressure room.

## USP Chapter <797> Guidelines for Hoods

Regardless of hood type, most hoods share a common design such that room air enters the cabinet through a **prefilter** that removes large particles that might damage the HEPA filter. As illustrated in Figure 2.2, the blower draws room air in through the prefilter and forces the air further into the hood, through the HEPA filter, and across the work surface. The blower should remain on at all times. If, for any reason, the blower is turned off, you must turn it back on and allow it to run for at least 30 minutes prior to cleaning the cabinet and using the hood for sterile compounding.

According to page 48 of the *USP <797> Guidebook*, the hood must be completely cleaned, at a minimum, "at the beginning of each work shift, before each batch preparation is started, every 30 minutes during continuous compounding periods of individual CSPs, when there are spills, and when surface contamination is known or suspected from procedural breaches."

**FIGURE 2.2**

**Cross Section of Horizontal LAFW (Side View)**

Room air is drawn into the cabinet through the prefilter and then through the blower, which forces the air upward, through the HEPA filter, and horizontally across the work surface toward the worker.

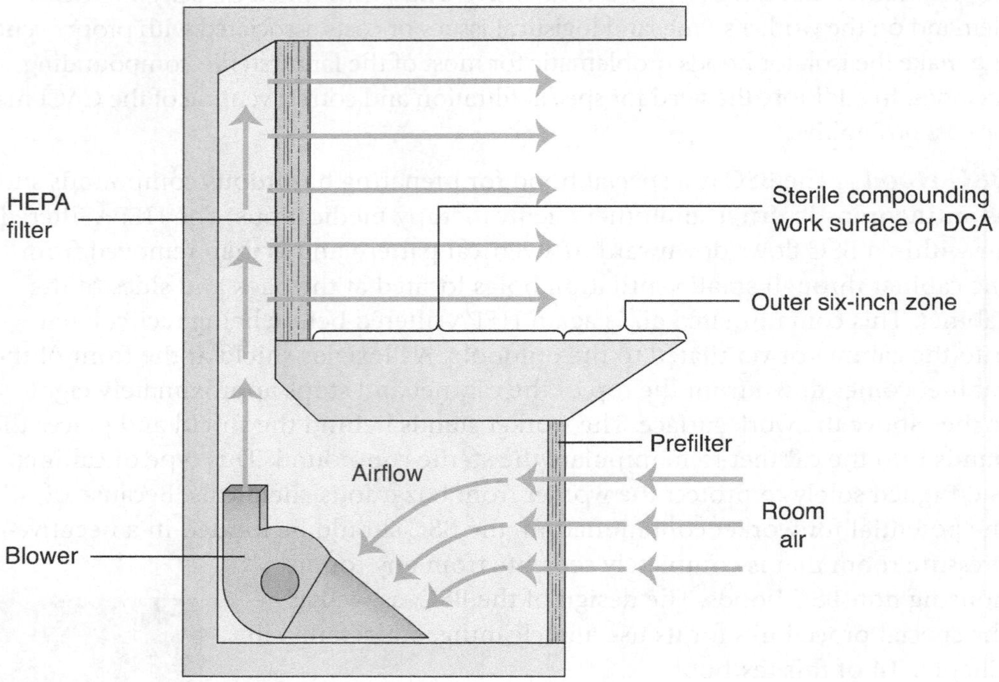


## Risk Levels in Sterile Compounding

USP Chapter <797> defines four microbial contamination risk levels associated with the creation of **compounded sterile preparations (CSPs)**. They include low-risk CSPs, medium-risk CSPs, high-risk CSPs, and immediate-use CSPs. The risk levels are provided as a guide for sterile compounding personnel to determine the potential for contamination in various compounding scenarios. The pharmacy supervisor is responsible for determining the risk level of CSPs, and for developing policies and procedures designed to reinforce USP Chapter <797> standards for all sterile compounding procedures and personnel. All pharmacy personnel hold the responsibility of following these policies and procedures to help ensure patient health and safety. USP Chapter <797> contains a provision for immediate-use CSPs, which may be used in certain emergency situations.

***Low-Risk CSPs*** Low-risk conditions involve the mixing of no more than three commercially packaged sterile products, and no more than two separate injections into the sterile container, all done aseptically, within an **ISO Class 5** workbench. This type of ISO Class 5 environment may also be referred to as a Class 100 work-bench or laminar airflow hood. The DCA is located in the section within the hood that is closest to the HEPA filter and receives uninterrupted laminar airflow. All sterile compounding must take place within the DCA. Many low-risk CSPs are prepared daily in every IV room. One example of a common low-risk CSP is dextrose 5% in water 1000 mL with 30 mEq of potassium chloride.

***Medium-Risk CSPs*** Medium-risk conditions meet all of the conditions associated with low-risk sterile product preparation and also involve other, more complex, sterile compounding procedures. For instance, multiple doses of sterile products that are combined or administered to multiple patients are considered medium-risk activities. In addition, the preparation of a **total parenteral nutrition (TPN)** solution is a medium-risk activity because it involves multiple injections of several medications into an IV bag that is designed to be administered over a 24-hour period.

**POINTER**

As an IV technician, you will prepare primarily low-risk and medium-risk CSPs.

***High-Risk CSPs*** High-risk CSPs meet all of the conditions of the low- and medium-risk groups and also involve the preparation of medications wherein one or more of the products being prepared is not sterile or the product is prepared in an environment that is less stringently controlled, or more risky, than ISO Class 5. Nonsterile medications must be sterilized before they are injected into the patient. The two most common sterilization methods include **filtration sterilization**, which is accomplished by passing the liquid medication through a 0.2-micron filter, and **heat sterilization**, which is achieved by **autoclaving** the compounded solution.

Pharmacy personnel do not commonly prepare high-risk CSPs in the sterile compounding environment. However, occasional manufacturer shortages of a commonly available product may necessitate the preparation of a high-risk CSP. One such example is compounded, injectable, caffeine citrate solution, which involves dissolving nonsterile caffeine citrate powder in sterile water. Personnel draw up the solution into a syringe and then inject it through a 0.2-micron filter into an empty evacuated container. Using a sterilizing filter provides some protection from microbial contamination, but because this compound is made with a nonsterile ingredient, it falls into the high-risk CSP classification.

***Immediate-Use CSPs*** Immediate-use preparations, according to page 12 of the *USP <797> Guidebook*, are "intended only for those situations where there is a need for emergency, or immediate, patient administration of a CSP. Such situations may include cardiopulmonary resuscitation, emergency room treatment, preparation of diagnostic agents, or critical therapy where the preparation of the CSP under conditions described for low-risk-level CSPs subjects the patient to additional risk due to delays in therapy." Immediate-use CSPs must be administered within one hour of preparation. One example of an immediate-use CSP is an epinephrine IV infusion, likely prepared by a nurse at the patient's bedside while the patient is undergoing emergency treatment for a cardiac arrest.

## *Potential Contaminants in the Sterile Compounding Environment*

The word *aseptic* means "without infection." Aseptic technique is a multi-part technique, or a set of practices and procedures specifically designed to not introduce any source of infection, such as a pathogen, into a sterile environment. Aseptic technique is performed under carefully controlled conditions with the goal of minimizing contamination by pathogens. **Pathogenic contaminants** may include bacteria, viruses, fungi, hair, dander, or particulate matter. For the purposes of sterile product preparation and aseptic technique, the sterile environment is the container or delivery vehicle, which can include items such as IV bags, IV piggyback bags, syringes, vials, medications, or solutions. The goals of aseptic technique are to protect the patient from infection and to prevent the spread of pathogens.

To help reach these goals, remember that some areas of each instrument, product, or supply item should never be touched, for **touch contamination** carries the potential for serious harm to the patient. For example, the tip of the syringe should never be touched by the IV technician. It should also never be left uncapped on the hood's surface because doing so significantly increases the potential for touch contamination. Chapter 3 of this textbook discusses in detail the critical sites of compounding supplies and further outlines techniques to avoid touch contamination.

Another form of contamination is **shadowing**. Shadowing is caused by incorrect technique, or incorrectly placing either objects or your hands within the laminar airflow hood. Shadowing jeopardizes product sterility. Consider that, in a horizontal LAFW, air flows horizontally through the HEPA filter and then across the work surface toward the worker. When that sterile air flows across the work surface, it also passes over and around the vials, syringes, and all products necessary for preparing sterile pharmaceuticals. The sterile air must not be disturbed as it flows across critical areas, such as the vial top, the injection port, the syringe tip, or the uncapped needle. Thus, you must carefully consider both the placement of your hands and of objects within the hood so that each item receives uninterrupted airflow and airflow to all critical areas is maintained. The area immediately behind an item within the hood is a **zone of turbulence** and is considered to be contaminated (see Figure 2.3).

The outermost edge of the hood (the edge closest to the worker and farthest from the origin of the flow) receives airflow of a lower velocity than the airflow that is closer to the hood filter. In addition, along the outer edge of the hood, room air mixes with the air blown through the HEPA filter. These facts determine that the six-inch band, or

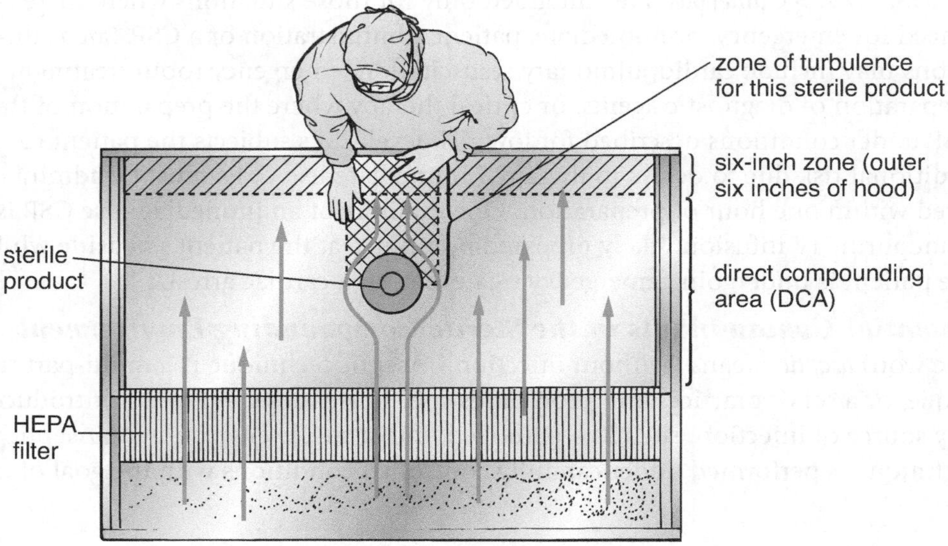


**FIGURE 2.3**

**Airflow in a Horizontal LAFW**
Downward view onto the hood's work surface, showing the direction of airflow moving horizontally from the HEPA filter toward the worker.

region, along the outer edge of the hood is a poor environment for preparing sterile products. You may hear this area referred to as the **six-inch zone** or the contamination zone of the hood. To help prevent contamination, you must prepare all products in the horizontal LAFW *at least six inches* inside of the hood.

You must consider numerous additional sources of potential contamination when preparing sterile products. Workers must avoid sneezing or coughing into the hood at any time. Needle sticks or cuts can lead to dangerous contamination. When any such situations occur, the worker should assume that everything on the hood's work surface (including all medications, supplies, etc.) is contaminated and must be disposed of in a designated waste receptacle. The worker must undergo a complete aseptic hand washing and don new sterile garb and gloves. Personnel must then clean the hood according to standard hood-cleaning procedures.

When you complete the compounding process, you must inspect all parenteral preparations for **precipitates** and **particulate matter**—any solid substance within an IV solution. Correct needle insertion technique, which Chapter 8 of this textbook discusses in detail, is essential to avoiding particulate matter because incorrect needle insertion can lead to **coring**, or the occurrence of tiny bits of a vial's rubber top entering a solution. Additives that are incompatible with an IV's base solution or with other additives might form a precipitate or show other evidence of **incompatibility**, such as crystallized particles, flakes, or a darkening or coloring of the solution.

Excellent aseptic technique is the foundation of sterile parenteral product preparation. As an IV technician, you must ensure that all policies and procedures are followed at all times. Failure to follow aseptic technique guidelines may lead to contaminated parenteral products that could transfer pathogens to patients. Appropriate conduct in the clean room, combined with correct technique and careful inspection of final products, will help to guarantee the sterility of CSPs.

**USP Chapter <797>**

Never prepare sterile compounds in the six-inch zone.

**USP Chapter <797>**

Failure to correctly clean your gloves with sterile foamed alcohol after touching a calculator, phone, or other potentially contaminated surface may lead to contamination.

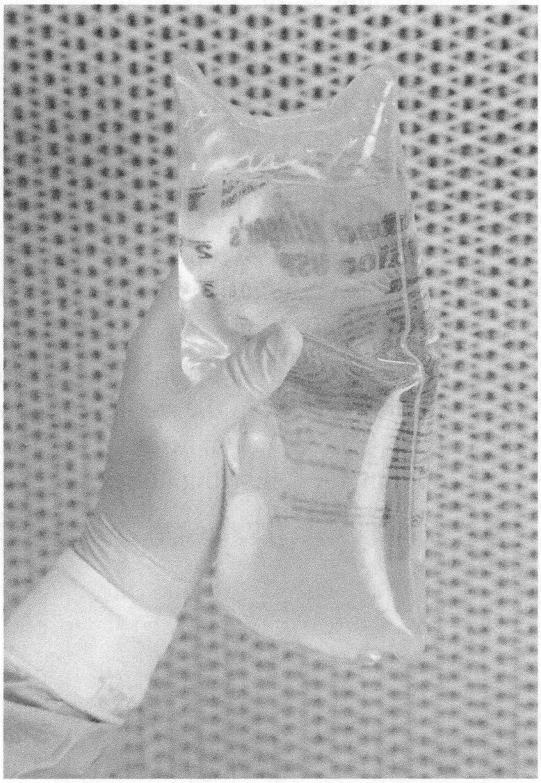

IV technician examining a CSP for leakage, precipitates, and evidence of incompatibility.

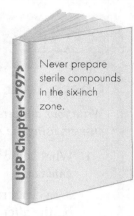

# Concepts Self-Check

## Check Your Understanding

*Write your answers on a separate sheet of paper, as modeled in these examples:* 1d; 2c; 3b; *etc. Check your answers using the Answer Key in Appendix A.*

**1.** What is the literal translation of the term *anteroom*?

a. a clean room
b. the after room
c. the before room
d. a preparation room

**2.** What are the four types of hoods used for sterile compounding?

a. LAFW, CAI, CACI, BSC
b. LAFW, CAI, BSC, PTCB
c. CACI, CAI, BSC, TPN
d. BSC, CACI, CAI, PTCE

**3.** The PEC is the same as which of the following?

a. anteroom
b. clean room
c. DCA
d. hood

**4.** What is the meaning of the acronym *CSP*?

a. critical sterile product
b. compounded sterile product
c. critical sterile preparation
d. compounded sterile preparation

**5.** Most sterile compounds prepared in the pharmacy fall into which risk levels?

a. low- and medium-risk
b. low- and high-risk
c. medium- and high-risk
d. high-risk and immediate-use

## Apply Your Knowledge

*On a separate sheet of paper, write your answer to the question posed in the paragraph below. Use complete sentences and take time to create a thorough and thoughtful response. Check your answer against the Answer Key in Appendix A.*

In Part 1 of this chapter, you learned that many different types and sources of potential contamination exist in the sterile compounding environment. With that in mind, what would be an appropriate course of action if an IV technician working near you in the compounding area was coughing or displaying flu symptoms?

# Examine the Resources and Supplies

## USP <797> Guidebook to Pharmaceutical Compounding – Sterile Preparations

As discussed in Chapter 1 of this textbook, USP Chapter <797> plays an important role in determining the setup of the anteroom and clean room, as well as the creation of policies and procedures related to all aspects of sterile compounding. In February 2008, the U.S. Pharmacopeia published the *USP <797> Guidebook to Pharmaceutical Compounding – Sterile Preparations*. The *USP <797> Guidebook* breaks down USP Chapter <797> into easy-to-understand terms, definitions, and policies and procedures. In addition, the *USP <797> Guidebook* contains appendices and an extensive commentary section that offers valuable information and a list of frequently asked questions and their answers. The *USP <797> Guidebook* is an invaluable resource for sterile compounding personnel.

## Hood-Cleaning Checklists

As noted earlier in this chapter, you must follow specific guidelines for the cleaning and maintenance of the anteroom and the clean room. You must maintain several checklists (often called log sheets) in the anteroom for sterile compounding personnel to record the completion of a number of required cleaning and maintenance activities. The hood-cleaning checklists must identify the date and time of the hood cleaning, as well as the name or initials of the person performing the cleaning (see Figure 2.4). Each hood should have its own, separate checklist that clearly identifies the particular hood being cleaned. To avoid confusion, number each hood and mark its corresponding hood-cleaning log sheets with that same number. Keep the checklists inside a plastic sleeve or sheet protector that can be wiped down to prevent dust buildup. Always place the checklists in the same designated location in the anteroom.

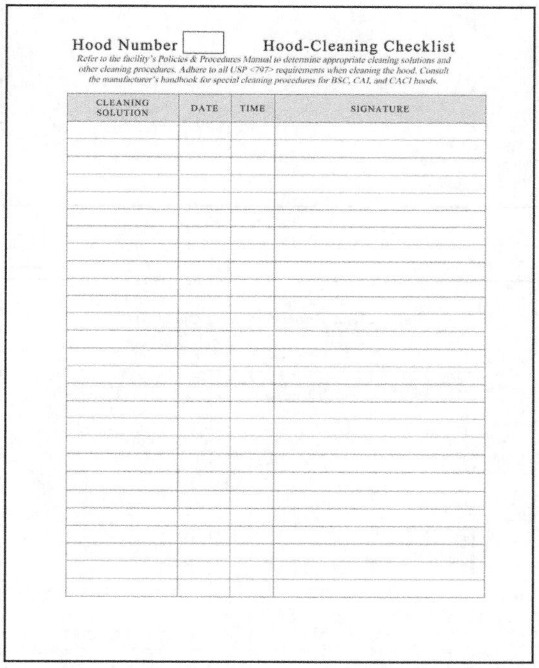
Hood Number ☐ Hood-Cleaning Checklist

*Refer to the facility's Policies & Procedures Manual to determine appropriate cleaning solutions and other cleaning procedures. Adhere to all USP <797> requirements when cleaning the hood. Consult the manufacturer's handbook for special cleaning procedures for BSC, CAI, and CACI hoods.*

| CLEANING SOLUTION | DATE | TIME | SIGNATURE |
|---|---|---|---|

**FIGURE 2.4**
**Hood-Cleaning Checklist**

**POINTER**
Because the hoods are cleaned many times each day, you should also store several blank log sheets in the plastic sleeve so that a fresh sheet is always available to replace a completed sheet.

## Anteroom-Cleaning and Clean-Room-Cleaning Checklists

You should record the daily and monthly cleaning procedures for the anteroom on anteroom-cleaning checklists or log sheets. You must record the same information about the clean-room-cleaning procedures as you record about anteroom-cleaning procedures, but you do so on separate clean-room-cleaning log sheets. In both cases, the checklists should state the cleaning frequency required by USP Chapter <797> (daily or monthly), the name of the equipment or area being cleaned, the type of cleaning solution used, the date and time of the cleaning, and the name of the person performing the cleaning procedure (see Figures 2.5 and 2.6).

**FIGURE 2.5**

**Daily and Monthly Anteroom-Cleaning Checklists**

**Daily Anteroom-Cleaning Checklist**

*Refer to the facility's Policies & Procedures Manual to determine appropriate cleaning solutions and other cleaning procedures. All of the following duties must be performed daily: empty trash containers, wipe down countertops, sweep floor, and mop floor.*

| EQUIPMENT OR AREA CLEANED | CLEANING SOLUTION | DATE | TIME | SIGNATURE |
|---|---|---|---|---|

**Monthly Anteroom-Cleaning Checklist**

*Refer to the facility's Policies & Procedures Manual to determine appropriate cleaning procedures. All of the following surfaces must be wiped down with sterile 70% IPA, or other approved cleaning solution, at least once each month: Ceiling, walls, shelves, furniture, countertops, storage bins, etc.*

| EQUIPMENT OR AREA CLEANED | CLEANING SOLUTION | DATE | TIME | SIGNATURE |
|---|---|---|---|---|

**FIGURE 2.6**

**Daily and Monthly Clean-Room-Cleaning Checklists**

**Daily Clean-Room-Cleaning Checklist**

*Refer to the facility's Policies & Procedures Manual to determine appropriate cleaning solutions and other cleaning procedures. All of the following duties must be performed daily: empty trash containers, wipe down countertops, sweep floor, and mop floor.*

| EQUIPMENT OR AREA CLEANED | CLEANING SOLUTION | DATE | TIME | SIGNATURE |
|---|---|---|---|---|

**Monthly Clean-Room-Cleaning Checklist**

*Refer to the facility's Policies & Procedures Manual to determine appropriate cleaning procedures. All of the following surfaces must be wiped down with sterile 70% IPA, or other approved cleaning solution, at least once each month: Ceiling, walls, shelves, furniture, countertops, storage bins, etc.*

| EQUIPMENT OR AREA CLEANED | CLEANING SOLUTION | DATE | TIME | SIGNATURE |
|---|---|---|---|---|

## Prefilter and HEPA Filter Maintenance

Despite the evident differences in function, most hoods share a common design. As described earlier and illustrated in Figure 2.2, room air enters the cabinet through a prefilter that removes large particles that might damage the HEPA filter. You must replace the prefilter every 30 days. Keep the prefilter-replacement checklist in a plastic sheet protector in the anteroom. This checklist should record the hood number, manufacturer's name, lot number of the replacement prefilter, date, time, and name of the technician who replaced the filter (see Figure 2.7).

In contrast to the prefilter, the HEPA filter is a permanent fixture within the hood. For two reasons, most HEPA filters are not able to be repaired or replaced. First, this filter is difficult to access because of its embedded placement within the hood. Second, the potential for damaging its sensitive components is high. Thus, users must take special care to ensure that a hood's HEPA filter is never touched or damaged. The hood and HEPA filter must be recertified every six months or whenever the cabinet is moved. The hood will not pass recertification if it is determined that, due to damage or wear, the HEPA filter no longer provides adequate airflow. In such cases, the entire hood must be replaced. Replacement can be problematic because LAFW hoods range in price from $15,000 to more than $100,000. You will learn more about correct hood procedures in Chapter 7 of this textbook.

Keep all records that provide evidence of hood maintenance procedures, as well as hood and HEPA filter certification and recertification, in a plastic-covered notebook for easy reference. As a general rule, keep all checklists and log sheets in the pharmacy for a minimum of two years. Keep all hood maintenance and recertification records in the pharmacy for the life of the equipment.

**POINTER**

Specific regulations regarding the record keeping of prefilter and HEPA filter maintenance may vary from state to state. Consult your State Board of Pharmacy to determine appropriate regulations for your facility.

Monthly Prefilter-Replacement Checklist

| HOOD NUMBER | PREFILTER MANUFACTURER | PREFILTER LOT NUMBER | DATE | TIME | TECHNICIAN'S NAME/SIGNATURE |
|---|---|---|---|---|---|
| | | | | | |
| | | | | | |
| | | | | | |
| | | | | | |
| | | | | | |
| | | | | | |
| | | | | | |
| | | | | | |
| | | | | | |
| | | | | | |
| | | | | | |
| | | | | | |
| | | | | | |
| | | | | | |
| | | | | | |
| | | | | | |
| | | | | | |
| | | | | | |
| | | | | | |
| | | | | | |
| | | | | | |
| | | | | | |
| | | | | | |
| | | | | | |
| | | | | | |
| | | | | | |
| | | | | | |
| | | | | | |

**FIGURE 2.7**

**Prefilter-Replacement Checklist**

# Exploratory Lab

This exploratory lab introduces you to additional sections of the *USP <797> Guidebook to Pharmaceutical Compounding – Sterile Preparations.* You also investigate the anteroom and clean room as well as a sterile compounding hood. In addition, you discover more information about the cleaning, maintenance, and record-keeping procedures necessary for sterile compounding.

***Note:** Some of the steps ask you to read and respond to one or more multiple-choice questions (marked by numbers containing dashes, such as **1–1** and **1–2**). Record your answers to these multiple-choice questions by either circling the correct answers on the pages or turning in your answers as directed by your instructor.*

## Supplies

- *USP <797> Guidebook to Pharmaceutical Compounding – Sterile Preparations*
- Hood-Cleaning Checklist
- Two Anteroom-Cleaning Checklists: Daily and Monthly
- Two Clean-Room-Cleaning Checklists: Daily and Monthly
- Access to anteroom or ante-area and clean room
- Access to a hood used for sterile compounding

## Procedure

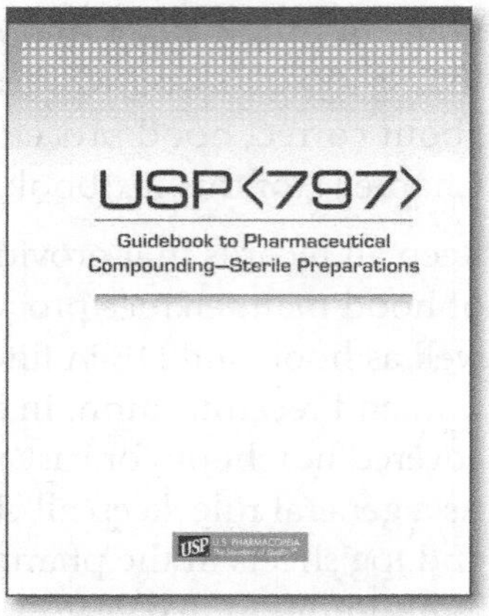


***USP <797> Guidebook to Pharmaceutical Compounding – Sterile Preparations***

1. Open the *USP <797> Guidebook* to the Introduction section.
2. Read the ISO Classification information in Table 1.
3. Answer the following multiple-choice question, recording your answer as directed by your instructor.

   **3–1.** According to Table 1 of the *USP <797> Guidebook,* which of the ISO classifications has a particle count of 352 per cubic meter of air?
   a. ISO Class 4
   b. ISO Class 5
   c. ISO Class 6
   d. ISO Class 7

4. Turn to the definitions section of the *USP <797> Guidebook* and read all of the definitions listed in boldface type.
5. Find Table 3 in the *USP <797> Guidebook* and read the information regarding the frequency of cleaning and disinfecting compounding areas.
6. Answer the following multiple-choice question, recording your answer as directed by your instructor.

6–1. According to Table 3 of the *USP <797> Guidebook*, at a minimum, how often must the PEC be cleaned during ongoing compounding periods?
   a. at least every day
   b. at least every shift
   c. at least every 60 minutes
   d. at least every 30 minutes

### *Hood-Cleaning Checklist*

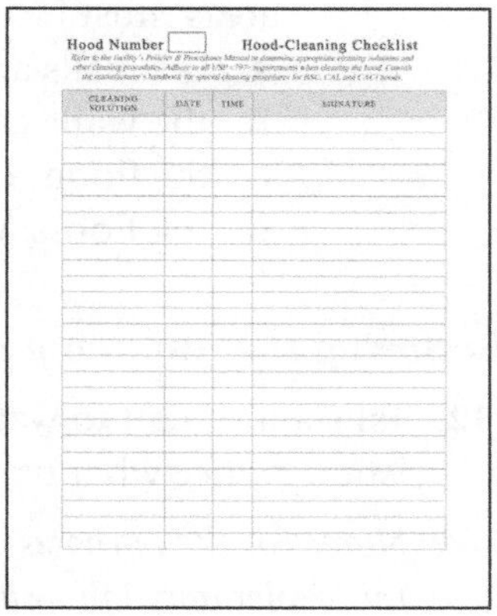


7. In the anteroom, remove the Hood-Cleaning Checklist from its protective covering.
8. Use the Hood-Cleaning Checklist to answer the following multiple-choice question, recording your answer as directed by your instructor. Once you have answered the question, return the checklist to its protective covering.

8–1. What information must be recorded on the Hood-Cleaning Checklist?
   a. the date, the name of the person cleaning the hood, and the solution used to clean the hood
   b. the date, the time, and the name of the person cleaning the hood
   c. the date, the name of the person cleaning the hood, the manufacturer's name, and the lot number of the prefilter
   d. the date, the time, the name of the person cleaning the hood, and the lot number of the prefilter

### *Anteroom-Cleaning and Clean-Room-Cleaning Checklists*

9. In the anteroom, remove the two Anteroom-Cleaning Checklists (Daily and Monthly) and the two Clean-Room-Cleaning Checklists (Daily and Monthly).
10. Find the appropriate Anteroom-Cleaning Checklist and use it to answer the following multiple-choice question, recording your answer as directed by your instructor.

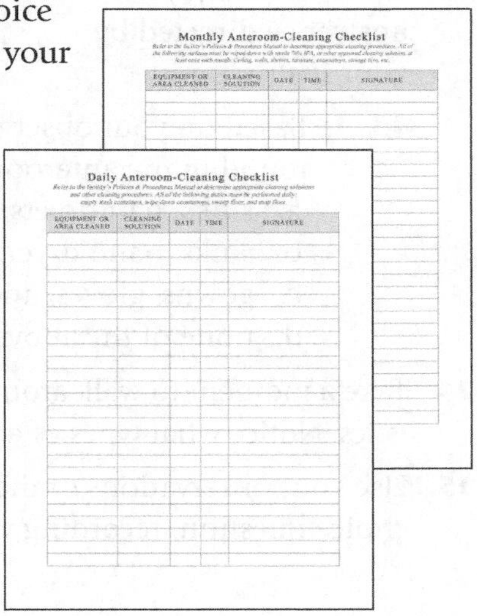


10–1. According to the appropriate Anteroom-Cleaning Checklist, which areas must be cleaned monthly?
   a. the prefilter and HEPA filter
   b. the hood and the floors
   c. the walls, ceiling, and floors
   d. the walls, ceiling, and storage shelving

11. Find the appropriate Clean-Room-Cleaning Checklist and use it to answer the following multiple-choice question, recording your answer as directed by your instructor. Once you have answered questions 10–1 and 11–1, return all checklists back to their protective coverings.

    11–1. According to the appropriate Clean-Room-Cleaning Checklist, which areas must be cleaned daily?
    a. the walls and ceiling
    b. the walls and floors
    c. the floors, counters, and work surfaces
    d. the floors, walls, and work surfaces

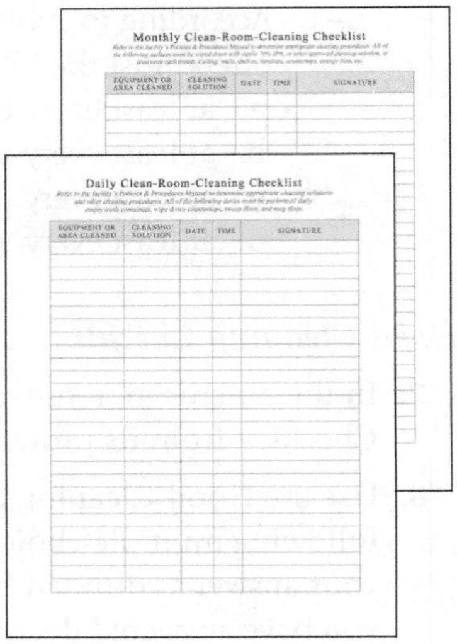


### *Exploring the Anteroom and Clean Room*

12. Take a moment to walk around the anteroom, carefully examining its characteristics. Notice what types of equipment and supplies are kept in the anteroom.

    ***Note:*** *For the purposes of this exploratory lab, you will not be required to don aseptic garb or perform aseptic hand washing as a part of this lab. You will be taught how to perform these procedures in Chapter 6 of this textbook.*

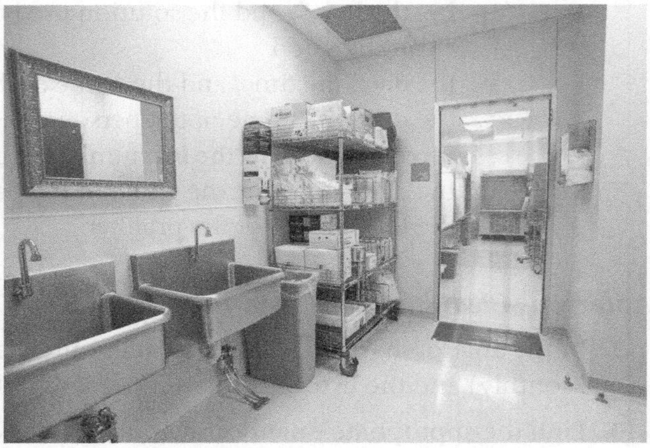

Modern pharmacy anteroom (foreground) and clean room (background).

13. Use your observations of the anteroom to answer the following multiple-choice question, recording your answer as directed by your instructor.

    13–1. Based on your observations, which of the following items might be found in the anteroom?
    a. sinks, hair dryers, and supplies stored in cardboard boxes
    b. sinks, hand dryers, and gowns
    c. gowns, gloves, and hood
    d. none of the above

14. Take a moment to walk around the clean room, carefully examining its characteristics. Notice what types of equipment and supplies are kept in the clean room.

15. Use your observations of the clean room to answer the following multiple-choice question, recording your answer as directed by your instructor.

15–1. Based on your observations, which of the following items might be found in the clean room?
   a. sinks, hand dryers, and gowns
   b. extra hood-cleaning supplies
   c. the sterile compounding hood
   d. gowns, gloves, and hood

### *Exploring the Sterile Compounding Hood*

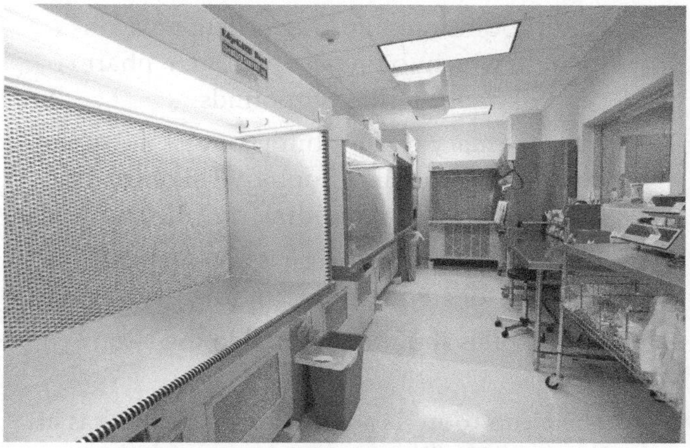

Modern pharmacy clean room with multiple horizontal LAFWs.

**16.** Examine the sterile compounding hood.

**17.** Determine where the prefilter is located and then open the compartment and examine the prefilter.

**18.** Close the compartment where the prefilter is kept.

**19.** Answer the following multiple-choice question, recording your answer as directed by your instructor.

19–1. Concerning the hood prefilter, which of the following statements is most accurate?
   a. It is similar to an air conditioner filter and must be replaced monthly.
   b. It is a permanent filter that must be recertified monthly.
   c. It is similar to an air conditioner filter and must be replaced every six months or whenever the cabinet is moved.
   d. It is a permanent filter that must be recertified every six months or whenever the cabinet is moved.

**20.** *Without touching it,* closely examine the hood's HEPA filter.

**21.** Answer the following multiple-choice question, recording your answer as directed by your instructor.

21–1. Concerning the hood's HEPA filter, which of the following statements is most accurate?
   a. It is similar to an air conditioner filter and must be replaced monthly.
   b. It is a permanent filter that must be recertified monthly.
   c. It is similar to an air conditioner filter and must be replaced every six months or whenever the cabinet is moved.
   d. It is a permanent filter that must be recertified every six months or whenever the cabinet is moved.

# Part 3: Assessment

## Chapter Summary

- Clean rooms and HEPA filters were the result of improvements in electronic, technology, and military manufacturing.
- Clean rooms provide an excellent environment in which to prepare biologics, pharmaceuticals, and sterile compounds.
- The pharmacy clean room is one of the tools for reducing the likelihood of contamination during sterile compounding procedures.
- The *USP <797> Guidebook* is an excellent resource for sterile compounding personnel.
- No supplies should be stored in the clean room.
- The clean room is an environment that has at least an ISO Class 7 rating.
- Laminar airflow hoods are usually located in the clean room.
- All supply items must be wiped with sterile 70% IPA before taking them into the clean room.
- No food, drink, gum chewing, or horseplay is allowed in the clean room or anteroom.
- The anteroom and clean room are designed, constructed, maintained, and cleaned to reduce the likelihood of surface contamination due to dirt and debris buildup.
- The anteroom is a low-traffic area for assembling supplies and preparing for entry into the clean room.
- The anteroom is an environment with at least an ISO Class 8 rating.
- The supplies stored within the anteroom should be limited to those items used in the direct preparation of sterile compounds.
- LAFWs provide the DCA in which sterile compounds are prepared.
- The PEC, or hood, has at least an ISO Class 5 (or Class 100) rating.
- The hoods used by sterile compounding personnel include the CAI, the CACI, the BSC, and the LAFW.
- The horizontal LAFW is the hood most commonly used by sterile compounding personnel.
- The primary components of all hoods are the prefilter, blower, HEPA filter, and work surface.
- The hood's prefilter is a standard air conditioner filter that filters large particles out of room air before the air enters the hood's HEPA filter; the prefilter must be replaced every 30 days.
- The HEPA filter within the hood must be recertified every six months or whenever the cabinet is moved.
- Documentation of anteroom cleaning and hood cleaning must be kept on hand in the pharmacy for a minimum of two years. Documentation of hood maintenance and recertification should be kept for the life of the equipment.
- USP Chapter <797> defines four risk levels associated with the creation of CSPs: low-risk, medium-risk, high-risk, and immediate-use.
- Most parenteral products prepared by the IV technician will fall in the low- and medium-risk levels for CSPs.
- Aseptic technique is specifically designed not to introduce any source of infection into the sterile environment. The goals of aseptic technique are to protect the patient from infection and to prevent the spread of pathogens through contaminated sterile products.
- Touch contamination carries the potential for serious harm to the patient.
- The critical sites are the areas of each instrument, product, or supply that should never be touched or shadowed.
- Objects within the hood must be placed such that the critical sites of each supply item receive uninterrupted airflow from the hood's HEPA filter.
- The outermost edge of the hood receives insufficient airflow velocity from the HEPA filter and is therefore not suitable for sterile compounding.

# Key Terms

**anteroom** a room or area, immediately before the clean room, in which CSP supplies are staged; an area with an ISO Class 8 environment or better

**antineoplastic drug** a type of medication that destroys neoplasms or tumors

**autoclaving** sterilizing certain medical supplies using pressurized steam heat in a piece of equipment called an autoclave

**barrier isolator** a device, such as a biological safety cabinet, that provides a physical barrier between the sterile compounder and the medication being compounded

**biological agent** a type of medicinal product created using biological processes; includes vaccines, allergy treatments, and gene therapy

**biological safety cabinet (BSC)** a vertical laminar airflow hood designed to protect the sterile compounder from exposure to antineoplastic drugs or other chemotherapy preparations

**chemotherapy** medication used to treat cancer

**clean room** a room in which the concentration of airborne particles is minimized by the use of HEPA filtration systems and aseptic technique; an ISO Class 7 environment or better

**compounded sterile preparations (CSPs)** the mixing of one or more sterile products using aseptic technique; subject to extensive USP Chapter <797> guidelines for determining the risk levels and appropriate procedures related to their preparation. Risk levels are:

- **low-risk CSP** a risk level that refers to sterile compounding situations that meet all of the following conditions: compounded entirely within an ISO Class 5 environment using aseptic technique, mixing no more than three commercially manufactured sterile ingredients, and using no more than two injections into any single container
- **medium-risk CSP** a risk level that refers to sterile compounding situations that meet all of the conditions associated with low-risk CSPs, as well as all of the following conditions: compounded entirely within an ISO Class 5 environment using aseptic technique, and involves the mixing of multiple sterile products using complex aseptic manipulations
- **high-risk CSP** a risk level that meets all of the conditions of the low- and medium-risk groups, as well as the following conditions: compounded in an environment worse than ISO Class 5, compounded by incorrectly garbed or gloved personnel, and/or compounded with one or more nonsterile ingredients
- **immediate-use CSP** a risk level intended only for CSPs prepared outside of the pharmacy in emergency situations; administration must begin within one hour of preparation; CSPs may not be stored for any length of time

**compounding aseptic containment isolator (CACI)** a type of enclosed isolator hood designed to protect the sterile compounder from exposure to airborne drugs or chemicals

**compounding aseptic isolator (CAI)** a type of isolator hood designed for mixing compounded sterile preparations

**coring** a small piece of rubber that is torn from the vial top and unintentionally ends up in the sterile solution; coring is caused by incorrect needle insertion into a vial

**direct compounding area (DCA)** within a hood, the area that is closest to the hood's HEPA filter, receives uninterrupted airflow, and is the location where sterile compounding procedures are performed; the area that extends from the hood's HEPA filter out to where the innermost part of the six-inch zone begins; may also be called first air

**filtration sterilization** a sterile compounding procedure in which a nonsterile fluid is passed through a 0.2-micron filter, thereby producing a sterile solution that may be administered intravenously

**heating, ventilation, and air conditioning (HVAC)** a ventilation system used in a sterile compounding laboratory

**heat sterilization** sterilization of a sterile compounding supply item such as an empty evacuated container by heating in an autoclave

**high-efficiency particulate airflow (HEPA) filter** a type of air filter that removes 99.97% of all contaminants within the DCA

**incompatibility** a sign that two or more solutions or ingredients within a solution are not suitable for use in combination, evidenced by the presence of precipitates, crystallized particles, flakes, or a darkening or coloring of a compounded solution

**industrial clean room** a large clean room used in the manufacturing of sensitive equipment such as computer microchips and radar equipment

**International Organization for Standardization (ISO)** an organization that creates worldwide industrial and commercial standards that often become law

**ISO Class 5** an environment appropriate for sterile compounding, containing no more than 3520 particles greater than 0.5 micrometers per cubic meter of air; may be called a Class 100 environment

**laminar airflow workbench (LAFW)** a type of hood, usually with a horizontal airflow, in which sterile products are prepared

**line of demarcation** a line that is taped or drawn on the floor of the anteroom or area that separates the anteroom from the clean room

**nonporous material** a type of material having a smooth, nonpermeable surface that is easy to clean and that does not provide cracks, holes, or pores in which contaminants might collect

**particulate matter** any unwanted solid substance within an IV solution; may be created by incorrect aseptic technique or from precipitates formed when mixing two incompatible solutions

**pathogenic contaminant** a type of contaminant capable of producing fever, infection, illness, or disease

**pharmaceutical** a drug manufactured for medicinal use

**pharmacy clean room** a room of a minimum ISO Class 7 environment in which CSPs are made; the room where PECs are located; may also be called the buffer area or clean room

**precipitate** particulate matter appearing within a compounded solution upon completion of the compounding process; may be caused by incompatible additives, such as a solution or an ingredient in a CSP

**prefilter** within a hood, the component that filters out debris and large particles of dust from room air so that they do not enter the hood; a filter such as that which is found in a home HVAC unit, which is a primary component of an LAFW; must be changed every 30 days

**primary engineering control (PEC)** a laminar airflow cabinet, workbench, or hood that provides an ISO Class 5 environment in which sterile compounds are prepared; may also be called a Class 100 environment

**shadowing** contamination caused by an interruption of airflow from the hood's HEPA filter to the critical site of any supply item

**six-inch zone** the outermost edge of the hood, closest to the worker and farthest from airflow origin at the HEPA filter; a poor environment for preparing sterile products because it receives lower velocity airflow than do areas closer to the hood filter; a zone wherein room air mixes with the air blown through the HEPA filter; a hood area that is considered to be contaminated; may also be called the contamination zone within the hood

**sticky mat** a mat comprising of multiple layers of sticky plastic; adheres to the floor in front of the door to the anteroom and/or clean room; helps to remove dirt and debris from the bottoms of shoes and shoe covers; topmost layer must frequently be removed and discarded

**total parenteral nutrition (TPN)** an advanced sterile compound that intravenously provides the patient with a 24-hour supply of all the fluid, protein, amino acids, calories, vitamins, minerals, and nutrients needed for life; an IV preparation for the patient who has long-term nutritional needs but cannot receive oral feedings

**touch contamination** contamination caused when the critical site of a supply item is touched by the preparer's finger, hand, the hood's surface, or any nonsterile item; the most common and dangerous form of contamination of CSPs

**zone of turbulence** the area behind any item (e.g., vial, IV bag, syringe) on the hood where sterile airflow from the HEPA filter is interrupted; the zone or area is thereby contaminated; sterile parenteral products should not be prepared within a zone of turbulence

## Make Connections

*On a separate sheet of paper, write your answers to the following three questions, using complete sentences and making sure your answers are thorough and thoughtful. Note that the third question requires Internet access.*

1. An emergency room physician prepared an IV bag for immediate administration to a patient. The nurse wants to know what type of beyond-use-date (BUD) or expiration date she should put on the IV label. When the pharmacist checks USP Chapter <797> to find an answer to this question, which risk level would be the most appropriate for the pharmacist to consult when determining the BUD or expiration date for this preparation?

2. List at least two components of the hood that are the same regardless of the type of hood.

3. Go to any Internet search engine and search for *ISO*. What are some of the other areas of standardization that the ISO is involved in? Why is standardization for airborne particulate matter so important to the field of sterile compounding?

## Meet the Challenge

***Scenario*** This "investigative" activity gives you the opportunity to examine a potentially septic clean room. Your instructor has placed a minimum of fifteen examples of incorrect aseptic technique within the "mock" clean room. As a clean room investigator, you must record every example of incorrect aseptic technique or procedure that you find.

***Challenge*** First, create a simple form for recording your observations about incorrect aseptic technique or procedures: Number from 1–15 on a sheet of paper, leaving yourself some writing space between numbers. Next, in small groups, enter the "mock" clean room. You have five minutes to record, on your numbered sheet, short observations regarding incorrect aseptic technique. This activity is a silent, independent activity. Please do not share your findings with other investigators unless and until directed to do so. Your instructor will direct you to either turn in the completed sheet or share your findings with classmates.

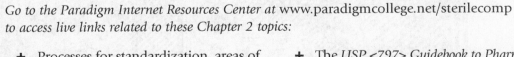

### ADDITIONAL RESOURCES

*Go to the Paradigm Internet Resources Center at* www.paradigmcollege.net/sterilecomp *to access live links related to these Chapter 2 topics:*

+ Processes for standardization, areas of standardization, and ISO ratings for airborne particulates according to the International Organization for Standardization
+ The ISO rating requirements for CSPs according to USP Chapter <797> of the *USP Pharmacists' Pharmacopeia*
+ The *USP <797> Guidebook to Pharmaceutical Compounding – Sterile Preparations,* an excellent resource for sterile compounding personnel

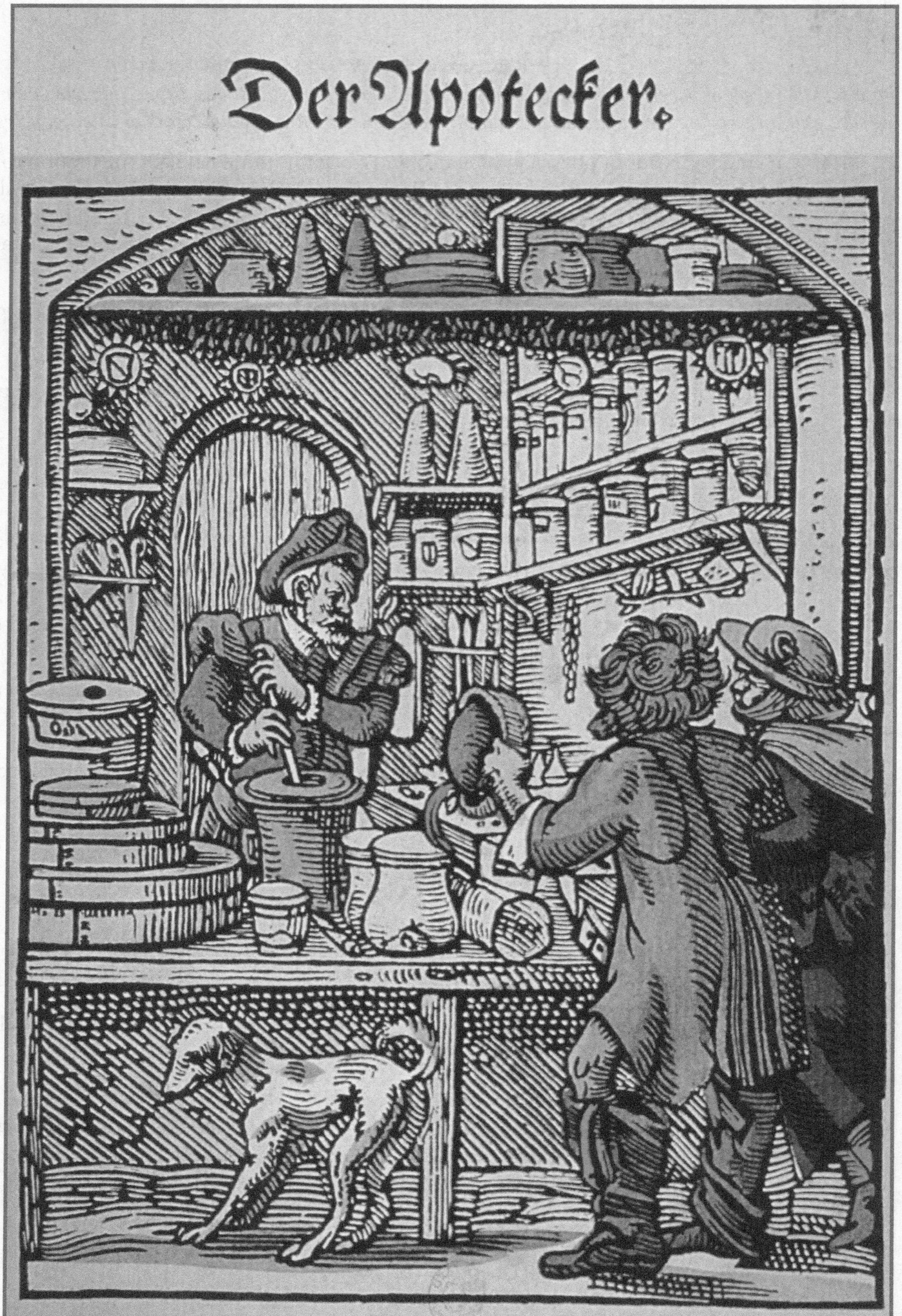
Der Apotecker.

# Chapter 3

# Sterile Compounding Supplies

## Learning Objectives

- Discover the origins of several sterile compounding supplies.
- Identify a variety of supplies used for preparing sterile compounds.
- Describe various components of the most frequently used sterile compounding supplies.
- Understand the rationale for using particular supplies in specific compounding situations.
- Identify the critical sites of commonly used sterile compounding supplies.

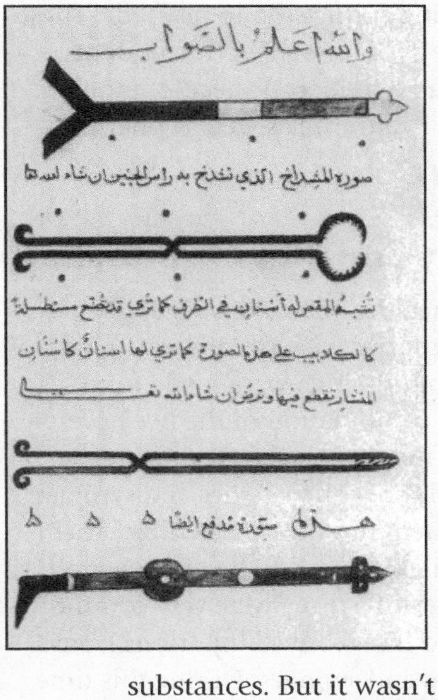


The syringe, which dates back to tenth-century medical practices, is one of the earliest sterile compounding supplies. Albucasis (circa 936–1013 CE), an Arab surgeon from the region of Andalusia in southern Spain, compiled a great mass of medical data, including information on pharmacology, over the several decades of his career. One of his thirty volumes outlines his surgical procedures, offering detailed illustrations of the instruments he used (many of which were his own inventions). Albucasis describes a bulb syringe that he created for the **irrigation** of wounds, the evacuation of the bowels, the extraction of bladder stones and cataracts, and the introduction of medications into the ears and nose. In fact, the word *syringe* comes from the Greek word *syrinx*, meaning "tube."

### Development of Syringe Types and Practices

By the fifteenth and sixteenth centuries, a particular syringe type based on a barrel and plunger became a common surgical tool for irrigating soldiers' battle wounds and infusing cuts with healing substances. But it wasn't until the seventeenth century that French physicist and mathematician Blaise Pascal applied his knowledge of **hydrostatics** toward devising a more advanced

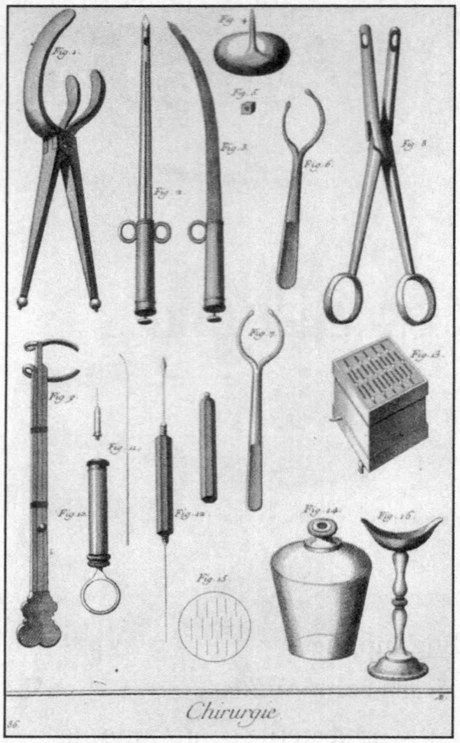


syringe. Pascal theorized that when pressure increases at any point in a confined fluid, an equal increase in pressure occurs at every other point in the container. His theory (now known as **Pascal's Law**) became the basis for not only the invention of the hypodermic syringe, but also the field of hydraulics.

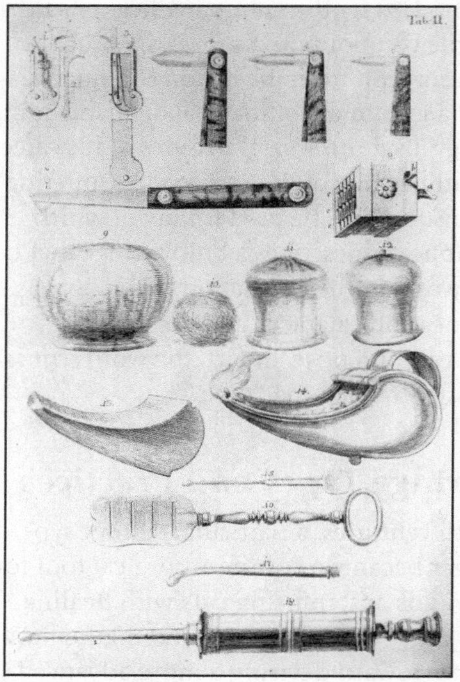


In the seventeenth century, physicians delivered most medications orally. They used crude metal syringes primarily for removing fluids rather than for injecting curative substances. For example, such syringes functioned in purging and **bloodletting** practices to rid the body of "bad **humors**." Nearly two centuries later, at the beginning of the nineteenth century, medical practitioners began to realize the advantages of delivering medications through the skin to access the circulatory system. This method allowed drugs to reach their targets more rapidly than when given orally. Practitioners performed experiments to test this drug delivery theory, including inserting medicinal pellets under the skin to create skin blisters and using incisions as access routes for medicinal treatments. However, the development of the needle-syringe device that most would recognize today was still to come.

By 1853, two doctors—Scottish physician Alexander Wood and French surgeon Charles Gabriel Pravaz—had independently invented two slightly different tools for administering injectable medications to their patients. Dr. Wood developed a hollow metal tube to which he attached a **hypodermic** needle. He used his new invention to administer **morphine** to patients suffering from **neuralgia**. Dr. Pravaz developed a hollow needle, to which he attached a glass syringe marked with graduated dose measures. The hollow needle was able to penetrate the skin without first requiring an incision to be made. These inventions were the predecessors of the modern syringe with attached hypodermic needle, a tool that revolutionized healthcare as well as pharmacy compounding.

## Syringe Safety and Mass Production

By the late 1800s, healthcare workers regularly administered medications with needles and syringes. But these early syringes, which were made from metal or glass (or a combination of the two), were used repeatedly on many patients. Healthcare personnel would simply soak the needles and syringes in alcohol or boil them in water to "sterilize" them. This process was quickly found to be inadequate because **nosocomial infections** were very common among patients who had received injections from these reused needles and syringes. During this time period, infection-control practices were only in their

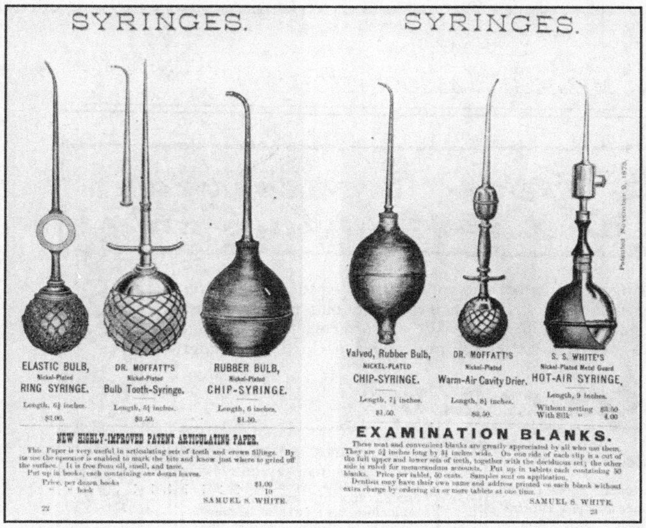


infancy, and a full understanding of the mechanisms by which nosocomial infections developed, and the procedures required to prevent them, was still many years away.

By the beginning of the twentieth century, glass syringes had become a popular medical product. In particular, many entrepreneurs and hospitals were eager to purchase the Luer glass syringe, manufactured by H. Wülfing Luer in Paris. By 1906, Becton, Dickinson, and Company (known as BD), an American medical device import company, acquired a half-interest in the patent rights of the Luer syringe and established production facilities to manufacture their own syringes. The company became highly successful, selling not only syringes but also thermometers, **sphygmomanometers**, and various surgical supplies.

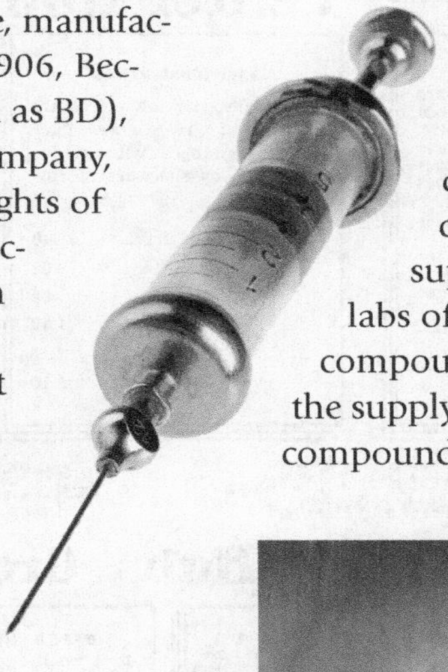

In the mid-twentieth century, BD created the first mass-produced, disposable glass syringe with an attached metal needle. They created this new device in response to two pressing challenges: the desire to reduce the number of infections caused by reusing needles and syringes, and the need to safely administer approximately 1 million doses of the polio vaccine that had just been developed by Dr. Jonas Salk in 1955. By 1961, BD had achieved another milestone in the history of the syringe: the introduction and mass production of the first disposable *plastic* syringe. BD is still one of the world's largest producers of sterile, disposable needles and syringes.

## Other Sterile Compounding Supplies

Needles and syringes are two of the oldest tools used in sterile compounding. Over time, as modern scientific knowledge developed and infection control practices were refined, additional supplies were invented. Vials, for example, were developed to provide a sterile, airtight container with a top that could accommodate needle insertion. Prior to using vials, practitioners kept liquid medications in glass bottles with screw tops. However, this design did not provide an airtight, antimicrobial environment and resulted in cases of medication contamination and patient infection.

Today, pharmaceutical supply companies have developed several sterile compounding supplies for specific use inside a laminar airflow hood. Pharmaceutical supplies are generally produced and packaged by the manufacturer so that they remain sterile until the outer packaging is opened. This chapter introduces some of the most commonly used sterile compounding supplies. Later, in Unit 2, the procedural labs of Chapters 8–14 present individual compounding supplies in greater detail when the supply item plays a particular role in the lab's compounding process.

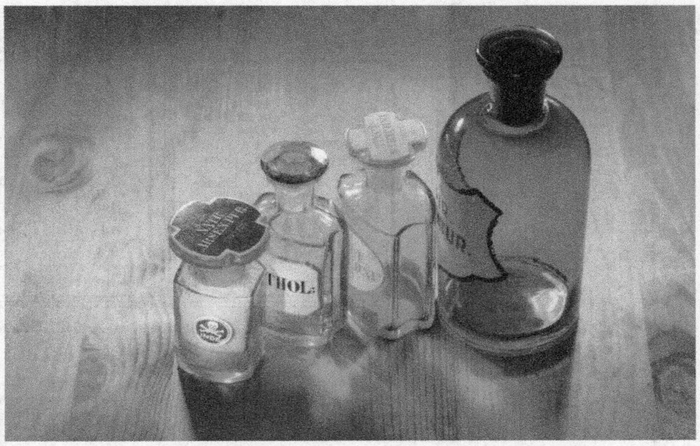

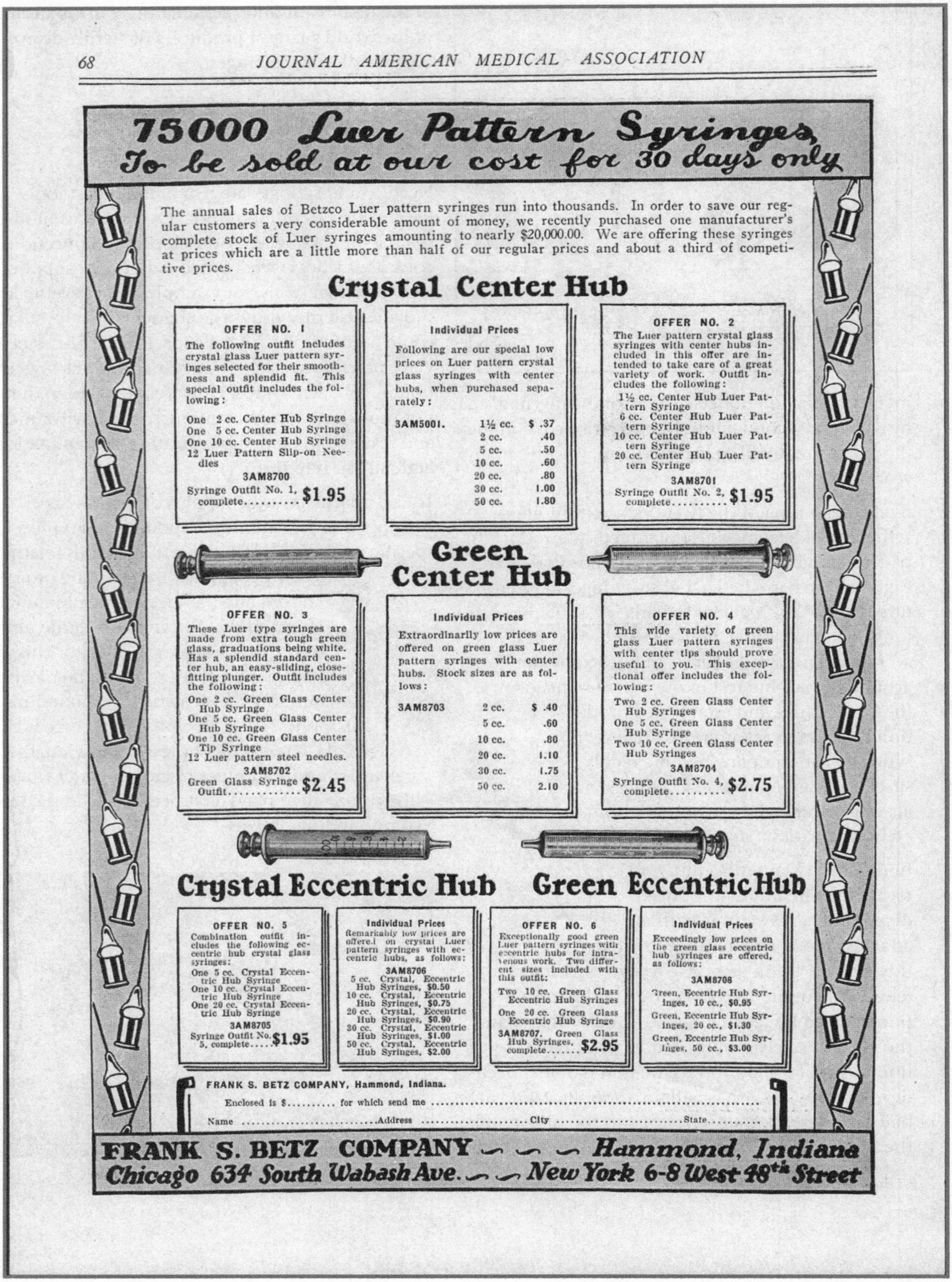

68 JOURNAL AMERICAN MEDICAL ASSOCIATION

# 75000 Luer Pattern Syringes
## To be sold at our cost for 30 days only

The annual sales of Betzco Luer pattern syringes run into thousands. In order to save our regular customers a very considerable amount of money, we recently purchased one manufacturer's complete stock of Luer syringes amounting to nearly $20,000.00. We are offering these syringes at prices which are a little more than half of our regular prices and about a third of competitive prices.

## Crystal Center Hub

**OFFER NO. 1**

The following outfit includes crystal glass Luer pattern syringes selected for their smoothness and splendid fit. This special outfit includes the following:

One 2 cc. Center Hub Syringe
One 5 cc. Center Hub Syringe
One 10 cc. Center Hub Syringe
12 Luer Pattern Slip-on Needles

3AM8700

Syringe Outfit No. 1, complete.......... **$1.95**

**Individual Prices**

Following are our special low prices on Luer pattern crystal glass syringes with center hubs, when purchased separately:

| | | |
|---|---|---|
| 3AM5001. | 1½ cc. | $ .37 |
| | 2 cc. | .40 |
| | 5 cc. | .50 |
| | 10 cc. | .60 |
| | 20 cc. | .80 |
| | 30 cc. | 1.00 |
| | 50 cc. | 1.80 |

**OFFER NO. 2**

The Luer pattern crystal glass syringes with center hubs included in this offer are intended to take care of a great variety of work. Outfit includes the following:

1½ cc. Center Hub Luer Pattern Syringe
6 cc. Center Hub Luer Pattern Syringe
10 cc. Center Hub Luer Pattern Syringe
20 cc. Center Hub Luer Pattern Syringe

3AM8701

Syringe Outfit No. 2, complete.......... **$1.95**

## Green Center Hub

**OFFER NO. 3**

These Luer type syringes are made from extra tough green glass, graduations being white. Has a splendid standard center hub, an easy-sliding, close-fitting plunger. Outfit includes the following:

One 2 cc. Green Glass Center Hub Syringe
One 5 cc. Green Glass Center Hub Syringe
One 10 cc. Green Glass Center Tip Syringe
12 Luer pattern steel needles.

3AM8702

Green Glass Syringe Outfit............ **$2.45**

**Individual Prices**

Extraordinarily low prices are offered on green glass Luer pattern syringes with center hubs. Stock sizes are as follows:

| | | |
|---|---|---|
| 3AM8703 | 2 cc. | $ .40 |
| | 5 cc. | .60 |
| | 10 cc. | .80 |
| | 20 cc. | 1.10 |
| | 30 cc. | 1.75 |
| | 50 cc. | 2.10 |

**OFFER NO. 4**

This wide variety of green glass Luer pattern syringes with center tips should prove useful to you. This exceptional offer includes the following:

Two 2 cc. Green Glass Center Hub Syringes
One 5 cc. Green Glass Center Hub Syringe
Two 10 cc. Green Glass Center Hub Syringes

3AM8704

Syringe Outfit No. 4, complete.......... **$2.75**

## Crystal Eccentric Hub

**OFFER NO. 5**

Combination outfit includes the following eccentric hub crystal glass syringes:

One 5 cc. Crystal Eccentric Hub Syringe
One 10 cc. Crystal Eccentric Hub Syringe
One 20 cc. Crystal Eccentric Hub Syringe

3AM8705

Syringe Outfit No. 5, complete..... **$1.95**

**Individual Prices**

Remarkably low prices are offered on crystal Luer pattern syringes with eccentric hubs, as follows:

3AM8706

5 cc. Crystal, Eccentric Hub Syringes, $0.50
10 cc. Crystal, Eccentric Hub Syringes, $0.75
20 cc. Crystal, Eccentric Hub Syringes, $0.90
30 cc. Crystal, Eccentric Hub Syringes, $1.00
50 cc. Crystal, Eccentric Hub Syringes, $2.00

## Green Eccentric Hub

**OFFER NO. 6**

Exceptionally good green Luer pattern syringes with eccentric hubs for intravenous work. Two different sizes included with this outfit:

Two 10 cc. Green Glass Eccentric Hub Syringes
One 20 cc. Green Glass Eccentric Hub Syringe

3AM8707. Green Glass Hub Syringes, complete....... **$2.95**

**Individual Prices**

Exceedingly low prices on the green glass eccentric hub syringes are offered, as follows:

3AM8708

Green, Eccentric Hub Syringes, 10 cc., $0.95
Green, Eccentric Hub Syringes, 20 cc., $1.30
Green, Eccentric Hub Syringes, 50 cc., $3.00

FRANK S. BETZ COMPANY, Hammond, Indiana.

Enclosed is $.......... for which send me ....................

Name .................... Address .................... City .................... State ..........

**FRANK S. BETZ COMPANY — Hammond, Indiana**
**Chicago 634 South Wabash Ave. — New York 6-8 West 48th Street**

# Part 1: Concepts

This chapter highlights many of the supplies that sterile compounding technicians use and provides an introduction to the critical sites for several of these items. The **critical site** is the part of the supply item that includes any fluid-pathway surface or fluid-pathway opening that is at risk for contamination by touch or airflow interruption. Critical sites include vial tops; ampule necks; needle hubs, shafts, and tips; syringe tips and plungers; tubing and dispensing pin spikes; and the injection ports of intravenous (IV) solutions or intravenous piggyback (IVPB) solutions. Manufacturer packaging determines whether critical sites are already sterile or will require sterilization. Packaged sterile items include syringe tips, all needle parts, the spike and syringe adaptor of the dispensing pin, and the spike and needle adaptor of IV tubing.

Because of the high potential for microbial contamination, critical sites must only be touched by a sterile tool such as a needle or spike, or a sterile supply item such as a sterile alcohol swab. Gloved hands or fingers, the hood surface, or other supply items, even though they may have been recently cleaned with sterile, foamed 70% isopropyl alcohol (IPA), must never touch the critical site because such an event would cause **touch contamination**. The critical sites of all supply items must also receive a continuous and uninterrupted flow of air from the high-efficiency particulate air (HEPA) filter. Anything that interrupts the airflow from the HEPA filter to the critical zone causes **shadowing**, another form of potential contamination.

## Correct Opening and Placement of Supplies

Aseptic technique procedures mandate that you take great care when opening the outer packages of all supply items. This helps you avoid injury and prevents contamination of the supply item. For example, when working in the hood, you must open the outer package of a supply item at least six inches inside of the hood to maintain aseptic technique. Keeping the sterile supply item within this **clean air zone**, also called the direct compounding area or DCA, ensures that the airflow from the HEPA filter to the supply item is at a sufficient velocity to maintain the product's effectiveness, provided the item is placed within the hood so that nothing interrupts the steady stream of airflow.

Along the entire outer edge of the hood's work surface, measuring six inches into the hood, sterile air from the hood's HEPA filter mixes with turbulent room air. This area is referred to as the **outer six-inch zone**, or the **zone of turbulence**. The outer six-inch zone is considered contaminated and is not an appropriate area in which to prepare sterile products. All sterile compounding procedures must take place at least six inches inside of the hood. Prior to performing a compounding procedure, keep all necessary supply items that are still in their outer packaging (sometimes called a **dust cover**), in the outer six-inch zone of the hood, the

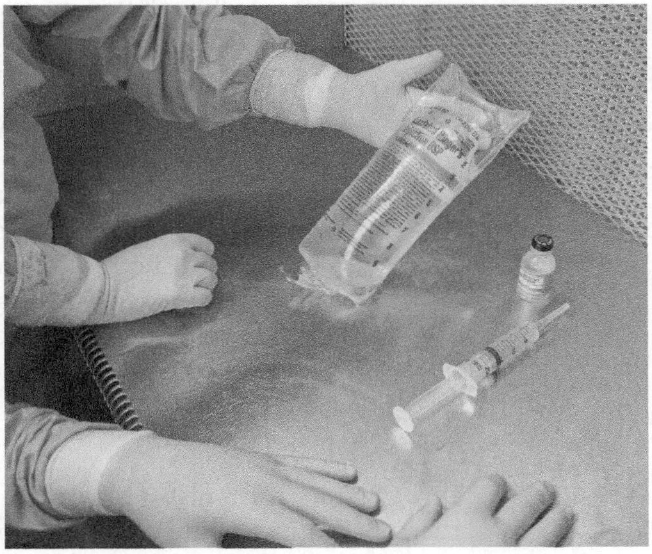

Pharmacist checking the IV technician's work; notice that sterile supply items are within the DCA of the hood.

> **POINTER**
> The outer six-inch zone is an area where small supply items can be kept immediately prior to bringing them into the DCA as they are needed for the procedure. Because of this, it is often referred to as the supply staging area of the hood.

edge closest to you. After you remove the outer packaging, you should keep the supply item at least six inches *inside* of the hood at all times. Even though the dust cover was wiped down with sterile 70% IPA prior to the item being brought into the clean room, this type of outer packaging is still considered a "dirty" item. Place any items still inside their dust covers onto the hood in the outer six-inch zone. Just prior to using the item, remove the dust cover and place the item into the "clean" section of the hood (not within the six-inch zone), which is used for sterile compounding. Then place the dust cover in the waste receptacle.

## Needles

Needles are one of the IV technician's most frequently used tools. The needle is attached to a syringe and is then used to either draw fluid into the syringe (also known as a **straight draw**) or push fluid out of the syringe and into an IV bag or bottle. Needles come in numerous sizes and lengths, and sterile compounding requires several different types of needles. An IV technician chooses needles by size, length, and type, depending on the task to be performed.

The length of the needle identifies the distance between the needle tip and needle hub. This measurement is an important consideration in the preparation of sterile products. For example, technicians use a long needle when injecting into an IV bag with a long neck. However, a short needle is more appropriate when preparing a skin test for intradermal (ID) administration. **Regular needles**, the most commonly used, are used specifically to withdraw or inject fluids for parenteral administration.

> **BE AWARE**
> A filter needle cannot be used to both withdraw and inject fluid. This in-needle filter only traps particulate matter successfully if used in one direction.

## Specialty Needles

Other needles are used to perform specialized functions in the IV room. The **filter needle** is a needle with a small, built-in filter (sometimes referred to as a **depth filter**) between the needle's shaft and hub. A filter needle is used to remove particulate matter from a solution, such as the glass shards that can enter a solution when an IV technician breaks the head off of a glass ampule to withdraw the liquid medication with a syringe. As the solution moves through the needle to the filter, the filter traps the particulate matter within the filter, thus removing any glass shards.

IV technicians also frequently use vented needles and transfer needles. Technicians use the **vented needle** primarily to dilute large-volume or multiple containers of parenteral medications in powdered form. These medications must be **reconstituted** prior to use. The needle is constructed to allow the fluid to be injected into the powder while simultaneously venting the positive-pressure air that has built up within the vial. The **transfer needle** transfers fluid from one vial or container to another. This needle type is rarely necessary but is most often used when the *entire volume* of fluid in one vial must be transferred into another vial containing a powder that is to be reconstituted for injectable use.

## Syringes

Syringes also play a major role in the sterile compounding process. Sterile compounding technicians use syringes to withdraw or inject solutions as part of the preparation of almost all sterile products. Most syringes are made of polyvinyl chloride (PVC) or plastic components and contain a rubber-tipped piston plunger that moves in and out along a sterile inner barrel. Several syringe sizes are commonly used during the compounding of sterile preparations, including 0.5 mL, 1 mL, 3 mL, 5 mL, 10 mL, 20 mL, 30 mL, and 60 mL. The size of the syringe indicates the maximum fluid volume it holds.

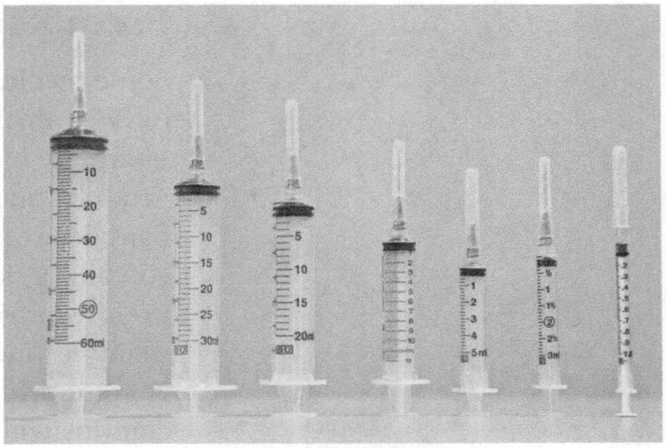

Various syringes used in sterile compounding; notice that they range in volume from 60 mL (left) to 1 mL (right).

**POINTER**

Glass syringes are required in some rare compounding scenarios, such as when a drug is incompatible with syringe components and when certain chemotherapy products are prepared. Chapter 14 further discusses these special glass syringes.

**POINTER**

The best syringe choice is the smallest syringe within which the total volume of desired fluid will safely fit.

## IV Base Solutions

An IV base solution is a large volume (usually 500 or 1000 mL) of sterile fluid that is delivered via sterile IV tubing to a patient. This IV base solution—also known as a **large-volume parenteral (LVP)**, base solution, primary IV, IV, or IV bag—is administered over an extended period ranging from one hour to twenty-four hours. The container that holds the IV fluid may be made of polyethylene, PVC, polyolefin, various other plastics, or even glass. The LVP is commonly the primary source of **hydration** for the patient and is run continuously while the patient is unable to take oral liquids. Most LVP solutions are made with varying concentrations of sodium and/or dextrose mixed with sterile water. The most common base solutions are provided to the pharmacy premade by their manufacturers. The pharmacy often keeps a supply of these solutions in each nursing unit to quickly and easily administer them to patients needing immediate hydration. During the sterile compounding process, personnel prepare IV solutions that require medication **additives**.

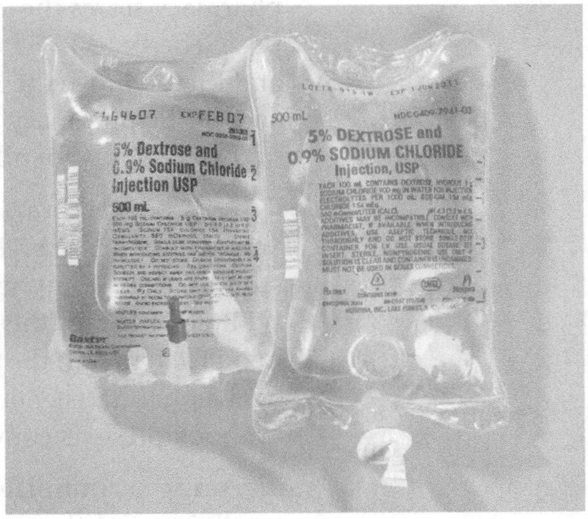


Two LVP base solutions.

## IVPB Solutions

An **IVPB solution** is a small volume (usually 25 mL, 50 mL, 100 mL, 150 mL, or 250 mL) of fluid mixed with an IV medication and administered to the patient via sterile IV tubing. IVPBs are a type of small-volume parenteral (SVP) product and are usually "piggybacked" through a primary IV line that contains the IV base solution. IV technicians administer the IVPB medication over a short period ranging from ten minutes to several hours. The IVPB medication is administered to the patient intermittently, based on the frequency ordered by the prescriber. Many intravenously administered antibiotics are delivered via an IVPB.

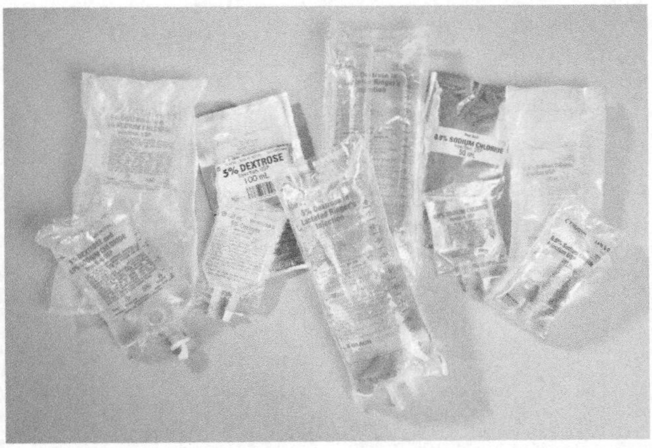


Various LVP and SVP solutions used in sterile compounding.

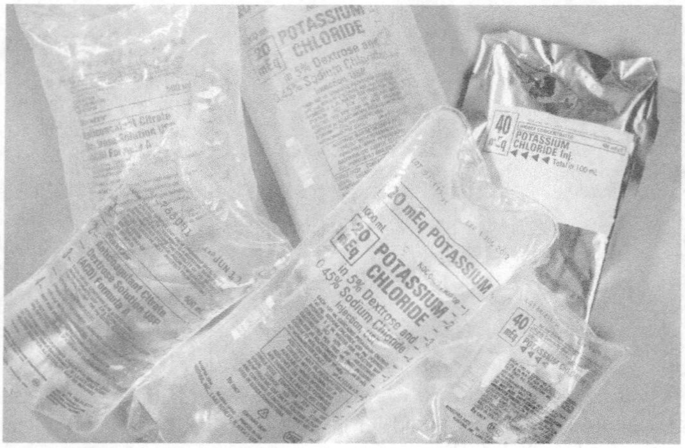

Various premixed, shelf-stable IV products.

## Premixed Parenteral Products

Some medications for administration by IV or IVPB are manufactured and supplied to the pharmacy in the form of premixed, **shelf-stable products** such as IV bags that contain a standard dose of potassium chloride, an IVPB that contains a standard dose of famotidine, or a **prefilled syringe** provided for **IV push** use. For example, one of the most commonly ordered IV solutions is dextrose 5% in 0.45% sodium chloride with twenty milliequivalents (mEq) of potassium chloride per liter ($D_5$ ½ NS w/20 mEq KCl), which is supplied as a premixed, shelf-stable solution by the manufacturer.

Many other premixed products are also available and widely used. Although some of these products are shelf-stable, others are kept frozen until ready for use. These premixed products include various IVPBs that are supplied in packages of 12, 24, or 48 and are shipped from the **wholesale supplier** in a container packed in dry ice. The pharmacy stores these products in a pharmacy freezer dedicated solely for this purpose. The IV technician must determine the usage for all of the hospitalized patients and then remove the IVPBs from the freezer and place them in a designated thawing area in the pharmacy. The technician typically thaws enough IVPBs to provide the necessary doses for all patients for 24 to 48 hours, based on usage.

Other products commonly used in the sterile compounding process are vial and bag systems such as **ADD-Vantage**, **MINI-BAG Plus**, and **Add-A-Vial**. These products require sterile compounding personnel to screw or snap a specially built vial onto an IVPB designed for this type of attachment. This connection process is performed in the hood to maintain the sterility of the IVPB contents. Then the device is labeled, checked by the pharmacist, and sent to the nurse for patient administration. Chapter 4 of this textbook presents correct procedures for labeling and checking parenteral products.

Just prior to administering these vial and bag system products, the nurse breaks a small, internal chamber located at the joint where the vial and IVPB are attached. This action opens the flow of fluid from the IVPB into the vial, which then allows the drug in the vial to mix with the fluid of the IVPB bag. Once the drug is mixed into the IVPB fluid, the nurse administers it to the patient through sterile IV tubing. One advantage of this type of IVPB is that it can be mixed just moments before the dose is required. This deferred mixing is helpful if the medication is not stable for long periods in its **mixed** form. Another advantage of the vial and bag system is that

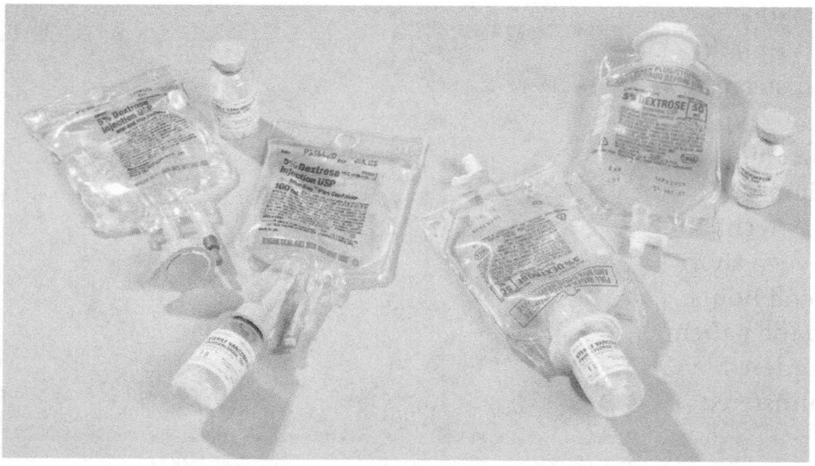

MINI-BAG Plus (left) and ADD-Vantage (right) IVPB and vial products.

personnel may return unused doses of medication to the pharmacy, where they are relabeled for use with other patients. Such reuse is possible because these systems are **stable** for up to 30 days, provided that the internal chamber has not been broken and the drug has not been mixed into the IVPB. Using vial and bag systems helps to decrease the wastage that would result from the relatively short stability of mixed IVPBs.

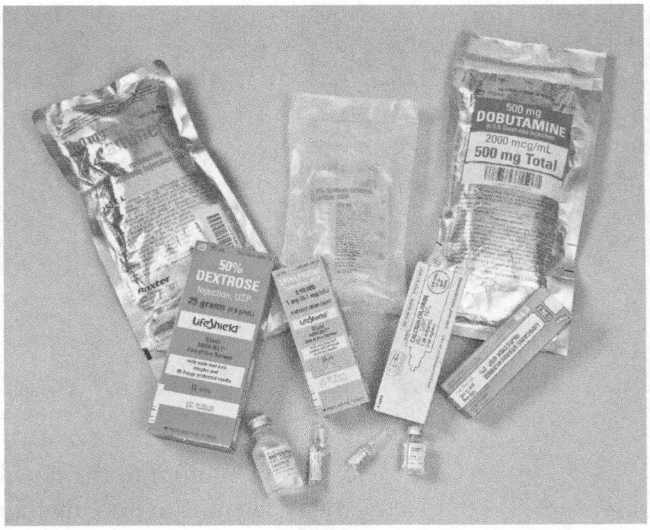

Various compounding supplies: premixed, shelf-stable, IV bags; prefilled syringes; vials; and an ampule.

The parenteral medications provided as prefilled syringes for IV push use contain the appropriate strength and amount of drug, in a form that the nurse can immediately administer either into the IV tubing or directly into the IV bag. Many of these medications are emergency drugs such as epinephrine or atropine. The prefilled syringe is provided by the manufacturer in an individual dose and packaged as a syringe with an attached needle plus a glass tube filled with the medication. The nurse assembles the two pieces by screwing the glass, medication-filled tube onto the end of the syringe and then pushing the tube into the barrel of the syringe. To inject the medication into the IV tubing or bag, the nurse pushes the glass tube deeper into the syringe.

## Vials

**Vials** are sealed, sterile containers made of plastic or glass, with a rubber top through which the IV technician draws fluid. Vials most often contain a sterile medication in a liquid or powdered form or a liquid **diluent** which is used to reconstitute a powder prior to injection. The most commonly used diluents are sterile water and normal saline. Medications from vials may be diluted by injecting them into an IV bag or IVPB, or they may be administered directly through the IV push or other routes of administration. The decision about how to dilute and administer a medication is made based on the prescriber's order, the patient's medical condition, information supplied by the drug's manufacturer, and the compounding facility's standard operating procedures.

The two main types of vials are **single-dose vials (SDVs)** that do not contain a preservative, and **multiple-dose vials (MDVs)** that do contain a preservative. The absence of a preservative in an SDV provides an ideal medium for the growth of microorganisms. Therefore, this type of vial is meant only for one-time use and should be discarded after puncturing the top and using the contents. MDVs are generally stable for up to 28 days from the initial use, unless otherwise specified by the manufacturer. The MDV contains a preservative, such as benzyl alcohol or methylparaben, to inhibit bacterial growth. Once opened, the MDV may be reused according to the manufacturer's instructions.

Another type of vial, called a **Mix-O-Vial**, is used infrequently by IV technicians due to the limited number of immediate-use medications supplied in this type of container. However, the vial's hourglass design makes it an easy tool for sterile compounding personnel to use when necessary. The upper chamber contains a diluent such as sterile

**POINTER**

Although not in vial form, ampules and medication-filled syringes are also considered SDVs and, therefore, are meant only for one-time use.

**BE AWARE**

Mix-O-Vial medications, once reconstituted, have a short stability period and therefore should only be activated just before administration.

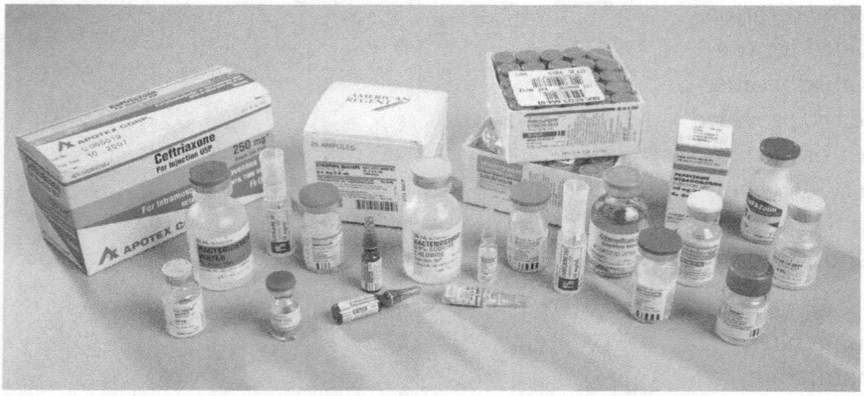


Various vials and ampules used in sterile compounding.

water; the lower chamber contains a drug in powdered form. A rubber plug separates the two chambers. When the IV technician is ready to prepare the sterile compound, she or he activates the medication by pressing down on a raised rubber stopper located at the top of the upper chamber. This action creates pressure that forces the rubber plug separating the chambers downward into the powder. Dislocating the plug releases the liquid into the powder, which dissolves and is then drawn up in solution by the IV technician for either an IV push or IVPB administration to a patient.

## Ampules

An **ampule** is a sterile, sealed container made entirely of glass with a tapered neck. IV technicians break the glass at this tapered, scored neck and aseptically remove the liquid with a needle and syringe. The ampule is an appropriate container for drugs that are not compatible with the rubber top or other components of a vial. Working with ampules requires specialized techniques, which Chapter 10 of this textbook covers in detail.

**USP Chapter <797>**

The saturated swab should be wiped once across the critical site. Avoid vigorously rubbing the swab back and forth across the critical site because this action may leave behind small fibers that could contaminate the sterile environment.

Medications from ampules may be diluted by injecting them into an IV bag or IVPB, or they may be administered directly through the IV push, IM, ID, Sub-Q, or other routes of administration. Sterile compounding personnel decide how to dilute and administer a medication based on the prescriber's order, the patient's medical condition, information supplied by the drug's manufacturer, and the compounding facility's standard operating procedures.

## IPA Swabs, Vented Dispensing Pins, IVA Seals, Sharps Containers

**USP Chapter <797>**

Alcohol swabs are for one-time use only and should be disposed of immediately after swabbing the critical site.

Many supplies are used on a frequent basis in the preparation of sterile compounds. Some such items include sterile 70% IPA swabs, vented dispensing pins, IVA seals, and sharps containers. **Sterile IPA swabs** are wiped across most critical sites, such as the vial top, ampule neck, and injection port, prior to aseptic compounding. Such steps help to ensure that the solution within the container remains sterile. According to USP Chapter <797>, appropriate alcohol swabs for use in the IV room must be individually packaged and presaturated with sterile 70% IPA. Be sure that the alcohol swab is completely saturated and has not dried out due to a hole or tear in the package. If you find a dry or semi-dry swab when you open a package, throw it away.

**Vented dispensing pins** are inserted into a vial or glass bottle and then attached to a syringe. These pins allow easy withdrawal of large volumes of fluids while equalizing the pressure within the container. The manufacturer's packaging provides a vented dispensing pin in which both of the critical sites—the syringe adaptor and the spike—are completely sterile, provided that they are handled aseptically. The sterile

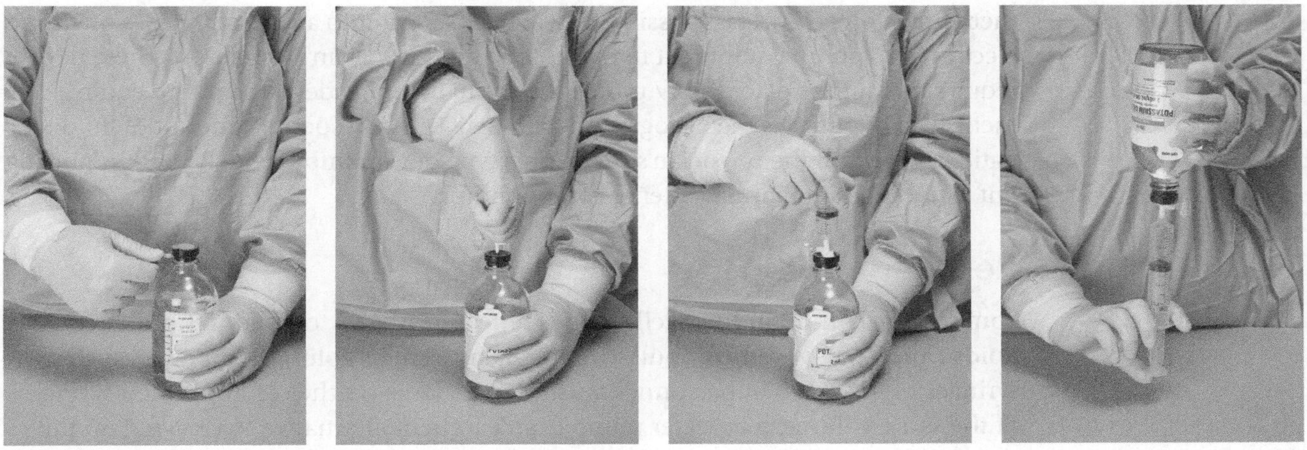

Sequence showing proper use of a vented dispensing pin; (left to right) removal of aluminum cap from EEC; insertion of pin into EEC; attaching the syringe to the dispensing pin; withdrawal of fluid from EEC, through dispensing pin, into the attached syringe.

nature of the critical sites of the vented dispensing pin requires that the sites never be touched or swabbed with alcohol before use.

**IVA seals** are small foil stickers that sterile compounding personnel place over the injection port of the prepared IV, IVPB, and various other compounded products. These sterile seals protect the injection port of a parenteral product and are designed to indicate needle puncture, which helps avoid accidental double-dosing. In addition, the seals self-destruct upon attempted removal, providing evidence of product tampering.

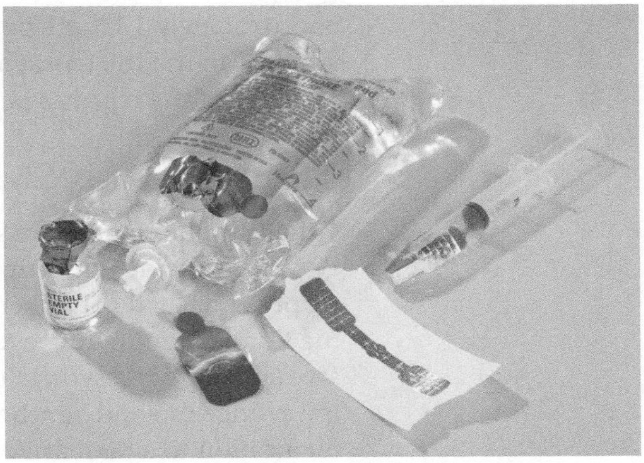

IVA seals used to cover an injection port, a vial top, and a filled syringe.

The **sharps container** is a large bucket, usually red in color, made of thick plastic and used to safely dispose of used needles, syringes, and broken glass. It is designed to prevent pharmacy personnel from reaching inside and accidentally injuring themselves with the contents.

## Sterile IV Tubing

Sterile IV tubing is a supply item frequently used throughout the hospital. Sterile compounding personnel use IV tubing to transfer solutions from one container into another. Nurses use IV tubing to administer IV fluids and IV push medications to the patient. **Primary IV tubing** is sterile IV tubing with multiple injection ports. Nurses use primary IV tubing to administer an IV base solution to the patient. **Secondary IV tubing** is short, sterile IV tubing that may or may not have an injection port. IV technicians use secondary IV tubing to transfer a solution from a source container to another bag or bottle. Nurses use secondary IV tubing to piggyback an IVPB medication through the primary IV line and into the patient's vein. The most important components of IV tubing are the same, whether you are using primary tubing or secondary tubing.

**POINTER**

Your facility may supply IV tubing with slide clamps rather than roll clamps. While slide clamps tend to cost less and are most commonly used in the IV room, roll clamps give you more control over the flow rate.

You control the flow rate of the IV solution by manipulating the clamp on the tubing. A clamp that is completely closed does not allow any fluid to flow from an IV bag into a patient; a clamp that is wide open provides no constriction upon the IV line and therefore allows the fastest possible flow rate of solution to a patient. Nurses often use electronic IV pump equipment to control the flow rate of an IV solution. These devices require that nurses place the IV tubing into a chamber inside of the pump equipment. The IV pump is then programmed to deliver a very specific amount of fluid to a patient, based on the physician's order. This type of IV pump is widely used in nursing but is not used in pharmacy sterile compounding.

## Repeater Pumps

Some sterile compounding facilities use **repeater pumps** to rapidly transfer sterile fluids from large-volume or bulk containers into small-volume containers such as syringes or vials. When personnel must prepare large batches of fluid-filled syringes of the same volume, a repeater pump is an excellent alternative to drawing up the syringes from a bulk container by hand. The repeater pump is calibrated to accurately and rapidly transfer a specific amount of fluid via an electronic pump. The pump can be programmed to deliver any volume between 0.2 mL and 999 mL at approximately 13.5 mL per second. In addition to batch preparation of syringes, personnel can use the repeater pump to dilute multiple vials of powder. The speed and accuracy of the repeater pump make it a valuable tool for an IV technician.

## Miscellaneous Sterile Compounding Supplies

Other supplies that are less frequently used but still important to the work of an IV technician include syringe caps, Luer-to-Luer connectors, membrane filters, and empty evacuated containers. A **syringe cap** is a small, plastic cap that attaches to the tip of a filled syringe. Adding a syringe cap is a precaution taken to allow the safe transport of a syringe to the nursing unit. After delivery, the nurse then removes the syringe cap and attaches a needle to the syringe just prior to administering the medication to a patient. A **Luer-to-Luer connector** is a plastic tube with Luer-lock hubs at both ends. This needleless system is used to transfer liquid from one syringe to another during certain compounding procedures. **Membrane filters** (0.2 micron or smaller) are used to sterilize solutions that have been prepared using nonsterile ingredients. The filter is attached to the tip of a syringe containing the nonsterile fluid. A needle is attached to the other side of the filter, and the fluid is pushed through the sterilizing filter and into a receptacle such as an **empty evacuated container (EEC)**. An EEC is a sterile, empty vial or glass bottle whose volume ranges from 2 mL to 1000 mL. EECs have a variety of purposes in sterile compounding: They can be used when transferring solutions from one container to another, for creating an IV base solution from scratch if the solution is not commercially available, and when administering an IV solution to a patient who is allergic to one of the plastic components of an IV bag.

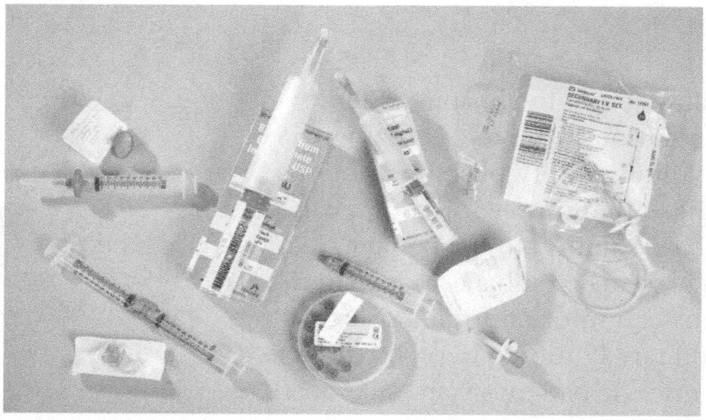

Miscellaneous sterile compounding supplies (clockwise from top left): membrane filter in package and attached to syringe; large and small prefilled syringes; secondary IV tubing; vented dispensing pin; package of syringe caps and capped syringe; syringes connected with Luer-to-Luer connector and connector in package.

# Concepts Self-Check

## Check Your Understanding

*Write your answers on a separate sheet of paper, as modeled in these examples: 1d; 2c; 3b; etc. Check your answers using the Answer Key in Appendix A.*

**1.** An IV technician most frequently uses these two solutions as diluents:

a. sterile water and alcohol
b. sterile water and normal saline
c. sterile water and $D_5W$
d. normal saline and $D_5W$

**2.** Which description reflects the qualities of an IVPB solution?

a. large volume, without additives, run continuously
b. large volume, with additives, run continuously
c. small volume, without additives, run intermittently
d. small volume, with additives, run intermittently

**3.** An ampule, a vial without preservatives, and a prefilled syringe are all considered to be which type of container?

a. SDV
b. MDV
c. LVP
d. none of the above

**4.** Which of the following scenarios would result in touch contamination?

a. blocking airflow to the prefilter by placing a sharps container in front of the filter
b. accidentally touching a syringe tip to your sterile, gloved finger
c. blocking airflow from the HEPA filter to a vial
d. failing to swab the needle before use

**5.** How far inside of the hood must you work in order to maintain adequate sterile airflow and correct aseptic technique?

a. four inches
b. five inches
c. six inches
d. It does not matter how far inside of the hood you work as long as the airflow is not blocked and you swab properly with alcohol.

## Apply Your Knowledge

*On a separate sheet of paper, write your answers to the questions posed in the paragraph below. Use complete sentences and take time to create a thorough and thoughtful response. Check your answers against the Answer Key in Appendix A.*

In Part 1 of this chapter, you learned that aseptic technique guidelines place a great deal of emphasis on avoiding contamination of the critical sites of every supply item. With that in mind, what would be an appropriate course of action if you realized, prior to injection, that the critical site of a vial was incorrectly positioned on the hood's work surface such that it did not receive adequate airflow from the HEPA filter? Would you take a different course of action if you realized this problem *after* injecting into the vial? Why or why not?

# Examine the Resources and Supplies

## Needles

In sterile compounding, needles are used to puncture containers and to inject or withdraw fluid. Needles are individually wrapped within one of two types of outer packaging: either a hard plastic cap covering the needle hub (designed to be twisted off and then discarded), or a paper wrapper (designed to be torn off and discarded). The most commonly used regular needle has a paper wrapper.

***Components*** Several components are common to every needle (see Figure 3.1). The **needle tip** is at the very end of the needle and is razor sharp. The tip of the needle has a slanted opening called the **bevel**. The **heel** is the rounded part of the bevel at the point where the slanted opening ends, opposite the needle tip. The **needle shaft** provides length to the needle and extends from the point where the colored needle hub attaches to the metal needle, to the needle tip. The inner core of the needle shaft is called the **lumen**, a hollow space through which fluid moves into or out of the syringe. The **needle hub** is the end point, which attaches to the syringe. A hard plastic cap covers the needle shaft and tip until the moment of use. The cap is the *only* place where you can aseptically touch or hold the needle.

**FIGURE 3.1**

**Needle Components**

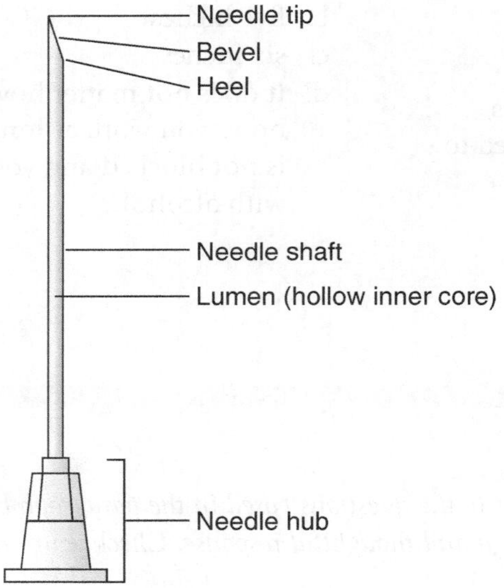


A needle's size is determined by its gauge and length. **Needle gauge** refers to the diameter of the opening, or lumen, of a needle. Sterile compounding needles range in size from 16-gauge to 25-gauge. The size of the gauge corresponds conversely to the size of the lumen: the larger the gauge number, the smaller the lumen and, consequently, the smaller the hole that the needle makes; the smaller the gauge number, the larger the lumen and, consequently, the larger the hole that the needle makes. For example, a 25-gauge needle makes a very small hole, whereas a 16-gauge needle makes a much larger hole (see Figure 3.2). Sterile compounding personnel choose a needle size based on the task they plan to perform.

**FIGURE 3.2**

**Common Needle Sizes Used by IV Technicians**

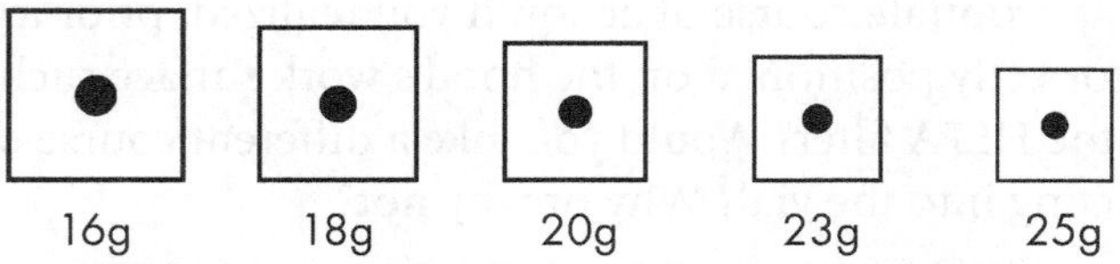

When drawing up a **viscous** liquid such as albumin, for instance, the IV technician would choose a needle with a large gauge size (indicated by a small gauge number). The technician would select a needle with a small lumen (indicated by a large gauge number) when providing an IM medication for a **neonate**. Most commonly, sterile compounders choose 18-gauge and 19-gauge needles. These gauge sizes enable easy drawing of fluid into the syringe without creating a large hole in the vial top or injection port.

IV technicians also choose **needle lengths** according to the task being performed (see Figure 3.3). For most sterile compounding procedures, the compounding personnel select a regular needle with a standard 1½" length. This needle length is necessary for removing fluid from large vials because shorter needles are not long enough to penetrate into the vial to reach the fluid.

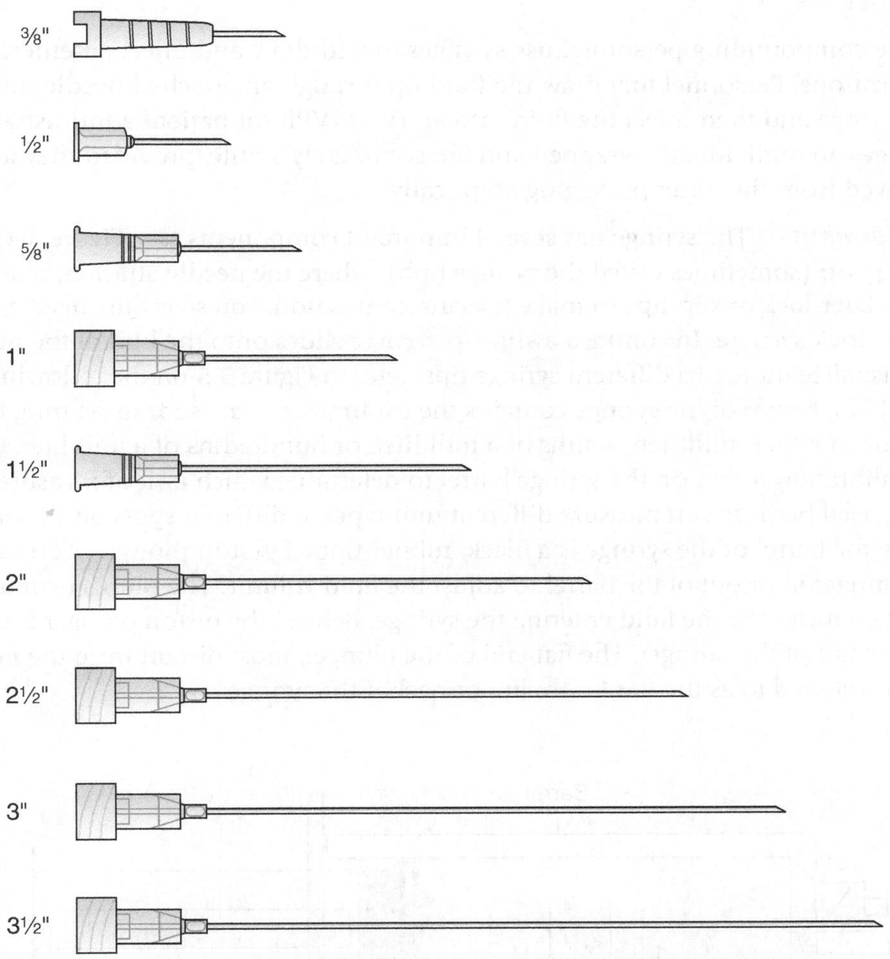


**FIGURE 3.3**

**Regular Needle Lengths**

***Handling*** Every component of the needle, except the needle cap, is considered to be a critical site and should never be subjected to touch contamination or shadowing. Needles are completely sterile, provided you remove them from the outer packaging aseptically.

**BE AWARE**

You should *not* swab the needle with alcohol prior to use. If you accidentally touch the hub, shaft, or tip of the needle, you must discard the contaminated needle in a sharps container.

**BE AWARE**

If you drop the needle or allow it to touch anything other than the tip of a syringe or a sterilized injection port (including the hood's work surface), you must dispose of the contaminated needle in a sharps container.

To safely recap a needle, an IV technician can use one of two methods. The **standard recapping method** requires the technician to hold the filled syringe as she or he would a dart and then recap the needle by holding the cap between the thumb and forefinger of the nondominant hand and carefully slipping it over the tip of the needle. The needle cap should then snap into place on the syringe. The standard method of needle recapping helps to prevent touch contamination of the needle-and-syringe unit but may lead to an inadvertent needle stick. The **scoop recapping method** involves placing the tip of the needle into the cap that is lying on an IPA swab on the hood's work surface. The IV technician uses the needle-and-syringe unit to scoop the needle cap onto the needle. This method helps prevent an accidental needle stick but increases the potential for contamination of the needle-and-syringe unit due to needle contact with the hood's work surface.

## Syringes

Sterile compounding personnel use syringes to withdraw and inject parenteral medications. Personnel first draw the fluid up through an attached needle into the syringe and then inject the fluid into an IV or IVPB for patient administration. Syringes are individually wrapped and are completely sterile, provided they are removed from the outer packaging aseptically.

***Components*** The syringe has several important components (see Figure 3.4). The **syringe tip** (sometimes called the syringe hub), where the needle attaches, may be either Luer-lock or slip-tip. To make a secure connection, you screw the needle onto a **Luer-lock syringe**. In contrast, a **slip-tip syringe** slides onto the hub of the needle. (To visualize these two different syringe tips, refer to Figure 3.5 on the following page.) The **barrel** of the syringe contains the **calibration marks** for measuring fluid volume in either milliliters, tenths of a milliliter, or hundredths of a milliliter. Check the calibration marks on the syringe barrel to determine which unit of measure is being used because you measure different unit types at different spots on the barrel. Inside the barrel of the syringe is a black, rubber-tipped **piston plunger**. You move the plunger in or out of the barrel to adjust the fluid volume. The plunger comes in direct contact with the fluid entering the syringe. Behind the piston plunger is the **inner shaft** of the plunger. The flat end of the plunger, most distant from the needle end, is referred to as the **flat knob**, lip, or heel of the syringe.

**FIGURE 3.4**

**Syringe Components**

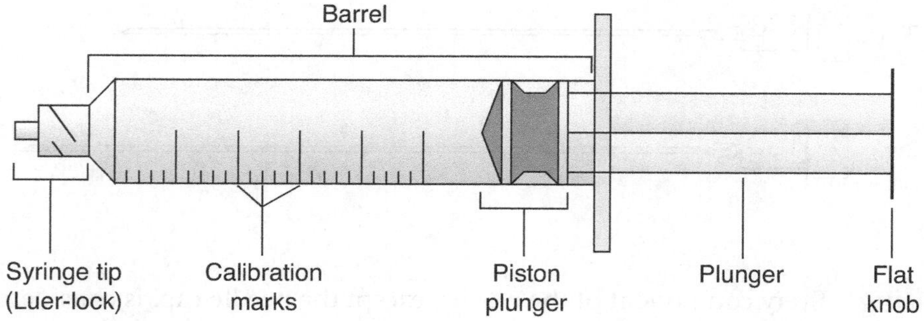

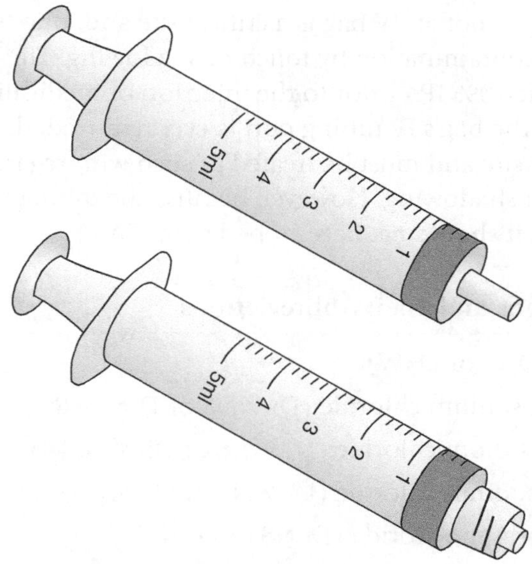


**FIGURE 3.5**

**Luer-Lock and Slip-Tip Syringes**

**POINTER**

In most sterile compounding situations, a Luer-lock syringe is preferable because the needle connection is secure. Although a slip-tip syringe is slightly more cost-effective, it can create a potentially hazardous situation if the needle inadvertently slips off of the syringe.

***Handling*** You can touch or hold the syringe only on the outer barrel or the flat knob. The critical sites of a syringe are the tip or hub, the piston plunger, and the inner plunger shaft. These critical sites should never be subject to contamination by touch or shadowing. Some syringes come with a plastic cap covering the syringe tip. You must remove this cap prior to attaching a needle. You should *not* swab the syringe with IPA prior to use. If you accidentally touch the hub, piston plunger, or inner plunger shaft of the syringe, you must dispose of the contaminated syringe in a sharps container. In addition, if you drop the syringe or allow it to touch anything other than the sterile hub of a needle (including the hood's work surface), you must dispose of the contaminated syringe in a sharps container.

## IV Base Solutions

IV base solutions, or LVPs, are frequently used in sterile compounding procedures. The majority of these solutions come in bags made from softened plastic products. The container is flexible and expands or collapses according to the volume of fluid that is added or removed from the bag.

***Components*** The top of an IV bag contains a small plastic **hang loop** for suspending the bag from the hang bar within the hood or from the IV pole at the patient's bedside. Calibration marks on the face of the bag help you determine the volume of fluid in the bag. The face of the bag also contains the manufacturer's information identifying the ingredients in the bag, such as the concentration of dextrose or sodium chloride. The injection port and the tubing port are on the bottom of the bag. The IV technician injects additives through the **injection port**, which self-seals once the needle is removed. In most facilities, standard operating procedure requires the IV technician to apply an IVA seal over the injection port prior to distributing the compounded IV solution to the nursing unit. When the nurse is ready to administer the IV solution to a patient, the nurse removes the rubber cap covering the bag's **tubing port** and inserts the tubing's **universal spike adaptor** (also known as the spike) into the tubing port.

***Handling*** The injection port of an IV bag is a critical site and, once swabbed, should never be subject to contamination by touch or shadowing. The injection port *must* be swabbed with sterile 70% IPA prior to the injection of medication. In addition, if the rubber cap over the bag's IV tubing port is ever removed, the tubing port is then considered a critical site and must be treated as such with regard to preventing touch contamination or shadowing. However, because the tubing port of an IV bag has a sterile, inner seal, it should *not* be swabbed with IPA.

| Common IV Base Solutions and Their Abbreviations |
|---|
| Dextrose 5% in water ($D_5W$ or D5W) |
| Dextrose 5% in 0.225% sodium chloride ($D_5$ ¼NS or D5 ¼NS) |
| Dextrose 5% in 0.33% sodium chloride ($D_5$ ⅓NS or D5 ⅓NS) |
| Dextrose 5% in 0.45% sodium chloride ($D_5$ ½NS or D5 ½NS) |
| Dextrose 5% in 0.9% sodium chloride ($D_5$ NS or D5NS) |
| 0.9% sodium chloride (NS) |
| Lactated Ringer's (LR or RL) |
| Dextrose 5% in lactated Ringer's ($D_5$ RL or $D_5$LR or D5RL or D5LR) |

## IVPB Base Solutions

IVPB base solutions are used solely for the dilution and administration of medications for intermittent IV administration to a patient. Similar to an IV base solution, an IVPB base solution is contained in an IV bag. However, because it is added or "piggybacked" into the tubing line of an LVP bag and administered as a single dose over a short period, the volume of the IVPB bag is smaller.

***Components*** IVPB bag components are similar to those of an IV base solution bag. The top of the bag has a hang loop; the face of the bag contains identifying information from the manufacturer; and the bottom of the bag contains both an injection port and a tubing port.

***Handling*** The injection port of an IVPB bag, like that of an LVP bag, *must* be swabbed with sterile 70% IPA prior to the injection of medication. In addition, if the rubber cap over the bag's IVPB tubing port is ever removed, the tubing port is then considered a critical site and must be treated as such with regard to preventing touch contamination or shadowing. However, because the tubing port of an IVPB bag has a sterile, inner seal, it should *not* be swabbed with IPA.

| Common IVPB Base Solutions and Their Abbreviations |
|---|
| 0.45% sodium chloride (½NS) |
| Dextrose 5% in water ($D_5W$ or D5W) |
| 0.9% sodium chloride (NS) |
| Sterile water (SW) |

## Vials

Vials are sterile, sealed containers that are used frequently in sterile compounding. Some vials may contain a sterile liquid medication that is ready to be drawn up into a syringe. Other vials many contain a powdered medication that requires reconstitution with a diluent such as sterile water or normal saline. An IV technician draws the diluent into a syringe and then injects it into another vial containing a powdered medication. Once the powder is reconstituted, the IV technician draws the liquid medication into a syringe and injects it into an IV or IVPB. Some common vial sizes are 5, 10, 20, and 30 mL. The choice depends on the volume of fluid or the amount of powder to be placed in the vial. However, while working in the IV room, sterile compounding personnel may encounter vial sizes from as small as 1 mL to as large as 250 mL.

**USP Chapter <797>**

An IV technician must always write the compounding date and time on the label of the reconstituted vial so that the expiration date (or beyond-use date) of the vial's contents may be determined.

***Components*** A hard plastic cap covers the top of a vial and must be removed prior to vial use. Under the cap is a rubberized, self-sealing port through which a needle or dispensing pin is inserted to inject or withdraw fluid.

***Handling*** The critical site of the vial is the self-sealing rubber top, also known as the injection port (see Figure 3.6). The vial top should never be subject to touch contamination or shadowing. The rubberized vial top *must* be swabbed with sterile 70% IPA prior to injection.

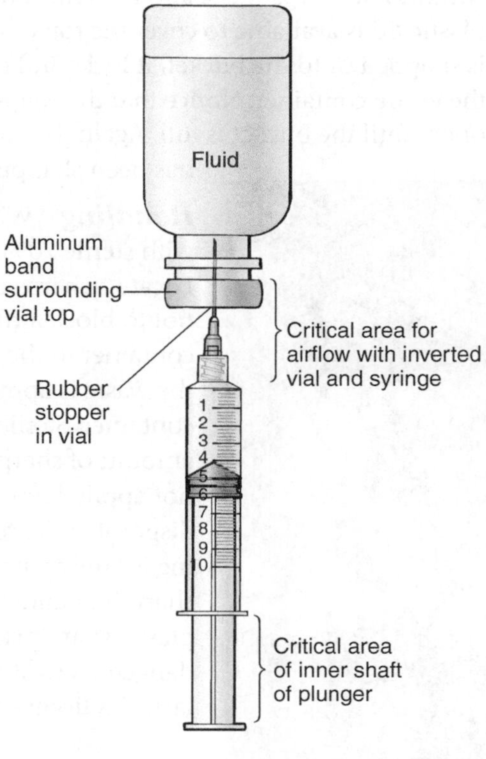


**FIGURE 3.6**

**Critical Areas for Vial, Needle, and Syringe**

## Sharps Containers

The red sharps container is used to safely dispose of all dangerous waste items, such as needles, syringes, and broken glass. Some facilities also prefer that used IV tubing be disposed of in the sharps container because the universal spike adaptor has a sharp point. Follow your facility's recommendations for disposing of IV tubing. No other items—including swabs, vials, empty IV bags, paper waste, and other nonsharps waste—should be placed in the sharps container. These items should be discarded in the regular trash. Chemotherapy waste must be disposed of in a special sharps container that is typically yellow in color. Chapter 14 of this textbook discusses the chemotherapy-specific sharps container.

Pharmacy-generated sharps containers, once filled, are retrieved and disposed of by a company that specializes in the disposal of medical waste. Medical waste disposal companies are regulated by the Environmental Protection Agency (EPA), the Department of Transportation (DOT), and the Drug Enforcement Agency (DEA). In most cases, pharmacy-generated sharps waste is autoclaved prior to being disposed of in a landfill. Best practice for sharps disposal involves incineration, instead of autoclaving and landfill disposal; however, this option is a more expensive alternative. Hazardous waste such as chemotherapy waste requires special high-temperature incineration procedures that are discussed in Chapter 14 of this textbook.

Note that most facilities use red sharps containers for their pharmacy-generated waste and yellow sharps containers for hazardous waste. However, a small number of states have implemented the use of "universal waste containers" that may be black or blue in color. Universal waste containers allow all medical, pharmacy, and hazardous waste to be disposed of by incineration without separating these waste categories into multiple bins. Consult your facility's Policy & Procedure (P&P) manual for information on disposal procedures for pharmacy-generated waste.

***Components*** The sharps container is made of a hard, plastic material that is impenetrable by needles and broken glass. Sharps containers come in several different sizes, ranging from a 0.5-gallon to an 8-gallon capacity. Patients with diabetes frequently use small-sized sharps containers to dispose of used insulin syringes. Clinic settings often use medium-sized sharps containers to dispose of waste from immunizations and other injections. Laboratories and sterile compounding environments generate large volumes of sharps waste and thus must use the large-sized sharps containers. A hard plastic lid is available to cover the top of each sharps container; however, once the lid is snapped onto the bucket, it locks and cannot be removed without visibly damaging the entire container. Notice that the snap-lock lid has a small opening that may be left open until the bucket is full. Again, be aware that once this smaller opening in the lid has been snapped shut, it locks and cannot be reopened.

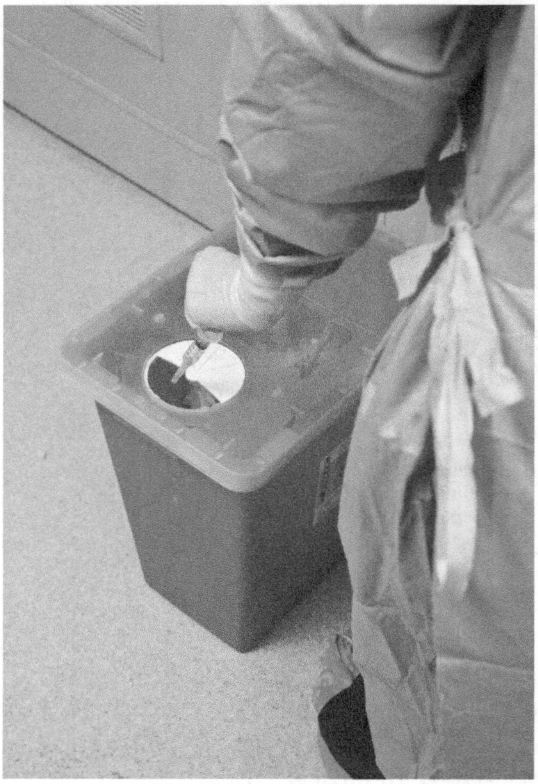

Correct disposal of needle-and-syringe unit into a sharps container.

***Handling*** Wipe down the exterior of the sharps container with sterile 70% IPA before bringing it into the clean room. Locate a sharps container next to each hood, positioned not to block airflow into the hood prefilter. Keep the sharps container in the clean room until it is full, which occurs when the waste is approximately two inches from the top of the container. Sterile compounding procedures produce a large amount of sharps waste. Thus, the hard plastic lid is usually not applied until the bucket is completely full, making sharps disposal easier for the IV technician because the bucket opening is larger with the lid off. An IV technician moves the full sharps container into the anteroom and attaches the hard plastic snap-lock lid onto the top, preventing access to the dangerous waste. Full sharps containers are sent to special facilities licensed to dispose of medical waste.

## Sterile IV Tubing

In a sterile compounding facility, personnel use sterile IV tubing to transfer solutions from one container into another. This type of tubing is called secondary IV tubing and differs from the primary IV tubing that nurses use to administer IV base solutions to patients. However, both types of tubing share some common components.

***Components*** The main components of sterile IV tubing include the universal spike adaptor (also called the tubing spike or spike), the drip chamber, the roll clamp, the tubing itself, and the needle adaptor. Sterile compounding personnel insert the universal spike adaptor into the tubing port on the IV source container. They observe the **drip chamber** to calculate the flow rate at which the IV is being infused. The **roll clamp** is used to regulate the flow rate of the IV from the source container into the receiving container or patient. The far end of the tubing is called the **needle adaptor**. The attached needle of the adaptor is inserted into the patient, the receiving container, or the primary tubing.

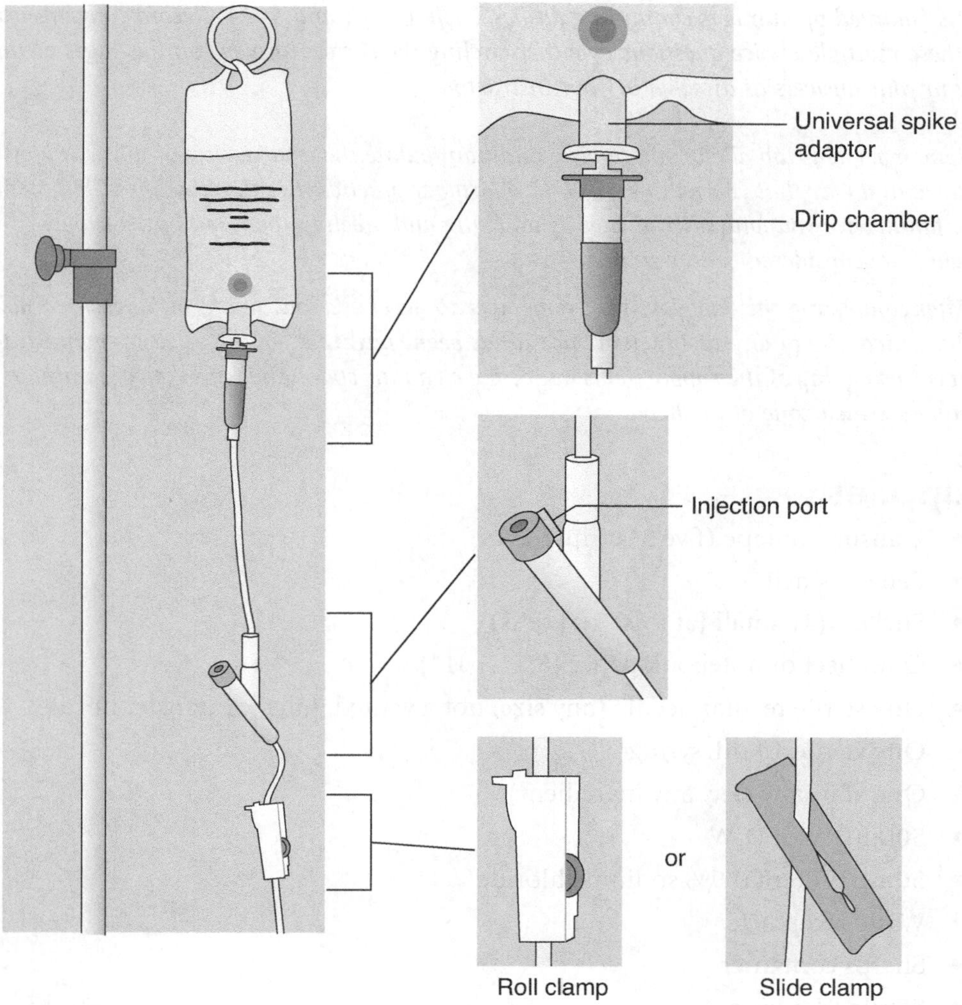


FIGURE 3.7

**Sterile IV Tubing and Components**

***Handling*** The critical sites of sterile IV tubing are the universal spike adaptor and the needle adaptor. Personnel must remove the protective plastic cap prior to using these adaptors. Because the spike adaptor and the needle adaptor are sterile, you should *not* swab these components with IPA prior to use. If you accidentally touch the spike or the needle adaptor, you must dispose of the contaminated IV tubing. In addition, if you drop the IV tubing, or allow it to touch anything other than the sterile tubing port or needle hub (including the hood's work surface), you must dispose of the contaminated IV tubing.

# Exploratory Lab

The purpose of this exploratory lab is to introduce you to some of the most important and commonly used sterile compounding supplies. In addition, this lab helps you to identify the critical sites of various compounding supplies. By knowing these sites well, you can more easily avoid touch contamination and shadowing when you compound sterile products—both while using this textbook and during your pharmacy IV technician practice. To complete this exploratory procedure most effectively, perform it while sitting at a desk or table in the classroom.

***Note:*** *Some of the steps ask you to read and respond to one or more multiple-choice questions (marked by numbers containing dashes, such as* **1–1** *and* **1–2***). Record your answers to these multiple-choice questions by either circling the correct answers on the pages or turning in your answers as directed by your instructor.*

*Remember, this lab allows you to view and manipulate the critical sites of many supply items in a way that you will never do in pharmacy practice. Because the lab is designed to familiarize you with critical sites by touching and labeling them, all of the supply items are considered contaminated.*

*After completing this lab, you must remember to never shadow, mark, or otherwise touch the critical site of any supply item once it has been sterilized. You must also remember to never bring any of the supply items out of the clean air space and into the contaminated outer six-inch zone of the hood.*

## Supplies

- Transparent tape (five 3" strips)
- Pen or pencil
- Stickers (11 small [at least ¾"] dots)
- One sheet of notebook paper (8.5" × 11")
- One sterile regular needle (any size; not a vented, filter, or transfer needle)
- One sterile 10-mL syringe
- One vial (any size, any ingredient)
- 500mL IV of $D_5W$
- 50mL IVPB of 0.9% sodium chloride
- Waste receptacle
- Sharps container
- Sterile IV tubing

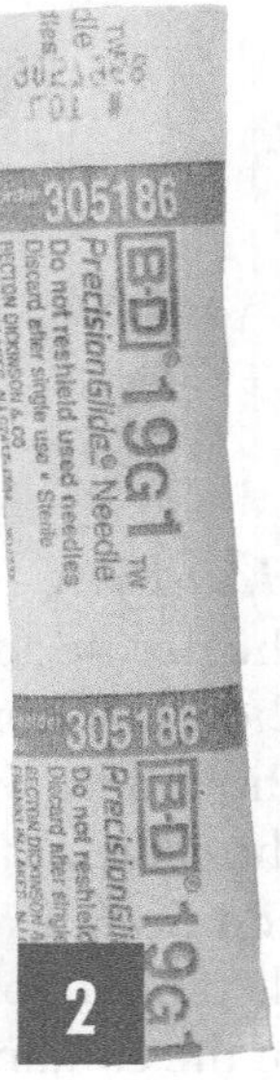


## Procedure

### *Opening, Identifying, and Labeling a Needle and Syringe*

1. Assemble all of the supplies at your desk.
2. Pick up the package that contains the sterile needle and note which end of the package contains the needle hub and which end contains the needle tip.

3. Slowly peel apart the paper wrapper that encases the needle, starting at the end that is slightly separated.
4. Grasp the hard plastic needle cap, with needle inside, with your nondominant hand. Use your dominant hand to remove the paper needle wrapper and put it in the waste receptacle.
5. Bring the capped needle close to you so that you may examine it and then grasp the hub of the needle with the thumb and forefinger of your dominant hand.
6. Carefully remove the needle cap by pulling it well away from the needle with your nondominant hand. Temporarily place the needle cap onto your desk.
7. Examine the needle thoroughly so that you can identify each of its components.
8. Carefully tape the uncapped needle to a piece of paper, using transparent tape. Use a pen or pencil to label the needle tip, bevel, heel, shaft, lumen, and hub of the needle once it is taped to the paper.
9. Answer the following multiple-choice question, recording your answer as directed by your instructor.

   **9–1.** Which of the following lists the critical sites of a needle?
   a. needle cap, hub, bevel, tip, heel, shaft, lumen
   b. needle hub, tip, shaft, lumen
   c. needle hub, bevel, tip, heel, shaft, lumen
   d. needle hub, bevel, tip, shaft, lumen, plunger
10. Draw an asterisk on the paper next to each labeled needle component that is considered a critical site.
11. Tape the needle cap to the paper and label it as such. Place the paper with the labeled needle temporarily onto your desk or tabletop.
12. Pick up the wrapped syringe. Identify the end of the syringe where the syringe tip is located.
13. Slowly peel apart the wrapper that encases the syringe, beginning at the end that is slightly separated.
14. Grasp the barrel of the syringe in your dominant hand. Remove the syringe wrapper and place it into the waste receptacle. If there is a plastic cap on the syringe tip, remove it and place it into the waste receptacle as well.
15. Bring the syringe close to you and examine it carefully while holding the barrel of the syringe in your nondominant hand. Using your dominant hand, pull down on the flat knob. Notice how this motion moves the plunger. Push up on the flat knob and notice how the plunger responds.
16. Tape the syringe to the piece of paper, next to the needle and needle cap. Use a pen or pencil to label the syringe tip, barrel, calibration marks, piston plunger, inner shaft, and flat knob on the paper.

**POINTER**
In several of the upcoming Unit 2 labs, you learn how to aseptically attach the needle hub to the syringe tip without touching the needle hub or shaft.

**BE AWARE**
Exercise caution when examining the razor-sharp needle.

**POINTER**
Identifying the locations of the critical sites now helps you to later avoid touching or shadowing them when removing the outer packaging.

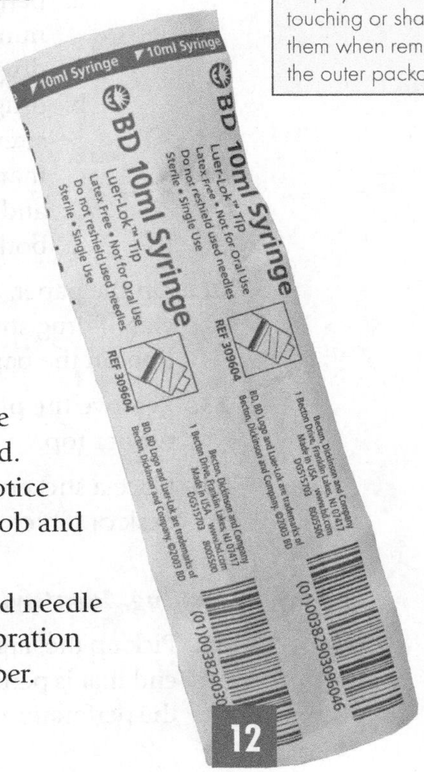

17. Answer the following multiple-choice question, recording your answer as directed by your instructor.

    17–1. Which of the following lists the critical sites of a syringe?
    a. syringe tip, piston plunger, inner shaft
    b. syringe tip, cap, piston plunger, inner shaft
    c. syringe tip, barrel, piston plunger, inner shaft
    d. barrel, piston plunger, inner shaft

18. Draw an asterisk on the paper next to each labeled syringe component that is considered a critical site.

19. Place the paper with the labeled needle and syringe temporarily onto your desk or tabletop.

### *Opening, Identifying, and Marking a Vial*

20. If necessary, remove the vial from its outer packaging. Place the outer packaging into the waste receptacle.

21. Bring the vial close to you so that you can examine it. Read the vial's label carefully and then answer the following multiple-choice question, recording your answer as directed by your instructor.

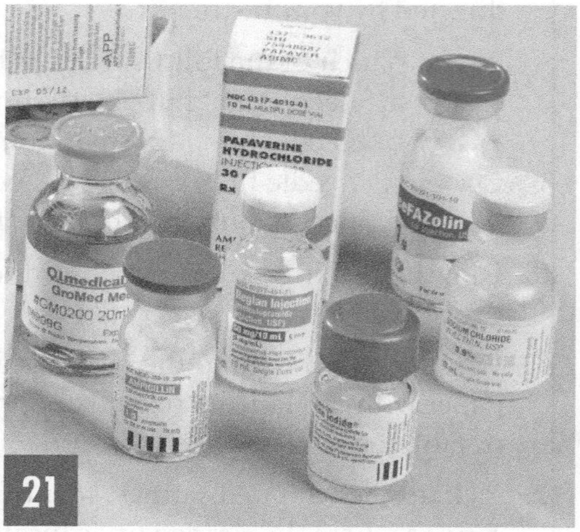


    21–1. Which of the following items are found on a vial's label?
    a. patient name, room number, drug name, and drug strength
    b. drug or solution name, strength, and/or amount
    c. manufacturer's name and expiration date
    d. both *b* and *c*

22. On the paper, write the name of the medication or solution contained in the vial. If drug strength or concentration is listed on the vial, record that information on the paper as well.

23. Remove the plastic cap that covers the top of the vial. Examine the vial's rubber top.

24. Place a sticker on the critical site of the vial. Place the stickered vial onto your desk or tabletop.

### *Opening, Identifying, and Labeling IV and IVPB Base Solutions*

25. Pick up the large-volume IV solution. Examine the outer dust cover to identify the end that is perforated for ease of opening. Tear the dust cover lengthwise, along the perforation.

26. Remove the IV bag from the dust cover. Put the dust cover into the waste receptacle.

27. Closely examine the IV bag to identify its five major components. Write the name of each one on a separate sticker and then add an asterisk on each of the stickers containing the name of a critical site.

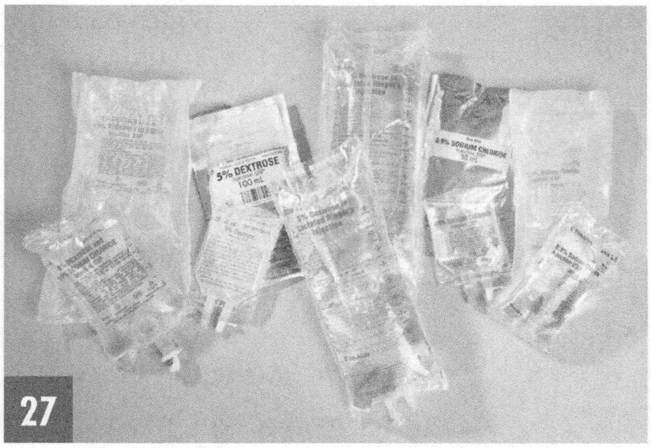


28. Place all of the stickers onto the IV bag in their correct locations and then place the stickered IV bag onto the tabletop.

29. Repeat steps 25–28 using the IVPB base solution in place of the large-volume IV solution.

30. Answer the following multiple-choice question, recording your answer as directed by your instructor.

 30–1. What are the five main components of both IV and IVPB bags?
 a. hang loop, calibration marks, manufacturer's identification information, injection port, tubing port
 b. hang bar, calibration marks, manufacturer's identification information, injection port, drip chamber
 c. hang loop, manufacturer's identification information, needle adaptor, injection port, tubing port
 d. hang loop, calibration marks, needle adaptor, injection port, tubing port

### *Opening, Identifying, and Labeling IV Tubing*

31. Tear open the outer packaging that contains the IV tubing and place the outer wrapping into the waste receptacle.

32. Closely examine the components of the sterile IV tubing.

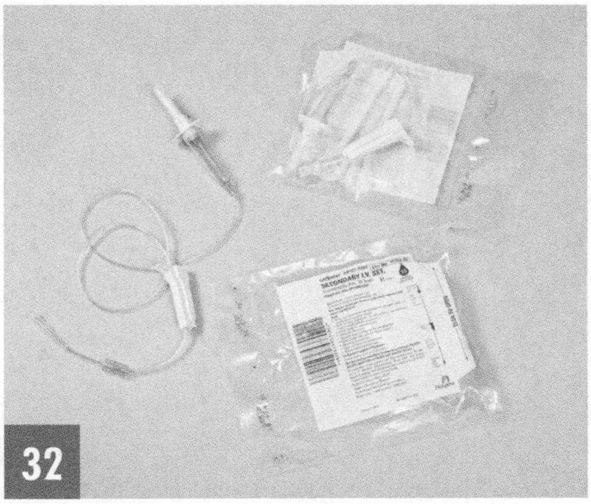

33. Roll the roll clamp down until the tubing is completely closed. Notice the protective cap covering the spike and needle adaptor.

34. Use the remaining pieces of tape to tape the tubing onto the paper and then answer the following multiple-choice questions, recording your answers as directed by your instructor.

 34–1. Which of the following identifies the five main components of sterile IV tubing?
 a. universal spike adaptor, drip chamber, tubing, roll clamp, needle hub
 b. universal spike adaptor, drip chamber, tubing, roll clamp, needle adaptor
 c. drip chamber, tubing, roll clamp, needle adaptor, syringe tip
 d. drip chamber, tubing, roll clamp, needle hub, syringe tip

34–2. Which part of the IV tubing controls the flow rate of the IV fluid?
   a. universal spike adaptor
   b. drip chamber
   c. roll clamp
   d. needle adaptor

**35.** Use a pen or pencil to label the five major components of the IV tubing on the paper, adding an asterisk on the paper next to components considered to be critical sites.

### *Concluding the Procedure*

**36.** Ask your instructor to verify that you have correctly identified all components and critical sites of the needle, syringe, vial, IV bag, IVPB bag, and IV tubing. Your instructor will also verify that you wrote down the correct medication or solution name and strength for the vial.

**37.** Once your instructor has checked your work, place the paper with the needle, syringe, and IV tubing into the sharps container. Return the vial, IV bag, and IVPB bag to your instructor for storage. Place any remaining trash in the waste receptacle. Return the sharps container and waste receptacle to their designated locations.

**Note:** *For the purposes of this lab only, you place the paper with the needle, syringe, and IV tubing taped to it, directly into the sharps container. In practice, paper items should be placed into the regular waste container, not the sharps container.*

# Part 3: Assessment

## Chapter Summary

- The development of disposable medical and pharmacy supplies was spurred by a need for infection control and mass immunizations.
- Needles and syringes are the primary tools for sterile compounding.
- The critical site is the part of the supply item that includes any fluid pathway surface or opening at risk for contamination.
- Critical sites include vial tops, opened ampules, needle hubs, needle shafts, syringe tips, tubing and dispensing pin spikes, and the injection ports of IVs and IVPBs.
- Critical sites must never be touched, other than by a sterile tool such as a needle or spike, or a supply item such as a sterile IPA swab.
- Critical sites that should never be swabbed with sterile IPA include the various components of the needle, syringe, tubing, dispensing pin and tubing port.
- Correct aseptic technique is essential for avoiding touch contamination or shadowing of compounded sterile preparations (CSPs).
- Airflow from the HEPA filter to the critical site(s) must never be interrupted.
- Sterile compounding must take place within the DCA of a hood.
- Needle components include the needle cap, tip, bevel, heel, shaft, lumen, and hub.
- The needle cap is the only component allowed to come into contact with your hand or the hood's work surface.
- Needle size is determined by length and gauge.
- The smaller the needle's gauge number, the larger the hole it makes.
- Specialty needles, such as vented needles and filter needles, are only used for designated procedures.
- The components of the syringe include the tip, the barrel with calibration marks, the piston plunger, the inner shaft, and the flat knob.
- IV base solutions are large-volume (usually 500 mL or 1000 mL) sterile solutions continuously administered intravenously over an extended period.
- IVPB solutions are small-volume (usually 50 mL, 100 mL, or 250 mL) sterile solutions with additives, which are piggybacked through an IV line extending from an LVP into the patient. IVPBs are administered intravenously on an intermittent basis.
- The components of both IV and IVPB bags include the hang loop, bag face with manufacturer's information and calibration marks, the injection port, and the tubing port.
- Some IV and IVPB products are supplied as premixed, shelf-stable, or frozen products.
- ADD-Vantage, MINI-BAG Plus, and Add-A-Vial products require the IV technician to aseptically attach a vial to a special IVPB, which a nurse activates just prior to patient administration.
- Vials are sealed, sterile containers having a rubber top through which fluid is withdrawn by the IV technician. Vials may contain a powder or liquid medication or liquid diluent.
- SDVs do not contain a preservative and are for one-time use. SDVs also include syringes and opened ampules.
- MDVs contain a preservative and may be reused for up to 28 days, as directed by the manufacturer.
- The components of IV tubing are the universal spike adaptor, drip chamber, roll clamp, sterile tubing, and needle adaptor.
- IPA swabs, vented dispensing pins, and IVA seals are frequently used in sterile compounding.
- Sharps containers are to be used for the disposal of needles, syringes, broken glass, and blood products only.
- Some of the less frequently used compounding supplies include repeater pumps, Luer-to-Luer connectors, membrane filters, and EECs.

# Key Terms

**Add-A-Vial** a brand of IVPB in which a specially designed vial and an IVPB either screw or snap together and are activated by the nurse just prior to patient administration

**additive** a medication or electrolyte that is injected into an LVP or SVP solution for administration to the patient; a drug that is injected into an IV solution

**ADD-Vantage bag** a brand of IVPB solution for which a specially designed vial and IVPB either screw or snap together and are activated by the nurse just prior to patient administration

**ampule** a small glass container for sterile liquid or powdered medication

**barrel** the inner part of the syringe into which fluid is drawn and held

**bevel** the slanted opening at the tip of the needle

**bloodletting** a medieval treatment designed to remove excess blood from the body, thereby bringing into balance the four humors

**calibration mark** a graduation mark on the outside of the barrel to indicate fluid volume

**clean air zone** the region wherein the sterile air that comes from the HEPA filter proceeds uninterrupted until it reaches the inner edge of the six-inch zone; sometimes called the direct compounding area (DCA); also known as "first air"

**critical site** part of the supply item that includes any fluid pathway surface or fluid pathway opening that is at risk for contamination by touch or airflow interruption

**depth filter** a small filter built into a specialty needle that removes particulate matter from a solution

**diluent** a fluid, typically sterile water or normal saline, that is used to dissolve or reconstitute a drug in powdered form or to dilute a liquid medication to a lesser concentration

**drip chamber** the small, open space just below the spike adaptor, into which the fluid from the IV bag drips before flowing into the tubing; nurses count the drops falling into this chamber to determine the flow rate of the IV solution

**dust cover** the outer packaging of a sterile supply item

**empty evacuated container (EEC)** an empty sterile vial whose slight negative pressure allows an easy transfer of solutions from a bulk container; often used for special preparations wherein both the base solution and additive are made from scratch

**filter needle** a needle that has an interior filter for filtering out large particles or glass from a solution

**flat knob** the flat end of the piston plunger that, when pulled out, allows fluid to fill the barrel and, when pushed in, allows fluid to be expelled from the barrel

**hang loop** the small, plastic loop at the top (most distant from the injection port) of an IV or IVPB bag that is used to suspend the IV bag on an IV pole or hood hang bar

**heel** the rounded part of the bevel opposite the needle tip

**humors** a medieval medical theory, often credited to Hippocrates, that believed optimal health may be attained only when the four elemental body fluids (blood, phlegm, black bile, and yellow bile) were in perfect balance

**hydration** fluid that is administered to the patient, often intravenously, to prevent or treat dehydration and restore electrolyte balance in the body

**hydrostatics** a branch of physics that deals with the characteristics of fluids at rest and the pressure they exert

**hypodermic** under or beneath the skin

**injection port** the area on an IV bag, IVPB bag, or vial into which a needle may be inserted to inject or withdraw fluids; the injection port is self-sealing to prevent post-injection leakage

**inner shaft** the inner surface of the syringe barrel, which comes in direct contact with fluid and into and out of which the rubber piston plunger moves

**intravenous piggyback (IVPB) solution** a small-volume parenteral solution (25 mL, 50 mL, 100 mL, 150 mL, or 250 mL) containing medications to be administered intravenously on an intermittent basis

**intravenous (IV) push** a sterile, injectable medication that is administered by direct injection through IV tubing into the patient's vein without further diluting the medication in an SVP or LVP solution

**irrigation** a form of parenteral administration in which a wound, tube, or catheter is flushed or rinsed with a sterile solution; irrigation solutions with additives (such as antibiotics) must be compounded in a laminar airflow hood

**IVA seal** a small, foil-backed adhesive seal that is applied to the injection port of an IV or IVPB bag or to the top of a vial after injection; it provides, if broken by unauthorized personnel, evidence of tampering

**large-volume parenteral (LVP)** any sterile solution of 250 mL or larger that is administered by the parenteral route of administration; an IV base solution ($D_5W$, NS, $D_5$ ½ NS, etc.) with or without additives that is administered intravenously

**Luer-lock syringe** a type of syringe onto whose tip the needle screws

**Luer-to-Luer connector** a needleless system that allows for the easy transfer of fluid from one syringe into another syringe

**lumen** the hollow, inner core of a needle

**membrane filter** a filter that attaches to the tip of a syringe that sterilizes fluid as it passes through its membrane; also known as a 0.2-micron filter or a sterilizing filter

**MINI-BAG Plus** a brand of IVPB bag in which a specially designed vial and an IVPB either screw or snap together and are activated by the nurse just prior to patient administration

**mixed** a pharmacy term meaning that an additive or a diluent has been added

**Mix-O-Vial** a small, hourglass-shaped container in which a diluent is separated from a powder by a rubber stopper; medication is activated when an IV technician presses on the rubber top, mixing the liquid and powder in preparation for patient administration

**morphine** a strong opiate analgesic classified as a CII narcotic

**multiple-dose vial (MDV)** a container of medication that can be used multiple times due to the presence of a preservative (such as benzyl alcohol or methylparaben) to inhibit bacterial growth; medication may be reused for up to 28 days based on manufacturers' recommendations

**needle adaptor** the end of the IV tubing that is farthest from the universal spike adaptor, and to which the needle is attached

**needle gauge** the diameter size of the lumen, or hollow space inside the needle; the lower the gauge number, the larger the hole

**needle hub** the part of the needle that attaches to the syringe tip

**needle length** the length of the needle from the needle hub to needle tip; needles used in sterile compounding typically range from ½" to 1½"

**needle shaft** the part of the needle that provides length

**needle tip** the razor-sharp end of the needle that is inserted into the patient; also known as bevel tip

**neonate** a newborn baby, generally less than 28 days old

**neuralgia** a condition of extreme pain (usually in the body's extremities) that travels along the path of a nerve or bundle of nerves

**nosocomial infection** an infection that originates in a hospital or healthcare facility; an infection transmitted to patients from healthcare workers

**outer six-inch zone** the contaminated area that runs along the entire outer six-inch edge of the hood; should not be used as an area for compounding sterile preparations; also known as the zone of turbulence

**Pascal's Law** law of physics stating that when pressure increases at any point in a confined fluid, an equal pressure increase takes place at every other point in the container

**piston plunger** the stopper at the bottom, interior part of the syringe; holds fluid in the barrel; moves up and down inside the barrel as fluid is drawn into or expelled from the syringe

**prefilled syringe** a manufacturer-provided parenteral medication (often an emergency drug) packaged as an individual dose for IV push use; contains appropriate drug strength and amount in a two-part form (syringe with attached needle plus glass tube of medication) for assembly and immediate administration into IV tubing or IV bag

**primary IV tubing** tubing used to administer IV fluids from an LVP to a patient

**reconstitute** the process of injecting sterile water, or other diluent, into a vial or an ampule that contains a powdered medication; solution is then drawn up into a syringe and injected into an IV or IVPB bag

**regular needle** a needle other than a specialty needle (such as a filter needle, transfer needle, or vented needle) that is commonly used in sterile compounding

**repeater pump** a pump used to rapidly and accurately make multiple fluid transfers from a bulk container to a vial or syringe

**roll clamp** a hard plastic device that provides compression on the tubing, thereby controlling the flow rate of the IV solution

**scoop recapping method** a method of recapping a needle that involves placing the tip of the needle into the cap that is lying on an IPA swab; the needle-and-syringe unit is then used to scoop the cap onto the needle, preventing accidental needle stick but increasing the potential for contamination of the needle-and-syringe unit

**secondary IV tubing** tubing that may be used to piggyback IVPB medications into a hydration solution for patient administration or to transfer fluid from one container into another container

**shadowing** contamination of the critical site of any supply item by interruption of the sterile airflow from the HEPA filter to the critical site; also known as shadow contamination

**sharps container** a hard plastic container, usually red in color, into which sharp or hazardous waste (such as needles, syringes, ampules, broken glass, spikes, blood products) is discarded

**shelf-stable product** a premade IV product, such as an LVP or IVPB solution, that is supplied by the manufacturer with the medication or electrolyte premixed into a parenteral solution; generally stable for several months without refrigeration

**single-dose vial (SDV)** a container of medication that lacks a preservative and therefore is intended for one-time use only

**slip-tip syringe** a type of syringe constructed so that the needle slips or pops onto the syringe tip

**sphygmomanometer** a device used to determine blood pressure that consists of an inflatable cuff that tightens to restrict blood flow and a manometer, an instrument that measures the pressure

**stable** refers to the beyond-use date of a product once it is opened, reconstituted, or mixed

**standard recapping method** a method of recapping a needle that requires an IV technician to hold the filled syringe like a dart and then recap the needle with the cap in the nondominant hand, being careful to avoid an inadvertent needle stick

**sterile isopropyl alcohol (IPA) swab** a small, cotton pad that is presaturated with 70% sterile IPA and is used to clean the critical sites of various supply items

**straight draw** the process of drawing fluid into a syringe using a regular needle

**syringe cap** a sterile, plastic cap that is temporarily attached to the tip of a syringe; the cap is removed and a sterile needle attached prior to patient administration

**syringe tip** the end of the syringe where the needle is attached; also called the syringe hub

**touch contamination** common form of product contamination caused by touching the critical site of any supply item or by introducing any contaminant into the ISO Class 5 compounding area

**transfer needle** a needle used to transfer fluid from one vial to another

**tubing port** a rubber-capped opening at the bottom of the IV or IVPB bag into which a tubing spike is inserted prior to patient administration

**universal spike adaptor** the sharp spike at the end of IV tubing; inserted into the tubing port of an IV bag

**vented dispensing pin** a needleless system that allows direct withdrawal from a vial into a syringe while simultaneously venting air pressure

**vented needle** a needle used to dilute powders that simultaneously vents air pressure out of the vial while injecting diluent into the vial

**vial** a container for sterile liquid or powdered medication

**viscous** any thick or sticky substance or medication used in sterile compounding

**wholesale supplier** a vendor who delivers large volumes of medications, IV solutions, and supplies to the pharmacy on a regular basis

**zone of turbulence** the area directly behind a supply item within the clean air zone, as well as the contaminated area that runs along the entire outer six-inch edge of the hood; should not be used as an area for compounding sterile preparations; also known as the outer six-inch zone

# Make Connections

*On a separate sheet of paper, write your answers to the following three questions, using complete sentences and making sure your answers are thorough and thoughtful. Note that the third question requires Internet access.*

1. IV technicians have a great deal of autonomy and often work alone—with the pharmacist only entering the IV room to perform the final check of the CSP. Considering the level of trust that is placed in an IV technician, what are some of the personal qualities that IV technicians must possess?

2. The injection port of an IV bag must be swabbed with sterile 70% IPA prior to use. The needle must never be swabbed with sterile 70% IPA. What is the rationale for using different procedures on the critical sites of various supply items?

3. Use any Internet search engine to look up the term "nosocomial infection." Read at least two articles on the many causes of nosocomial infections. Based on what you have read, do you think that supply innovations such as the development of disposable syringes and needles play an important role in reducing these types of infections? Why or why not? What sort of impact might the aseptic technique of an IV technician have on nosocomial infections?

# Meet the Challenge

***Scenario*** This scavenger activity is designed to help you become more familiar with common IV compounding supplies and their locations in the laboratory or pharmacy facility.

***Challenge*** Your instructor has a *Scavenger Hunt* handout for an interactive activity that allows you to learn about sterile compounding supplies through lab exploration. To meet this challenge, ask your instructor for the handout. Once your instructor distributes the handout, you have 20 minutes to answer as many of the scavenger hunt questions as possible. Go!

## ADDITIONAL RESOURCES

*Go to the Paradigm Internet Resources Center at* www.paradigmcollege.net/sterilecomp *to access live links related to these Chapter 3 topics:*

+ A history of the development of sterile, disposable needles and syringes
+ A complete listing and photographs of current sterile compounding supplies
+ Information on infection control and the prevention of nosocomial infections

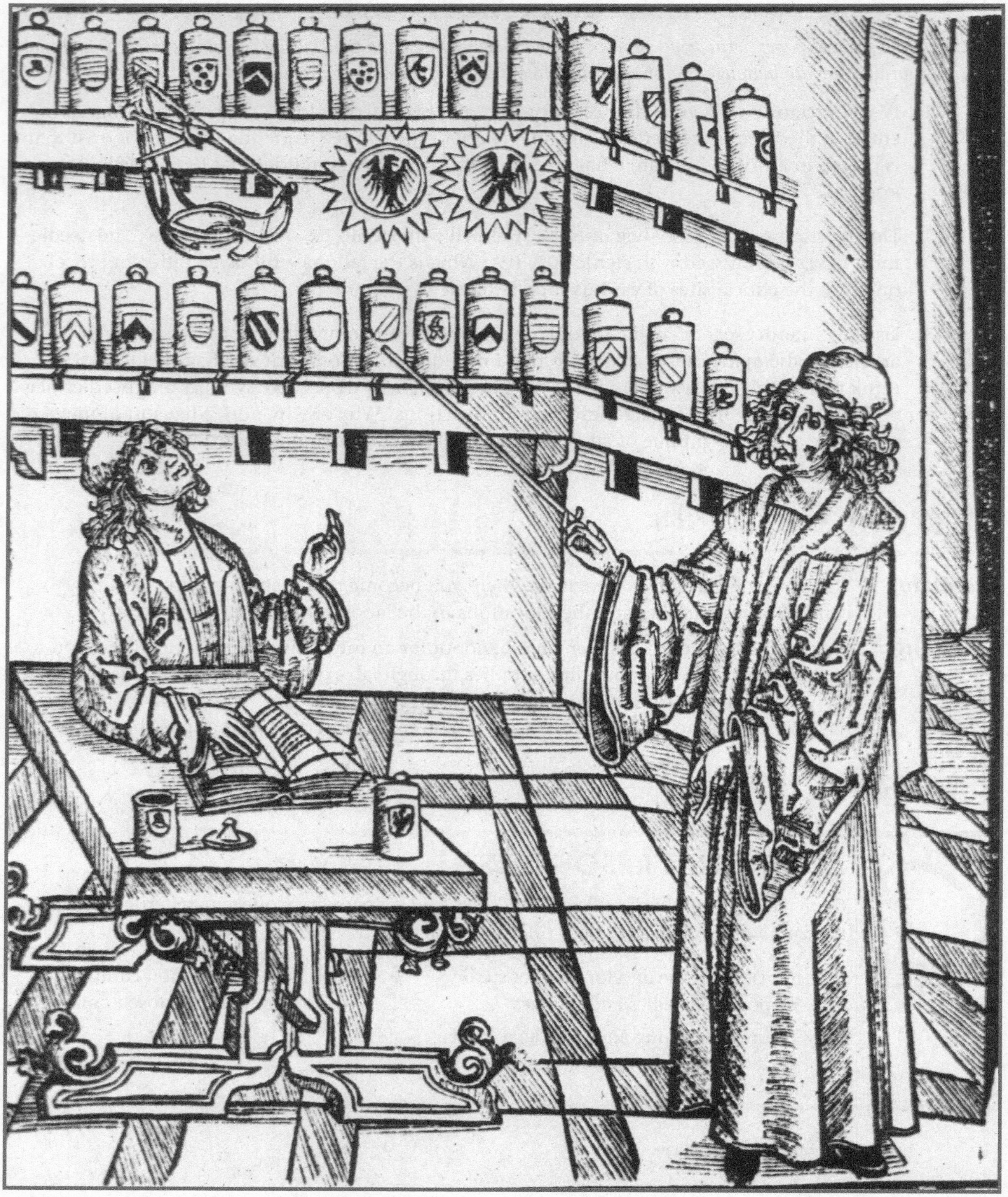

# Chapter 4

# Medication Orders and Labeling

## Learning Objectives

- Gain an awareness of the historical roots of prescriptions, the Rx symbol, and the signa.
- Recognize the influence of early Greek and Roman healthcare practitioners on current medical terminology and abbreviations.
- Understand the difference between a prescription and a medication order.
- Understand common medical and pharmacy terminology, abbreviations, acronyms, and symbols.
- Identify pharmacy directions written in signa language.
- Recognize physician instructions and other pertinent information on a medication order.
- Identify the various components of a compounded sterile preparation label.

During numerous excavations in the Middle East and Far East, archaeologists have uncovered the precursors to modern-day **prescriptions** recorded on a variety of objects (clay tablets, papyrus, silk, and birch bark leaves) and in seemingly odd places (on a sarcophagus and on grotto walls). These ancient recordings followed a recipe-like format, typically listing many ingredients drawn from nature, including flowers, herbs, tree resins and fruits, minerals, and animal parts. The compounded remedies combined these substances to address specific symptoms of an illness or a disease. The amount of each ingredient was often tailored to a patient's gender and age, and some early prescriptions varied according to the annual growth cycles of their natural ingredients. To treat the illnesses and abate the suffering of early civilizations, ancient healers straddled the realms of the practical and magical, coupling their limited knowledge of anatomy and physiology with their beliefs in the healing powers of nature and the human spirit.

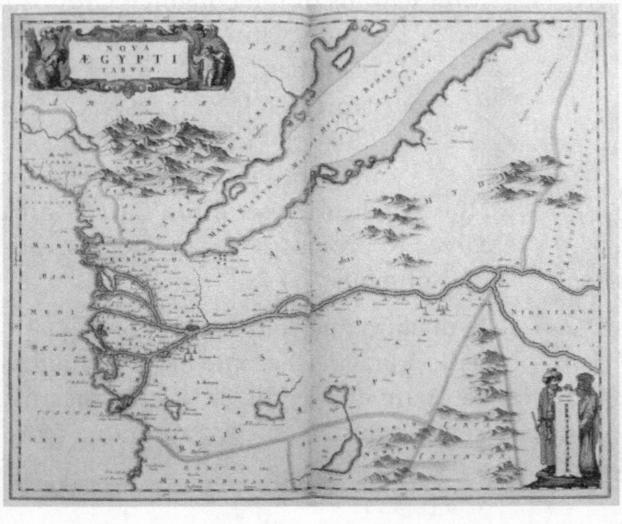

## Ancient Prescriptions and Herbal Medicines

One of the earliest known recordings of medical prescriptions was discovered by archaeologists in Mesopotamia and dates back to around 3000 BCE. The artifact does not specify ingredient quantities, nor the illnesses or diseases being addressed, but it does contain a series of more than 15 prescriptions written in cuneiform on a Sumerian clay

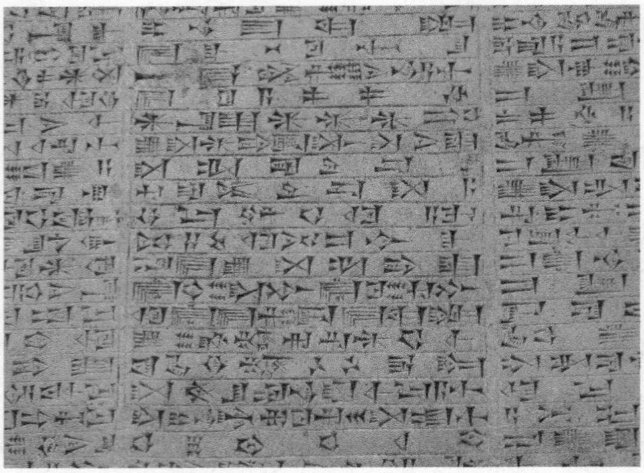

tablet. **Cuneiform** is an ancient type of writing common to many early cultures. It began as a series of pictographs but, over time, the communication transformed into a series of specific characters with meanings. To record cuneiform characters, ancient scribes wielded a **stylus**, or a sharp-ended reed, to carve wedge-shaped impressions into a wet clay tablet. Below is a translation of one of the prescriptions on the Sumerian clay tablet:

*Sift and knead together, all in one turtle-shell, the sprouting naga plant and mustard; wash the sick spot with quality [fermented barley] and hot water; scrub the sick spot with all of the kneaded mixture; after scrubbing, rub with vegetable oil and cover with pulverized fir.*

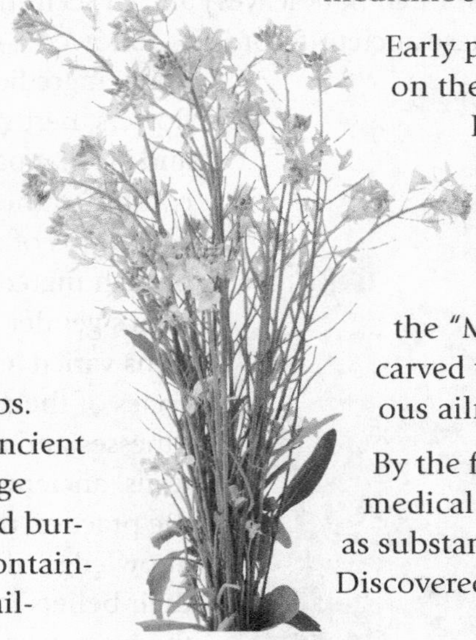

Other ancient prescriptions from around 1534 BCE were recorded on **papyrus** and buried in Egyptian tombs. The most well-known document of ancient Egyptian pharmacology is the 110-page **Ebers Papyrus**, supposedly discovered buried between the legs of a mummy. Containing more than 700 prescriptions for ailments that beset early Egyptian cultures, the Ebers Papyrus addresses many common troubles: ophthalmic conditions from the dry and sandy environment, gastrointestinal parasites from drinking and bathing in unclean water, and insect-borne diseases such as malaria and trachoma. Egyptians believed in the curative powers of plants, and at least one-third of the plants referenced in their prescriptions (such as the aloe plant to treat burns) are still part of modern **pharmacopeia**.

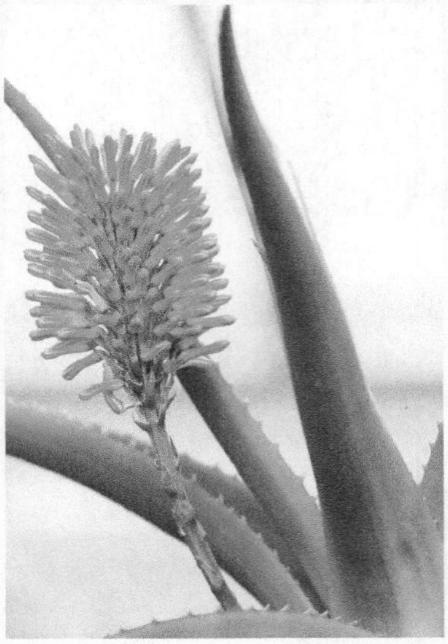

In the Far East, archaeologists found early prescriptions in the Han tombs at Mawangdui, which date back to the Western Han dynasty (206 BCE to 25 CE). Of particular significance was the discovery, in Tomb No. 3, of a silk scroll entitled *Wu Shi Er Bing Fang*, or *Prescriptions for Fifty-Two Diseases*. This document lists 283 prescriptions for treating the 52 noted conditions or diseases, with skin ulcers, urinary problems, and hernias being most frequently addressed. More than 240 herbal drug remedies are included on this silk document, and **traditional Eastern medicine** still relies on many of them.

Early prescriptions were also discovered on the walls of the Longmen Grottos in Luoyang, China. Buddhists occupied these grottos during the Northern Wei dynasty (386 to 534 CE). The entrance walls of one grotto in particular—dubbed the "Medical Prescription Cave"—are carved to present 140 remedies for various ailments.

By the fifth and fourth centuries BCE, medical practice became more formalized, as substantiated by the **Bower Manuscript**. Discovered during an excavation in a remote

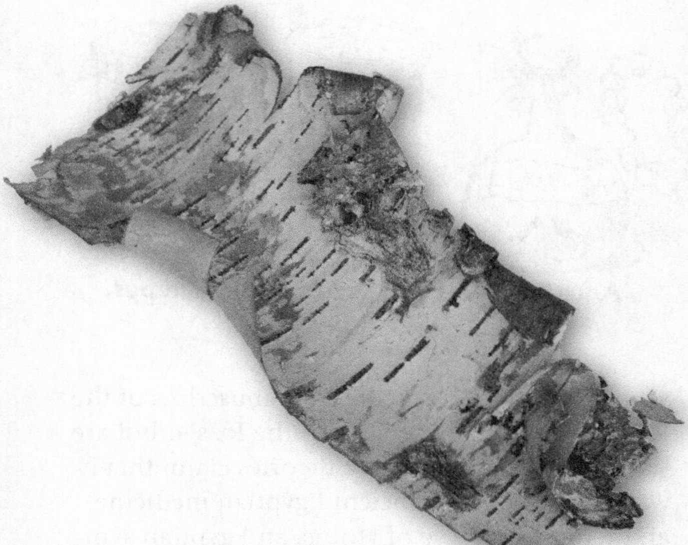

region of China, the manuscript was written on birch bark and lists 1,120 illnesses plus 760 herbal medicines for treating them. The Bower Manuscript's author, the East Indian shaman Sushruta, divided the body into three parts—the spirit, the phlegm, and the bile—laying the foundation for **ayurvedic medicine**, a holistic approach to healing that is still practiced today.

## Greek and Roman Influences on Medicine

During this same period in Greece, medical practice began to shift from a spiritual-based approach to a more scientific, logic-based approach. The Greek physician Hippocrates, now known as the "Father of Modern Medicine," played a significant role in this movement. Hippocrates published more than 70 medical texts, categorizing diseases, symptoms, physical findings, and treatments. His works provided the Greek lexicon for a majority of today's medical terminology. Hippocrates also developed the diagnostic concept of the four **humors** (blood, phlegm, yellow bile, and black bile) within the body, claiming that all four must be in the right balance to maintain optimal health. His hypothesis formed the beginnings of **traditional Western medicine**.

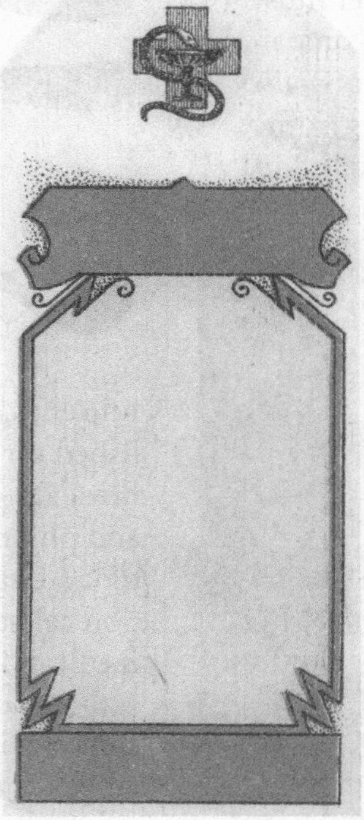

With the rise of the Roman Empire, medical practices grew more formalized and specialized. The many Greek physicians who were Roman prisoners of war during this time agreed to set up medical practices within the Roman Empire in exchange for their freedom. Their practices, based on the knowledge of anatomy and physiology and of diseases and associated herbal remedies that they had learned in their homeland, brought Greek medical insights into the Empire. The Roman healthcare practitioners, known as *medici*, had many roles—including those of physician, surgeon, pharmacist, and herbalist—and recognized the particular importance of public health and hygiene practices. Many *medici* became adept at surgical procedures by tending to the battle wounds of the Roman soldiers.

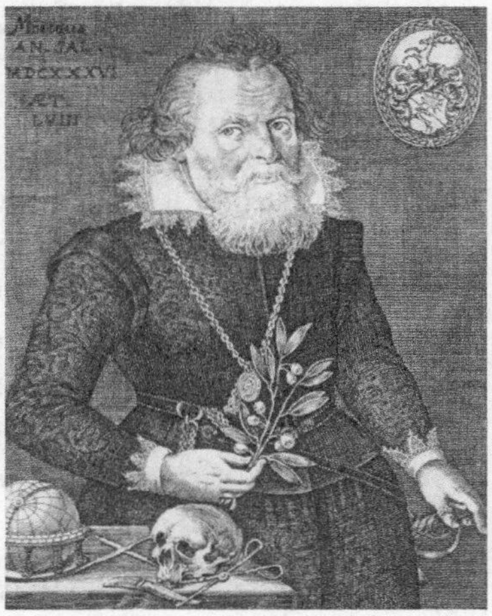

The influence of these early Greek and Roman medical practitioners is evident in today's medical vocabulary. Specialized medical terms and abbreviations stem from the Greek and Latin languages spoken by ancient practitioners. In fact, as Latin spread across Europe in the Middle Ages, communication among healthcare practitioners became standardized, and simple written labels often marked ordinary glass or ceramic containers of herbal medicines. Prior to this period, the physician was responsible for all three treatment phases: diagnosing a patient's malady, preparing a remedy, and also administering that remedy. However, with the emergence of medieval **apothecaries**—merchants who compounded and dispensed spices, herbs, and other cures

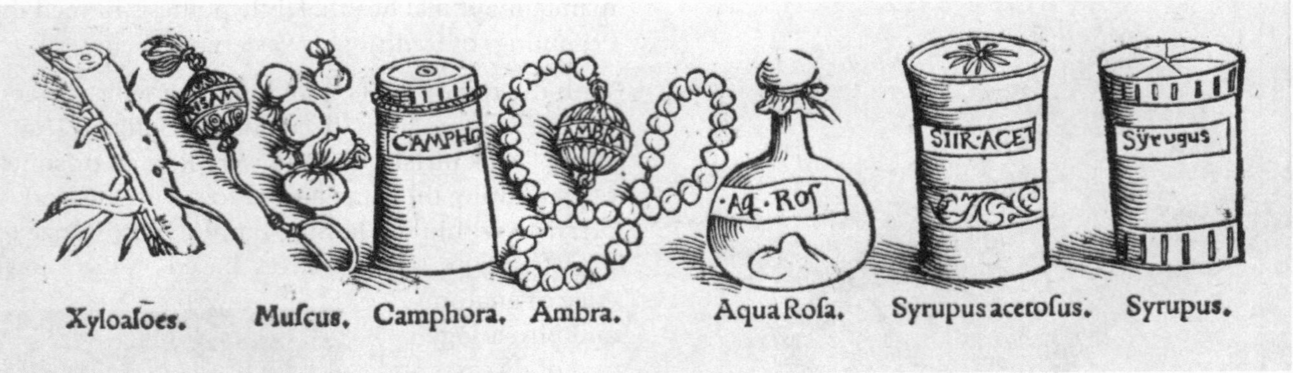


from their storefronts—the physician was able to focus more on patient care, working collaboratively with an apothecary to prepare and label necessary medications. Once Latin became commonly spoken across the European continent, physicians used it to communicate with the apothecary *and* the patient. Consequently, the early prototype of today's handwritten prescription can be traced to its Latin roots.

## The Origins and Evolution of "Prescription," the Rx Symbol, and the Signa

The word "prescription" comes from the Latin word *praescriptus*, with the prefix *pre* meaning "before" and the root word *script* meaning "written." Thus, the word *prescription* means "to write before," alluding to the fact that an order must be written down before a medication is prepared. The prescription symbol—the **Rx symbol**—also has its roots in Latin. The symbol comes from the Latin word *recipere*, meaning "to take," and was first seen in the medieval manuscripts of the Roman Empire. The origins of the Rx symbol are not as clear-cut. Some folk theories claim that it was borrowed from ancient Egyptian medicine and refers to the Eye of Horus, an Egyptian symbol for protection and good health. Still others believe that the Rx symbol is derived from the ancient symbol for the Roman god Jupiter, upon whom they called for protection from illness and disease. The written symbols for both the Eye of Horus and the god Jupiter bear a striking resemblance to the Rx symbol. Today, the Rx symbol continues to be printed on written prescriptions, implying that the patient must "take thus."

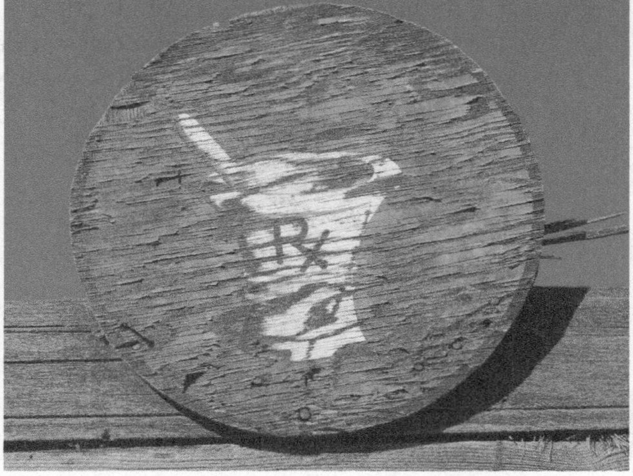

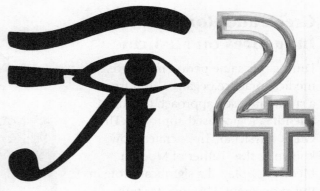

Ancient Greek and Latin cultures not only established the foundations for traditional Western medicine and influenced the medical terminology and pharmacy abbreviations central to healthcare today, but also impacted the part of a prescription called the **signa**, often referred to as the *sig* in medical documents. *Signa* comes from the Latin verb *signare*, meaning "to mark, write, or indicate." The signa is the section of the prescription language that directs the patient in how to use the medicine. Working within this language, physicians

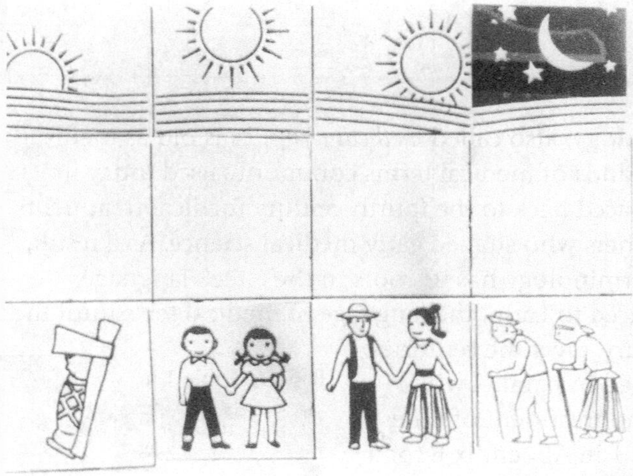

rely on Latin abbreviations to indicate the dosage and route of medication administration, a practice stemming from medieval times.

Over the centuries, the written prescription served as a primary communication vehicle for the triad of physician, apothecary, and patient. The physician would write the order, and the patient would carry it to the apothecary or pharmacy, which compounded and dispensed it. The pharmacy would then often direct the patient orally or provide symbol-based instructions for taking the medication, or if the patient could read, provide a written directive or label. Today, this prescription-to-labeled-product process has been slightly altered due to specialization within the pharmaceutical industry and increasing reliance on computer technology.

Pharmacy technicians now handle different types of patient prescriptions, depending on their work setting. Sterile compounding personnel will frequently encounter a type of prescription known as a **medication order**. A medication order specifies patient medications within the institutional or hospital setting. Personnel enter the prescription into a computer system using specialized pharmacy software designed to increase medication safety. The computer then transfers the prescription information onto a printed label. Labels for compounded sterile preparations (CSPs) may contain signa information about the preparation, its storage requirements, and its administration guidelines.

To perform the vital duties of an intravenous (IV) technician, you must become familiar with pharmacy prescriptions, medication orders, and labels—as well as the specialized terminology and abbreviations that make up these healthcare communications.

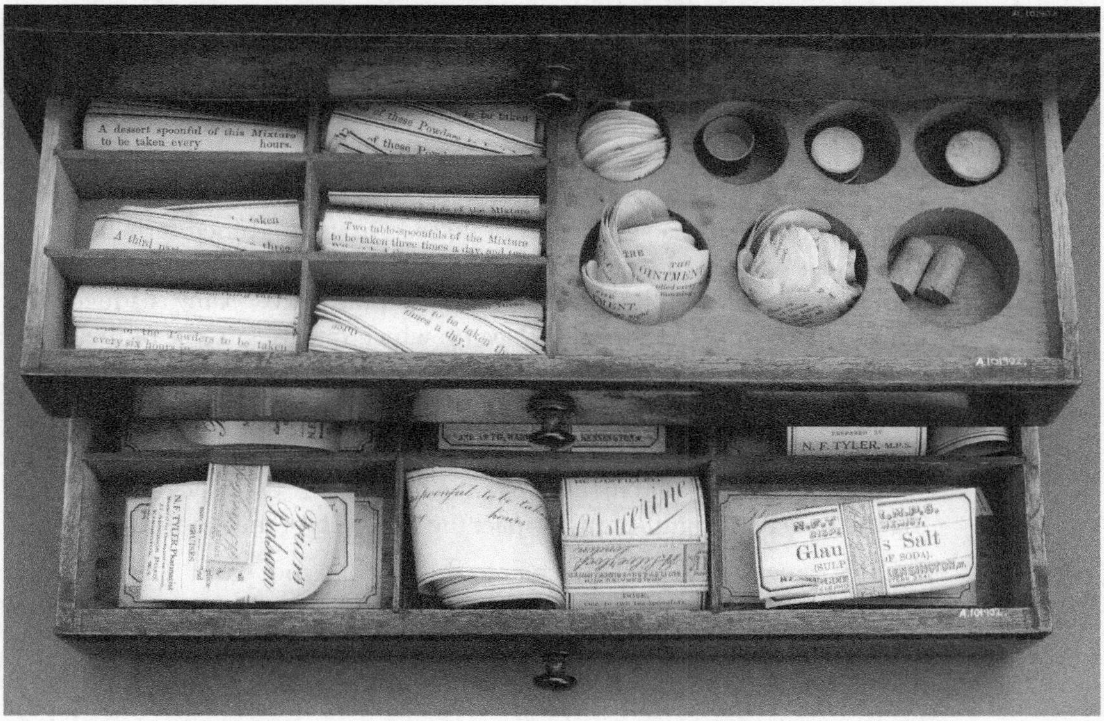

# Part 1: Concepts

The origin of **medical terminology**, also called *medical terms*, is as old as medicine itself. Many of the thousands of medical terms commonly used today in medicine and pharmacy can be traced back to the fourth-century medical treatments developed by Hippocrates and others who shaped early medical science. As a result, approximately 75% of medical terminology has its roots in the Greek language. Much of the remainder can be traced to Latin, the language of medical texts until the beginning of the eighteenth century. Over the centuries, medical terminology has developed in parallel with advancements in the diagnosis and treatment of illness, injury, and disease. Refer to Table 1 in Appendix B for a listing of common medical terms.

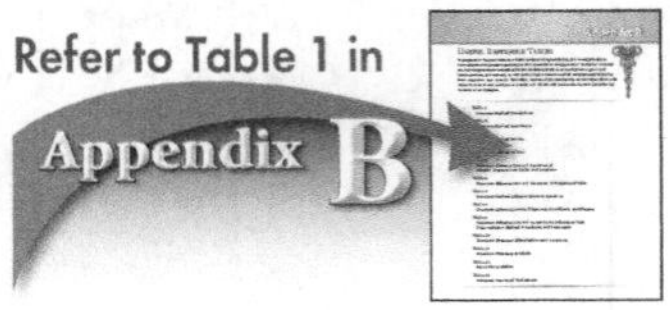
Refer to Table 1 in
Appendix B

*In preparation for your work as a sterile compounding technician, it is essential that you memorize the information provided in the tables of Appendix B. Table contents are not comprehensive but, rather, list the most frequently used medical terms (plus root words, prefixes, and suffixes), as well as the most common medical and pharmacy abbreviations, acronyms, and symbols. One effective method for learning this crucial information is to create flash cards and use them as a study tool. Check with your instructor and classmates to discover other strategies.*

## Medical Root Words, Prefixes, and Suffixes

Most medical terminology is based on a combination of medical **morphemes**, or root words, prefixes, and suffixes. A word's meaning is derived from the **root word** (sometimes called the word root). All medical terms have at least one root word, and these roots typically refer to regions or organs of the body or to pathological processes or conditions. To make pronunciation of the root word easier and to assist with the root word's connection to the suffix, a **combining vowel** is sometimes added to the end of the root word. The vowel most commonly added for this purpose is *o*; however, *i* or *e* may also be used. When a root word contains this combining vowel, the word is said to be in its **combined form**. For example, the root word *gastr*, meaning "stomach," is most often seen in its combined form as *gastr/o* or *gastro*. This combined form of the root word facilitates the English-language spelling and pronunciation of the medical term when the suffix *–pathy* is added. The medical term in its combined form is *gastropathy*, which means "disease of the stomach."

A **prefix** is a word element attached to the beginning of a root word. In medical terminology, a prefix often indicates time, location, direction, or number. Some common prefixes include *pre–* meaning "before," *post–* meaning "after," *hypo–* meaning "under" or "below," and *hyper–* meaning "above" or "excessive." Notice how changing the prefix can significantly impact the meaning of the medical term.

A **suffix** is a word element attached to the end of a root word. The addition of a suffix further defines the meaning of a root word. Some common suffixes include *–ectomy* meaning "surgical removal," *–tomy* meaning "surgical incision," and *–pathy* meaning "disease."

In order to read, understand, and carry out medication orders and medication label instructions, pharmacy personnel must have a thorough understanding of medical terminology. Memorizing the most common root words, prefixes, and suffixes, as well as frequently utilized medical terminology, will help prepare you for clear communication at work and aid your performance in the sterile compounding environment. Refer to Tables 2–4 in Appendix B for a listing of common medical root words, prefixes, and suffixes.

Refer to Tables 2–4 in Appendix B

## Medical Abbreviations, Acronyms, and Symbols

Approximately 35,000 abbreviations, acronyms, and symbols are used in medicine and pharmacy. Collectively, these abbreviations, acronyms, and symbols are referred to as **medical abbreviations**, or simply **abbreviations**. Most abbreviations are developed to shorten the length of words and word combinations related to health, medicine, laboratory procedures or tests, and pharmacy. Healthcare professionals communicate with each other quickly, easily, and effectively with these abbreviated forms. For example, it is faster and more convenient for a physician to write the abbreviation *TPN* on a medication order than to record the words *total parenteral nutrition*. To provide safe and effective healthcare, all sterile compounding personnel must have a thorough understanding of medical and pharmacy abbreviations, acronyms, and symbols. Although learning these common abbreviations can be a challenging task for pharmacy technicians, the importance of knowing this specialized "language" cannot be overestimated.

> **BE AWARE**
>
> Exercise caution when using and interpreting abbreviations, acronyms, and symbols. Several abbreviated forms are ambiguous or nonstandard. The convenience of using abbreviations must never outweigh the potential risk for medication error that may result from their misinterpretation.

***Common Medical Abbreviations*** Abbreviations refer to many components of healthcare. For example, abbreviations may indicate specific patient care facilities, units, or departments (e.g., *ICU* for intensive care unit) or the titles of individual team members (e.g., *RN* for registered nurse). Abbreviations also refer to specific medical diagnoses and conditions, procedures, treatments, patient directives/activities, equipment/supplies, and tests. Some examples of abbreviations include *CVA* for cerebrovascular accident, *CBC* for complete blood count, and *NC* for nasal cannula. In fact, most of the hundreds of laboratory and diagnostic procedures and tests performed in a medical setting have corresponding abbreviations that are more frequently used than the longer word(s) to which they refer. For instance, people with no training or knowledge specific to the medical field may be familiar with the term *CAT scan*, but few of those same people know that *CAT* is an abbreviation for *computer-aided tomography*.

Becoming familiar with these common abbreviations is an important aspect of your role as an IV technician. To begin memorizing these medical abbreviations and acronyms, as well as their corresponding meanings, refer to Tables 5–9 in Appendix B.

Refer to Tables 5–9 in Appendix B

***Common Pharmacy Abbreviations*** Abbreviations are also prevalent in pharmacy practice. They are typically seen on medication orders or other written communications between providers and pharmacies. Many of these abbreviations are derived from their Latin roots. For example, *q.i.d.* comes from the Latin words *quater in die*, meaning "four times a day"; *PO* is from the Latin words *per os*, meaning "by mouth."

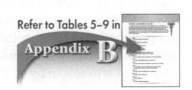

For an IV technician, pharmacy abbreviations provide important information, such as the name of a certain medication or the name of a specific IV base solution that is necessary for preparing a sterile compound. For example, physicians often write orders for CSPs using the abbreviations *NTG* (for nitroglycerin) and *PCN* (for penicillin). They may also include abbreviations when ordering IV base solutions, such as this physician's medication order: $D_5W$ *w/KCl 20 mEq/L @ TKO*. To understand this order, you would need to know what the abbreviations mean before beginning the compounding process. In this case, the physician wants you to compound a 1000 mL bag of dextrose 5% in water with 20 milliequivalents of potassium chloride, which would then be administered at an IV rate that provides just enough fluid to keep the patient's vein from collapsing.

A medication order might also include abbreviations to communicate specific compounding directives. For example, a physician may order *PF gentamicin* for a neonate. As an IV technician, you would need to know that *PF* means "preservative-free" before preparing the medication for patient administration. Lack of familiarity with this abbreviation could lead to patient endangerment.

Pharmacy abbreviations are also common for indicating the **route of administration** and the **dosing intervals** for prescribed medications. For example, a medication order that contains the abbreviations *IM* and *b.i.d.* asks that a medication be administered intramuscularly, twice a day. Knowing these important abbreviations ensures the correct administration directives for medications. To begin memorizing these common pharmacy abbreviations and acronyms, as well as their corresponding meanings, refer to Table 10 in Appendix B.

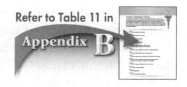


***Common Pharmacy Symbols*** In addition to knowing pharmacy abbreviations, you need to recognize and understand a number of symbols specific to pharmacy practice. Symbols such as ↑ and ↓ are frequently placed on medication orders to indicate "increase" and "decrease," respectively. For example, a physician may order a change in an IV flow rate to increase the dose of a medication, such as ↑ *heparin to 1000 units per hour*. Another common symbol is the Greek delta symbol (Δ), which is used to indicate a desired change. For example, the medication order *famotidine 20 mg Δ from IV to PO* communicates that the physician wants to change the route of administration from intravenous (IV) to oral (PO). Because symbols are drawn by hand, and handwriting may be poor or at least vary significantly among personnel, the symbols could easily be misinterpreted. Therefore, take extra care when using or interpreting pharmacy symbols. Typewritten or computer-generated symbols are preferred over handwritten symbols, whenever possible. To help you recognize and interpret common pharmacy symbols, refer to Table 11 in Appendix B.

***The Official "Do Not Use" List of Abbreviations*** In 2004, the Joint Commission was driven to create **The Official "Do Not Use" List of Abbreviations** in response to a number of **sentinel events** that had been noted across the United States. Due to the overwhelming evidence that certain frequently used abbreviations led to an increased incidence of medication errors, the Joint Commission integrated its "Do Not Use" List into the **Performance Standards for Healthcare Accreditation**.

The **nonstandard** and potentially dangerous abbreviations on the Joint Commission's list should not be used in any healthcare application. Healthcare personnel need to recognize these abbreviations, so that in the event a medication order arrives containing one of these abbreviations, personnel may pursue additional clarification to ensure that the patient receives the correct medication or treatment.

> **POINTER**
> To view the most up-to-date "Do Not Use" List, find the website for the Joint Commission and then search for this specific listing from the home page. Be aware that new items are frequently added to this list.

## Signa Interpretation

All sterile compounding personnel must possess an extensive knowledge of the components of medication orders. The signa component is a specialized language that physicians or other prescribers place on a medication order. The specialized signa language provides the pharmacy with specific directions for administering the medication order. These directions may include dosage information, the route of administration, the amount to be dispensed, the time schedule or dosing interval, and any special instructions. Signa language combines an assortment of abbreviations, acronyms, and symbols, all of which inform and direct the pharmacy, nursing staff, and other members of the healthcare team to take specific actions in the treatment of the patient. Table 4.1 presents examples and interpretations of medication orders written in signa language.

**Table 4.1 Sample Signa and Interpretations**

| Signa | Interpretation of Signa |
|---|---|
| i packet in 2 oz. OJ PO q.i.d. ut dict | Mix one packet in two ounces of orange juice and give by mouth four times daily as directed. |
| aaa b.i.d. prn itching | Apply to affected area twice daily as needed for itching. |
| SSI Sub-Q p.c. and h.s. | Sliding scale insulin, inject subcutaneously after meals and at bedtime. |
| iii gtts au q8h | Instill three drops into both ears every eight hours. |

You encounter signas on medication orders, prescriptions, and sterile compound labels, as well as in pharmacy computer and labeling programs. Transcribing or interpreting a signa requires you to seek the portions of the directive that address the following questions:

- What is the route of administration of the medication?
- How much of the medication is the patient supposed to take and how often?
- What special instructions need to be followed when taking the medication?

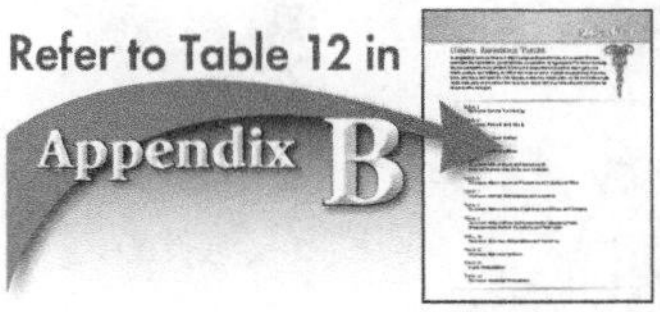
Refer to Table 12 in
Appendix B

For guidance on interpreting signas, refer to Table 12 in Appendix B.

> **POINTER**
> Because healthcare practitioners use medication orders (not prescriptions) to order CSPs, only medication orders are covered in this textbook. To reference basic community pharmacy prescription information, you may wish to consult your State Board of Pharmacy's website or refer to Paradigm Publishing's *Pharmacy Practice for Technicians* textbook, by Don Ballington and Robert Anderson.

## Medication Orders

Medication orders are similar to prescriptions but are exclusive to the institutional or hospital setting. Medication orders may also be referred to as *med orders, medical orders, physician orders, medication administration records,* or *MARs*. Medication orders entered directly into a computer by the physician are often called **eMARs** (electronic medication administration records). Physicians use medication orders to communicate patient care directives to all members of the healthcare team. In addition to delivering instructions to the pharmacy, medication orders may also provide directions for the laboratory, radiology, dietary, physical therapy, and other departments within the hospital.

Physicians or other prescribers write up medication orders using signa as well as a combination of medical terminology, abbreviations, acronyms, and symbols. Upon receipt of the medication order, the pharmacy determines what medications and dosages have been ordered and then interprets the signa directions. The medication order is then transcribed, or interpreted, and then entered into the pharmacy's computer system through a process called **order entry**. The pharmacist usually performs order entry, but specially trained pharmacy technicians may also complete this task. A label is then prepared for each of the medications. As a sterile compounding technician, you will likely receive medication orders for parenteral products regularly. Refer to Table 13 in Appendix B for a list of such medications.

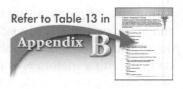


Just like other types of prescriptions, medication orders are legal documents that must be filed, usually based on the date the order was written, and kept on hand for up to two years. Consult the State Board of Pharmacy as well as your pharmacy's Policy & Procedure (P&P) manual for specific requirements for record storage.

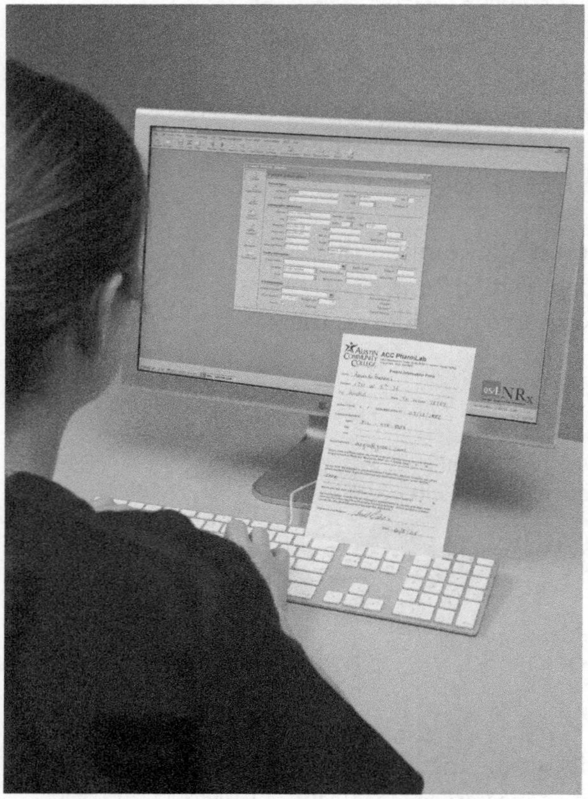
Pharmacy technician entering a medication order into the pharmacy computer system.

## CSP Labeling

Upon completion of sterile compounding and checking procedures, personnel must appropriately label the sterile compound in its final container. This container may be an IV bag, intravenous piggyback (IVPB), syringe, vial, cassette, or bottle, depending on what the physician ordered. Labels will most often be affixed by the IV technician but may also be affixed by the pharmacist. Federal laws require that pharmacy labels accurately identify the ingredients and the amount of each ingredient in the final sterile compound. The CSP label must also include the product's administration and storage requirements, expiration date, and preparer identification. Part 2 of this chapter describes CSP labeling requirements in greater detail and lists them in Table 4.2.

# Concepts Self-Check

## Check Your Understanding

*Write your answers on a separate sheet of paper, as modeled in these examples:* 1d; 2c; 3b; *etc. Check your answers using the Answer Key in Appendix A.*

**1.** What is the meaning of the Latin word *recipere,* from which the abbreviation Rx is believed to have originated?

a. to reciprocate
b. to make
c. to compound
d. to take

**2.** What is the medical term that means *disease of the stomach*?

a. gastrostomy
b. gastrology
c. gastropathy
d. gastroanastomosis

**3.** What is the meaning of the abbreviation *au*?

a. right ear
b. left ear
c. both ears
d. both eyes

**4.** What is the name of the type of prescription used in an institutional setting?

a. physician order
b. medication order
c. physician-entered computer order
d. all of the above

**5.** Which of the following lists of information includes items that are *all* required on a sterile compound label?

a. product administration, storage requirements, and expiration date
b. patient admit date, physician's name, and ingredient amounts
c. product administration, additives, and physician's name
d. additives, expiration date, and patient's release date

## Apply Your Knowledge

*On a separate sheet of paper, write your answer to the question posed in the paragraph below. Use complete sentences and take time to create a thorough and thoughtful response. Check your answer against the Answer Key in Appendix A.*

In Part 1 of this chapter, you learned that approximately 35,000 abbreviations, acronyms, and symbols are used to communicate in the healthcare setting. With that in mind, what are the advantages and disadvantages of relying on this shorthand type of communication?

# Examine the Resources and Supplies

## Types of Medication Orders

During hospital treatment, a physician examines a patient and then writes the first medication order on the patient's **medical chart**. The medical chart is commonly called the *medication administration record, the patient's chart* or, simply, *the chart*. The physician's initial order is called the **admission order** and is often written while the patient is in the emergency department or has just been admitted to a hospital room (see Figure 4.1). Typically, an admission order includes requests for lab tests, radiology exams, dietary requirements, and medication orders, as well as instructions for the nursing staff.

If applicable, the admission order includes a list of the medications, including dosages and dosing intervals, that the patient has been taking at home. These medications are commonly referred to as **home medications** or *home meds.* In many instances, the physician orders the pharmacy to *continue home meds* so that the patient will receive these same medications while he or she is hospitalized. To guarantee the integrity and safety of these medications, the patient is not generally allowed to bring them from home. Instead, the pharmacy dispenses new prescriptions for the medications for hospital administration.

A physician usually examines the patient on a daily basis, but this frequency varies based on patient need. Critically ill patients may be examined several times a day. Patients may also be seen by numerous physicians, according to their particular health issues. Every time a physician examines a patient, new orders, or changes to existing medication orders, are written. These orders may be referred to as **daily orders** (see Figure 4.2).

Other healthcare team members may also write orders or record information in the patient's chart. In most states, the authority to write prescriptions lies solely with the licensed physician. Some states may allow limited prescribing authority for nurse practitioners, physician assistants, and registered pharmacists. Refer to the State Board of Pharmacy and your pharmacy's P&P manual for guidance.

Some physicians whose specialties involve commonly prescribed medical treatments take advantage of preprinted order forms called **standing orders**, or **routine orders** (see Figure 4.3). For instance, an orthopedic surgeon who specializes in knee replacement surgery may order the same IV base solutions, IVPB antibiotics, and nursing or laboratory instructions for all patients having that procedure. Because each patient receives a similar medical regimen, the physician relies on a preprinted form that lists all medications, dosages, dosing intervals, nursing orders, and other treatments commonly prescribed for that procedure. The physician may then either simply sign the bottom of the form or slightly modify the standing orders by crossing out or adding items before signing the form. Standing order forms provide a convenient method for prescribing treatment regimens for patients with similar medical conditions, procedures, or surgeries. In addition, these typewritten forms help to ensure clear communication between the prescriber and other healthcare team members, avoiding treatment errors that may result from misinterpreting handwriting.

**FIGURE 4.1**

## Admission Order

A physician typically creates an admission order after examining a newly admitted patient.

PHARMACY

B 427687

IN DOSAGE FORM AND THERAPEUTIC ACTIVITY MAY BE ADMINISTERED UNLESS CHECKED

Patient Information Below

**START EACH NEW SERIES OF ORDERS BELOW**

Check one: (FOR NEW PATIENTS OR CHANGE IN STATUS)

❑ OBSERVATION: short stay expected

☑ Admit – in patient; longer stay expected Height: 5'3" Weight: 251

Diagnosis: (L) Leg DVT, Fe deficiency anemia

Activity: Bed rest c̄ bedside commode × 24° then ad lib

Diet: cardiac

Allergies: NKDA Reactions:

(1) Admit to Medicine – Dr. Galangal

(2) Condition – stable

(3) Vitals per routine

(4) Labs – PT/INR q AM – call c̄ results of PT/INR tonight

– guaiac stools × 3

– Fe/Ferritin next lab draw

(5) IV – HL flush q shift

NURSE'S SIGNATURE DATE TIME

ID#: S1008994566
Name: Hayashi, Amy
DOB: 08/24/1950
Room: 420
Dr.: Rashmi Galangal

PHARMACY

B 427687

**START EACH NEW SERIES OF ORDERS BELOW**

(6) Meds – Lovenox 1 mg/kg SQ q 12

– Coumadin 10 mg PO tonight × 1̄ dose

– Fe-Tinic 150 mg PO b.i.d.

– Vicodin 1–2 PO q6h prn

– Colace 100 mg PO b.i.d. – hold per loose stool

– LOC prn

– Benadryl 50 mg PO qHS prn insomnia

(7) Call per acute changes

(8) Nutrition consult re: vitamin K diet

Dr. Galangal

NURSE'S SIGNATURE DATE 11/16/2012 TIME

ID#: S1008994566
Name: Hayashi, Amy
DOB: 08/24/1950
Room: 420
Dr.: Rashmi Galangal

7ØØ781 (2-97)
H-NSO781B **MERCY HOSPITAL**

**PHYSICIAN'S INITIAL ORDERS SHEET**

FIGURE 4.2

**Daily Order**

A physician creates a daily order following each patient examination, or to change orders or make new orders.

**ID#:** J1008912345
**Name:** Echeverria, Begonia
**DOB:** 12/01/1939
**Room:** 804
**Dr.:** Yuka Sun, MD

**MEMORIAL HOSPITAL**
**PHYSICIAN'S MEDICATION ORDER**

**BEAR DOWN ON HARD SURFACE WITH BALLPOINT PEN**

GENERIC EQUIVALENT IS AUTHORIZED UNLESS CHECKED IN THIS COLUMN

ALLERGY OR SENSITIVITY TO Ø
NONE KNOWN ☐ SIGNED:

DIAGNOSIS: S/P Hernia Repair

COMPLETED OR DISCONTINUED

| DATE | TIME | ORDERS | PHYSICIAN'S SIG. | NAME | DATE | TIME |
|---|---|---|---|---|---|---|
| 6/24 | 4 PM | Routine Orders | | | | |
| | | Height 5'7" Weight 186 lbs | | | | |
| | | Condition – stable | | | | |
| | | VS: q4° × 2, then q shift | | | | |
| | | Diet: Regular | | | | |
| | | | | | | |
| | | D5 ½ NS w/20 mEq KCl/Liter | | | | |
| | | run at 100 mL/hr, DC when taking PO well | | | | |
| | | Meds: | | | | |
| | | meperidine 50 mg IM q3h prn pain | | | | |
| | | Vistaril 25 mg IM q3h prn pain | | | | |
| | | Halcion 0.25 mg PO q hs prn | | | | |
| | | LOC prn | | | | |
| | | cefazolin 1 gram IVPB q6h | | | | |
| | | Lance wound on foot in am | | | | |
| | | Call H.O. for: T > 101.5 | | | | |
| | | BP > 180/100, or < 80/60 | | | | |
| | | | Yuka Sun, MD | | | |
| | | | 06/24/2013 | | | |

PHARMACY COPY

FIGURE 4.3

**Standing Order**

A physician saves time and aids hospital efficiency and communication when using a preprinted Standing Order form.

**ID#:** M03822015669
**Name:** Cruz, Nestor
**DOB:** 05/11/1955
**Room:** 400
**Dr.:** Gary R. Smith, MD – Standing Orders

DR. GARY R. SMITH

STANDING ORDERS FOR POST-OP DISCECTOMY

1. VS q2h × 4, then q4h overnight.
2. Turn q2h.
3. May stand to void.
4. Bathroom privileges with assistance, if tolerated.
5. Ambulate with assistance ~~in A.M.~~ *today* if tolerated.
6. Heat lamp to ~~back~~ *neck* 20 minutes q.i.d.
7. Reinforce dressing PRN.
8. Diet as tolerated after nausea subsides.
9. Percocet one or two q3h PRN pain.
10. M.S. 10 mg or 15 mg IM q3h PRN more severe pain.
11. Restoril 15 mg hs PRN sleep. MR × 1.
12. Tylenol gr X PO q4h PRN temperature elevation above 101 degrees.
13. Tigan 100 mg IM q4h PRN nausea.
14. Peri-Colace 1 capsule PO PRN or M.O.M. 30 cc PO PRN.
15. Laxative of choice.
16. Decadron 4 mg IV or PO q6h × 24 hrs. Then start Medrol dosepak and label for home use.
17. ~~Tagamet 300 mg IV or PO b.i.d.~~ *Pepcid 20 mg IV × 1*
18. Intermittent cath. q 4–6h PRN.
19. R/L 90 cc q.h. DC after nausea subsides. × 1
20. *Resume home dosage of prozac post nausea.*
21.
22.
23.

*DOB: 05/11/55*
*5'6"*
*217#*
*NKDA*
*Rm 400*

**DATE:** *August 21st, 2013*

**SIGNATURE:** *Gary R. Smith, MD*

Dr. Gary R. Smith, MD
711 W. 30th Street, Suite 200
Kalamazoo, MI 49001
Phone 269-555-0423
Fax 269-555-0566

## Medication Order Contents and Processing

The medical chart contains both patient identification information and copies of all treatment orders prescribed during the patient's stay. Standard patient identification information—name, identification number, hospital room number, date of birth, gender, height, weight, and allergy information—is either handwritten on the order, provided on a computer-generated patient ID label affixed to the order, or preprinted at the top of each medication order by using an **addressograph**.

**POINTER**
You are required to strictly follow all federal and state regulations regarding access to PHI.

Much of the patient's identification and treatment information is strictly private. Access to **protected health information (PHI)**, such as that found on a medication order or in a patient chart, is restricted and the information may be viewed only by those departments that must see the data in order to correctly treat the patient. Examples of hospital departments permitted access to PHI include the pharmacy, laboratory, and nursing departments. However, even pharmacy employees and other authorized personnel must only access PHI in the course of performing their required job duties. Healthcare practitioners who access PHI in order to obtain patient information for anything other than their professional responsibilities are considered to be in breach of laws that restrict access to PHI. Ancillary departments, such as laundry, central supply, and maintenance, do not need to see this type of patient information to perform their essential functions and are therefore prohibited from accessing PHI.

The treatment orders kept in the medical chart are carbon copies of all medication, diagnostic, laboratory, dietary, and other orders prescribed by the physician and other members of the healthcare team while the patient is hospitalized. The top copy of the carbon, called the **original copy**, remains in the chart, while the other carbon copies are hand-delivered, faxed, scanned electronically, or sent via **pneumatic tube system** to the pharmacy or other relevant hospital departments. On the medication administration record within the patient's medical chart, nurses record all pharmacy items and medications administered to the patient. The chart may be kept at the **nursing station** or maintained on a computer record.

During the patient's hospitalization, the physician and other healthcare team members continue to assess the patient, review any prior nursing notes and test results, and record new orders in the patient's medical chart. These orders are most often written by hand, using a combination of medical terminology and signa instructions, but they may also be entered directly into a hospital computer. Facilities that depend on an eMAR system provide computer terminals at the nursing station or near the patient's room. Physicians use these terminals for direct order entry, commonly referred to as **computerized physician order entry (CPOE)**.

Once the pharmacy receives the medication order, a pharmacist or technician based in either the **central pharmacy** or a **satellite pharmacy** enters the order into the pharmacy's computer system. Most institutional and sterile compounding pharmacies install specialized pharmacy software that assists with the identification of patient medication allergies and **cross-sensitivities**, **drug–drug** or **drug–food interactions**, **appropriate medication dosage**, **duplicate therapy**, **contraindications**, and other information pertinent to the medications the physician ordered. If an issue or potential problem arises with the ordered medication, a flashing caution or warning screen (sometimes called a **warning flag**) appears on the computer monitor.

The pharmacist must resolve all relevant computer-generated warnings by contacting the physician to request either an adjustment to the medication form or dose, or a complete change of medication. But if the flagged issue is insignificant in nature, the pharmacist may simply override the warning flag in the computer. *Only the pharmacist* is allowed to resolve potential medication issues, an area of pharmacy practice requiring professional judgment.

Once all of the patient's medication orders have been entered into the system, personnel generate labels for each medication on the printer attached to the pharmacy computer. If the medication requires sterile compounding, the computer generates a separate label for each dose of medication. The IV technician then compares the sterile compound label to the medication order prior to performing calculations, gathering supplies, and, ultimately, compounding the medication. Once compounding procedures are complete, the pharmacist compares the sterile compounding label and the medication order to the final CSP to verify the accuracy of the preparation. The IV technician then affixes the computer-generated CSP label to the product.

## Sterile Compound Label Components

The CSP label provides general information, such as the patient's name and **identification (ID) number** as well as the room or department number of the facility where the patient is admitted. In addition, the CSP label must also contain very specific information about the product, its administration and storage requirements, expiration date, and preparer (see Table 4.2).

Product information on the CSP label specifies the name, **concentration**, and amount of each base solution used to prepare the compound. For instance, the base solution $D_5W$ 1L indicates the type of solution (dextrose) as well as the concentration of the solution (5% or 5 grams of dextrose per 100 mL of fluid) and the amount of the solution (1L or 1000 mL). The label must also clearly identify each **additive**, or medication or ingredient that has been added to the base solution during the sterile compounding process, as well as the amount. A CSP may have one or more

**POINTER**

Most facilities require the CSP label to have a unique, computer-generated number called the prescription or Rx number, which links the CSP label with the medication order in the patient's records. Review your facility's P&P manual to determine prescription numbering requirements.

**Table 4.2 CSP Labeling Requirements**

- The name and ID number of the patient for whom the medication is prescribed
- The name, concentration, and amount of each solution contained in the compound (e.g., *$D_5W$ 500 mL*)
- The name and amount (or concentration) of each medication or additive in the compound (e.g., *potassium chloride 2 mEq*)
- The administration time or infusion rate of the compound (e.g., *100 mL/hr or infuse over 20 min*)
- The time, schedule, or dosing interval for medication administration (e.g., *q6h* or *t.i.d.*)
- The route of administration (e.g., *for intramuscular administration; for intrathecal administration*)
- The beyond-use date (date and time of expiration of the compound)
- Storage requirements (e.g., *keep refrigerated* or *protect from light*)
- Auxiliary labels or special instructions (e.g., *shake well before administering; warm to room temperature before administering; or for wound irrigation only*): auxiliary information may be included in the preprinted CSP label or may be added to the CSP label as a small sticker.
- Device-specific instructions (e.g., *MINI-BAG Plus must be activated and mixed prior to administering*)
- The preparer's and pharmacist's identification (may be initials or signature)

*Note: To determine additional state-based labeling requirements, consult your State Board of Pharmacy. For your institution's specific labeling requirements, consult your pharmacy's P&P manual.*

additives. For example, a TPN solution may have as many as 15 additives. (For more information about additives in TPN solutions, see Chapter 13 of this textbook.) Some of the most common additives are electrolytes such as potassium chloride, or antibiotics such as cefuroxime.

**POINTER**
Many pharmacy computer systems have predetermined administration times for each drug and dose and are automatically printed onto the CSP label when the label is generated.

The CSP label should also indicate the administration time or infusion rate for the medication. In general, only IV push and IVPB medications require an **administration time**, which is the length of time over which the drug is to be given (see Figure 4.4). For instance, furosemide 20 mg IV push is administered by a nurse who slowly injects the solution into the patient's IV line over a two-minute period, whereas a gentamicin 100 mg IVPB may be administered using an IV pump, over a period of 60 minutes. The administration time varies widely among different types of medications and may also vary depending on the route of administration or dosage of the drug. The medication administration time may be indicated by the physician, or it may be determined by consulting the package insert provided by the medication's manufacturer. If the medication's administration is not ordered by the physician and the package insert is unavailable, the pharmacist may find this information by consulting one of the pharmacy reference manuals, such as the ***Handbook on Injectable Drugs***, or a computerized pharmacy reference source, such as **Micromedex**.

In contrast to an administration time, an **infusion rate** is specified for large-volume parenteral (LVP) products, such as IV bags and TPN solutions (see Figure 4.5). The physician usually orders an infusion rate in milliliters per hour, such as *100 mL/hour*. Occasionally, the physician will order the IV infusion rate based on the drug concentration in the CSP. For instance, the infusion rate of a heparin drip is often ordered in *units* per hour, such as *1000 units/hour*. Once the administration time or infusion rate of the CSP has been established, the pharmacy is then responsible for ensuring that this information is placed on the CSP label.

The CSP label must also provide the physician's directions for the medication's dosing interval, such as *t.i.d.*, *q6h*, or *qDay*, and route of administration. In some instances, the route of administration is printed within the body of the CSP label (see Figure 4.6), but in others, it is identified by an **auxiliary label** or sticker affixed to the CSP. Sterile compounding personnel generally choose the auxiliary label method because such labels are often brightly colored and call attention to uncommon or infrequently used routes of administration, such as when

**FIGURE 4.4 IVPB Label**

****IV Piggyback****

**Pt. Name:** Andreachi, Azar **Room:** ICU-9
**ID#:** S1143367722 **Rx#:** 12249648

Gentamicin 100 mg
$D_5W$ 100 mL
Rate: over 60 min

Keep refrigerated – warm to room temperature before administration.

Expiration Day/time: ____________ Tech ______ RPh ______

**FIGURE 4.5 Large-Volume Parenteral (LVP) Label**

****Large-Volume Parenteral****

**Pt. Name:** Li, Oscar **Room:** ICU-8
**ID#:** S1147872252 **Rx#:** 14839511

$D_5NS$ 1000 mL
Potassium Chloride 20 mEq
Rate: 100 mL/hour

Keep refrigerated – warm to room temperature before administration.

Expiration Day/time: ____________ Tech ______ RPh ______

a CSP is to be used for irrigation. Personnel also add auxiliary labels to clarify special instructions or highlight physician directions for the nursing staff. Table 4.3 presents some examples of the many auxiliary labels available.

**FIGURE 4.6 Syringe Label**

****Syringe****

**Pt. Name:** Decoteau, Kaya **Room:** ICU-7
**ID#:** S114971441 **Rx#:** 17725909

Ceftriaxone 250 mg/2.5 mL
for IM administration only

Expiration Day/time: ________ Tech ______ RPh ______

Another required component on the CSP label is the **expiration date** of the sterile compound, sometimes referred to as the **beyond-use date (BUD)**. The expiration date is the date *and* time after which the CSP may not be used and is determined from the day and time the sterile compound was prepared. Several factors determine the expiration date, including the **stability** of the drug in its compounded form. Note that some sterile compounds may be stable for as little as one hour, whereas other sterile compounds may be stable for up to 45 days. The expiration date on the CSP label must reflect this stability information.

**POINTER**
The BUD should automatically be printed on the CSP label when it is generated. If you encounter a situation that requires you to write the expiration date for a CSP, consult your pharmacy's P&P manual to determine the appropriate date.

Other factors affecting the expiration date are the number of ingredients in the compound, the risk level within which the compound was prepared, and the conditions under which the compound will be stored. Typically, sterile compounds stored in a refrigerator or freezer have a longer beyond-use date than those CSPs stored at room temperature. **Storage requirements**, such as *refrigerate, keep frozen — thaw immediately prior to administration,* or *do not refrigerate,* must also be included on the label. You may find information about a CSP's expiration date on the manufacturer's package insert for the drug, within various pharmacy reference materials, and in the USP Chapter <797> guidelines for beyond-use dating.

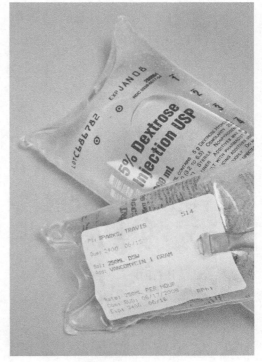

Beyond-use-dating (BUD) refers to the expiration date of a CSP, beyond which the product must not be used.

Every CSP label must also identify the pharmacy personnel who prepared the compound. Sterile compounders identify themselves by writing their name or initials in the provided blanks. The headings next to the identification blanks may vary widely among institutions, depending on the pharmacy's labeling system. In some facilities, the label may provide separate blanks: one blank for the preparer or IV technician (preceded by the terms *prep by* or *preparer* or *tech*) and one blank for the pharmacist verifying the accuracy of the CSP (preceded by the terms *checked by* or *RPh*). Some labels have a blank space where both the IV technician and the pharmacist must sign their names instead of using their initials. In other facilities, the name of the hospital or facility is also included on the pharmacy label. Despite these noted differences, all CSP labels require the same basic content. Consult the State Board of Pharmacy and your pharmacy's P&P manual for labeling requirements specific to your facility.

**Table 4.3 Auxiliary Labels Commonly Used in Sterile Compounding**

| Label | Description |
|---|---|
| ***Auxiliary Labels with Blanks for Required Information*** | |
| Drug Name ________ <br> ______ mg/ ______ ml <br> Date ______ Tech ______ <br><br> Drug Name Kefzol (Cefazolin) <br> 1000 mg/ 10 ml <br> Date 2/10/13 Tech LMC | Labels for powdered drug vials: one label is blank and one is completed by the sterile compounding technician, who attaches the label to the powdered drug vial upon dilution; in addition to recording the drug name, final drug concentration, and the date and time of dilution, the technician diluting the powered drug records her or his initials |
| ______ MGM = ______ ML <br> (dose) (liquid) <br><br> VIAL OPENED <br> EXPIRES ______ <br> DATE ______ INITIALS ______ | Some facilities use two auxiliary labels to provide information similar to that provided on the larger labels above |
| ***Preprinted Auxiliary Labels*** | |
| "STAT" <br> "NOW" | Labels indicating that this CSP should be delivered to the nursing unit and administered to the patient immediately |
| P.R.N. | Label indicating that this medication is to be used as needed |
| KEEP IN REFRIGERATOR <br> REMOVE 30 MINUTES PRIOR TO USE | Label indicating that this CSP should be kept in a refrigerator prior to use |
| CAUTION <br> High Concentration | Label indicating that this medication has a dangerously high concentration (most often used as a warning label on bulk potassium chloride bottles used in sterile compounding) |
| FOR IRRIGATION ONLY | Label indicating that this CSP is to be administered only for irrigation of a wound, dressing, tube, etc. |
| DO NOT REFRIGERATE | Label indicating that this CSP should not be stored in a refrigerator |
| KCL ADDED | Label alerting handlers that this CSP contains potassium chloride, a potentially dangerous drug |

***Note***: This table presents but a small sample of some of the most frequently used CSP auxiliary labels. Many other auxiliary labels are used in sterile compounding.

## Sterile Compound Label Verification and Application

With the completed CSP label in hand, IV technicians must compare it to the medication order to verify the label's accuracy and determine what compounding procedures must next be performed. Some pharmacy labeling programs provide mixing instructions directly on the CSP label. For instance, the label might contain mixing instructions that direct the IV technician to draw up 15 mL of a 2 mEq/ml concentration of potassium chloride, in order to provide a 30 mEq dose of the medication. However, in many instances, mixing instructions are not provided on the label. The IV technician is then responsible for determining the desired volume of each ingredient by comparing the dose ordered by the physician with the concentration of the drug they will use to prepare the CSP. It is vital to patient health and safety that the IV technician always double-check the label and related calculations to ensure the correct dose is administered to the patient. Chapter 5 of this textbook presents information on pharmacy calculations.

**POINTER**

In some facilities, the verification of the CSP label against the medication order is performed by the pharmacist. She or he then gives the CSP label to the IV technician in order to begin the sterile compounding process.

Verifying the accuracy of the medication order and the CSP label is one of the most important components of ensuring the Five Patient Rights, previously discussed in Chapter 1. During the verification procedure, you should ensure that the CSP label displays the right patient, right drug, right dose, right route, and route time.

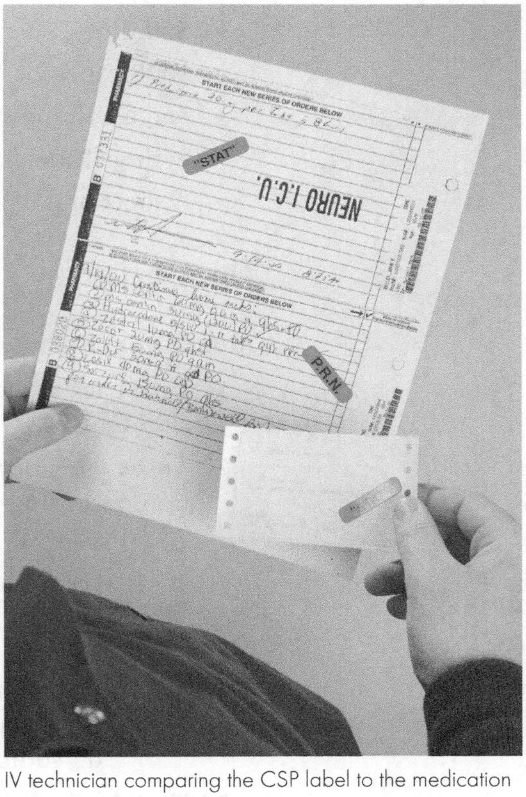


IV technician comparing the CSP label to the medication order to verify accuracy.

After verification of the medication order and the CSP label, the IV technician places the order and label in separate, clear plastic bags. The bags allow the sterile compounder to maintain the integrity of the printed information while providing a surface that can be easily sprayed with sterile 70% IPA or wiped down with an aseptic cleaning wipe before transport into the clean room. That way, aseptic technique is not compromised.

Once the compounding process is completed (as described in the specific compounding chapters of Unit 2) and the pharmacist has checked the final compound, the IV technician or pharmacist may affix the label to the CSP. The label should be applied to the CSP so that it does not obstruct the volume calibration marks or interfere with the administration of the preparation. Sterile product labels must be legible, **pharmaceutically elegant**, and complete, containing all of the requirements outlined in Table 4.2.

# Exploratory Lab

The purpose of this exploratory lab is to help you to identify and interpret the different components of medication orders and labels that you will typically encounter in a sterile compounding facility.

***Note:*** *Some of the steps ask you to read and respond to one or more multiple-choice questions (marked by numbers containing dashes, such as* ***1–1*** *and* ***1–2****). Record your answers to these multiple-choice questions by either circling the correct answers on the pages or turning in your answers as directed by your instructor.*

## Supplies

- Admission Order for Hayashi (Figure 4.1)
- Daily Order for Echeverria (Figure 4.2)
- Standing Order for Cruz (Figure 4.3)
- IVPB Label for Andreachi (Figure 4.4)
- Large-Volume Parenteral (LVP) Label for Li (Figure 4.5)
- Syringe Label for Decoteau (Figure 4.6)
- A sheet of notebook paper and a pen

## Procedure

### *Admission Order for Hayashi*

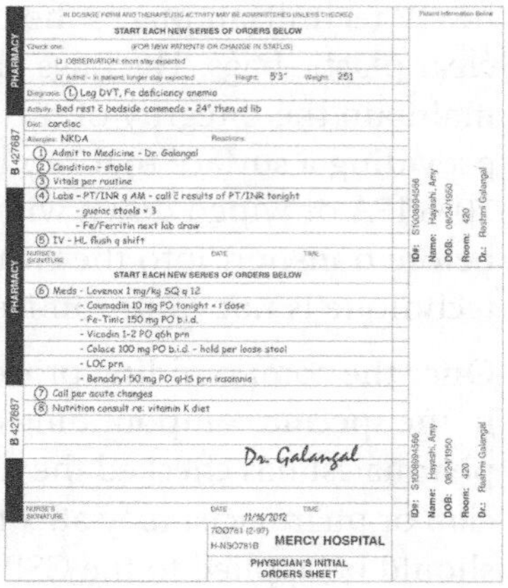
PHARMACY

IN DOSAGE FORM AND THERAPEUTIC ACTIVITY MAY BE ADMINISTERED UNLESS CHECKED

START EACH NEW SERIES OF ORDERS BELOW

Check one: (FOR NEW PATIENTS OR CHANGE IN STATUS)

☐ OBSERVATION: short stay expected

☐ Admit – in patient; longer stay expected Height: 5'3" Weight: 251

Diagnosis: (1) Leg DVT, Fe deficiency anemia

Activity: Bed rest c̄ bedside commode × 24° then ad lib

Diet: cardiac

Allergies: NKDA Reactions:

(1) Admit to Medicine - Dr. Galangal

(2) Condition - stable

(3) Vitals per routine

(4) Labs - PT/INR q AM - call c̄ results of PT/INR tonight

- guaiac stools × 3

- Fe/Ferritin next lab draw

(5) IV - HL flush q shift

NURSE'S SIGNATURE DATE TIME

START EACH NEW SERIES OF ORDERS BELOW

(6) Meds - Lovenox 1 mg/kg SQ q 12

- Coumadin 10 mg PO tonight × 1 dose

- Fe-Tinic 150 mg PO b.i.d.

- Vicodin 1-2 PO q6h prn

- Colace 100 mg PO b.i.d. - hold per loose stool

- LOC prn

- Benadryl 50 mg PO qHS prn insomnia

(7) Call per acute changes

(8) Nutrition consult re: vitamin K diet

Dr. Galangal

NURSE'S SIGNATURE DATE 11/16/2012 TIME

B 427687

ID#: S1008894566 Name: Hayashi, Amy DOB: 08/24/1950 Room: 420 Dr.: Rashmi Galangal

7DO781 (2-97) H-NSO781B MERCY HOSPITAL

PHYSICIAN'S INITIAL ORDERS SHEET

1. Turn back to Figure 4.1 and read the Admission Order for Hayashi in its entirety.
2. Answer the following multiple-choice question, recording your answer as directed by your instructor.

   **2–1.** According to the medication order, what are the patient's allergies?

   a. no known allergy
   b. sodium, potassium, and Demerol
   c. no known drug allergy
   d. sodium and potassium chloride

3. Find the circled number 5 on the order.
4. Answer the following multiple-choice question, recording your answer as directed by your instructor.

   **4–1.** List the three abbreviations and their corresponding meanings.

   a. IV (intravenous), HL (heparin lock), q (every)
   b. IV (four), HL (heparin lock), q (every)
   c. IV (intravenous), HL (half-liter), q (every)
   d. IV (intravenous), HL (heparin lock), q (quantity)

5. Find the heading "Meds" on the order. Scroll down to the sixth medication on the list.

6. Answer the following multiple-choice question, recording your answer as directed by your instructor.

**6–1.** What is meant by the order "LOC prn"?

a. treat for loss of consciousness as needed
b. laxative of choice in the evening
c. laxative of choice as needed
d. none of the above

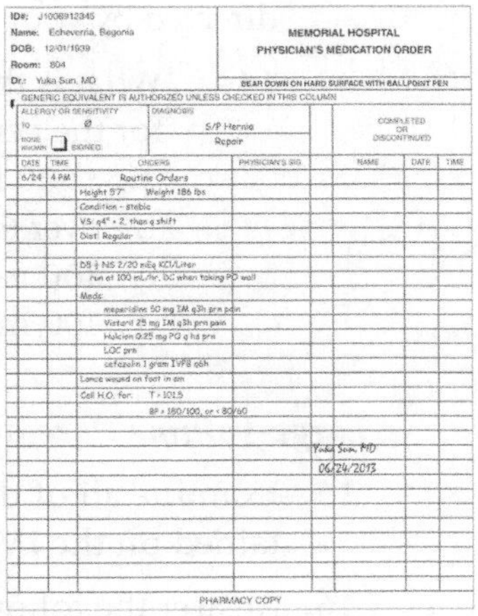


## *Daily Order for Echeverria*

7. Turn back to Figure 4.2 and read the Daily Order for Echeverria in its entirety.

8. Answer the following multiple-choice question, recording your answer as directed by your instructor.

**8–1.** What is the patient's condition?

a. postop
b. stable
c. regular
d. S/P hernia repair

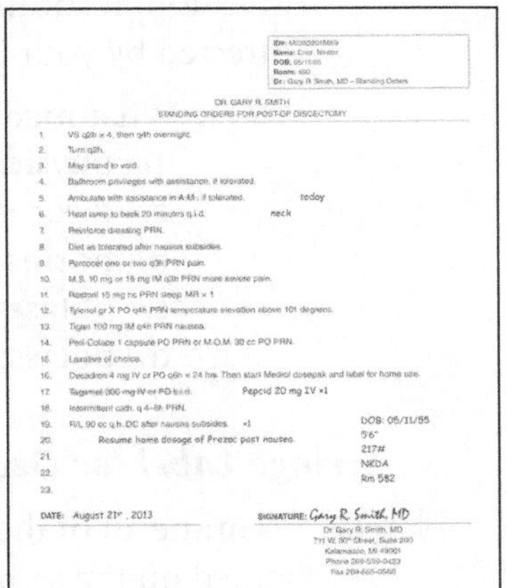

## *Standing Order for Cruz*

9. Turn back to Figure 4.3 and read the Standing Order for Cruz in its entirety.

10. Answer the following multiple-choice questions, recording your answers as directed by your instructor.

**10–1.** What is the patient's height, weight, and date of birth?

a. 67 inches, 217 kg, 09/11/00
b. 67 inches, 217 pounds, 12/20/95
c. 5 feet and 6 inches, 217 pounds, 09/11/00
d. 5 feet and 6 inches, 217 pounds, 05/11/55

**10–2.** How many pharmacy items has the physician ordered?

a. 10
b. 11
c. 12
d. 13

11. Find number 19 on the order.

12. Answer the following multiple-choice question, recording your answer as directed by your instructor.

**12–1.** What IV solution and infusion rate has the physician ordered?

a. lactated Ringer's solution to be infused at 90 mL/hour
b. Ringer's lactate to be infused at 90 mL/day
c. Ringer's lactate to be infused at 90 mL/hour
d. both *a* and *c*, for they are identical
e. none of the above

### *IVPB Label for Andreachi*

**13.** Examine all of the information contained on the IVPB label for Andreachi.

**IV Piggyback**

**Pt. Name:** Andreachi, Azar **Room:** ICU-9
**ID#:** S1143367722 **Rx#:** 12249648

Gentamicin 100 mg
$D_5W$ 100 mL
Rate: over 60 min

Keep refrigerated – warm to room temperature before administration.

Expiration Day/time: __________ Tech _____ RPh _____

**14.** Answer the following multiple-choice question, recording your answer as directed by your instructor.

**14–1.** What is the administration time for the gentamicin IVPB?

a. 1600 hours
b. over 60 minutes
c. 100 mg
d. 100 mL

### *Large-Volume Parenteral (LVP) Label for Li*

**15.** Examine all of the information contained on the LVP label for Li.

**Large-Volume Parenteral**

**Pt. Name:** Li, Oscar **Room:** ICU-8
**ID#:** S1147872252 **Rx#:** 14839511

$D_5NS$ 1000 mL
Potassium Chloride 20 mEq
Rate: 100 mL/hour

Keep refrigerated – warm to room temperature before administration.

Expiration Day/time: __________ Tech _____ RPh _____

**16.** Answer the following multiple-choice question, recording your answer as directed by your instructor.

**16–1.** What medication and dose has the physician ordered?

a. dextrose 5%
b. normal saline 1000 mL
c. potassium chloride 20 mEq
d. potassium chloride 100 mL/hour

### *Syringe Label for Decoteau*

**17.** Examine all of the information contained on the syringe label for Decoteau.

**Syringe**

**Pt. Name:** Decoteau, Kaya **Room:** ICU-7
**ID#:** S114971441 **Rx#:** 17725909

Ceftriaxone 250 mg/2.5 mL
for IM administration only

Expiration Day/time: __________ Tech _____ RPh _____

**18.** Answer the following multiple-choice question, recording your answer as directed by your instructor.

**18–1.** What dose of medication has the physician ordered?

a. 100 mg
b. 250 mg
c. 250 g
d. 250 mL

# Part 3: Assessment

## Chapter Summary

- Medical terminology, abbreviations, and symbols, many of which have Greek or Latin origins, have communicated prescription and medical information for centuries.
- Most medical terminology is based on a combination of medical morphemes, or root words, prefixes, and suffixes.
- The root word, sometimes called the word root, is the foundational element of the medical term and provides the term's meaning.
- The prefix is a medical word element attached to the beginning of a root word and may indicate time, location, direction, or number.
- The suffix is a medical word element attached to the end of a root word and helps to define the root word's meaning.
- Medical abbreviations, acronyms, and symbols provide a convenient method for healthcare personnel to communicate information related to health, medicine, laboratory procedures or tests, and pharmacy.
- Abbreviations are common for terms related to patient care facilities, professional titles, diagnoses and conditions, procedures, treatments, patient directives/activities, equipment/supplies, and tests.
- Abbreviations in pharmacy practice communicate information about a medication's dosage, route of administration, administration time, parenteral preparation base solution and ingredients, and other pertinent information.
- Abbreviations, acronyms, and symbols may be easily misinterpreted, resulting in dangerous medication errors; therefore, they should be used with caution.
- The Joint Commission published The Official "Do Not Use" List of Abbreviations due to a number of medication errors that led to patient injury or death.
- Medication orders are generated by physicians in the institutional setting to prescribe medications and treatments for patients.
- Medication orders are written by physicians using a combination of medical terminology and signa.
- Medication orders are often written or modified by physicians on a daily basis, based on the patient's condition and treatment requirements.
- Medication orders are part of the patient's medication administration record, which may include admission orders, daily orders, and standing orders.
- Medication orders are entered into the pharmacy computer system, and a label is generated for each dose of a parenteral medication.
- CSP labels should be clear, accurate, and pharmaceutically elegant.
- CSP labels must contain the name and ID number of the patient; the name, concentration, and amount of each solution in the CSP; the additive name and amount; the administration rate or infusion rate of the CSP; the CSP's expiration date and time; the storage requirements of the CSP; any auxiliary labels or special instructions; any device-specific instructions; the dosing schedule of the CSP; and the preparer's and pharmacist's identification.
- IV technicians must compare the sterile compound label to the medication order to verify accuracy and determine which compounding procedures must be performed.
- IV technicians must determine the desired volume of each ingredient by comparing the dose ordered by the physician with the concentration of the drug required to prepare the CSP.
- The pharmacist must check the CSP ingredient types and amounts and verify the accuracy of all CSP solutions and ingredients.
- The CSP label is affixed to the CSP's final container once compounding procedures are complete.

# Key Terms

**abbreviations** characters, acronyms, or symbols used by healthcare professionals to communicate medical information; see also *medical abbreviations*

**additive** a medication, electrolyte, or other ingredient that is injected into a parenteral solution

**addressograph** a machine in the institutional healthcare setting that stamps the patient's name, identification number, hospital room number, date of birth, and other information onto a medication order

**administration time** the length of time (usually prescribed in mL per hour) over which a parenteral medication is to be administered to a patient; see also *infusion rate*

**admission order** the first medication order written by a physician; often occurs while a patient is in the emergency department or just after she or he has been admitted to a hospital room

**apothecary** a merchant who compounded and dispensed spices, herbs, and other cures from a storefront; this community position began in the Middle Ages and continued well into the nineteenth century

**appropriate medication dosage** a dose of medication that is appropriate for the treatment of a patient's medical condition, based on the manufacturer's dosing recommendation; a dose of medication that may be determined based on the patient's body weight, age, gender, liver and kidney functions, and various other factors

**auxiliary label** a small label affixed to a primary CSP label; this label provides additional information or special instructions relating to the administration or storage of the CSP

**ayurvedic medicine** a form of East Indian medicine that involves spiritual and whole body well-being and employs changes in diet and lifestyle in its treatment modalities

**beyond-use date** the date beyond which a parenteral preparation, medication, or ingredient is no longer suitable for patient use; see also *expiration date*

**Bower Manuscript** an ancient manuscript written by East Indian shaman Sushruta that listed 1,120 illnesses and the herbal medicines for treating them; manuscript that laid the foundation for ayurvedic medicine

**central pharmacy** the main or primary pharmacy that serves the needs of an entire hospital and provides backup support for the facility's satellite or decentralized pharmacies

**combined form** the form of a medical word element that is created when a root word is linked to a combining vowel

**combining vowel** a vowel (typically an *o*, but sometimes an *i* or *e*) added to the end of a root word that aids the pronunciation of the root word and its connection to a suffix

**computerized physician order entry** medication orders entered directly into the pharmacy-networked computer system by the physician; also called CPOE

**concentration** the strength of a medication; may be defined as percent strength (%), or units/mL, mg/mL, mEq/mL, etc.

**contraindication** a medical condition or symptom that makes a particular line of treatment inadvisable; a condition for which treatment with a specific drug is not recommended

**cross-sensitivity** a sensitivity to one substance that predisposes an individual to having the same reaction to other analogous substances; this type of allergic reaction can be seen with similar classes of antibiotics

**cuneiform** an ancient form of writing composed of a series of pictographs or symbols impressed into a wet clay tablet

**daily order** new or changed medication order written by a physician after every patient examination

**dosing intervals** the time intervals between the administration of medication dosages, such as *b.i.d.*, *t.i.d.*, *q.i.d.*, *q8h*, etc.; also known as dosage intervals or dosing schedule

**drug–drug interaction** an unintended and adverse modification in a drug's strength or action when combined with a drug with which it is physically incompatible

**drug–food interaction** an adverse modification in the effect or strength of a drug when it is administered with a food with which it is physically incompatible

**duplicate therapy** unintended administration of two or more drugs with the same or similar pharmacological action

**Ebers Papyrus** a well-known ancient Egyptian document, written on papyrus, that contains more than 700 prescriptions for ailments that beset early Egyptian cultures

**eMAR** an abbreviation for electronic medication administration record; a computerized patient medical record or chart

**expiration date** the date beyond which a parenteral preparation, medication, or ingredient is no longer suitable for patient use; see also *beyond-use date*

***Handbook on Injectable Drugs*** a comprehensive reference manual that provides pharmacy and other healthcare professionals with compatibility, stability, and administration information about parenteral drugs

**home medications** a medication order while the patient is hospitalized that indicates the physician wishes to continue the same medications and doses the patient was taking at home; a list of medications the patient was taking prior to admission to the hospital

**humors** the four body fluids—blood, phlegm, yellow bile, and black bile—whose relative proportions were thought to determine an individual's general health and disposition

**identification (ID) number** a unique number, usually computer-generated, that a healthcare facility relies on for identifying and tracking a patient

**infusion rate** the length of time (usually prescribed in mL/hour) over which a parenteral medication is to be administered to a patient; see also *administration time*

**medical abbreviations** abbreviations, acronyms, or symbols used by healthcare professionals to communicate medical information; see also *abbreviations*

**medical chart** a patient healthcare record that includes diagnostic and treatment procedures, medication orders, medical administration records, and other instructions; commonly called the patient's chart or, simply, the chart

**medical terminology** vocabulary used by medical professionals to describe the human body and associated conditions, diseases, and treatments; often consists of a prefix/root word/suffix combination

**medication order** a type of order form generated by a physician to prescribe medications, diagnostic tests, and other treatments for a patient in an institutional or hospital setting; may be called the medication administration record or medical order

***medici*** ancient Roman healthcare practitioner; Italian word meaning "medical doctor or medic"

**Micromedex** an Internet-based reference resource widely consulted in hospital pharmacy settings to gain real-time access to drug information and clinical pharmacy knowledge

**morpheme** a root word, prefix, or suffix

**nephrologist** a doctor who specializes in the treatment of kidney disease or dysfunction

**nonstandard** an abbreviation or acronym that is not well known or commonly used among healthcare facilities

**nursing station** the central area on the nursing unit or department that acts as the unit's command center; the place on the nursing unit where supply items and equipment are stored

**order entry** a term describing the process of data entry of medication orders into a pharmacy computer system

**original copy** the top copy of a multi-layered, carbon-copy medication order form

**papyrus** an ancient form of paper made from the spongy tissue of a papyrus, a marshy plant native to the Nile River

**Performance Standards for Healthcare Accreditation** the minimum standards that a healthcare facility must uphold in order to achieve and maintain accreditation with the Joint Commission

**pharmaceutically elegant** a method of preparing and applying pharmacy labels that ensures the label information is legible, uniform, and orderly in appearance; pharmacy labels must be free from erasures and strike-throughs and should be prepared using an easy-to-read font

**pharmacopeia** an official compendium that lists medications and their uses

**pneumatic tube system** a system for transporting medication orders, as well as certain medications and supply items, between the pharmacy and the nursing unit; a series of containers that carry items through an air-driven system of interconnecting tubes

**prefix** a word element that, when attached to the beginning of a root word, changes the meaning of the term

**prescription** an order written by a physician or other qualified healthcare practitioner for a medication or medical device; a type of medication order within the community pharmacy setting

**protected health information (PHI)** any individually identifiable health information including diagnosis, treatment, prescription information, etc., as defined by the 1996 Health Insurance Portability and Accountability Act (HIPAA); any information about health status, provision of health care, or payment for health care that can be linked to a specific individual

**root word** the foundational element of the medical term that provides the term's meaning; may or may not be attached to a prefix and/or suffix; also known as a word root

**route of administration** the way a drug is introduced into the body; examples include oral, topical, intravenous, intramuscular, sublingual, etc.

**routine order** a medication order written by the physician on a daily or regular basis; a standard medication order; see also *standing order*

**Rx symbol** a symbol having varied possible origins and referring to either a pharmacy, a prescription, or a medication

**satellite pharmacy** a small, secondary pharmacy that serves a specific unit or department within a hospital

**sentinel event** a term used by the Joint Commission to identify an event that has an unexpected and unintended outcome leading to serious harm or death of a patient; a medical or medication error that causes death or serious harm to a patient

**signa** the physician's instructions for use or administration of a prescribed medication; a form of communication composed of a combination of abbreviations, acronyms, and symbols to communicate medical information among healthcare professionals

**stability** a period of time a parenteral preparation, medication, or ingredient maintains its full efficacy and is therefore suitable for patient administration

**standing order** a type of medication order in which the same set of medications and treatments applies for each patient who receives a similar treatment or surgery; a preprinted set of orders and treatments used for each patient; see also *routine order*

**storage requirements** the conditions under which a CSP or an ingredient must be maintained prior to administration; the temperature at which a CSP must be stored in order to maintain its stability; includes such label directives as *refrigerate, do not refrigerate, keep frozen until use, protect from light*, etc.

**stylus** a sharp-ended reed that produces wedge-shaped impressions onto a wet clay tablet

**suffix** a medical word element that, when attached to the end of a root word, changes the meaning of the medical term

**The Official "Do Not Use" List of Abbreviations** a list of medical abbreviations that the Joint Commission has deemed unsafe to use due to their high potential for error

**traditional Eastern medicine** medical treatment based on ancient East Indian or Asian philosophies that blend various healing modalities in order to bring balance and harmony to the body; herbal-based treatments that may be prescribed, prepared, and administered by practitioners other than medical doctors

**traditional Western medicine** medical treatment by a licensed professional, usually a medical doctor; treatment with various natural and synthetic medicinal products or drugs

**warning flag** a computer-generated warning or alert screen that automatically appears during medication order entry in pharmacy software in cases where the physician-ordered medication may be inappropriate due to patient allergy, drug interaction, or unsuitable dosage; a computer-generated warning that directs the pharmacist to consult with the ordering physician about the prescribed medication

# Make Connections

*On a separate sheet of paper, write your answers to the following three questions, using complete sentences and making sure your answers are thorough and thoughtful. Note that the third question requires Internet access.*

1. Handwriting quality and legibility on medication orders vary greatly among healthcare professionals. Considering these variations in handwritten documentation and the important role that accuracy plays in medication safety and error prevention, what are some possible advantages and disadvantages of using an eMAR system for computerized physician order entry?

2. Considering what you have learned so far about CSP labeling, why is it important for the label to be *pharmaceutically elegant*?

3. On the Web, find the home page for the Joint Commission and then search for "*sentinel event statistics.*" Read the report on sentinel event statistics between 2004 and 2010. Which setting reports the largest number of sentinel events? What is a possible reason for such a large number of sentinel events in this setting?

# Meet the Challenge

***Scenario*** This puzzling activity challenges you to decipher the components and medical terminology of several medication orders.

***Challenge*** Your instructor has three handouts (Medication Orders 1, 2, and 3) that address the correct interpretation of medication orders. To successfully complete this challenge, ask your instructor for the handouts and use your knowledge of medical morphemes, abbreviations, acronyms, and signas to help you respond to the critical-thinking questions. For additional assistance, you may also refer to resources such as a brand-generic handbook, the Internet, any pharmacy reference materials in your lab, and your textbook. When you are finished, turn in your answers to your instructor.

## ADDITIONAL RESOURCES

*Go to the Paradigm Internet Resources Center at* www.paradigmcollege.net/sterilecomp *to access live links related to these Chapter 4 topics:*

+ Listings for medical terminology, abbreviations, acronyms, and symbols
+ The Joint Commission's accreditation standards and The Official "Do Not Use" List of Abbreviations
+ Medication safety information, including sentinel events and the National Patient Safety Goals
+ Regulations related to the Health Insurance Portability and Accountability Act (HIPAA)
+ Identification of generic drugs and their brand name counterparts

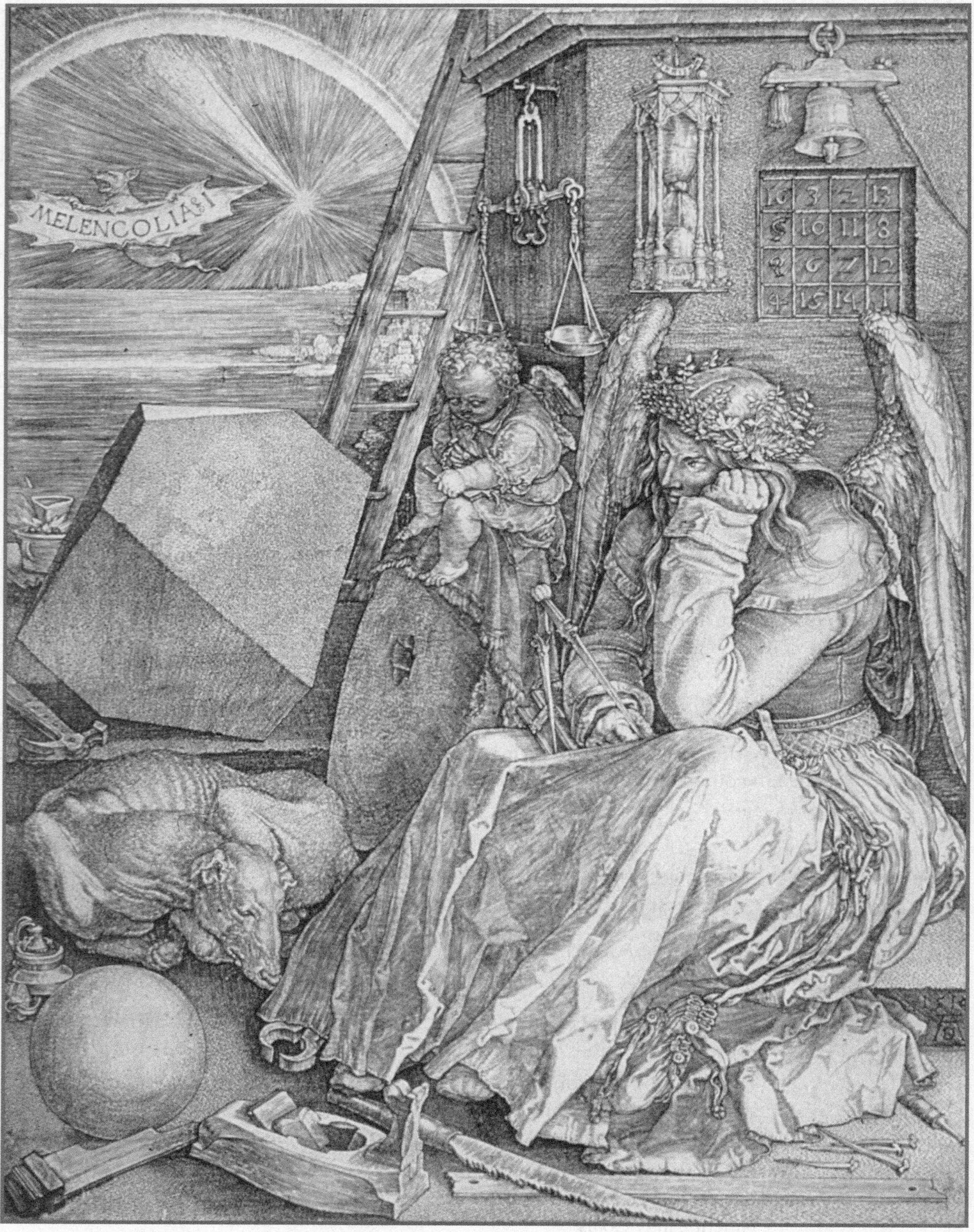
MELENCOLIA I
16 3 2 13
5 10 11 8
9 6 7 12
4 15 14 1

# Chapter 5

# Calculations for Sterile Compounding

## Learning Objectives

- Explore the evolution of mathematical formulas used in sterile compounding.
- Understand the principles of pharmacy dosage calculations.
- Practice several types of pharmaceutical calculations using a basic formula, ratio and proportion, dimensional analysis, intravenous flow rates, intravenous drip rates, and alligations.
- Determine the best method of solving pharmaceutical dosage questions based on the medication labeling and sterile compounding procedure required.

In ancient cultures, the formulas used to prepare medicinal compounds were based on recipes that had been passed down orally through the generations. Apothecaries, alchemists, and other healers prepared many of these recipes from memory, although some were written down and stored in medicine books. Early compounding procedures were based on the **trial-and-error mixing** of **crude drugs**, such as opium, with other plant-based products or homemade tinctures. The ingredients used in compounding recipes, along with the mixed compounds themselves, were **unregulated** for quality, purity, strength, and **side effects**, and the methods used to measure the ingredients tended to vary greatly based on who was preparing them.

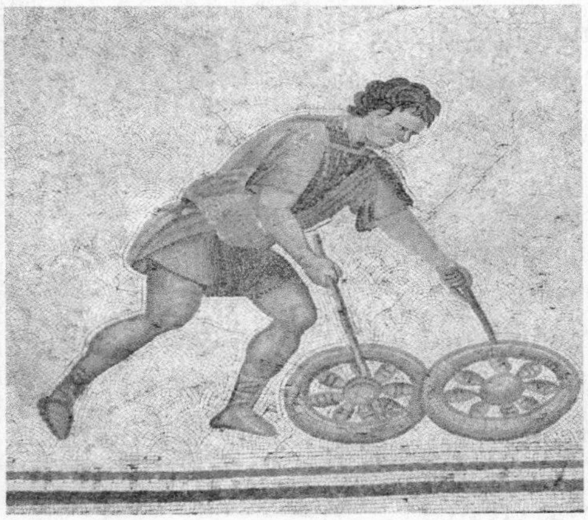

## Origins of Measurement

Units of measurement are one of humankind's oldest tools. To measure length, the ancient Egyptians created a unit called the **cubit**, which was equal to the length of a forearm from the elbow to the middle finger. To the same end, the Romans created the *mille passus*, a unit of length equal to a thousand paces (where each pace was the length of five human feet). To measure weight, many ancient civilizations relied on a measurement known as the **talent**, which was based on the weight of the water required to fill a large ceramic vessel

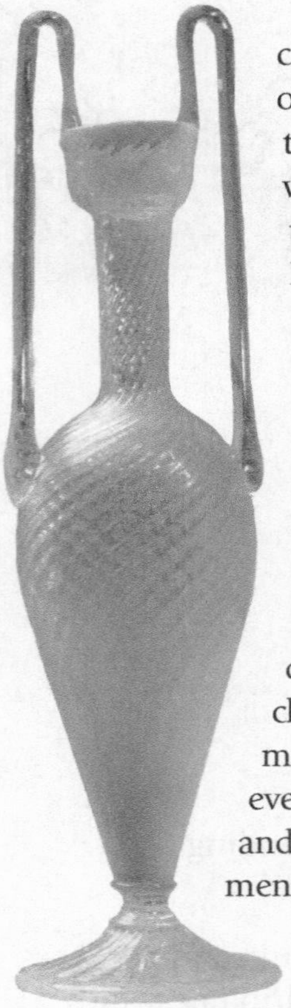

called an *amphora*. Depending on the culture, the weight of the talent varied: The Greek talent weighed 57 pounds; the Egyptian equivalent weighed 60; the Babylonian, 67; and the Roman, 71. When it came to weighing lighter objects, stones and seeds were common reference points, whereas gourds and other containers were often used to measure volume. While inconsistent measurement units may not have toppled empires, disciplines such as medicine and chemistry that required precise measurements did suffer, both in everyday compounding practices and in sharing consistent measurement information across cultures.

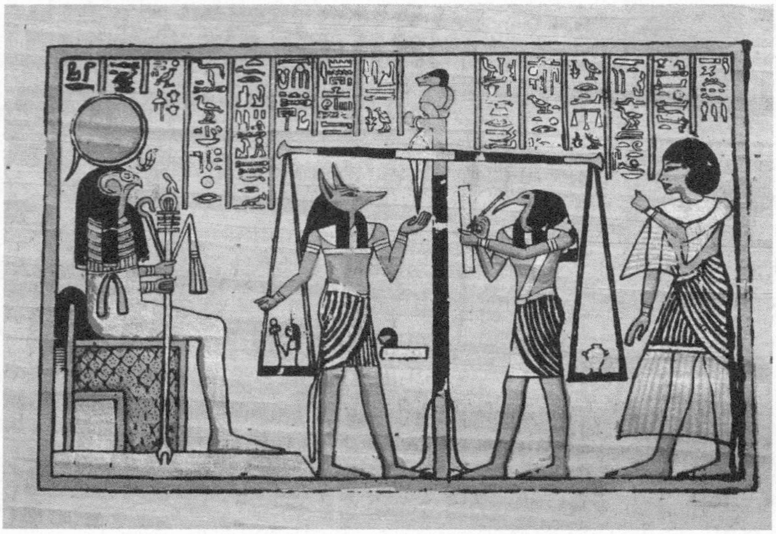

## Early Systems of Pharmaceutical Measurement

Prior to the late 1700s, it was common for apothecaries, pharmacists, physicians, and other healthcare professionals to use several different systems of measurement when compounding medications—the most well-known of which are the apothecary, avoirdupois, and household systems. These systems are virtually obsolete in the practice of modern dosage calculation. However, the household system is still occasionally used by prescribers, and many of the original terms from these early systems are still in use today.

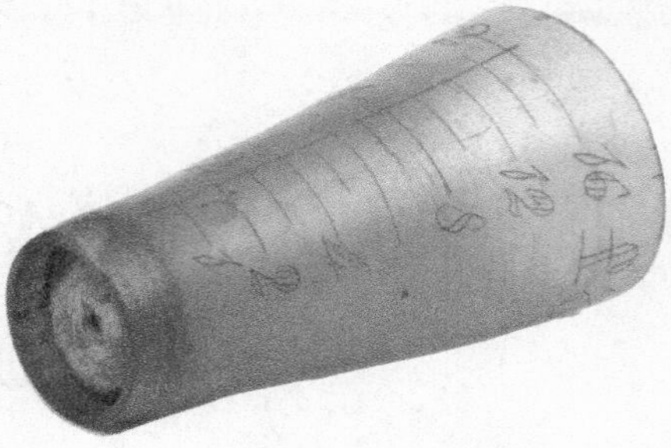

The **apothecary system** is one of the oldest systems of measurement and is based on the classical weight system developed by the Romans. The apothecary system includes units of measurement such as the **dram**, which is roughly equivalent to 4 milliliters, and the **scruple**, which is roughly equivalent to 1.3 grams. Although the apothecary system did help establish some terms of measurement still in use today—such as the ounce, pint, quart, and gallon—the modern equivalencies of these measurements have changed.

The **avoirdupois system**, which originated in France, has been used in the United States to varying degrees since colonization and remains the "everyday" measurement system in this country. The name of the system comes from the French term *aveir de peis*, or "goods of weight," which referred to products sold in bulk that had to be weighed to determine their value. The avoirdupois system is based on units such as feet, miles, and pounds but also contains more obscure units of measure, such as the **grain**. The **pound**, a unit weighing 16 **ounces**, was created

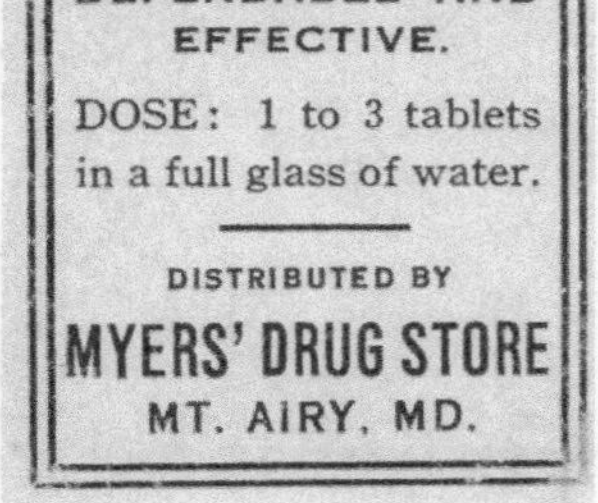
100 TABLETS
ASPIRIN
5 GRAINS
THIS ASPIRIN IS OF HIGHEST PURITY, DEPENDABLE AND EFFECTIVE.
DOSE: 1 to 3 tablets in a full glass of water.
DISTRIBUTED BY
MYERS' DRUG STORE
MT. AIRY, MD.

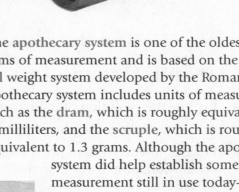

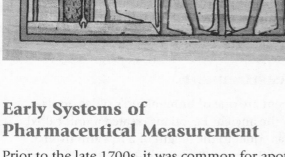

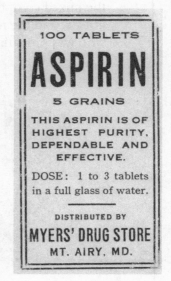

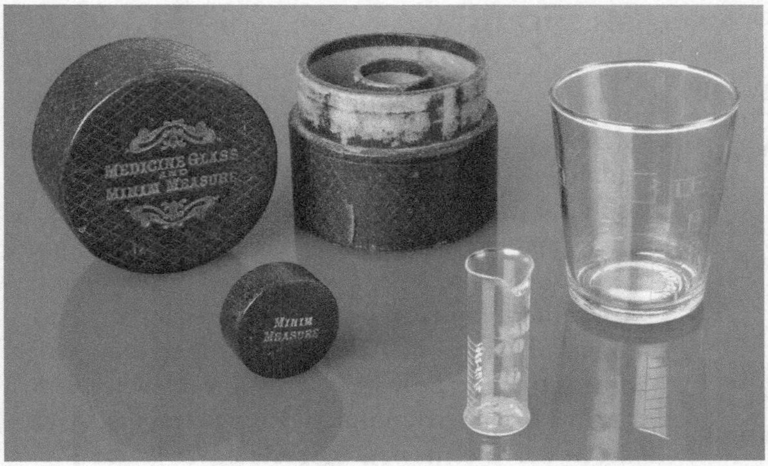


in London in 1303 and then standardized as 7,000 grains by Henry VIII in the 1500s. The grain, as its name suggests, is based on the weight of a single seed from grains such as wheat or barley. Some form of this unit has been used by nearly every culture in recorded history.

The **household system** of measurement is based on the apothecary system and was created to assist patients taking medications at home. Common dry units of this system are the ounce and pound; common liquid units include the drop, teaspoon, tablespoon, and cup; and obscure volume units include the jigger and the hogshead. In the United States, the food industry and some areas of pharmacy still use the household system, despite its insufficiently small units and lack of uniformity.

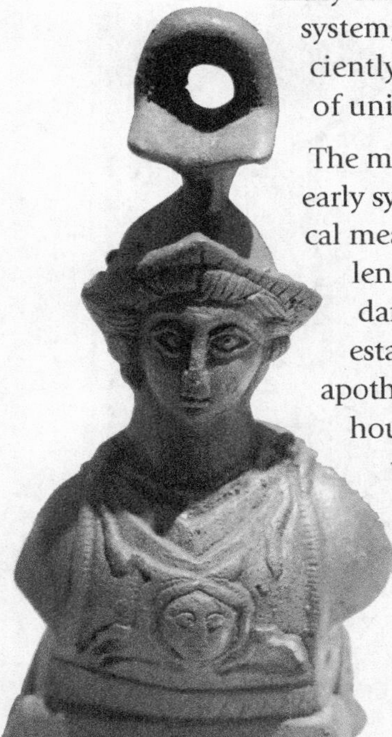

The major problem for most early systems of pharmaceutical measurement was equivalency. Because no standard equivalencies were established between the apothecary, avoirdupois, and household systems prior to the nineteenth century, pharmacies relying on different measurement systems tended to produce widely differing doses. For instance, if a pharmacy received an order to compound 1 pound of a cream, the pharmacist would prepare 12 ounces under the apothecary system, 16 ounces under the avoirdupois system, and "a pound" if she or he was following the household system. These inconsistencies often led to dangerous differences between the physician's prescription and the product prepared by the pharmacy.

## Pharmaceutical Measurement Tools

Another source of dosage inaccuracies stemmed from the measurement tools used by early apothecaries and healers. Scales have been used for thousands of years to assist in the weighing and calculation of compounding ingredients, and they are still being used in pharmacy practice today. However, the accuracy of this measurement device is dependent on several variables.

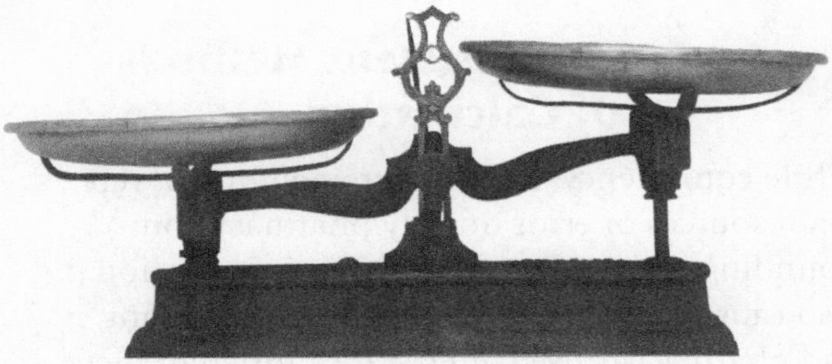

The simple **balance scale** has been in use since at least 2400 BCE, and its descendant models are still relied on today. A balance scale consists of a horizontal beam placed across a point, or fulcrum, so that the scale sits perfectly level. Plates are attached to either side of the beam. The object to be weighed is placed on one plate, and weight references (objects whose weight is known) are added to the other plate until the two sides of the beam are balanced. Although highly effective and extremely accurate when properly maintained, a balance scale requires a perfectly frictionless fulcrum to move accurately. Another drawback to a balance is that it only works as a reference scale, meaning it only gives a measurement relative to the weights used to balance the scale, and the measurement is accurate only to the extent that the reference weights are.

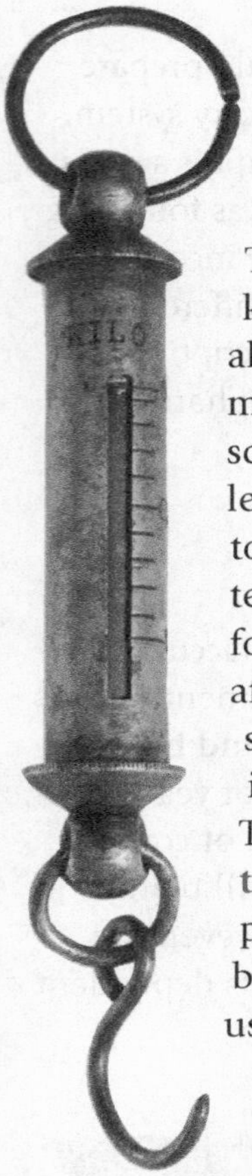


The **spring scale**, which measures the weight of an object hanging from the bottom of a spring, gained popularity in the 1800s. The spring's stretch, combined with knowledge of elasticity and gravity, allows weights to be measured much more quickly than with a balance scale. However, the spring scale is less accurate and more susceptible to environmental influences, such as temperature and even gravitational force, which vary across regions and affect the spring's strength. Today, spring scales are used mainly in industrial settings for large loads. The medical field currently uses **electronic scales** to accurately deliver precise measurements, though the balance scale is still occasionally used as a substitute, if necessary.

## Inconsistent Methods of Calculation

While equivalency and measurement tools were main sources of error in early pharmacy compounding, inconsistent methods of calculation also caused problems. For example, physicians and pharmacists used at least four different methods to calculate children's dosages (some of which were still in use in the twentieth century). These calculation methods, based on simple equations, were known as "rules" and included Clark's Rule, Cowling's Rule, Fried's Rule, and Young's Rule. For example, **Clark's Rule** took a child's weight in pounds, divided it by 150, and then multiplied that fraction by the adult dosage. **Fried's Rule** was nearly identical but, since it was designed for infants, it required the child's age in months rather than the child's weight in pounds. Both **Cowling's Rule** and **Young's Rule** used the child's age for their equations. These rules were inconsistently applied and also used variables such as age that were not appropriate for determining dosage (see Table 5.1 for a comparison of these four obsolete children's dosing rules).

## Metrication

The **metric system** was introduced in France in 1799 in response to the need for a standardized system of measurement that could be used internationally. The main advantage of the metric system is that it uses a group of base units (such as meters, liters, and grams) in conjunction with a set of prefixes (such as *deci–*, *centi–*, and *milli–*) that represent different powers of ten. The prefixes are used to modify all of the base units in the system, which means the user only needs to know a few terms to be able to understand many measurements. Over the next two centuries, the system was gradually adopted by countries across the world, and today it standardizes and greatly simplifies international commerce and communication, especially in the areas of science and technology (although many countries still use traditional measurements in areas such as construction, plumbing, and human weight). The United States is one of three

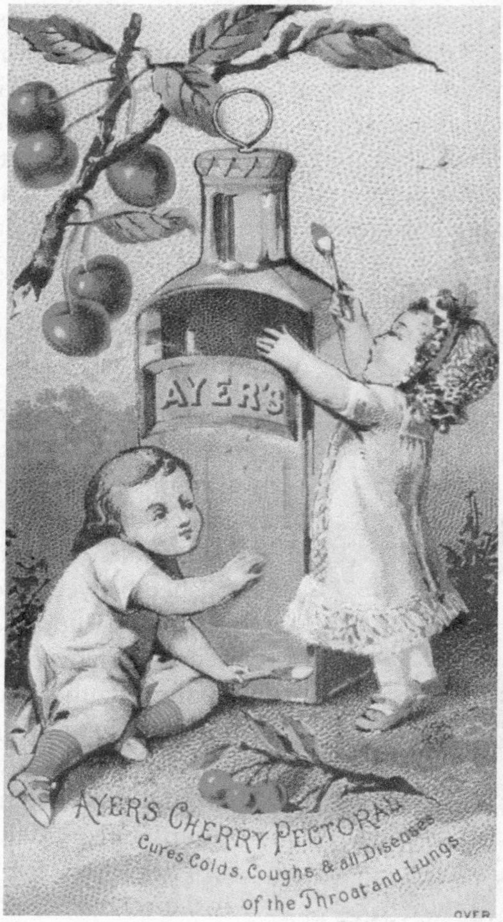

**Table 5.1** Dosage Variation Based on Obsolete Children's Dosing Rules

To compare the four obsolete children's dosing methods, or "rules," provided below, consider the patient to be a six-year-old child who weighs 50 pounds and consider the initial adult dose to be 600 mg. Each of the four rules determines the child's dose by modifying the adult dose based on either the child's weight or age. Compare the variation in resulting dosage among the four rules.

| | | | |
|---|---|---|---|
| **Clark's Rule** | **States:** | $\frac{\text{Child's weight (in lbs.)} \times \text{adult dose}}{150}$ | = Child's dose |
| | **And for this example, results in:** | $\frac{50 \times 600 \text{ mg}}{150}$ | = ***200 mg*** |
| **Cowling's Rule** | **States:** | $\frac{\text{Child's age (in years) at next birthday} \times \text{adult dose}}{24}$ | = Child's dose |
| | **And for this example, results in:** | $\frac{7 \times 600 \text{ mg}}{24}$ | = ***175 mg*** |
| **Fried's Rule** | **States:** | $\frac{\text{Child's age (in months)} \times \text{adult dose}}{150}$ | = Child's dose |
| | **And for this example, results in:** | $\frac{72 \times 600 \text{ mg}}{150}$ | = ***288 mg*** |
| **Young's Rule** | **States:** | $\frac{\text{Child's age (in years)} \times \text{adult dose}}{\text{Child's age (in years)} + 12}$ | = Child's dose |
| | **And for this example, results in:** | $\frac{6 \times 600 \text{ mg}}{6 + 12}$ | = ***200 mg*** |

countries that, despite sporadic efforts over the course of 200 years, does not use the metric system as the standard, though it has adopted this international system for a variety of specific purposes, including pharmacy practice.

## Regulation and Standardization in Pharmacy Practice

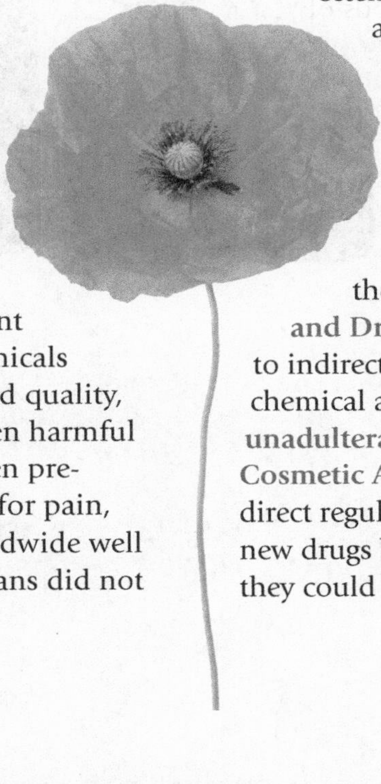

Prior to the 1800s, the practice of pharmacy was unregulated. Pharmacists were not required to complete any formal education or training programs, and the substances and methods they used to create medications were uncontrolled. Differences in systems of measurement and calculation, combined with chemicals and drugs of inconsistent strength and quality, led to inaccurate, ineffective, and often harmful medication dosing. For instance, when prescribing opium—a common remedy for pain, sleeplessness, and diarrhea used worldwide well into the nineteenth century—physicians did not distinguish between the various plant species, or by what methods the extract would be created. As a result, pharmacists often prepared and administered doses that were too weak or, worse, too strong.

In the 1800s, pharmacy began to transform from an art, or a subjective science based on old and often unproven or imprecise recipes, into a more exact discipline. In 1821, the Philadelphia College of Pharmacy became the first U.S. college to offer an advanced degree in pharmaceutical science. By 1880, individual states had begun to create pharmacy boards to oversee pharmacists and their practice. In 1906, the **Pure Food and Drug Act** became the first federal law to indirectly affect pharmacy. This law required chemical and drug labeling to be "truthful and **unadulterated**." In 1938, the **Food, Drug, and Cosmetic Act (FDCA or FD&C)** provided the first direct regulation of pharmacy by requiring that new drugs be proven safe and effective before they could be marketed to the public. Since then,

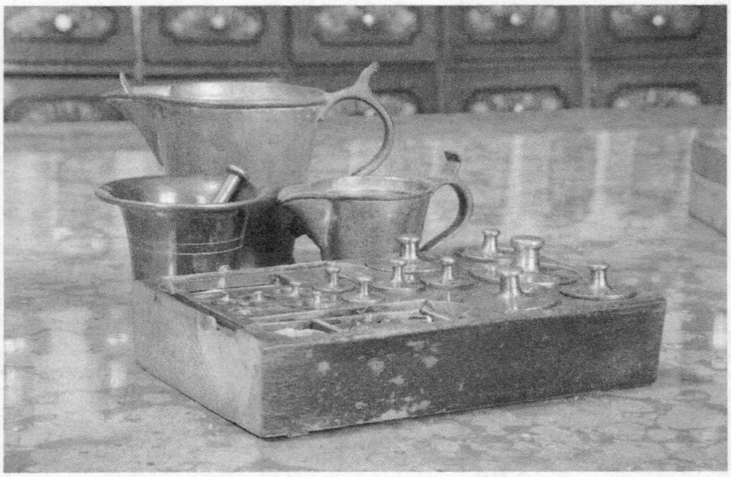

numerous amendments to the FDCA have helped standardize drug formulations and labeling as well as ensure the purity and quality of medications.

In 1890, the United States Pharmacopeia (USP) adopted the metric system of weights and measures as its primary system of measurement, although some of the approximate equivalents from other systems of measure continue to be used in pharmacy practice to this day.

Advancements in medicine and pharmacy, supplemented by the implementation of strict federal laws governing the creation, preparation, and compounding of medications, also led to the standardization of medication dosing. The mathematical formulas discussed in this chapter are a major part of this standardization. Note that the "rules" that caused problems with children's doses are now considered obsolete and have been replaced by more accurate methods of dosing. Today, physicians determine the desired dose of each parenteral medication based on either the patient's body weight or **body surface area (BSA)**. In particular, prescribers use BSA when writing medication orders for chemotherapy—a topic addressed in Chapter 14 of this textbook. However, pharmacy technicians do not routinely perform BSA calculations.

Today's sterile compounding personnel are provided with medication orders, ingredient information on manufacturers' labels, and pharmacy-printed compounded sterile preparation (CSP) labels. They then use streamlined formulas, some of which are based on **conversion factors**, to determine the amount of each ingredient needed to prepare various sterile compounds. Intravenous (IV) technicians use calculation methods such as ratio and proportion, dimensional analysis, and alligation to determine quantities such as diluent volumes, **drug concentrations**, and the amount of each drug that must be drawn up in order to prepare each CSP. The precise nature of these calculation methods, in conjunction with the use of standard systems of measurement and controlled, regulated ingredients, ensure that each patient receives the safest and most beneficial dosage of medication.

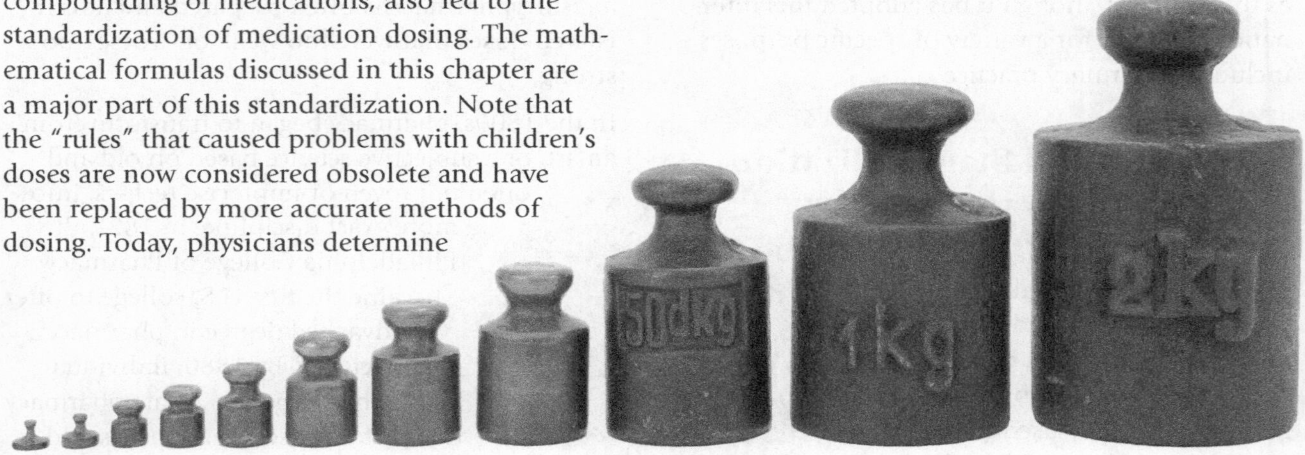

# Part 1: Concepts

The majority of the CSPs assembled by an IV technician will require the application of one or more pharmacy calculation methods in order for the technician to determine the volume of the medication, additive, or solution component needed to prepare a CSP or to resolve the number of CSPs necessary for a 24-hour supply. The decision about which calculation method to use is often based on the personal preference of the IV technician; however, the compounding scenario should also factor into the technician's choice.

The most commonly used pharmacy calculation methods include basic formula, ratio and proportion, dimensional analysis, IV flow rate, IV drop factor, and alligation. Regardless of the calculation method used, the IV technician should double-check all calculations to verify the accuracy of the process as well as the final answer. Accurate pharmacy dosage calculations ensure safe and effective CSPs for patient recipients.

The calculations and formulas presented in this chapter are specific to the compounding work of institutional pharmacy and are commonly used in the sterile compounding environment. Numerous other calculation methods applicable to the retail pharmacy setting are used by pharmacy personnel to determine information such as **day's supply**, **quantity to be dispensed**, and **average wholesale price (AWP)**.

## Calculations as Part of the Anteroom Protocol

In an institutional setting, a prescriber writes medication orders for all aspects of the care and treatment of a patient. These orders typically include several medications, such as oral and topical agents, that are dispensed by the pharmacy but do not require sterile compounding. However, most medication orders also include directives to administer one or more sterile compounds. The prescriber includes the names of the desired medications, the desired doses, and the dosing intervals as part of the CSP order. The prescriber also determines the desired base solution and **infusion rate** for large-volume parenterals (LVPs). Most small-volume parenterals (SVPs), however, are prepared using standard base solutions and volumes and are administered using standard administration times. See Chapters 3 and 4 for information on standard intravenous piggyback (IVPB) base solutions and administration times.

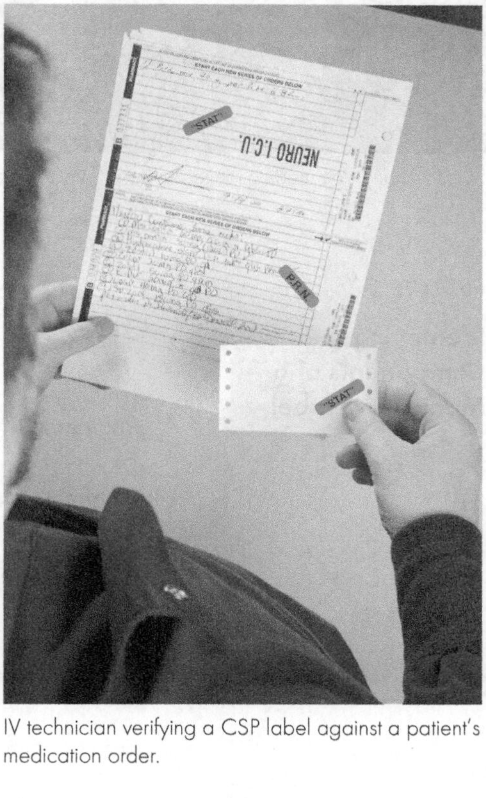

IV technician verifying a CSP label against a patient's medication order.

As discussed in Chapter 4 of this textbook, once the medication order is received in the pharmacy, personnel then enter the information into the computer system and generate a label for each CSP. The pharmacist and IV technician must verify that the CSP label matches the medication order and is 100% accurate, to ensure patient safety. The IV technician then performs one or more calculations to determine the volume of the

**POINTER**
Some facilities require pharmacist verification of the CSP label and the medication order. Consult your facility's P&P manual to determine the policy for your pharmacy.

CSP ingredients to be drawn up to prepare the sterile compound. Once the correct drug volumes of each medication are determined, the IV technician gathers the necessary supplies and then wipes down the exterior surfaces of all supply items. Prior to entering the clean room, she or he dons aseptic garb, performs an aseptic hand washing, and dons a sterile gown.

## Dosage Calculations

The calculations that an IV technician must perform are based on information on the CSP label and the label on the **stock medication** (also called *stock drug*) container. This container may be either a vial or an ampule and may be supplied in either a powdered or readily injectable form.

The IV technician begins the calculation process by determining the **concentration** of the medication. This information can be found on the **medication label** of the stock medication's container. She or he then uses the medication's concentration and the ordered dose from the CSP label to perform a calculation or series of calculations based on one of the calculation methods provided in this chapter. These calculations determine the drug **volume** of each medication needed to prepare the CSP.

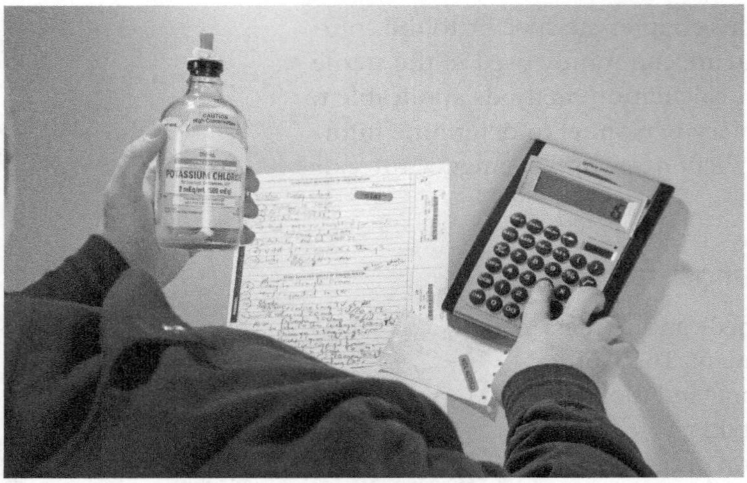

IV technician using medication label to perform calculations.

To help with these calculation tasks, Figure 5.1 identifies the components of a medication label, including the printed guidelines that identify the concentration or strength of the drug, which is necessary for the preparation of a CSP. Locating and understanding label information is an important initial step in ensuring accuracy in pharmacy calculations and in sterile compounding.

**FIGURE 5.1**

**Identifying the Components of a Medication Label**

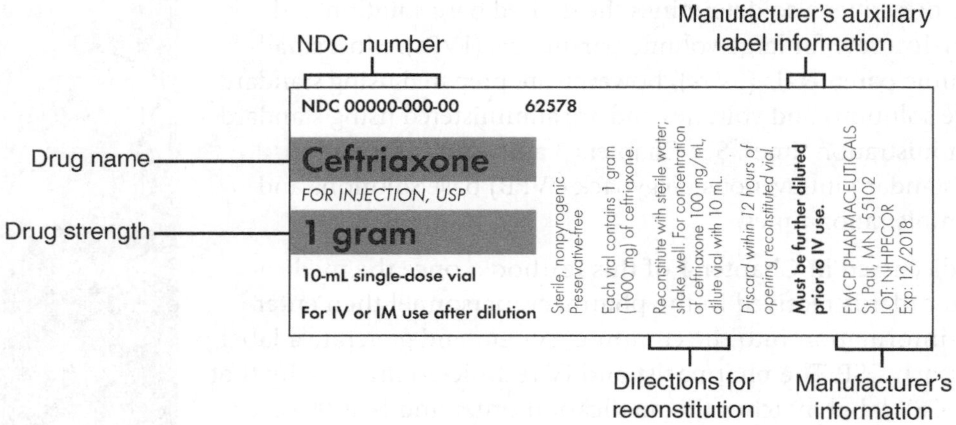

## Special Considerations

When performing calculations, sterile compounding personnel must be aware of some special considerations. One consideration is that the volume (in milliliters [mL] or liters [L]) and strength (in percent [%]) of the base solution are not to be included in any equation in which personnel are asked to determine the amount or volume of drug that is to be drawn up for a desired dose. In most pharmacy sterile compounding situations, an IV technician will *not* include any of the base solution information in the calculation. On rare occasions, the technician may be asked to determine how long an IV bag will last, or the number of bags needed (such as in the calculation of IV flow rates), in which case she or he must use the volume of the base solution in the calculations. However, in this scenario, the strength of the base solution is not needed in the calculation. For the most part, the only time a technician will ever need to include the strength of the base solution in a calculation is during the preparation of a total parenteral nutrition (TPN) solution. For specific information on TPN preparation, refer to Chapter 13 of this textbook.

Another consideration when performing pharmacy calculations is that an IV technician chooses a method or formula based on the type of CSP being prepared as well as a personal calculation preference. With that in mind, this chapter presents several common methods for solving pharmacy calculations as well as the types of compounding scenarios in which each type of calculation is typically applied.

***Note:*** *Many possible methods may be used to solve pharmacy calculation problems in the sterile compounding environment. In practice, the best method to use is whichever you, as an IV technician, are most comfortable with, given the information provided by the medication order, the CSP label, and the medication label. Only the most commonly used pharmacy sterile compounding calculation methods are presented in this chapter; you may encounter other methods for solving pharmacy calculations.*

## Common Pharmacy Equivalents and Conversions

In addition to understanding basic math principles, the IV technician must memorize the most commonly used equivalents and metric conversions. In order to learn the pharmaceutical calculations presented later in this chapter, you will need to memorize all of the liquid and solid measurement equivalents as well as their metric conversions provided in Tables 5.2 and 5.3. Doing so will enable you to quickly and accurately perform calculations without having to stop to locate pharmacy reference materials for looking up the common equivalents and conversions. Working in the fast-paced sterile compounding environment requires the IV technician to work quickly while maintaining 100 percent accuracy.

In addition to memorizing the equivalents and metric conversions provided in Tables 5.2 and 5.3, sterile compounding personnel must also memorize the conversions from **standard time** (clock time) to **military time** (see Table 5.4). This knowledge is especially pertinent in the institutional setting in which all time references are based on military time.

After memorizing the commonly used pharmacy equivalents and conversions, an IV technician may choose to employ one of the calculation methods discussed in the following pages: basic formula, ratio and proportion, dimensional analysis, IV flow rate, IV drip rate, or alligation.

**Table 5.2 Commonly Used Liquid and Solid Measurement Equivalents**

| | Apothecary, Household, or Avoirdupois (used by some physicians) | Exact Metric Equivalent (sometimes used in pharmacy practice) | Approximate Metric Equivalent (commonly used in pharmacy practice) |
|---|---|---|---|
| Liquid Measurement Equivalents | 15 drops | 1 mL | 1 mL |
| | 1 teaspoon | 5 mL | 5 mL |
| | 1 tablespoon | 15 mL | 15 mL |
| | 1 fluid ounce (1 fl) | 29.57 mL | 30 mL |
| | 4 fluid ounces | 118.28 mL | 120 mL |
| | 8 fluid ounces | 236.56 mL | 240 mL |
| | 16 fluid ounces (1 pint) | 473 mL | 480 mL |
| | 2 pints (1 quart) | 946 mL | 960 mL |
| | 1 gallon (4 quarts) | 3784 mL | 3840 mL |
| Solid Measurement Equivalents | 2.2 pounds | 1 kg | 1 kg |
| | 5 grains | 325 mg | 325 mg |
| | 10 grains | 650 mg | 650 mg |
| | 1 pound | 453.59 g | 454 g |

**Table 5.3 Commonly Used Liquid and Solid Metric Conversions**

| Liquid and Solid Metric Conversions | |
|---|---|
| 1 L (liter) | 1000 mL (milliliter) |
| 1 cc (cubic centimeter) | 1 mL (milliliter) |
| 1 g (gram) | 1000 mg (milligram) |
| 1 mg (milligram) | 1000 mcg (microgram) |
| 1 kg (kilogram) | 1000 g (gram) |

**Table 5.4 Standard Time and Military Time Equivalents**

| Standard Time | Military Time |
|---|---|
| 1:00 a.m. | 0100 hours |
| 2:00 a.m. | 0200 hours |
| 3:00 a.m. | 0300 hours |
| 4:00 a.m. | 0400 hours |
| 5:00 a.m. | 0500 hours |
| 6:00 a.m. | 0600 hours |
| 7:00 a.m. | 0700 hours |
| 8:00 a.m. | 0800 hours |
| 9:00 a.m. | 0900 hours |
| 10:00 a.m. | 1000 hours |
| 11:00 a.m. | 1100 hours |
| 12:00 p.m. | 1200 hours |

| Standard Time | Military Time |
|---|---|
| 1:00 p.m. | 1300 hours |
| 2:00 p.m. | 1400 hours |
| 3:00 p.m. | 1500 hours |
| 4:00 p.m. | 1600 hours |
| 5:00 p.m. | 1700 hours |
| 6:00 p.m. | 1800 hours |
| 7:00 p.m. | 1900 hours |
| 8:00 p.m. | 2000 hours |
| 9:00 p.m. | 2100 hours |
| 10:00 p.m. | 2200 hours |
| 11:00 p.m. | 2300 hours |
| 12:00 a.m. | 2400 hours |

## Basic Formula Calculations

The **basic formula method** is a simple process to calculate most parenteral medication dosages and may be used when the concentration on the drug label is provided in units per *one* milliliter (usually mg/mL). This commonly used method is based on the following formula:

D/H = $x$ mL

D = Desired dose (the dose ordered by the prescriber on the medication order)

H = The concentration on hand (the concentration or strength of the drug *per milliliter*, found on the medication label [either a vial or an ampule])

$x$ = The unknown volume of drug needed to be drawn up for the preparation of the CSP

The basic formula method for solving pharmacy dosage calculations is best used in sterile compounding scenarios that meet any of the following criteria:

- The prescriber has ordered a CSP with a single medication additive. *Examples:* The medication order indicates an IV bag with 40 mEq of potassium chloride or an IVPB with 120 mg of gentamicin.
- The drug is in an injectable form (i.e., does not require reconstitution prior to use).
- The medication label provides you with the concentration of the drug in the form of number of units (i.e., milligrams [mg] or milliequivalents [mEq]) per *one* milliliter.

**POINTER**
The slash mark, when used between numbers, indicates division and is frequently used in pharmacy sterile compounding calculations.

**POINTER**
To make the various sterile compounding calculation formulas easier to work with and remember, each component of the formula is typically represented by a corresponding letter. Be sure to review each letter and its corresponding meaning before beginning the calculation process.

***Performing a Basic Formula Calculation*** Find the desired dose (D) on the CSP label, and record that number. Next, locate the concentration of the medication (identified in mg/mL) on the medication label; this number (H) represents the dose on hand. Divide the desired dose (D) by the concentration of the medication (H) to determine the volume of drug ($x$) needed to be drawn up for the preparation of the CSP. You have then determined the proper dose ($x$) in milliliters. To recap:

1. Find the desired dose (D), as described above.
2. Determine the concentration on hand (H), as described above.
3. Divide D by H; the resulting answer equals $x$ mL.

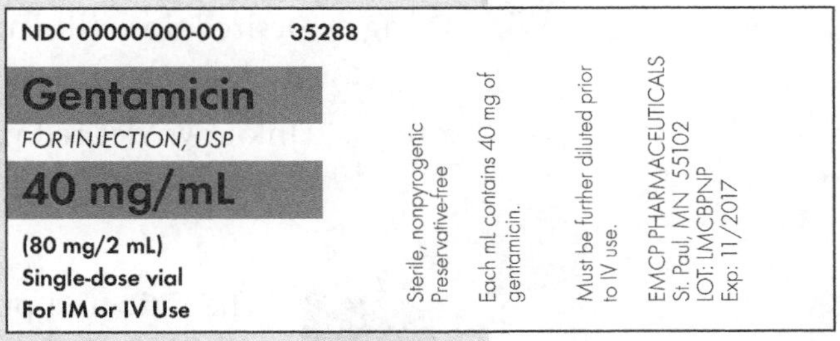

NDC 00000-000-00 35288
Gentamicin
FOR INJECTION, USP
40 mg/mL
(80 mg/2 mL)
Single-dose vial
For IM or IV Use
Sterile, nonpyrogenic
Preservative-free
Each mL contains 40 mg of gentamicin.
Must be further diluted prior to IV use.
EMCP PHARMACEUTICALS
St. Paul, MN 55102
LOT: LMCBPNP
Exp: 11/2017


**FIGURE 5.2**
**Medication Label for Gentamicin**

BASIC FORMULA EXAMPLE The prescriber has written a medication order to administer 80 mg of gentamicin IVPB. The label on the vial of gentamicin states that the stock medication has a concentration of 40 mg/mL (see Figure 5.2).

In this scenario, the desired dose (D) is 80 mg, and the concentration on hand (H) is 40 mg/mL. The IV technician must determine the unknown volume of drug ($x$) needed to be drawn up for the preparation of the CSP.

Divide the desired dose (80 mg) by the concentration on hand (40 mg/mL) to determine the volume of drug needed to prepare a CSP delivering 80 mg of gentamicin.

D = 80
H = 40
$x$ = ?

80/40 = 2
**$x$ = 2 mL**

***Answer:*** *The answer to this pharmacy calculation using the basic formula method is 2 mL.*

## Ratio and Proportion Calculations

The ratio and proportion method is another frequently used technique for solving pharmacy sterile compounding calculations. An equation that states two ratios are equal is called a "proportion." The ratio and proportion method may be used whenever three of the four values in a proportion are known, thus allowing the IV technician to solve for the fourth, unknown value of the proportion. This commonly used method is based on the following formula:

$$\frac{\text{H mg}}{\text{Y mL}} = \frac{\text{D mg}}{x\ \text{mL}}$$

**H mg** = Number of milligrams on hand (per the given number of milliliters on hand; from the concentration stated on the stock medication's label)

**Y mL** = Number of milliliters in the concentration on hand (per the given number of milligrams on hand; from the concentration stated on the stock medication's label)

**D mg** = Desired dose (the number of milligrams in the dose ordered by the prescriber)

***x* mL** = Unknown desired volume (in milliliters) of the drug needed to be drawn up for the preparation of the CSP

The ratio and proportion method for solving pharmacy dosage calculations is best used in sterile compounding scenarios that meet any of the following criteria:

- The stock drug is already in a liquid, injectable form (does not need to be reconstituted). However, the medication label identifies the concentration of the drug in a form other than the form milligrams per *one* milliliter (i.e., the concentration is identified as the amount of milligrams per *multiple* milliliters—i.e., anything *other than x* mg/1 mL or *x* mg/mL [e.g., 500 mg/5 mL or 40 mEq/20mL]).

*Example*: The medication label for cefazolin indicates that the concentration is 1000 mg/5 mL, and the CSP label indicates that the patient needs a 750-mg dose.

- The stock drug is in a powdered form and requires reconstitution prior to drawing it up for injection.
- Either a liquid or powdered drug requires the completion of several additional steps to solve the problem.

> **POINTER**
> To be accurate and clear when using the ratio and proportion method, sterile compounding personnel should always write down the abbreviations for the units (mg, mEq, mL, etc.) when recording numbers.

***Performing a Ratio and Proportion Calculation*** Find the concentration of the reconstituted drug on the medication label, and write that number down, in fraction form, so that the concentration of the drug in milligrams (H mg) is above the concentration of the drug in milliliters (Y mL). Next to this concentration, or ratio, place an equal sign, and then write out another fraction; this time, write the desired dose (D mg) in milligrams above the unknown desired volume (*x* mL).

You have created a proportion that communicates that one ratio is equivalent to the other ratio. You can now cross-multiply (Y × D), and then divide that answer by H to solve for *x*. You have then determined the proper dose (*x*) in milliliters. To recap:

1. Set up the ratio, as described above.
2. Cross-multiply Y × D.
3. Divide the answer from step 2 by H. The resulting answer equals *x* mL.

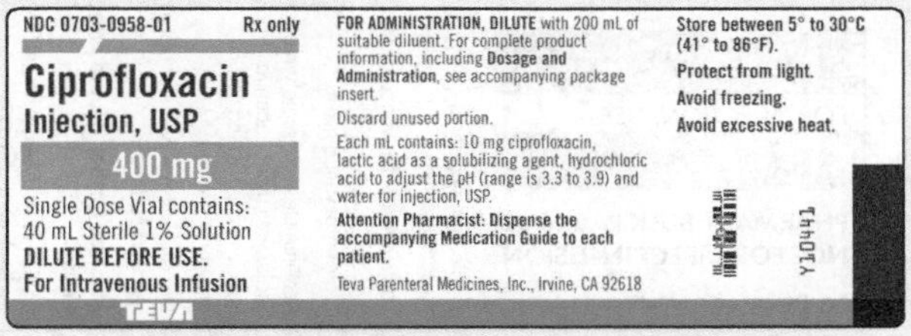


**FIGURE 5.3**

**Medication Label for Ciprofloxacin**

### Ratio and Proportion Example—Scenario One

The prescriber has written a medication order to administer 200 mg of ciprofloxacin IVPB. The label on the vial shows that you have a stock medication of ciprofloxacin with a concentration of 400 mg of ciprofloxacin in 40 mL of solution (see Figures 5.3 and 5.4).

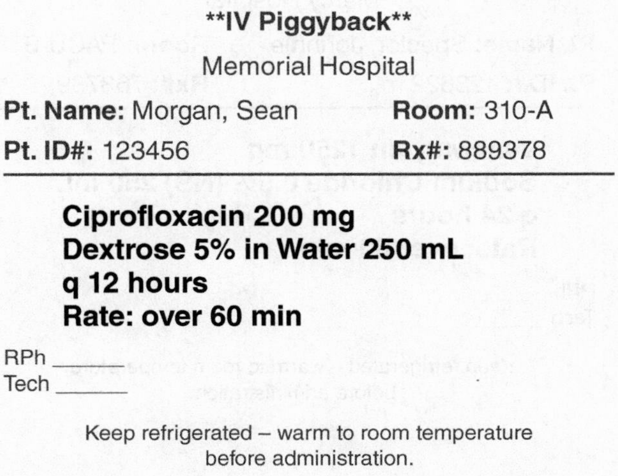

**IV Piggyback**
Memorial Hospital
Pt. Name: Morgan, Sean
Room: 310-A
Pt. ID#: 123456
Rx#: 889378
Ciprofloxacin 200 mg
Dextrose 5% in Water 250 mL
q 12 hours
Rate: over 60 min
RPh ______
Tech ______
Keep refrigerated – warm to room temperature before administration.


**FIGURE 5.4**

**CSP Label for Ciprofloxacin**

In this instance, the concentration on hand (H mg/Y mL) is 400 mg per 40 mL. The desired dose (D mg) is 200 mg. The unknown volume of the desired dose is $x$ mL. Using this information, set up a proportion:

$$\frac{400 \text{ mg}}{40 \text{ mL}} = \frac{200 \text{ mg}}{x \text{ mL}}$$

$H$ = 400 mg
$Y$ = 40 mL
$D$ = 200 mg
$x$ = ? mL

$40 \times 200 = 8000$
$8000/400 = 20$
**$x$ = 20 mL**

*Answer:* *The amount of ciprofloxacin that must be drawn up to provide a 200-mg dose is 20 mL.*

**Ratio and Proportion Example—Scenario Two** The prescriber has written a medication order to administer 1250 mg of vancomycin IVPB. You have on hand a 5-gram vial of vancomycin, and the label shows that, after reconstitution with 100 mL of sterile water, the concentration will be 500 mg/10 mL (see Figures 5.5 and 5.6).

*Note: For drugs that require reconstitution, you must first reconstitute the powder according to the manufacturer's directions. This information is provided on the medication label or in the drug's package insert. You should then use the concentration of the drug in its reconstituted (injectable) form to perform the calculation.*

**FIGURE 5.5**

**Medication Label for Vancomycin**

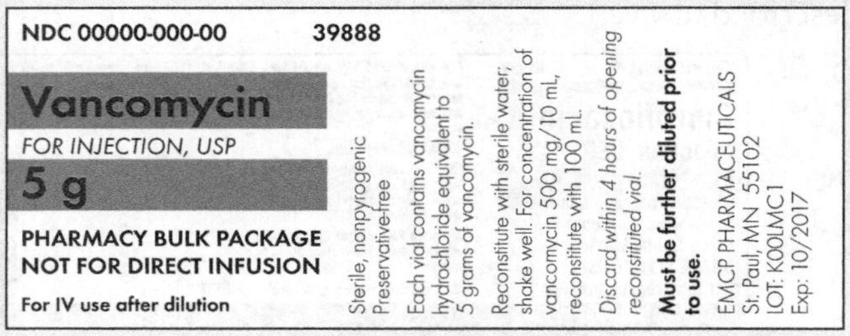


**FIGURE 5.6**

**CSP Label for Vancomycin**

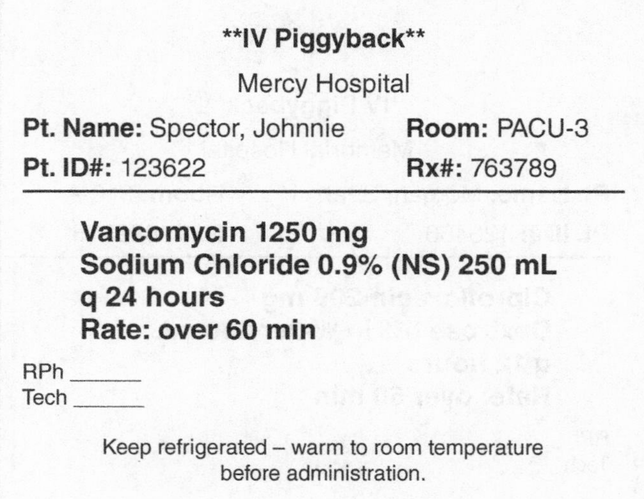

In this instance, the concentration on hand (H mg/Y mL) is 500 mg per 10 mL. The desired dose (D mg) is 1250 mg. The unknown volume of the desired dose is $x$ mL. Using this information, set up a proportion:

$$\frac{500\text{ mg}}{10\text{ mL}} = \frac{1250\text{ mg}}{x\text{ mL}}$$

$$H = 500\text{ mg}$$
$$Y = 10\text{ mL}$$
$$D = 1250\text{ mg}$$
$$x = ?\text{ mL}$$

$$1250 \times 10 = 12{,}500$$
$$12{,}500/500 = x$$
$$x = 25\text{ mL}$$

*Answer: The amount of vancomycin that must be drawn up to provide a 1250-mg dose is 25 mL.*

**Ratio and Proportion Example—Scenario Three** The prescriber has written a medication order to administer a single dose of tobramycin that is to be 2 mg/kg of the patient's body weight. The medication order indicates that the patient weighs 150 pounds. The label on the vial of tobramycin indicates that the concentration of the drug is 80 mg/2 mL (see Figures 5.7 and 5.8).

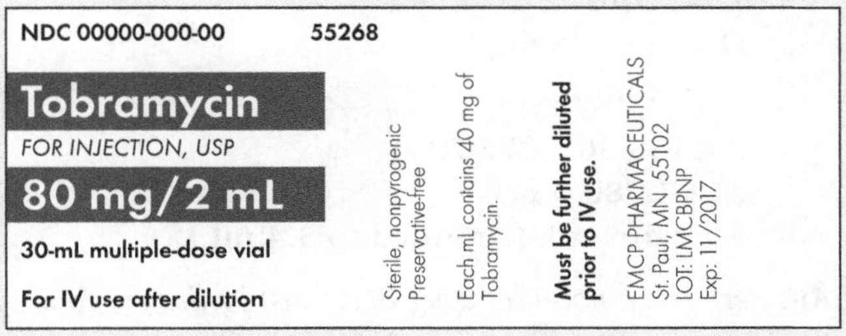


**FIGURE 5.7**

**Medication Label for Tobramycin**

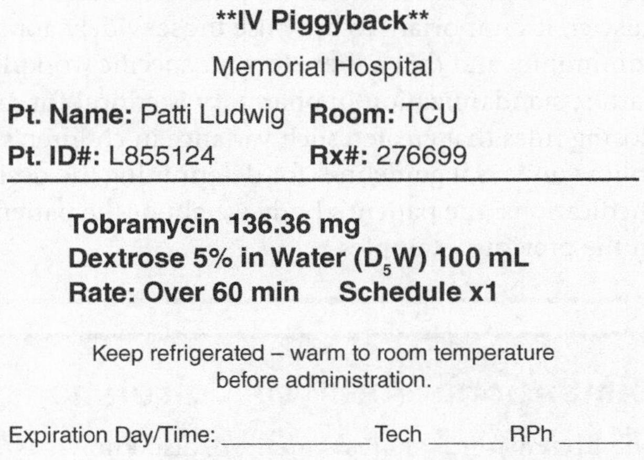
**IV Piggyback**
Memorial Hospital
Pt. Name: Patti Ludwig Room: TCU
Pt. ID#: L855124 Rx#: 276699
Tobramycin 136.36 mg
Dextrose 5% in Water (D5W) 100 mL
Rate: Over 60 min Schedule x1
Keep refrigerated – warm to room temperature before administration.
Expiration Day/Time: ________ Tech ______ RPh ______

**FIGURE 5.8**

**CSP Label for Tobramycin**

In order to determine this dose, you must perform several calculations to resolve the final amount of drug to draw up to prepare the CSP. First, you must determine the patient's weight in kilograms (kg). (Refer to Table 5.2 for the conversion factor from pounds [lbs] to kilograms [kg].) Then, you must determine the desired dose based on the patient's weight in kg. Finally, you must determine the amount of tobramycin to draw up to prepare a CSP that delivers the correct dose.

**POINTER**

To provide greater ease in calculating and preparing CSPs for adult patients, prescribers will often round medication dosages to the nearest tenth. For example, the dosage on the CSP label for tobramycin (see Figure 5.8) would be rounded to 140 mg. However, for the purposes of learning about ratio and proportion calculations, the CSP medication dosage will be exact and not rounded.

1. Solve for $x$ to determine the patient's weight in kilograms:

$$\frac{1 \text{ kg}}{2.2 \text{ lb}} = \frac{x \text{ kg}}{150 \text{ lb}}$$

$1 \times 150 = 150$
$150/2.2 = x$
**$x$ = 68.18 kg** (the patient's weight in kilograms)

2. Determine the desired dose by multiplying the prescriber-ordered amount (2 mg) by the patient's weight (68.18 kg).

$2 \times 68.18 =$ **136.36 mg** (the desired dose)

3. Finally, use ratio and proportion calculation to determine the amount of drug to be drawn up for the CSP:

$$\frac{80 \text{ mg}}{2 \text{ mL}} = \frac{136.36 \text{ mg}}{x \text{ mL}}$$

H = 80 mg
Y = 2 mL
D = 136.36 mg
$x$ = ? mL

$2 \times 136.36 = 272.72$
$272.72/80 = x$
**$x$ = 3.409 mL (rounded to 3.4 mL)**

***Answer:*** *The amount of drug that must be drawn up to prepare a CSP delivering 80 mg of tobramycin is 3.4 mL.*

Although there are many calculations that can be used to arrive at the same answer, it's important to only use those widely approved by the pharmacy community and that adhere to your specific workplace standards. As stated earlier, standardization in pharmacy is critical for safe practice. Unlike the past dosing rules that created such variance in children's doses, prescribers now follow universal guidelines for determining the desired dose of parenteral medications: the patient's body weight or the patient's BSA, as demonstrated in the previous examples.

## Dimensional Analysis Calculations

The **dimensional analysis method**, also known as "calculation by cancellation," is another approach that some IV technicians prefer to use when a dosage calculation involves multiple steps. This method is based on the principle that any number can be multiplied by one without changing its value.

Unlike the basic formula and ratio and proportion methods, the dimensional analysis method is not based on a set formula. To solve a pharmacy calculation problem using this method, IV technicians must first determine the answer that is needed, and then use the values provided in the text to perform a series of calculations. This mathematical process reveals the missing values necessary to arrive at a solution.

The dimensional analysis method for solving pharmacy dosage calculations is best used in sterile compounding scenarios that meet either of the following criteria:

- To determine the volume of drug needed to prepare the CSP, the IV technician must answer several questions by performing multiple calculations.
- The IV technician must make one or more conversions between various units of measure.

  *Example:* The prescriber has written a medication order that asks for a vancomycin dose of 100 mg/kg for a patient who weighs 150 lbs, requiring a conversion from a household system of measurement to a metric system of measurement.

***Performing a Dimensional Analysis Calculation*** A typical way to set up a dimensional analysis equation is to put the unknown quantity (the *x* you want to define) on its own on the left side of the equation, followed by an equal sign. On the right side, record a series of ratios, using both standard equivalents from Table 5.2 and information provided by the medication label (such as the drug concentration in mg/mL) and the CSP label (such as the desired dose in mg). You then multiply the ratios together to provide the answer to the problem.

**POINTER**

To be accurate and clear when using the dimensional analysis method, sterile compounding personnel should always write down the abbreviations for the units (mg, mEq, mL, etc.) when recording numbers.

The unit of measure in the **numerator** of the first ratio must be the same as the unit of measure you are solving, and the unit of measure in each successive numerator must match the unit of measure in the preceding **denominator**. As a result of this setup, the units of measure in each alternate numerator–denominator will cancel out, such that the only unit of measure remaining is the one you must solve. To illustrate how to solve a problem using dimensional analysis, look at the following example, which uses the information presented in the Ratio and Proportion Example—Scenario Three but performs the calculations using this alternative method.

**DIMENSIONAL ANALYSIS EXAMPLE** The prescriber has written a medication order to administer a single dose of tobramycin, to be dosed at 2 mg/kg of the patient's body weight. The medication order also indicates that the patient weighs 150 lbs. The label on the vial of tobramycin states that the concentration of the drug is 80 mg/2 mL.

1. In this scenario, the unknown quantity is *x* mL. Set that up on the left side of the equation, followed by the equal sign:

   $x \text{ mL} =$

2. The first ratio on the right must have mL in its numerator. Looking at the problem, you see that the concentration in the vial is 80 mg/2 mL. Enter that information by inverting the fraction so that mL appears in the numerator.

   $$x \text{ mL} = \frac{2 \text{ mL}}{80 \text{ mg}}$$

3. The next ratio must contain mg in its numerator. Look at the problem again. The ordered dose is 2 mg/kg, so plug in those numbers and units to form the next ratio:

$$x \text{ mL} = \frac{2 \text{ mL}}{80 \text{ mg}} \times \frac{2 \text{ mg}}{1 \text{ kg}}$$

4. Now continue plugging in more ratios. First, turn to Table 5.2 to determine the conversion factor used to convert pounds to kilograms; plug that ratio into the formula. Next, place the remaining information (in this case, 150 lbs) into the formula.

$$x \text{ mL} = \frac{2 \text{ mL}}{80 \text{ mg}} \times \frac{2 \text{ mg}}{1 \text{ kg}} \times \frac{1 \text{ kg}}{2.2 \text{ lbs}} \times \frac{150 \text{ lbs}}{1}$$

5. Now, cancel out like terms:

$$x \text{ mL} = \frac{2 \text{ mL}}{80 \cancel{\text{mg}}} \times \frac{2 \cancel{\text{mg}}}{1 \cancel{\text{kg}}} \times \frac{1 \cancel{\text{kg}}}{2.2 \cancel{\text{lbs}}} \times \frac{150 \cancel{\text{lbs}}}{1}$$

6. Multiply all numerators together and all denominators together, which results in the following equation:

$$x \text{ mL} = \frac{600 \text{ mL}}{176}$$

7. Divide the numerator by the denominator.

$x$ **= 3.4 mL**

***Answer:*** *The amount of drug that must be drawn up to prepare a CSP delivering 80 mg of tobramycin is 3.4 mL.*

## IV Flow Rate Calculations

In addition to compounding newly ordered CSPs, the IV technician is also responsible for preparing all of the CSPs needed for all patients in designated facilities for a specified period of time. This responsibility may be called the **daily IV run**, or the **batch**, and typically requires the IV technician to compound a 24-hour supply of CSPs for each patient.

To determine how many LVPs are needed for a 24-hour batch period for an individual patient, the IV technician frequently uses one of several types of IV flow rate calculations to determine the answer to one or more of the following questions:

- How long will this bag last (i.e., how many hours before this bag runs dry and a new one is needed)?
- What time will the next bag be needed?
- How many bags will be needed for the patient for a 24-hour period?

These questions may all be solved using IV flow rate calculations that employ simple addition, division, and/or multiplication. The answers provide the information that the IV technician needs to prepare the correct number of CSPs for a 24-hour batch period.

Unlike the basic formula and ratio and proportion methods, IV flow rate calculations are not based on a set formula. To solve a pharmacy calculation problem using this method, IV technicians must first determine the answer needed and then use the values provided in the text to perform a series of calculations. This mathematical process reveals the missing values necessary to arrive at a solution.

The three methods for solving IV flow rate questions are best used in sterile compounding scenarios that meet the following criteria:

- The infusion rate in mL/hour is provided on the medication order or CSP label.
- The total volume is provided on the medication order or CSP label.
- The current time is known or may be easily determined.

***Performing an IV Flow Rate Calculation*** The answers to the three questions posed on the previous page can be determined by setting up a division or multiplication problem. When calculating IV flow rates, you must know the total volume of the LVP and either 1) the infusion rate in milliliters per hour (mL/hr) or 2) the number of hours over which the LVP is to be infused. This information can be found on the medication order or the CSP label.

*Note:* Depending on the medication order, you may need to convert from liters (L) to milliliters (mL) prior to performing the calculations below.

**POINTER**

As a general rule, complete any necessary metric conversions so that you are working with similar units when performing pharmacy calculations.

IV Flow Rate Example Use this example to answer each of the following questions: The medication order indicates that the prescriber has ordered a continuous infusion of dextrose 5% in water ($D_5W$) at 125 mL/hour, and the pharmacy will provide the solution in 1000-mL bags.

**How long will this bag last?** To answer this question, perform the following calculation: Divide the total volume (TV) by the infusion rate (IR). The total volume of the LVP in this scenario is 1000 mL. The infusion rate is 125 mL/hour.

TV = 1000 mL
IR = 125 mL/hour
$x$ = number of hours the bag will last

$1000/125 = x$
**$x$ = 8 hours**

***Answer:*** *The answer to the question—"How long will this bag last?"—is 8 hours.*

**What time will the next bag be needed?** To answer this question, perform the following calculations:

1. First, determine how long the bag will last. Do this by performing the same calculation you did to answer the first question: Divide the total volume (TV) by the infusion rate (IR). The total volume of the LVP is 1000 mL. The infusion rate is 125 mL/hour.

   TV = 1000 mL
   IR = 125 mL/hour
   $x$ = number of hours the bag will last

   $1000/125 = x$
   **$x$ = 8 hours**

2. Then add the number of hours that you calculated in step 1 (8 hours) to the current standard time. For the purposes of this example, assume that the current time is 1:00 p.m.

   1:00 p.m. + 8 hours = 9:00 p.m.

***Answer:*** *The answer to the question—"What time will the next bag be needed?"—is 9:00 p.m. (2100 hours in military time).*

**How many bags will be needed for the patient in a 24-hour period?** To answer this question, perform the following calculations:

1. First, determine how long the bag will last. Do this by performing the same calculation you did to answer the first question: Divide the total volume (TV) by the infusion rate (IR). The total volume of the LVP is 1000 mL. The infusion rate is 125 mL/hour.

   TV = 1000 mL
   IR = 125 mL/hour
   $x$ = number of hours the bag will last

   $1000/125 = x$
   **$x$ = 8 hours**

2. Then, divide 24 (the number of hours in a day) by your answer to the previous question (the number of hours the bag will last).

   $24/8 = x$
   $x = 3$

***Answer:*** *The answer to the question—"How many bags will be needed for the patient in a 24-hour period?"—is 3 bags.*

## IV Drip Rate Calculations

To determine an IV rate calculation utilizing an IV tubing drop factor, sterile compounding personnel frequently use the IV drip rate method, more commonly known as the **drop factor method**. This method relies on the specific **drop factor** (gtts/mL), or the number of drops per milliliter, that a certain type of IV tubing delivers. Each of the different types of IV tubing delivers a different drop factor. For instance, **macrodrip IV tubing** may deliver either 10 gtts/mL or 20 gtts/mL, whereas **microdrip IV tubing** delivers 60 gtts/mL. An equation using drop factor is sometimes called an **IV drip rate calculation**.

Unlike the basic formula and ratio and proportion methods, IV drip rate calculations are not based on a set formula. To solve a pharmacy calculation problem using this method, IV technicians must first determine the answer that is needed and then use the values provided in the text to perform a series of calculations. This mathematical process reveals the missing values necessary to arrive at a solution.

The drop factor method for solving pharmacy dosage calculations is best used in sterile compounding situations that meet the following criteria:

- The total volume to be infused is known (i.e., provided by the medication order or CSP label).
- The total infusion time (the amount of time, in minutes, over which the entire volume of the LVP will be administered to the patient) is known.
- The drop factor of the IV tubing is known.
- The desired answer is to be provided in drops per minute (gtts/min).

***Performing an IV Drip Rate Calculation*** An IV drip rate calculation can be determined by setting up a modified ratio and proportion equation using information provided in the medication order. Answers to IV drip rate questions also require the IV tubing's drop factor, which is provided on the tubing's outer packaging. When calculating IV drip rates, you must know the total volume of the LVP, the infusion time (in minutes), and the IV tubing's drop factor. Your answer determines how many *drops per minute* will be administered to the patient.

IV drip rate problems can be solved using the following drop factor calculation:

$$\frac{\text{total volume in mL}}{\text{infusion time in minutes}} \times \text{drop factor} = \frac{\text{drops}}{\text{minute}}$$

*Note:* Depending on the medication order, you may need to convert from hours to minutes prior to performing the calculations below.

**IV Drip Rate Calculation Example** Use the following example to answer each of the following questions: The medication order indicates that the prescriber has ordered normal saline (NS) 500 mL with 25,000 units of heparin to be infused over 8 hours. The IV tubing's outer packaging indicates that the tubing is microdrip and has a drop factor of 60 gtts/mL (see Figures 5.9 and 5.10 on the following page).

**FIGURE 5.9**

**Medication Label for Heparin**

NDC 00000-000-00 54568

**Heparin**

FOR INJECTION, USP

**10,000 units/mL**

**5-mL multiple-dose vial**

**NOT FOR IV PUSH USE**

**For IV use after dilution**

Sterile, nonpyrogenic
Bacteriostatic solution

Each mL contains 10,000
units of heparin for injection.

**Must be further diluted
prior to IV use.**

EMCP PHARMACEUTICALS
St. Paul, MN 55102
LOT: BPNPLMC1
Exp: 09/2017

**FIGURE 5.10**

**CSP Label for Heparin**

****IV Drip****

Memorial Hospital

**Pt. Name:** McQueen, Tina **Room:** 511

**Pt. ID#:** 9883722 **Rx#:** 676399

**Heparin 25,000 units**
**Sodium Chloride 0.9% (NS) 500 mL**
**Rate: 62.5 gtts/minute**

Keep refrigerated – warm to room temperature before administration.

Expiration Day/Time: ________ Tech ______ RPh ______

1. First, convert from hours to minutes:
   8 (hours) × 60 (minutes in one hour) = 480 minutes
2. Next, set up the equation using the information provided in the medication order and on the IV tubing's outer packaging:

$$\frac{500}{480} = 1.042$$

$$1.042 \times 60 = x$$

$$\mathbf{x = 62.5 \text{ gtts/min}}$$

***Answer:*** *The number of drops per minute needed to administer this dose of heparin at the prescribed rate using microdrip tubing with a drop factor of 60 gtts/mL is 62.5 (62.5 gtts/min).*

## Alligation Calculations

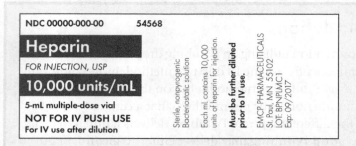

Occasionally, a prescriber will write a prescription for a medication strength that is not commercially available, or that is not kept on hand in the pharmacy. In these instances, the pharmacy may be required to mix two different strengths of the same active ingredient of a drug or solution to make the **desired strength**. A **higher-percent strength** of a drug or solution is mixed with a **lower-percent strength** of a drug or solution in order to make the desired strength, which falls somewhere between the two extremes. This scenario requires you to employ a calculation called the **alligation method**, or simply *alligation*. Alligations are rarely performed by IV technicians, but you will need to carry out this kind of calculation from time to time.

The alligation method of solving pharmacy dosage calculations is best used in compounding situations that meet the following criteria:

- Two or more strengths of the same active ingredient or solution *must* be used to prepare the desired strength of a drug or solution.
- The desired strength of the drug or solution is known (from the medication order or CSP label).
- The total volume of the CSP is known (from the medication order or CSP label).

***Performing an Alligation Calculation*** To understand how to set up an alligation problem, refer to Figure 5.11 below. Use this grid as your template for the scenario that follows.

| | | |
|---|---|---|
| A | | D<br>(the difference of B – C) |
| | B | |
| C | | E<br>(the difference of A – B) |

**FIGURE 5.11**

**Tic-Tac-Toe Alligation Grid**

KEY
A = higher concentration or strength (stated as a percent [%])
B = desired concentration or strength (stated as a percent [%])
C = lower concentration or strength (stated as a percent [%])

#### Alligation Example

The CSP label shown in Figure 5.12 indicates that the prescriber has ordered 250 mL of dextrose 7% in water ($D_7W$). In your pharmacy, you have both dextrose 5% in water ($D_5W$) and dextrose 70% in water ($D_{70}W$). Since the value of 7 falls between 5 and 70, you can use these two strengths to make the 7% you need.

****IV Solution – LVP****

Mercy Hospital

**Pt. Name:** Werekela, Francis **Room:** PICU-4
**ID#:** 543678 **Rx#:** 420883

**Dextrose 7% in Water ($D_7W$) 250 mL**
**Rate: 10 mL/hr**

Keep refrigerated – warm to room temperature before administration.

Expiration Day/Time: __________ Tech ______ RPh ______

**FIGURE 5.12**

**CSP Label for Dextrose**

The problem asks you to determine how much $D_5W$ (dextrose concentration of 5% [see Figure 5.13]) and $D_{70}W$ (dextrose concentration of 70% [see Figure 5.14]) must be combined to make a solution of $D_7W$ (dextrose concentration of 7%) and a total volume of 250 mL for IV administration.

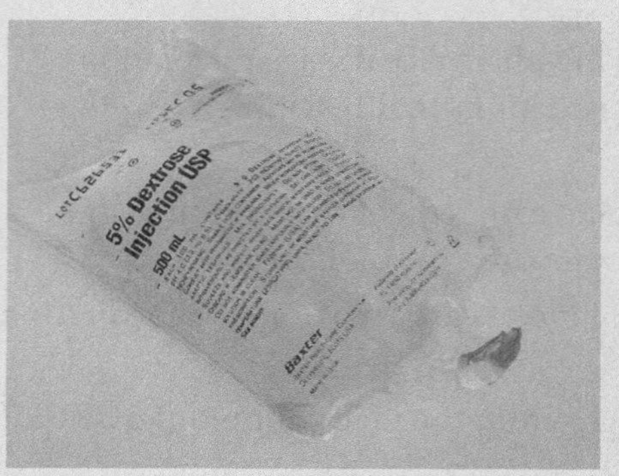


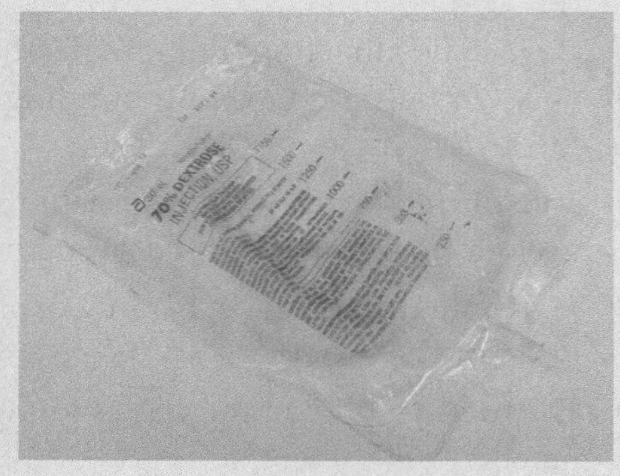

**FIGURE 5.13** (left)
**$D_5W$ 500-mL bag**

**FIGURE 5.14** (right)
**$D_{70}W$ 2000-mL bag**

1. Identify the variables by determining the component concentrations: The desired concentration (B%) is what the prescriber has written on the medication order and, therefore, is indicated on the CSP label. The higher concentration (A%) and lower concentration (C%) are determined by the stock IV base solution strengths on hand in your pharmacy. In this case, the desired concentration is 7%; the higher concentration is 70%; and the lower concentration is 5%.
2. Using the alligation template from Figure 5.11, fill in the concentration strengths (given as percentages) in the Key section below the tic-tac-toe grid. Place those same strengths in their designated squares on the grid.

| | | |
|---|---|---|
| A (higher %)<br>70 | | D (parts of higher %; the difference of B – C) |
| | B (desired %)<br>7 | |
| C (lower %)<br>5 | | E (parts of lower %; the difference of A – B) |

KEY
A% = 70
B% = 7
C% = 5
D (parts of 70% solution) =
E (parts of 5% solution) =

3. To find the value of D in the upper right square, set up the equation B – C = D. Then fill in the values for B and C (found in step 2) in the equation, as shown below:

7 – 5 = D
D = 2 (or the number of parts of 70% dextrose)

Record the number 2 in the key and in the upper right square.

4. To find the value of E in the lower right square, set up the equation A – B = E. Then fill in the values for A and B (found in step 2) in the equation, as shown below:

   70 – 7 = E
   E = 63 (or the number of parts of 5% dextrose)

   Record the number 63 in the key and in the lower right square.

5. Check that your completed grid now resembles the grid shown below:

| | | |
|---|---|---|
| A (higher %)<br>70 | | D (parts of higher %)<br>2 |
| | B (desired %)<br>7 | |
| C (lower%)<br>5 | | E (parts of lower %)<br>63 |

   KEY
   A% = 70
   B% = 7
   C% = 5
   D (parts of 70% solution) = 2
   E (parts of 5% solution) = 63

6. Set up a ratio using the values of D and E as shown in the right-hand column of your completed grid:

$$\frac{D}{E} = \frac{2}{63}$$

   This ratio indicates that in order to prepare the desired concentration (in this case, a D7% solution), dextrose 70% ($D_{70}W$) and dextrose 5% ($D_5W$) must be mixed in a 2:63 ratio: 2 parts of D70% and 63 parts of D5%.

7. Using the ratio from step 6, add together D and E to obtain the total number of parts (TP):

   D + E = TP

   2 + 63 = TP

   65 = TP

8. Now you need to determine the exact volume of each component needed to prepare 250 mL of $D_7W$. Because you already know the ratio in which the parts must be combined and the total number of parts, you can set up a ratio and proportion problem.

   To find the volume of $D_{70}W$ needed for the CSP, use the following formula:

$$\frac{D}{TP} = \frac{x}{TV}$$

D = parts of the higher % solution
TP = total number of parts
TV = total volume of desired concentration

$$\frac{2}{65} = \frac{x}{250 \text{ mL}}$$

Cross-multiply: $2 \times 250 = 500$
Divide: $500/65 = x$
$x = 7.69$ mL (rounded to 7.7 mL) of $D_{70}W$

9. To find the volume of $D_5W$ needed for the CSP, use the following formula:

$$\frac{E}{TP} = \frac{x}{TV}$$

E = parts of the lower % solution

TP = total number of parts

TV = total volume of desired concentration

$$\frac{63}{65} = \frac{x}{250 \text{ mL}}$$

Cross-multiply: $63 \times 250 = 15750$
Divide: $15750/65 = x$
$x = 242.30$ mL (rounded to 242.3 mL) of $D_5W$

10. To verify the volume of each component (determined in steps 8 and 9), add the volumes of the two components. Your answer should equal the total volume of the desired concentration.

    7.7 mL ($D_{70}W$) + 242.3 mL ($D_5W$) = 250 mL (total volume of desired concentration)

## Calculation Skills in the Sterile Compounding Environment

In sterile compounding, accurate calculation and measurement of the components or ingredients of the formulation are critical, for even minor errors could lead to potentially harmful medication errors. In order to achieve consistent, accurate CSPs, the pharmacy technician must have an understanding of historical practices and a working knowledge of current systems of measurement and pharmacy calculations. She or he must also have an excellent understanding of basic math principles—including addition, subtraction, multiplication, and division of fractions, decimals, and percentages—and should have completed a course in pharmaceutical mathematics. Having this math background is necessary before taking a class or workshop in sterile compounding and aseptic technique, an area of pharmacy that requires advanced knowledge in pharmacy calculations and formulas.

# Concepts Self-Check

## Check Your Understanding

*Write your answers on a separate sheet of paper, as modeled in these examples:* 1d; 2c; 3b; *etc. Check your answers using the Answer Key in Appendix A.*

**1.** Which of the following scenarios best describes the criteria in which ratio and proportion might be used to solve a sterile compounding calculation question?

a. The drug is supplied in a powdered form that must be reconstituted prior to use.
b. The drug's concentration is 1000 mg/10 mL.
c. The dosage calculation problem requires that more than one calculation must be performed in order to determine the dose.
d. any of the above

**2.** Which of the following scenarios best describes the criteria in which the basic formula might be used to solve a sterile compounding calculation question?

a. The drug is in an injectable form.
b. The concentration of the drug is 100 mg/1 mL.
c. The concentration of the drug is 100 mg/2 mL.
d. both *a* and *b*
e. both *a* and *c*

**3.** Which of the following items on a medication order is the best indication that dimensional analysis is an appropriate method for solving the pharmacy equation?

a. The technician must convert between various units of measure.
b. The drop factor is 20 gtts/mL.
c. The infusion rate is 50 mL/hr.
d. The drug must be reconstituted prior to use.

**4.** Which two pieces of information are necessary to determine how long an IV bag will last?

a. the LVP's total volume and the infusion rate
b. the LVP's total volume and the dosing interval
c. the drug's dosage and strength
d. the drug's dosage and volume

**5.** Which two items must be compared to verify for accuracy, prior to the start of the sterile compounding process?

a. the medication order and the CSP label
b. the medication order and the manufacturer's drug label
c. the manufacturer's drug label and the CSP label
d. the CSP label and the SVP label

## Apply Your Knowledge

*On a separate sheet of paper, write your answers to the questions posed in the paragraph below. Use complete sentences and take time to create a thorough and thoughtful response. Check your answers against the Answer Key in Appendix A.*

In Part 1 of this chapter, you learned that verifying and double-checking the accuracy of pharmacy calculations help to ensure patient health and safety. With that in mind, what would you do in the following scenario: You have received an order for $D_5NS$ 1 L with 40 mEq of KCl. Because potassium chloride is a common additive used in sterile compounding, you know that the concentration of potassium chloride is 2 mEq/mL. Having this familiarity with the medication, you wonder if you should still check the medication label to verify its concentration. Should you verify the medication's concentration? Why or why not?

# Part 2: Training

## Examine the Resources and Supplies

### Identifying Drug Information on the Medication Order

**POINTER**
Be sure to memorize all the information in Appendix B. You must know this information to accurately read and interpret medication orders, CSP labels, and medication labels.

Prior to performing the pharmacy calculations needed for the sterile compounding process, an IV technician must draw upon his or her knowledge of medication orders and labeling. Chapter 4 provides an in-depth introduction to medical terminology, abbreviations and acronyms, pharmacy symbols, signa language, and the components of the medication order. To accompany this background information, Appendix B offers a series of tables that list examples of the specialized pharmacy "language" seen on medication orders and labeling and in the communications among pharmacy personnel. IV technicians should become familiar with the information on these tables in order to perform sterile compounding tasks safely and effectively.

Moreover, the IV technician must also be familiar with the brand and generic names of the drugs frequently used in sterile compounding (see Table 13 of Appendix B) as well as the common IV base solutions and IVPB fluids central to the compounding procedures (see Chapter 3). Memorizing these parenteral medications and solutions helps in the identification and understanding of these drugs on a medication order.

In addition to identifying common parenteral drugs and solutions, sterile compounding personnel need to be familiar with other components of the medication order, including dosage, dosing interval, and route of administration for each medication on the order. Looking for words or abbreviations that identify a number, dose, volume, amount, or route can help in identifying the medications needed for sterile compounding (see Tables 5.5 and 5.6).

**Table 5.5 Words, Abbreviations, and Symbols that Identify Drug Dose**

| | |
|---|---|
| Gram | g, G |
| Liter | L |
| Microgram | mcg |
| Milliequivalent | mEq |
| Milligram | mg |
| Milliliter | mL |
| Millimole | mm |
| Million units | MU* |
| Percent | % |
| Units | U |

*As an IV technician, you should be familiar with this abbreviation. However, be aware that the Joint Commission has placed this abbreviation on its Official "Do Not Use" List of Abbreviations due to its high potential for medication error. If you receive a medication order with this abbreviation, seek clarification from the prescriber to ensure accuracy.

**Table 5.6 Words, Abbreviations, and Symbols that Identify Routes of Administration**

| | |
|---|---|
| Intramuscular | IM |
| Intrathecal | IT |
| Intravenous | IV |
| Intravenous piggyback | IVPB |
| Intravenous push | IVP |
| Irrigation | Irr. |
| Subcutaneous | SQ; sub-Q; SC |

Once the IV technician identifies the medications on the order that require sterile compounding, he or she enters the information into the pharmacy computer system. A label is then printed for each dose of the CSP.

***Note:** Pharmacy order entry and label generation may be done by the pharmacist or a specially trained technician. For the purposes of this lab, you will practice with the medication order and labels included in the lab portion of this chapter.*

## Comparing the CSP Label to the Medication Order

To help ensure patient safety, every CSP label must be compared to the medication order to verify that the label is 100% accurate. The IV technician usually completes this comparison just prior to gathering the necessary sterile compounding supplies. However, this step is sometimes done by a pharmacist prior to giving the verified CSP label to the IV technician for compounding. It is considered best practice to have both the pharmacist and the IV technician confirm that the CSP label matches the medication order. Involving two people in this verification process provides a valuable double check, which greatly reduces the possibility of a medication error.

In order to verify that the CSP label and the medication order match exactly, the IV technician should perform the verification process using the same method, in the same order, each time the verification process is performed. First, the IV technician should verify that the patient's name (including the spelling) and room number (location) are identical on both the medication order and the CSP label. Next, the IV technician should confirm that the drug name and desired dose match exactly. The IV technician must then confirm that the route of administration and either the dosing interval (for IVPB, IM, SQ, or IV push administration) or the infusion rate (for IV administration) are the same on both the medication order and the CSP label. Once all of the parenteral medications on the medication order have been matched and verified with the corresponding CSP label, the IV technician should retrieve the medication or medications in order to proceed to the next step in the procedure: reading the information on the medication label.

**POINTER**

If the medication label does not provide reconstitution information, consult the package insert provided by the manufacturer.

## Reading the Medication Label

Manufacturers most often provide the medications used in sterile compounding in either a vial or an ampule. Medications in these types of containers may be in liquid or powdered form. Parenteral medications in liquid form are considered to be injectable and do not need reconstitution, whereas parenteral medications in a powdered form are not injectable and must be reconstituted prior to use.

Regardless of the type or content of the medication's container, each drug used in sterile compounding has a label that identifies the drug name, strength, concentration, manufacturer's name, expiration date, and lot number. In addition, some powdered medications will include instructions for reconstituting the powder. As an IV technician, review the information in Figure 5.1 to identify the components of a medication label. You must carefully read the medication label information to determine the concentration (usually in mg/mL) of the drug in order to perform the necessary calculations.

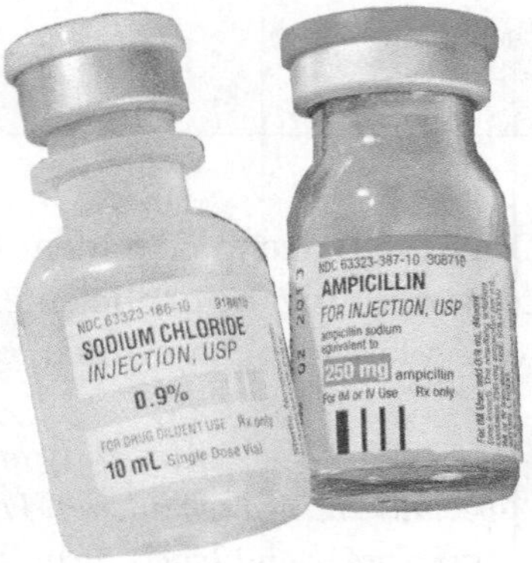


## Choosing a Calculation Method

Once you have identified the medications that require sterile compounding, verified that the CSP label is accurate, and determined the concentration of the medication that you need to use in preparing the CSP, you must then choose a calculation method. The calculation method used depends on the information provided in the medication order, on the CSP label, and on the medication label. In most cases, you will be required to determine the number of milliliters of injectable medication you must draw up to provide the desired dose.

Refer to the criteria for each calculation method (outlined in Part 1 of this chapter) to determine which method should be used to perform the calculation. Possible methods for calculating pharmacy sterile compounding problems include the basic formula, ratio and proportion, dimensional analysis, IV flow rate, IV drop factor, and alligations. For the purpose of this exercise, you will use the medication order, CSP label, and medication label provided in the lab section of this chapter to determine which calculation method to use.

## Performing the Calculation

In pharmacy, you must use the information provided by the prescriber to determine the required volume needed to prepare the CSP. You also need to review the medication and CSP labels.

Once you have determined the best method for solving this calculation, write the calculation down on a piece of paper. In order to perform accurate calculations, you must write down the equation and verify that you have the correct information in the correct place within the formula. Perform the calculation using the method that is most appropriate based on the criteria outlined in this chapter.

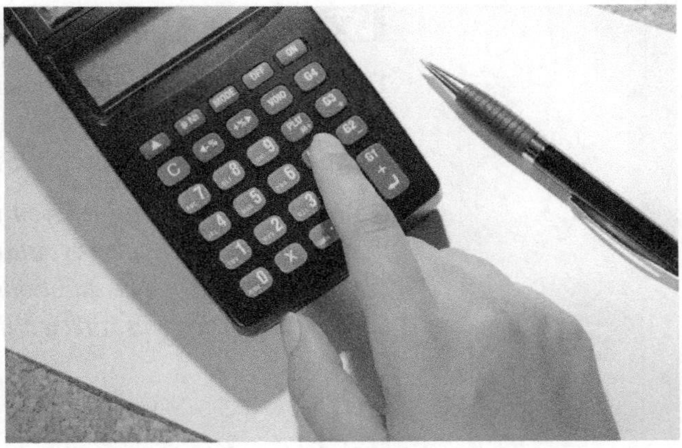

In the following lab scenario, you must determine the volume of potassium chloride that must be drawn up into a syringe in preparation for injection into a base solution of lactated Ringer's with a total volume of 1000 mL. In practice, once the volume of potassium chloride has been drawn up into a syringe and has been verified by a pharmacist, you will use aseptic technique to inject the medication into an IV bag. You will learn more about this part of the sterile compounding process in Chapters 8, 9, and 10 of this textbook.

**POINTER**

Many pharmacy computer programs automatically print the desired dosage volume of drug (i.e., the amount to draw up) on the CSP label. However, you must still verify the accuracy of the dosage volume by performing your own calculations. Never rely solely on the dosage volume information (sometimes called the mixing instructions) provided on the CSP label.

# Exploratory Lab

This exploratory lab helps you to identify and verify important medication information as well as perform pharmacy calculations to determine the amount of drug you must draw up to prepare a CSP.

*Note: Some of the steps ask you to read and respond to one or more multiple-choice questions (marked by numbers containing dashes, such as 1–1 and 1–2). Record your answers to these multiple-choice questions by either circling the correct answer on the page or turning in your answers as directed by your instructor.*

## Supplies

- Sample medication order (Figure 5.15)
- Sample CSP label (Figure 5.16)
- Sample drug vial label (Figure 5.17)
- Basic calculator
- Scratch paper and pencil

## Procedure

***Cross-checking the Medication Order and the CSP Label***

1. Review the medication order (see Figure 5.15) to determine the patient's name and room number (or location).
2. Check the CSP label (see Figure 5.16) to verify that the spelling of the patient's name and the patient's room number match the medication order exactly.
3. Scan the medication order to find the following order: IVF: LR w/KCl 20 mEq/L @ 150 mL/hr × 3 L.
4. Check the CSP label to verify that the label clearly indicates the drug name, strength, base solution name and volume, and infusion rate.

FIGURE 5.16

**CSP Label for Potassium Chloride (KCl) in Lactated Ringer's**

****IV Solution – LVP****

Mercy Hospital

**Pt. Name:** Tang, Phuong　　**Room:** 2235
**ID#:** D89257887901　　**Rx#:** 102387

**Potassium Chloride 20 mEq**
**Lactated Ringer's 1000 mL**
**Rate: 150 mL/hr**

Keep refrigerated – warm to room temperature before administration.

Expiration Day/Time: ____________ Tech ______ RPh ______

FIGURE 5.15 **Lab Procedure Medication Order**

**ID#:** D89257887901
**Name:** Tang, Phuong
**DOB:** 06/25/1950
**Room:** 2235
**Dr.:** Llewellyn, Douglas

**MERCY HOSPITAL**
**PHYSICIAN'S MEDICATION ORDER**

**BEAR DOWN ON HARD SURFACE WITH BALLPOINT PEN**

GENERIC EQUIVALENT IS AUTHORIZED UNLESS CHECKED IN THIS COLUMN

ALLERGY OR SENSITIVITY TO Bactrim, EES. Shellfish

NONE KNOWN ☐ SIGNED:

DIAGNOSIS: DKA, HTN

COMPLETED OR DISCONTINUED

| DATE | TIME | ORDERS | PHYSICIAN'S SIG. | NAME | DATE | TIME |
|---|---|---|---|---|---|---|
| | | **Routine Orders** | | | | |
| | | **Height** 5' 7" **Weight** 218 **lbs** | | | | |
| | | Labs: | | | | |
| | | Blood Glucose per home schedule | | | | |
| | | $O_2$ Sat per shift | | | | |
| | | CBC, chem. -7, lytes - NOW | | | | |
| | | | | | | |
| | | Resp. Care to evaluate in AM | | | | |
| | | I/S per shift | | | | |
| | | T.E.D. Stockings | | | | |
| | | | | | | |
| | | Temp, B/P, pulse q shift | | | | |
| | | | | | | |
| | | **Meds:** | | | | |
| | | Pepcid po bid (may give IVPB if not taking p.o. well) | | | | |
| | | SSI per home schedule | | | | |
| | | Norvasc 5 mg po bid (call HO for orders if NPO) | | | | |
| | | | | | | |
| | | IVF: LR w/ KCl 20 mEq/L @ 150 mL/hr × 3 L | | | | |
| | | | | | | |
| | | | Douglas Llewellyn | | | |

PHARMACY COPY

**5.** Answer the following multiple-choice questions, recording your answers as directed by your instructor.

**5–1.** Looking at the medication order, what base solution has the prescriber ordered?

a. potassium chloride
b. lactated Ringer's
c. 20 mEq
d. 150 mL/hr

**5–2.** Looking at the medication order, what is the volume of the base solution that the prescriber has ordered?

a. 150 mL
b. 1000 mL
c. 1 L
d. both *b* and *c* are correct

**5–3.** Looking at the CSP label, what is the name of the drug that the prescriber has ordered?

a. potassium chloride
b. lactated Ringer's
c. both *a* and *b* are correct
d. none of the above

**5–4.** Looking at the CSP label, what is the dose of the drug that the prescriber has ordered?

a. 150 mL
b. 1000 mL
c. 1 L
d. 20 mEq

**5–5.** Looking at the CSP label, what is the infusion rate that the prescriber has ordered?

a. 20 mEq per liter
b. lactated Ringer's 1000 mL
c. 150 mL per hour
d. 20 mL per liter

### *Reading the Drug Vial Label*

**6.** Carefully read the drug vial label, also known as the medication label, to determine the concentration of the medication in the container (see Figure 5.17).

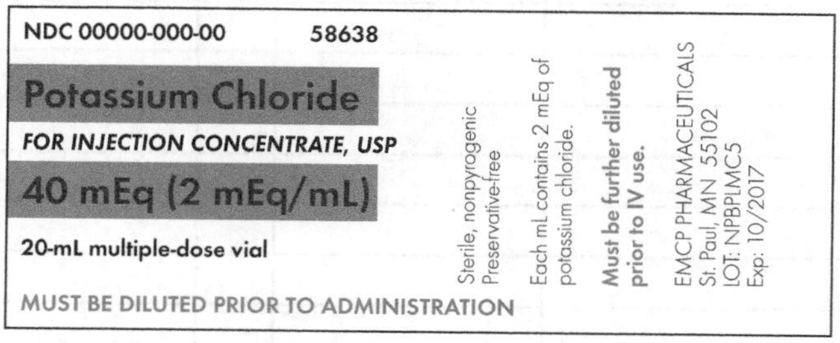


FIGURE 5.17
**Medication Label for Potassium Chloride**

7. Answer the following multiple-choice questions, recording your answers as directed by your instructor.

   7–1. Looking at the drug vial label, what is the name of the medication in the container?
   a. EMCP
   b. lactated Ringer's
   c. potassium chloride
   d. all of the above

   7–2. Looking at the drug vial label, what is the concentration of the medication in the container?
   a. 2 mEq/mL
   b. 20 mL
   c. 40 mEq
   d. all of the above

### *Determining Which Calculation Method to Use*

8. Review the criteria (provided earlier in this chapter) for using the following calculation methods: basic formula, ratio and proportion, dimensional analysis, IV flow rate, IV drop factor, and alligation.

9. Use the information provided on the CSP label and the medication label—along with the criteria for the various calculation methods—to determine which method is most appropriate for determining how much potassium chloride must be drawn up for this dose.

10. Answer the following multiple-choice question, recording your answer as directed by your instructor.

    10–1. Based on the criteria identified for each of the calculation methods, which calculation method is most appropriate for determining the volume of potassium chloride that must be drawn up to deliver a 20 mEq dose?
    a. ratio and proportion
    b. dimensional analysis
    c. IV drip rate
    d. basic formula

### *Performing the Calculation*

11. Once you have determined which method you will use, write the equation on a piece of paper.

12. Use a calculator to perform the calculation(s).

13. Answer the following multiple-choice questions, recording your answers as directed by your instructor.

13–1. Based on the medication label, what is the concentration on hand?

a. 2 mEq/mL
b. 20 mEq/mL
c. 4 mEq/mL
d. 40 mEq/mL

13–2. Based on the calculation that you performed, what is the volume of potassium chloride 2 mEq/mL that must be drawn up to prepare a CSP that delivers 20 mEq of potassium chloride?

a. 40 mL
b. 30 mL
c. 20 mL
d. 10 mL

# Part 3: Assessment

## Chapter Summary

- Prior to the 1800s, pharmacists and other practitioners mixed crude drugs on a trial-and-error basis often using unproven and imprecise formulas for drug compounding.
- The 1906 Pure Food and Drug Act was the first law that affected the practice of pharmacy by helping to ensure quality and purity of drug products.
- The 1938 Food, Drug, and Cosmetic Act set forth laws that required new drugs to be proven safe and effective prior to marketing. This law also established the Food and Drug Administration, which is the federal entity that oversees drug regulation in the United States.
- The apothecary, avoirdupois, and household systems of measure are now considered virtually obsolete for use in the area of pharmacy and medicine.
- Although the balance scale and spring scale have been used as measurement devices in medicine for centuries, today's healthcare practitioners rely on electronic scales to accurately deliver precise measurements.
- Clark's Rule, Fried's Rule, Cowling's Rule, and Young's Rule are no longer used in pediatric dosing due to the inconsistency of dosages determined by using these rules.
- The metric system is the preferred system of measurement used in pharmacy practice. This system is based on the decimal system and measures in increments of ten.
- In current practice, most medicine is ordered by the prescriber based on a patient's body weight or BSA.
- The primary use of BSA is for the calculation of chemotherapy doses by prescribers. In general, a pharmacy technician will not have to determine a dose based on BSA.
- The system used to solve any pharmacy calculation is determined by the compounding situation and the type of information that is desired, as well as the personal preference of the technician performing the calculation.
- Many pharmacy dosage calculations may be solved using the basic formula method, provided that the drug concentration on the label is in mg/1 mL (or units/1 mL). The basic formula is: D/H = $x$ mL.
- The ratio and proportion method is one of the most frequently used pharmacy calculation methods. This method is used whenever three of the four values in a proportion are known, thus allowing the technician to solve for the fourth, unknown value. The ratio and proportion formula is set up as:

$$\frac{\text{H mg}}{\text{Y mL}} = \frac{\text{D mg}}{x\text{ mL}}$$

$$\frac{\text{Y} \times \text{D}}{\text{H}} = x\text{ mL}$$

- Dimensional analysis is a modified ratio and proportion formula based on the understanding that multiplying any number by one does not change the value of the original number.
- Nurses sometimes calculate IV drip rates using the drop factor provided by the primary IV tubing.
- Most IV flow rate questions may be solved using simple addition, division, and/or multiplication.
- To determine how long an IV bag will last before it runs empty and a new bag is needed, use the following formula: TV/IR = $x$ hours.
- To determine what time the next IV bag will be needed, use the following formula:
  TV/IR = $x$ hours
  Determine the current time and count forward from that time the number of hours determined in $x$.

- To determine how many IV bags will be needed for an individual patient in a 24-hour period, use the following formula: TV/IR = $x$, then 24/$x$ = the number of bags needed for a 24-hour period.
- Most IV drip rate problems may be solved using the drop factor method, which is a modified ratio and proportion equation:

$$\frac{\text{total volume in mL}}{\text{infusion time in minutes}} \times \frac{\text{drop factor}}{\text{(of the tubing)}} = \frac{\text{drops}}{\text{minute}}$$

- The alligation method is rarely used by pharmacy technicians but serves to determine the volume (D, E) of two or more strengths (A, C) of a solution in order to create a different, desired strength (B). The alligation formula is:

| | | |
|---|---|---|
| Stronger % (A) | | B – C = D |
| | Desired % (B) | |
| Weaker % (C) | | A – B = E |

## Key Terms

**alligation method** a method of problem solving that may be used to find the amount of each ingredient needed to make a mixture of a given quantity of drug; a method of solving math problems related to the mixture of two ingredients; also called, simply, *alligation*

**apothecary system** a virtually obsolete system of measurement used predominantly by pharmacies prior to the metric system

**average wholesale price (AWP)** the average price that a drug wholesaler charges the pharmacy for a particular drug

**avoirdupois system** a virtually obsolete system of measurement predominantly used by pharmacies prior to the metric system

**balance scale** a device that measures powder or other solid ingredients; used in some extemporaneous pharmacy compounds

**basic formula method** a simple method to calculate most parenteral medication dosages; may be used when the concentration on the drug label is provided in units (usually mg per 1 mL); based on the formula: D/H = $x$ mL

**batch** multiple, uniform doses of a CSP mixed in anticipation of future need; batch CSPs are sometimes stored in the pharmacy refrigerator or freezer before preparing medication orders

**body surface area (BSA)** a method of patient-specific dosing that is determined based on the patient's weight and height; BSA dosing is expressed in mg/$m^2$

**Clark's Rule** an outdated formula once used to determine a pediatric dose; weight in pounds multiplied by the adult dose, and then divided by 150 to equal the pediatric dose

**concentration** the amount or weight of drug in a given volume of solution; usually expressed in mg/mL

**conversion factor** an expression of the equivalency between two different systems of measurement; often used to solve ratio and proportion problems

**Cowling's Rule** an obsolete formula once used to determine a pediatric dose; the adult dose multiplied by the age of the child (in years), and then divided by 24

**crude drug** a drug, plant, or herb in its natural, unrefined state

**cubit** an ancient unit of measurement based on the length of the forearm from the elbow to the tip of the middle finger

**daily IV run** the entire number of CSPs needed for all patients in designated facilities for a specific period; all of the CSPs for a 24-hour period that are often prepared by the IV technician during a single compounding period

**day's supply** the number of doses of a particular drug needed for patient administration over a 24-hour period; an inventory management method calculated as the value of inventory divided by the average daily cost of products sold

**denominator** the part of the fraction below the line that is divided into the number above the line (numerator); the divisor

**desired strength** the percent strength or concentration ordered by the prescriber, which must be compounded by an IV technician

**dimensional analysis method** a problem-solving method based on the fact that any number can be multiplied by one without changing its value; a conversion method

**dram** an apothecary unit of measure, approximately equivalent to 4 mL

**drop factor** the number of drops that an IV tubing delivers in order to provide 1 mL; also called "drop set" or "drip set"; may be used by the nursing staff to calculate the IV flow rate when using certain types of primary IV tubing

**drop factor method** a method of determining how long an LVP or IV drip will last given a specified concentration and the IV drop factor rate; IV flow rate calculation based on the number of drops delivered through microdrip or macrodrip tubing

**drug concentration** the strength of a drug usually expressed in mg/mL; an expression of the number of units per a given amount, volume, or weight of a drug

**electronic scale** an electronic or digital device that weighs a powdered or solid ingredient; used in some extemporaneous pharmacy compounds

**Food, Drug, and Cosmetic Act (FDCA)** a federal law enacted in 1938 that gave the federal government oversight over the safety of food, drug, and cosmetics within the United States; brought the FDA into existence; also known as the Federal Food, Drug, and Cosmetic Act (FFDC) and the FD&C

**Fried's Rule** an obsolete formula once used to determine a pediatric dose; adult dose multiplied by the child's age (in months), and then divided by 150 to equal the child's dose

**grain** an apothecary measurement of weight equivalent to 65 milligrams in the metric system

**higher-percent strength** an ingredient or a solution with a higher mass or concentration (number of grams/100 mL) than that of the desired concentration or any of the other solution components or ingredients; placed in the upper left corner in an alligation calculation; may be defined as percent (%) or number of grams per 100 mL

**household system** a system of measurement used in homes, generally for cooking and baking; a system of measurement using volumes such as teaspoon, tablespoon, cup, pint, quart, and gallon; uses weight such as ounce and pound

**infusion rate** the IV flow rate; the rate, usually provided in mL/hr, at which the IV solution is to be administered to the patient based on the prescriber's medication order

**IV drip rate calculation** an equation used to calculate an IV flow rate based on the drop factor of a particular type of IV tubing

**IV flow rate calculation** the use of addition, division, and/or multiplication to determine the following values: how long an IV bag will last, when a new bag will be needed, or how many bags are needed for a 24-hour period

**lower-percent strength** an ingredient or a solution with a lower mass or concentration (number of grams/100 mL) than that of the desired concentration or any of the other solution components or ingredients; placed in the lower left corner in an alligation calculation; may be defined as percent (%) or number of grams per 100 mL

**macrodrip IV tubing** a type of IV tubing constructed to administer approximately 10 or 20 drops per milliliter

**medication label** the drug vial label

**metric system** an internationally recognized system of measurement based upon the decimal system (multiples of ten)

**microdrip IV tubing** a type of IV tubing constructed to administer approximately 60 drops per milliliter

**military time** a system of measuring time with hours from 0100 to 2400; based incrementally on the 24-hour day

***mille passus*** an ancient Roman unit of distance measurement; equivalent to approximately a mile

**numerator** the number in a fraction located above the line, into which a denominator is divided; the dividend

**ounce** a unit of measure roughly equivalent to 30 milliliters (fluid) or 28.35 grams (mass)

**pound** a unit of measure equivalent to 0.453 kilogram (mass)

**Pure Food and Drug Act** the first federal law enacted in 1906 to require accurate labeling of contents and dosing; prohibited the sale of drugs with secret ingredients or misleading labels

**quantity to be dispensed** the number of doses of a particular drug for an individual patient, to be dispensed by the pharmacy based on the prescriber's medication order; in the hospital setting, this quantity is usually equal to the day's supply; in the retail setting, this quantity may be enough for 30 days or more

**ratio and proportion method** a way of comparing a complete ratio to an incomplete ratio with a missing component (the variable *x*); in other words, a ratio with both a numerator and a denominator compared with a ratio with either a numerator or a denominator and with a missing variable (*x*); a conversion method

**scruple** an apothecary unit of measure; approximately equivalent to 1.3 grams

**side effect** an undesirable effect of a drug or treatment; may include nausea, diarrhea, headache, etc.

**spring scale** a type of scale used to measure the mass of certain chemicals and compounding ingredients prior to 1900

**standard time** a system of measuring time related to the cycle of the natural day; 12 hours of a.m. and 12 hours of p.m. within each 24-hour cycle

**stock medication** a drug, medication, ingredient, or additive used in the preparation of a CSP; also called a *stock drug*

**talent** an ancient and inaccurate method of measuring volume no longer used in pharmacy compounding

**trial-and-error mixing** a system employed by early physicians, pharmacists, and chemists whereby drugs and drug compounds were mixed in varying amounts and tested on animal and human subjects

**unadulterated** describes a method of drug labeling that is clear and truthful

**unregulated** describes a drug or chemical whose uniformity, strength, or purity is not controlled by a set of standards; term applies to drugs and drug compounds prior to FDA regulation

**volume** the capacity or amount of space that a liquid occupies; often identified in milliliters or liters (metric system); often identified in teaspoon, tablespoon, ounce, pint, or gallon (household system)

**Young's Rule** an obsolete formula once used to determine a pediatric dose; child's age (in years) multiplied by the adult dose, and then divided by the child's age (in years) plus 12 to equal the pediatric dose

# Make Connections

*On a separate sheet of paper, write your answers to the following three questions, using complete sentences and making sure your answers are thorough and thoughtful. Note that the third question requires Internet access.*

1. In addition to nursing, laboratory, radiology, and dietary orders, a medication order often contains orders for numerous drugs. Many of the medication orders will require sterile compounding. Considering what you have learned about the importance of accuracy, how might the CSP label verification procedure be affected if, instead of a single label that requires verification, you are presented with numerous CSP labels reflecting the multiple medications and doses that the prescriber has written on the medication order?

2. An IV technician receives a medication order and CSP label for verification, and both the order and the label are affixed with "stat" stickers. Should the presence of these stickers affect the verification process of the CSP label? Why or why not? If the pharmacist were to mention to the technician that a nurse was awaiting the compounding of the medication, should this knowledge affect the technician's procedure for verifying the CSP label? Why or why not?

3. Go to the Institute for Safe Medication Practices (ISMP) website (www.ismp.org) and search for high-alert medications. Notice the specific medications listed on this page. What does this information indicate about the medication referred to in the procedural lab section of this chapter?

# Meet the Challenge

***Scenario*** This "calculated" activity challenges you to become more proficient at using medication orders, CSP labels, and medication labels to accurately perform pharmacy sterile compounding calculations.

***Challenge*** Your instructor has a handout with a series of questions based on the correct interpretation of a medication order and its corresponding medication and CSP labels. This activity provides you with "real-world" practice in the medication verification procedures that you will be required to perform—with 100% accuracy—in the sterile compounding environment. To meet this challenge, ask your instructor for the handout and corresponding labels for this activity and, on your own, complete the worksheet. When finished, turn in the handout to your instructor.

## ADDITIONAL RESOURCES

*Go to the Paradigm Internet Resources Center at* www.paradigmcollege.net/sterilecomp *to access live links related to these Chapter 5 topics:*

- Reducing medication errors in pharmacy, a resource from the Institute for Safe Medication Practices
- Obtaining generalized math tutoring
- Obtaining math tutoring specific to pharmacy

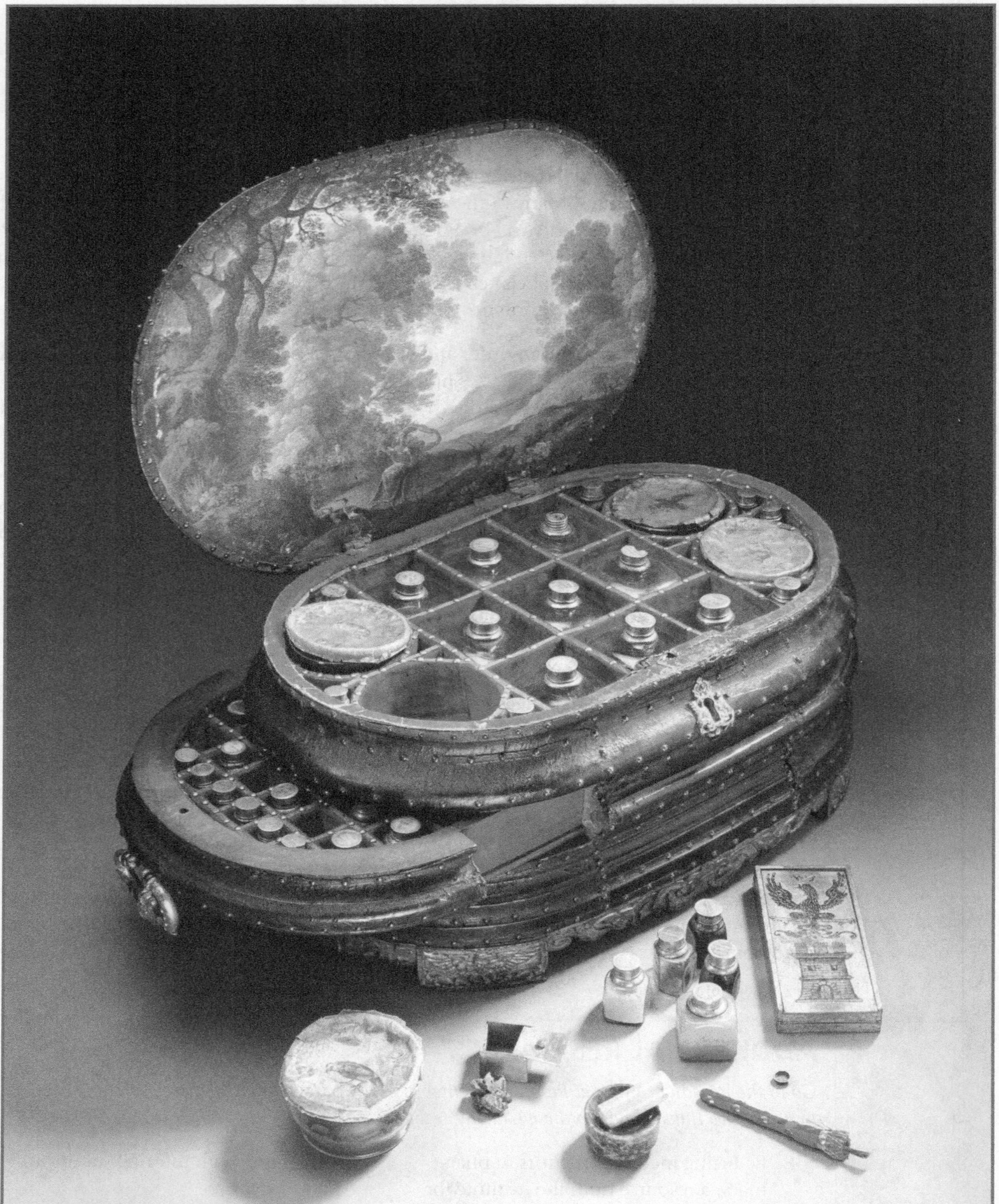

# Unit 2

# COMPOUNDING STERILE PREPARATIONS



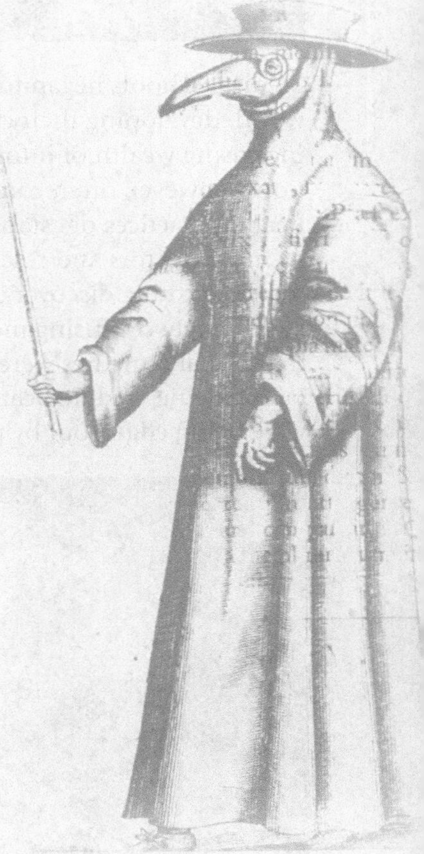

## Changing Healthcare Environment

Prior to the nineteenth century, healthcare practices were guided by the knowledge and expertise of a variety of local individuals: shamans, healers, alchemists, herbalists, apothecaries, and—of course—physicians. Their treatments for illness and disease were confined to the rural neighborhoods and villages where they resided and were subsequently passed down among generations of families. As a result, most citizens relied on the opinions and skills of a small group of individuals, including some with questionable medical expertise and motives. Those who were affluent had the advantage of access to institutions of higher learning, published medical resources, and transportation to seek out cures from well-known medical practitioners or healing sites.

During the Industrial Revolution in Europe and North America in the eighteenth and nineteenth centuries, population growth surged. With more citizens came a greater need for access to a formal system of healthcare information and treatment.

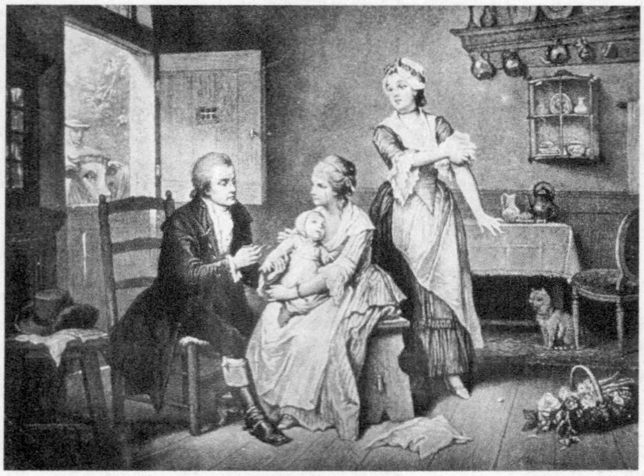

Medical schools began to sprout up around the world, developing their curricula based on an increasing wealth of information. These institutions, however, often competed with the traditional healing practices of established community leaders. As more doctors and researchers joined the race for the next big discovery, citizens were left with an increasingly confusing medical environment where traditional remedies were at odds with experimental medicine, and dedicated medical professionals were being edged out by profit-driven quacks.

## Rise of Unregulated Medicine

In the United States, the rapid expansion of both large cities and isolated rural communities became a gold mine for small-time con men and big-time drug companies. Consumers became the victims of these fraudulent practices, buying into the miracle drugs and bogus vaccines that were advertised. At one point, fraudulent versions of the smallpox vaccine were being manufactured and distributed nationwide by multiple companies. To curb this unethical behavior, U.S. lawmakers passed the Vaccine Act of 1813, the first federal law addressing consumer protection and pharmaceutical production. To ensure vaccine quality, the federal government assigned an agent to monitor and oversee the distribution of the genuine vaccine. Unfortunately, the Vaccine Act was limited in its

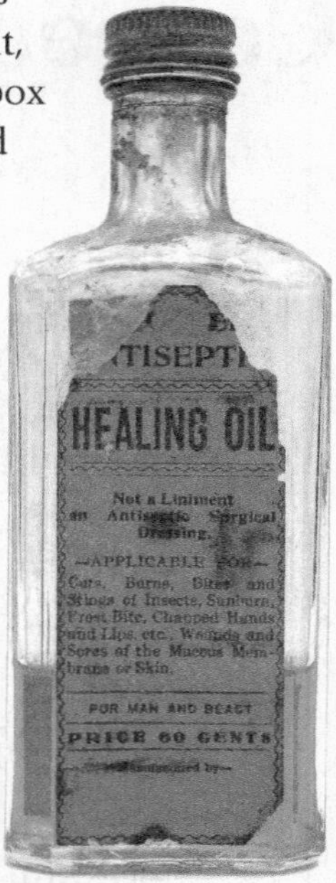


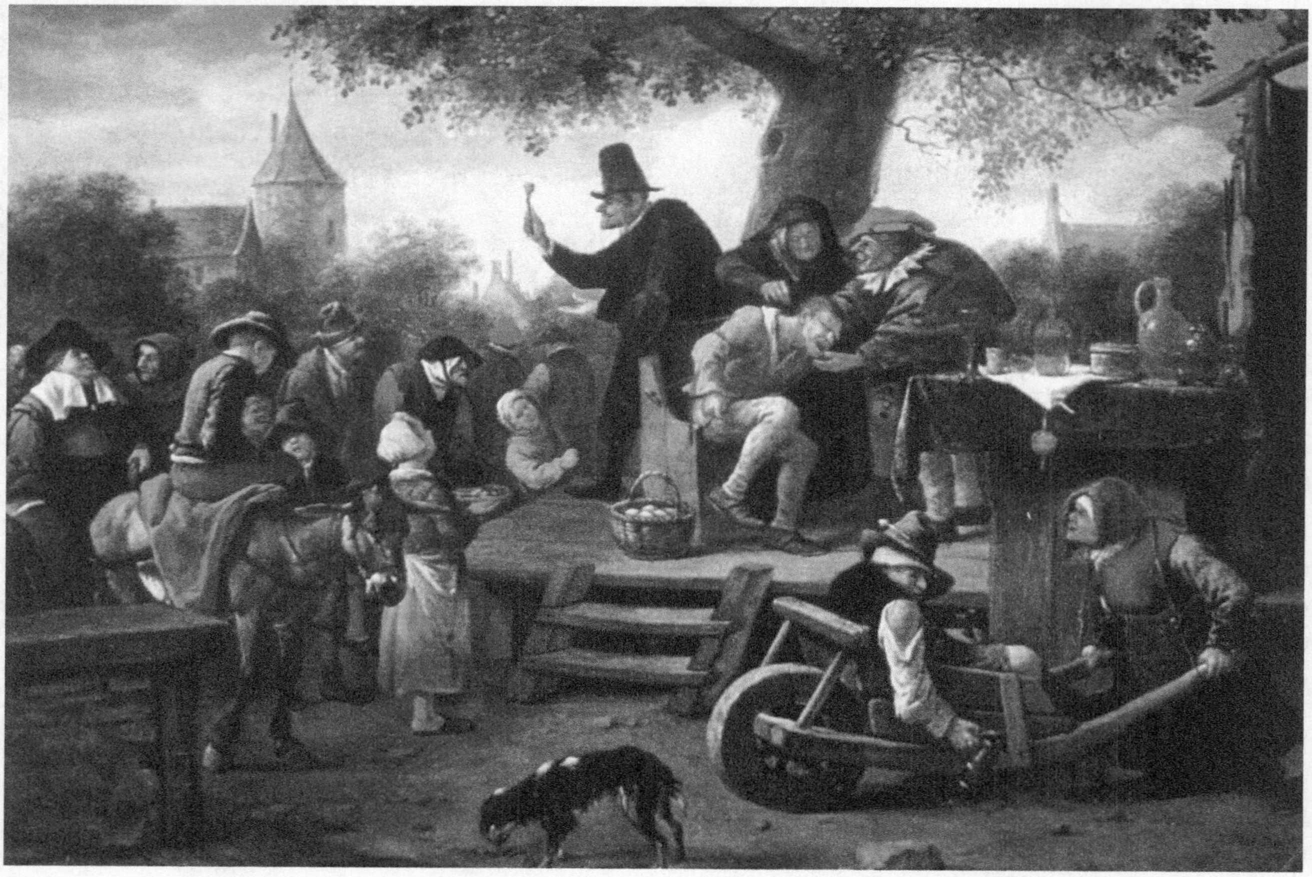

language and scope and was repealed less than a decade later in response to a smallpox outbreak in North Carolina. The cause of the outbreak was traced to ineffective vaccines created by a pharmacist working under a government representative.

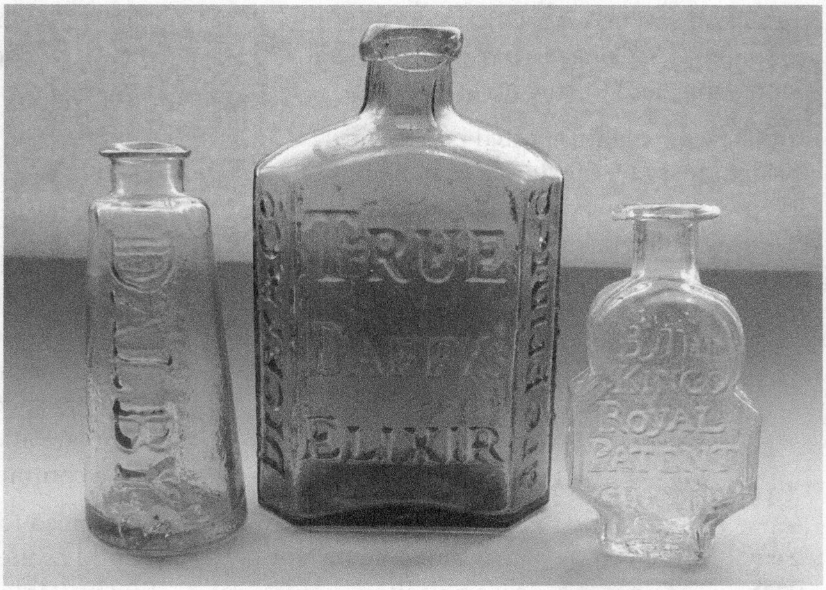


Even with the First Transcontinental Telegraph linking the coasts in 1861, information traveled slowly, and medical regulation was virtually nonexistent. Factories could produce and distribute medicines in huge quantities without quality control or inspection and claim medicinal properties based on faulty research or outright lies. Small-time hucksters crisscrossed the country promoting fabulous cure-alls, such as Hamlin's Wizard Oil (a remedy for rheumatism) and Reanimating Solar Tincture (a liquid to "restore life in the case of sudden death"). Often, traveling salespeople would be accompanied by performers. These traveling medicine shows wowed audiences with circus-like entertainment, musicians, and celebrities while promoting particular drugs. These quack medicines were usually elixirs comprised of large amounts of alcohol or opium, often laced with random herbs or "secret ingredients." Some of these hawked remedies actually possessed minor medicinal qualities, but most were a simple sedative, an ineffective antidote, or even a poisonous substance. Still, a hundred years would pass before the U.S. government would begin to implement controls for the production and distribution of medicine.

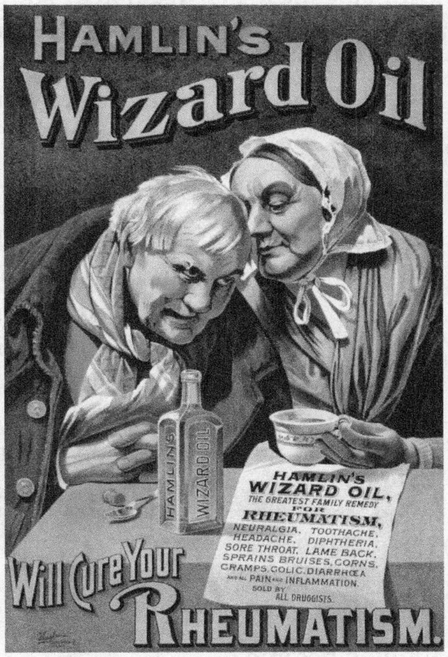


## Institution of Quality Standards for Medications

By the beginning of the twentieth century, a more-educated public, fueled by the investigative reports of journalists known as muckrakers, demanded that the U.S. government set sanitation and manufacturing standards for the food industry. One muckraker in particular, Upton Sinclair, exposed the corruption of the meat-packing industry and the appalling working and living conditions of America's poor in his novel *The Jungle*. As a result of this public outcry, lawmakers passed the Pure Food & Drugs Act in 1906, setting standards for both the food *and* drug industries. This act established federal inspection of meat products and forbid the manufacture, sale, and transportation of adulterated food products and poisonous patent medicines. It also mandated accurate content and dosage labeling of certain drugs and established, from previously existing organizations, the Bureau of Chemistry. This organization would later become the Food and Drug Administration (FDA).

Although the intentions of the Pure Food & Drugs Act were laudable, the act was limited in its power to regulate trade and enforce quality standards across the country. Once again, citizens were outraged at being victimized—first by unscrupulous peddlers and now by unregulated drug companies. Lawmakers too realized that stronger, more comprehensive legislation was necessary. Consequently, in 1938, the U.S. Congress passed the Federal Food, Drug, and Cosmetic (FD&C) Act.

This act was, in part, spurred by a tragic incident in 1937: the deaths of more than 100 people poisoned by an antimicrobial drug called Elixir Sulfanilamide. The raspberry-flavored drug utilized diethylene glycol, a poisonous compound used

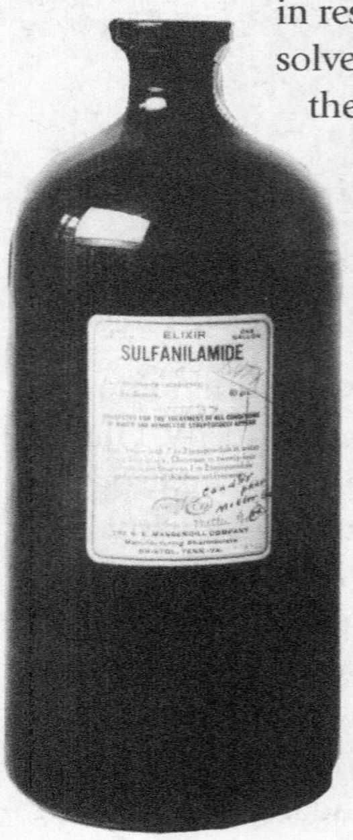


in resins and dyes, as a solvent. Although many in the medical community knew of the danger of this compound, the chief chemist at S.E. Massengill Company was unaware of diethylene glycol's poisonous nature and subsequently promoted the product without testing it on animals. Under the existing Pure Food & Drugs Act, the company only had to pay a minimal fine for labeling a product as an elixir when it contained no alcohol.

Since that event, diethylene glycol has been at the center of several public poisoning controversies (as recently as 2008) as it continues to be used in unregulated medicines and toothpastes, contributing to hundreds of deaths in more than 30 countries. This finding confirms the need for both national and international health and safety regulations.

The FD&C Act greatly increased the strength of regulating bodies, requiring animal testing on all new drugs and recognizing the United States Pharmacopeia–National Formulary (USP–NF) as the official compendium of drug standards. As the USP–NF developed and evolved, the need for specific procedures for sterile compounding became more evident. Prior to the introduction of regulatory and safety standards, incidences of patient injury or death associated with sterile compounding were relatively commonplace.

During the 1960s and 1970s, many hospital pharmacy departments began integrating intravenous (IV) admixture services into their facilities.

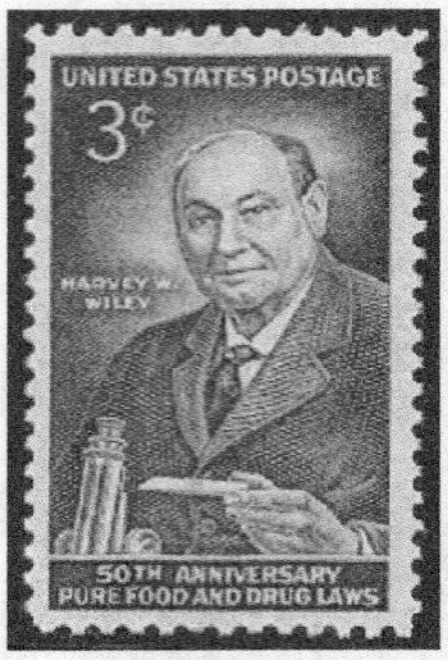


In previous decades, most sterile compounds were made by nurses and physicians immediately before patient administration. In the 1980s and 1990s, the increasing demand for specialized parenteral products led to a greater demand for compounded sterile preparations. These specialized medications are sometimes needed for total parenteral nutrition (TPN), pain management, pediatric preparations, and for those patients who require specialized dosing, or formulations, or who are allergic to one or more of the ingredients in a commercially available product.

The need for such preparations continues to build as the number of requests for commercially unavailable medications grows. However, the training of personnel for aseptic technique and sterile product preparation has not always kept up with marketplace demand. Prior to 1995, few guidelines existed for sterile compounding personnel, and standards of practice were not well defined or regulated. The growing complexity of drug products as well as an increased need to compound medications according to patients' needs have also contributed to increased numbers of medication errors and pharmacy-related nosocomial infections. In fact, in 2004, the American Society of Health-System Pharmacists (ASHP) declared that "since 1990, the FDA has become aware of more than 55 quality problems associated with compounded preparations, many of which have resulted in recalls, patient injury, and deaths." In light of these relatively recent safety issues, both training and

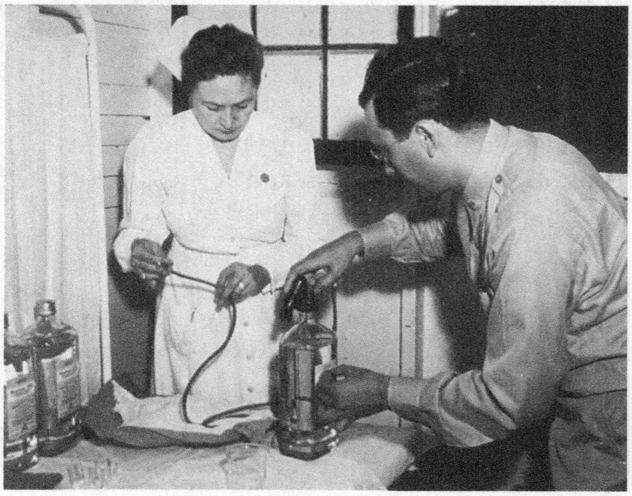

practice standards for sterile compounding personnel must continue to be examined and refined.

In the early 1990s, pharmacy organizations such as the ASHP, the USP, the National Coordinating Committee on Large Volume Parenterals (NCCLVP), and the National Association of Boards of Pharmacy reviewed policies related to sterile product preparation and eventually issued several recommendations regarding the compounding of sterile preparations. In 1993, the ASHP issued the Technical Assistance Bulletin, "Quality Assurance for Pharmacy-Prepared Sterile Products." This bulletin helped to identify and delineate the parameters of information that would eventually be incorporated into USP <797> *Pharmaceutical Compounding – Sterile Preparations*. In 1997, the U.S. Food and Drug Administration Modernization Act (FDAMA) set into motion the development of official sterile compounding standards. In 2004, the first official version of USP Chapter <797> was adopted. The revised standards for USP Chapter <797>, often referred to as USP <797>, became effective on June 1, 2008.

Because of the recommendations of the aforementioned pharmacy organizations, USP Chapter <797> has become a requirement for all pharmacies that perform sterile compounding. By law, these pharmacies may be inspected for compliance with the standards set forth by USP Chapter <797>, the State Boards of Pharmacy, the FDA, and accreditation organizations such as the Joint Commission (formerly known as the Joint Commission on Accreditation of Healthcare Organizations or JCAHO). The most important aspects of USP Chapter <797> center on the guidelines that sterile compounding personnel must follow during sterile compounding and aseptic technique procedures.

℞ We absolutely guarantee that this prescription has been filled exactly as prescribed by your physician from pure and fresh drugs.

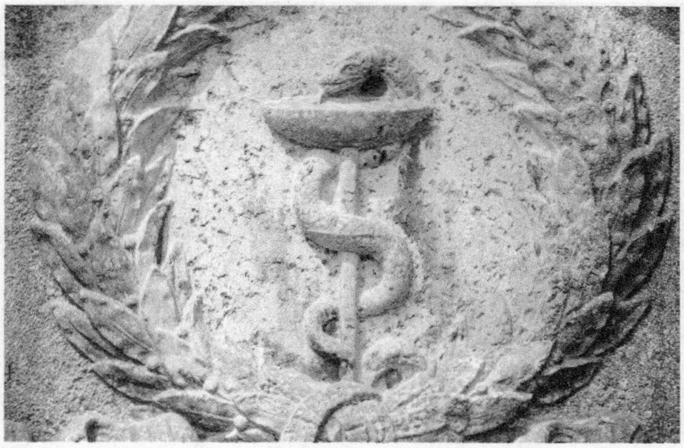

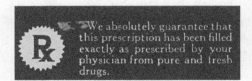

## Unit 2 Overview: Nine Procedural Labs

Unit 2 of this textbook broadens your understanding of the roots and concepts that reinforce your understanding of sterile compounding regulations and guides you through the aseptic technique and step-by-step procedures you must master. As you work from Chapter 6 to Chapter 14, you progress from the most basic concepts in aseptic technique to more advanced procedures, such as TPN and chemotherapy preparation. All information and procedures presented in this textbook are based on real-world experience, are considered best practice, and are in full compliance with the current regulatory standards.

As you complete the nine "Procedural Labs" contained in Unit 2, you will find that they require more traditional lab work than did the "Exploratory Labs" of Unit 1. Indeed, in the Unit 2 labs, you either prepare yourself and your working environment for product preparation (Chapters 6 and 7) or produce a tangible product (Chapters 8–14). The labs are designed to reinforce your sterile compounding training, offering plentiful practice to hone your skills toward mastering the work. Your instructor will evaluate your sterile compounding and aseptic technique, ensuring that they adhere to the revised regulations of USP Chapter <797> that became effective on June 1, 2008.

## Sterile Compounding Area Procedures

### Anteroom Procedures

#### *Physical Appearance and Behavior*

- Assess your appearance and remove any restricted items, including cosmetics, hair spray, nail polish, perfume, jewelry, or artificial nails.
- Abstain from food, drink, and gum chewing while working in the sterile compounding area.

#### *Calculations and Supplies*

- Whenever possible, perform calculations prior to gathering supplies.
- Gather supplies at the beginning of the lab to avoid the airflow disturbance caused by entering and exiting the clean room frequently.
- Wipe down all supplies with an aseptic cleaning wipe.

#### *Aseptic Garbing, Hand Washing, and Gloving*

- Don correct attire including shoe covers, hair cover, face mask, and beard cover (if necessary).
- Cleanse hands according to aseptic hand-washing procedures.
- Don a sterile gown.

### Clean Room Procedures

#### *Restrictions of Working in the Hood*

- Cleanse hands with sterile, foamed 70% IPA and put on sterile gloves.
- Do not bring potentially septic items such as pens, pencils, calculators, paper supplies, product overwrap, etc. into the hood.
- Cleanse gloved hands frequently using a product such as sterile, foamed 70% IPA.
- Avoid touching the face, hair, eyeglasses, or trash container. If inadvertent touch contamination occurs, cleanse hands with sterile, foamed 70% IPA.
- Avoid talking, sneezing, coughing, and whistling.

#### *Compounding in the Hood*

- Leave the hood on for at least 30 minutes before using it.
- Clean the hood according to standard protocol, both prior to making sterile products and at the intervals designated by USP Chapter <797>.
- Perform all manipulations at least six inches inside the outer edge of the hood to maintain good airflow over critical sites (the needle, tip of the syringe, vial tops, injection port, etc.). Also, avoid placing items anywhere on the hood's work surface where they may obstruct horizontal airflow to the critical sites of supply items.

# Sterile Compounding Area Procedures

## Clean Room Procedures *(continued)*

### *Manipulation of Supplies*

- Avoid touch contamination of supplies, including the uncapped needle; the tip or inner plunger of the syringe; the hub of the needle; the tubing or dispensing pin spike; or the injection port of the vial, IVPB, or IV bag.
- Prior to needle insertion, use sterile 70% IPA to swab the critical sites of supply items that do not come presterilized from their manufacturers. These items include the vial top, ampule neck, and IV or IVPB injection ports. Do *not* swab the critical sites of the supplies that come presterilized from their manufacturers. These items include the syringe tip, all parts of the needle, the spike and syringe adaptor of the dispensing pin, and the spike and needle adaptor of the IV tubing.
- Perform a correct needle insertion by following these steps: With the bevel of the needle face up, place the tip of the needle onto the swabbed rubber top of the vial. Using a slight rounded motion of the wrist, penetrate the vial top with the needle. (The needle will bend slightly upon penetration due to the gentle downward pressure.)
- When withdrawing fluid from a vial, create positive pressure by injecting a volume of air that *is equal to* the desired volume being withdrawn. (When too little air has been added, withdrawing the fluid is difficult; when too much air has been added, aspiration, excess fluid in the syringe, or the spraying of droplets upon needle removal will occur.)
- Verify that the measurement of fluid in the syringe is exact by observing the area where the top of the inner syringe plunger meets the barrel.
- Confirm that no air bubbles are present in the syringe. If air bubbles are present, remove the bubbles by tapping the barrel of the syringe so that they flow upward toward the capped needle. Once bubbles are at the tip of the syringe, gently pull down on the plunger approximately ½ mL. Next, carefully push up on the plunger to expel excess air. Watch the fluid slowly come up to the hub of the needle and then immediately release the plunger. This action will help decrease the potential for inadvertent fluid injection into the needle cap.
- Inject fluid into an IV bag by inserting the needle directly into the port without puncturing the stem, neck, or bag. There is no need to inject air into a bag as the flexible container expands and contracts itself so that air pressure is not an issue.

### *Completion of Compounding*

- Inspect the IV bag or IVPB for leaks, incompatibility, and particulate matter.
- Place needles, syringes, and broken glass into a sharps container for disposal. Place all other trash into a regular trash receptacle unless directed otherwise by your instructor.

### *Maintenance of Hood*

- Change the prefilter every 30 days.
- Arrange to have the HEPA filter certified by a hood certification company every six months or whenever the cabinet is moved.
- Maintain careful record keeping of hood cleaning, prefilter replacement, and HEPA filter/hood recertification, as well as the daily, weekly, and monthly cleaning of the sterile compounding area.

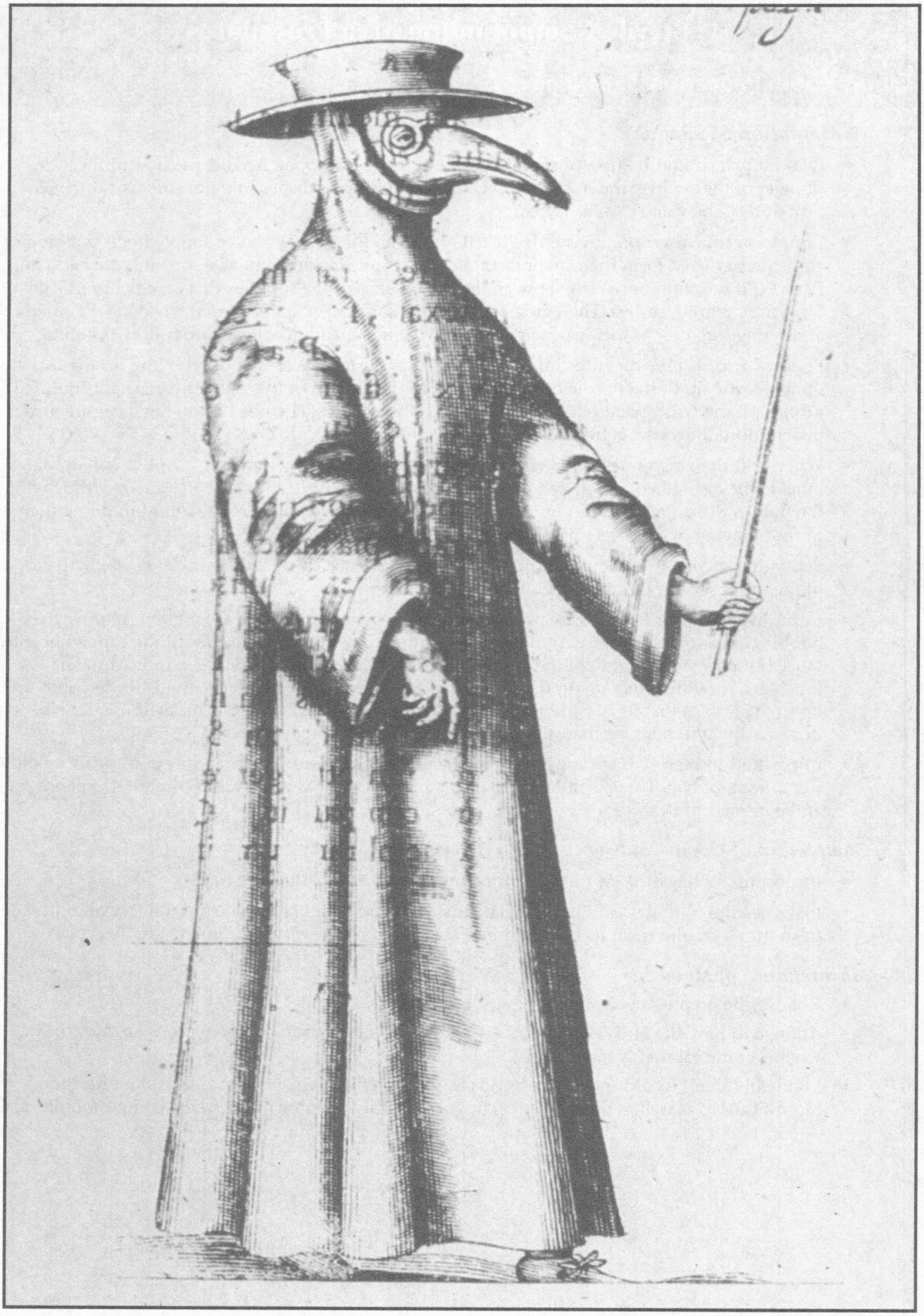

# Chapter 6

# Aseptic Garbing, Hand Washing, and Gloving

## Learning Objectives

- Gain an awareness of the connections between early concepts of germ transmission and current procedures for aseptic garbing, hand washing, and gloving.
- Understand the procedures for aseptic garbing, hand washing, and gloving according to USP Chapter <797> guidelines.
- Identify ways that aseptic garbing, hand washing, and gloving protect the patient from infection.
- Recognize and respond appropriately to actions that compromise asepsis during aseptic garbing, hand washing, and gloving procedures.
- Demonstrate excellent technique in aseptic hand washing, garbing, and gloving.

Today's healthcare practitioners are well-versed in the methods of germ transmission and their role in preventing the spread of illness and disease. Scientific evidence has proven that, in the healthcare setting, **microorganisms** can be transmitted by direct contact with an infected individual, by indirect contact with contaminated clothing or objects (**fomites**), or by airborne transmission. Consequently, healthcare personnel follow strict cleanliness and **infection-control** mandates when providing both direct and indirect patient care. These mandates include aseptic **garbing**, hand washing, and gloving procedures that form a protective barrier against **contagion**.

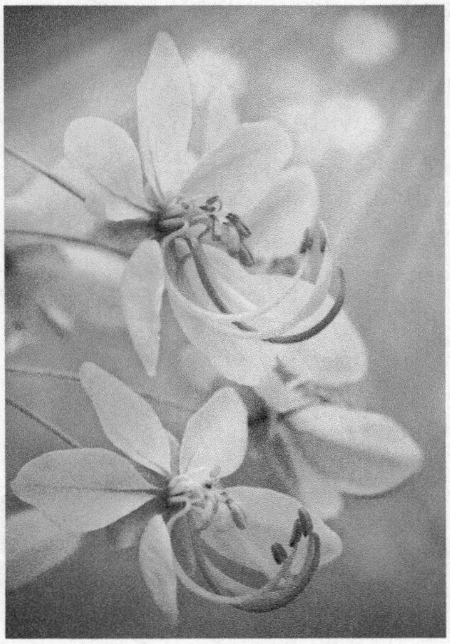

Recognizing the relationship between personal cleanliness and germ transmission, however, is not a recent development. In fact, many primitive cultures developed logical and sophisticated methods to decrease the spread of illness and ensure healthful living. For example, a Babylonian clay tablet from 2200 BCE provides a formula for soap that combines water, alkaline salts, and cassia oil. Ancient Egyptians used a similar recipe in their bathing rituals but substituted animal oils instead. Although many of these early cleansing practices were limited in effectiveness, they did provide some degree of protection against illness and infection in cultures where germs and disease were not understood.

## Early Hand-Washing Practices

Like medical practices, early cleanliness and sanitation methods were taught primarily through spiritual beliefs and religious doctrines. Islam's holy book, the Koran, demands hand washing multiple times daily, including before prayer. Other religions also followed this practice of hand washing before prayer and provided fonts of water at the entrances to their sanctuaries. Participating in this ritual supposedly cleansed not only the body but the soul as well.

The ritual of bathing was popular among early Greek and Roman cultures. The ancient Greeks used pieces of clay and a curved metal tool called a **strigil** (a crude prototype of the surgical scrub tool used in sterile preparatory procedures today) to scrape the dirt from their skin. Early Romans could often be found in public bathhouses, participating in elaborate cleanliness rituals with their fellow citizens. For these early cultures, personal cleanliness—including hand washing—was a sign of civility and respectfulness.

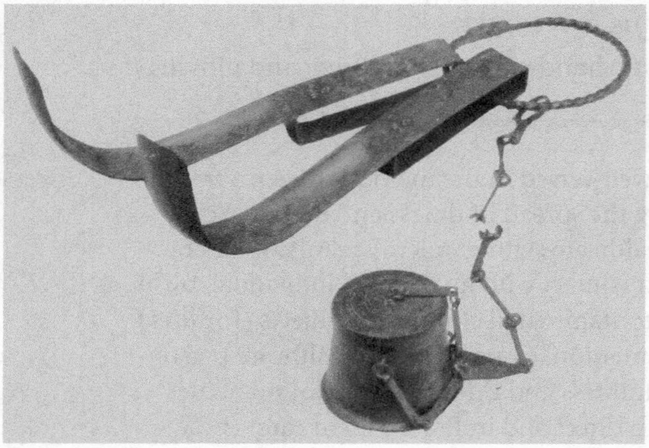

## Decline of Personal Cleanliness

By the beginning of the Middle Ages, ancient medical practitioners began to see hand-washing practices as a possible preventive measure against the transmission of disease and prescribed for their patients the use of warm water, wine, or vinegar to slow the spread of the **Black Plague**. Surprisingly, soap making was a booming trade during this period, although soaps were used mainly for aromatic purposes and often without water. However, this early understanding of the relationship between cleanliness and disease was dismissed by the Christian church, which condemned bathing and led its followers to believe that washing the body allowed disease to creep into the body's pores. Consequently, personal cleanliness practices began to decline, and this lack of hygiene coupled with poor living conditions only accelerated the spread of the Plague, nearly obliterating the population of the European continent. Ironically, the body parts that were regularly cleansed were the hands, mainly because they were exposed to others and therefore became an outward symbol of gentility. The remainder of the body was often covered by a layer of filth, emanating a stench that was regularly cloaked by ample doses of perfumed oils.

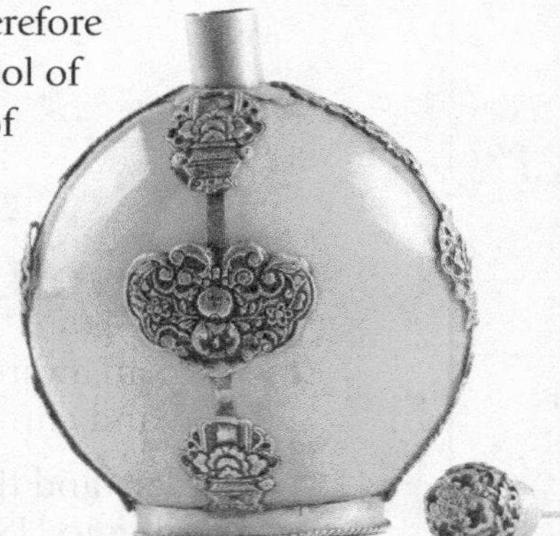

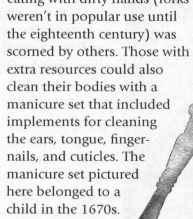

At the beginning of the Renaissance, cultures continued to avoid bathing for fear of contracting the Plague. Many physicians, in fact, recommended that a layer of dirt would offer protection from the scourge of disease. Yet, hand-washing rituals before and after meals were conducted regularly as a social grace. Wealthy citizens, in fact, typically employed a Laverer, a servant who would provide water and towels for invited guests to use before they dined. No matter the social status of a citizen during this historical period, any individual who was observed eating with dirty hands (forks weren't in popular use until the eighteenth century) was scorned by others. Those with extra resources could also clean their bodies with a manicure set that included implements for cleaning the ears, tongue, fingernails, and cuticles. The manicure set pictured here belonged to a child in the 1670s.

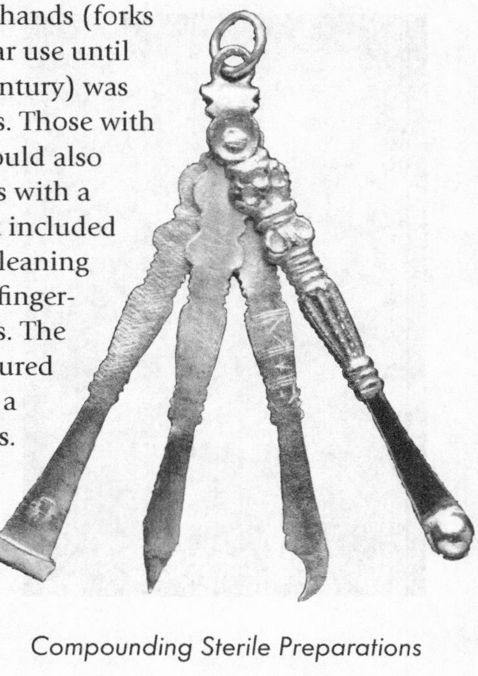

## Lack of Healthcare Cleanliness Standards

Bathing continued to be shunned throughout the eighteenth century. This lack of personal hygiene crossed over into the healthcare arena as physicians and surgeons would treat patients without regard for their own cleanliness or that of their environment. Doctors in hospitals and in private practice would assess patients sequentially, without pausing to wash their hands. Surgeries were performed by physicians with unclean hands in unsanitary conditions. With little understanding of germ transmission, patient mortality rates climbed.

Nowhere was the connection between germ transmission and mortality rates more apparent than with expectant mothers, many of whom held a supernatural charm or **amulet** to protect themselves against infection. An amulet's powers came from its symbols and the organic materials it was made from. The Bavarian amulet shown here is comprised of three objects: the white, bone fist, an ancient Roman protective symbol; a circular shell, a symbol of fertility; and a filigree chamber, a symbol for a container of special oil extracted from the bones of an eighth-century missionary. It would take another century, however, for medicine to recognize that infection control was—literally and figuratively—in the hands of humans.

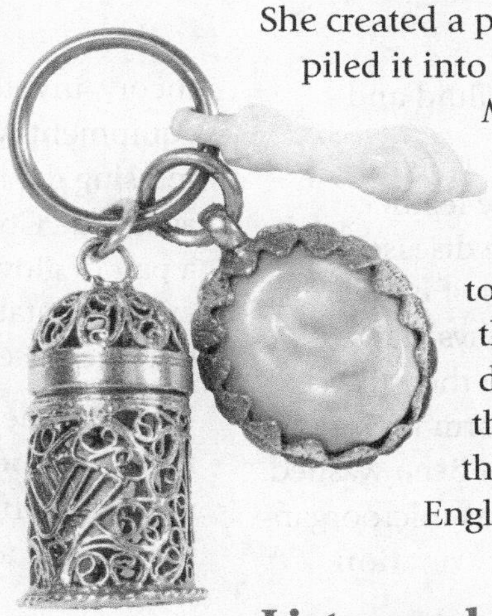

## Rise of Infection-Control Practices

In the nineteenth century, the work of Hungarian obstetrician Ignaz Semmelweis influenced hospital awareness of infection control. At Vienna General Hospital in Austria, Semmelweis recognized the role that hand cleansing played in reducing infection and mortality among maternity patients. To encourage such results, Semmelweis insisted that all obstetric interns wash their hands with chlorinated lime before they examined patients. By enforcing these antiseptic practices, the hospital saw mortality rates for new mothers in the maternity ward decline by more than 10 percent.

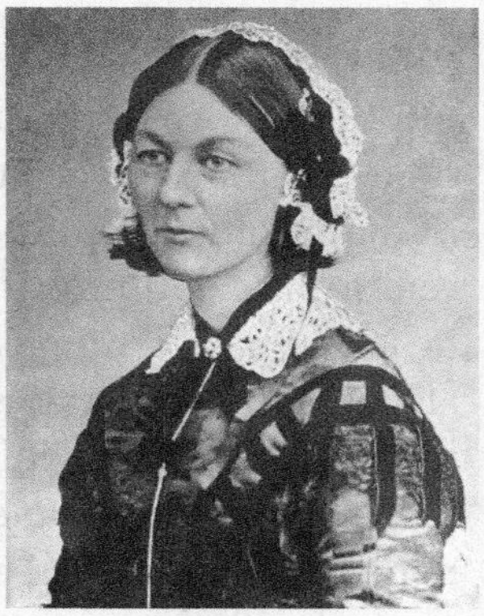

By the 1850s, the understanding of the importance of cleanliness and sanitary conditions to curbing the spread of contagion was slowly building momentum. Notable English nurse Florence Nightingale observed this connection firsthand as she provided care and treatment for wounded soldiers during the Crimean War. Upon her return to England, Nightingale conducted an exhaustive study of the health of the British Army and provided documented statistics that reinforced the connection between poor hygiene and the deaths of thousands of soldiers. She created a plan for healthcare reform and compiled it into a 500-page report titled *Notes on Matters Affecting the Health, Efficiency, and Hospital Administration of the British Army* (1858). Nightingale submitted this confidential report to the British government. Although the report was poorly received, the document was eventually leaked to the British populace, providing the catalyst for healthcare reform in England.

## Lister and the Germ Theory

The sterile practices set forth by Semmelweis and Nightingale influenced the research of nineteenth-century British surgeon Dr. Joseph Lister. Lister explored the **germ theory** of disease by building upon the microorganism theories of French chemist Louis Pasteur. Lister's experiments with sterilization techniques proved that cleansing the hands, donning gloves, and using germicides on surgical instruments greatly reduced the incidence of infection. His sterile practices were met with skepticism by many surgeons, who found the presurgical preparations time-consuming and the caustic disinfecting agents irritating to the skin and eyes. However, Lister's pioneering work in aseptic technique laid the foundation for the importance of gloving and garbing in the healthcare field.

## Emergence of Gloving

Although gloves did not become official garb in the healthcare field until the end of the nineteenth century, the donning of gloves can be traced back centuries to when alchemists, apothecaries, and healers wore gloves while preparing **elixirs** and other medicinal remedies. Ancient herbalists who worked with these healthcare practitioners, such as balsam harvesters, often wore gloves to gather the tree's medicinal sap. The sap—as well as the needles, inner bark, and branches—was used to treat health concerns such as skin rashes, throat irritations, and ulcers. The gloves both protected the harvesters' hands from the sticky fluid and helped keep the sap clean.

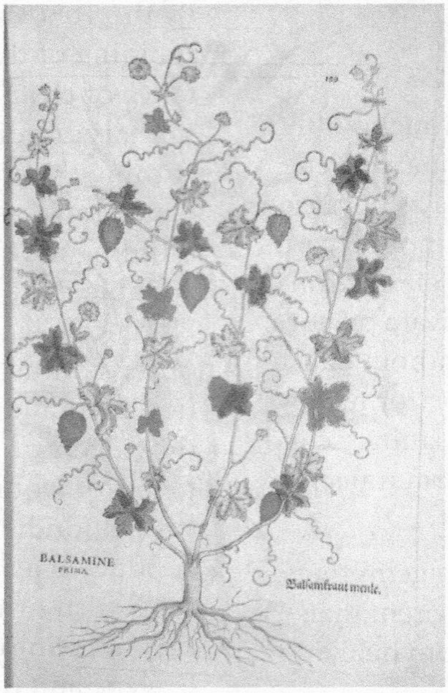


During the Black Plague, doctors wore leather gloves to protect their hands from the disease-ridden "bad air" that filled the houses of its victims. However, in the eighteenth century, physicians and surgeons were not using gloves in their direct patient care, choosing instead to perform their procedures using bare hands that had not been washed. As a result, the transmittal of infectious microorganisms via direct contact, or **cross contamination**, was rampant among patient populations.

With increased trepidation among practitioners as to contracting disease from patient examinations, several scientists and physicians conducted experiments to create some type of physical barrier to protect their hands. Gloves at that time were made of dense materials, making tactile sensitivity difficult for physicians during patient examination. One such experiment, conducted by Dr. Richard Cooke in the 1830s, used spirit of turpentine to paint on a "pseudo glove" before he examined his patients. He would then rub off the coating upon completion of the assessment. Recognizing the drawbacks of this process, Cooke turned his attention to experimenting with different types of glove materials, ultimately suggesting to the medical community that "a pair of India rubber gloves would be perfectly impenetrable to the most malignant virus."

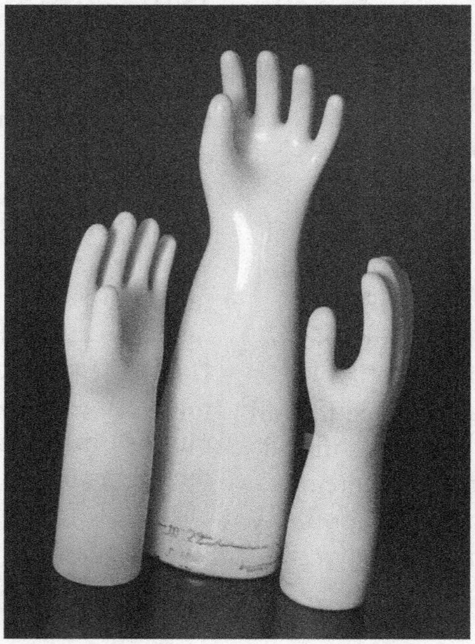

However, it wasn't until late in the nineteenth century that rubber medical gloves first appeared as part of surgical attire. In 1889, Dr. William Stewart Halstead, a physician at Johns Hopkins University who supported Lister's germ theory, insisted on the disinfection of his surgical equipment. When his nurse expressed reluctance to using the harsh disinfecting chemicals, Halstead asked the Goodyear Rubber Company to make a pair of gloves that would protect the skin. The experimental thin rubber gloves proved so effective that their use spread throughout the healthcare field.

By 1905, the Ansell Company had developed the first **latex medical glove**. Practitioners sterilized these early rubber and latex gloves by dipping them in **carbolic acid** or steaming them in an **autoclave**. Sterilizing gloves in this way was labor-intensive and time-consuming, and evidence was growing that glove sterilization methods failed to render the gloves bacteria-free. These concerns wouldn't be entirely addressed until decades later when, in 1964, the Ansell Company manufactured the first presterilized, disposable, latex medical gloves.

Currently, USP Chapter <797> mandates that all sterile compounding personnel wear sterile, disposable gloves while preparing **compounded sterile preparations (CSPs)**.

## Importance of Garbing

Like gloving, garbing became an important practice in the healthcare field during the late nineteenth and early twentieth centuries. Prior to this time, heavy cloth lab aprons were worn by surgeons, who modeled their attire after the leather aprons worn by early craftspeople and inventors. These cloth aprons provided a surface for surgeons to wipe their bloody hands as well as a covering to protect their street clothes from the patient's body fluids.

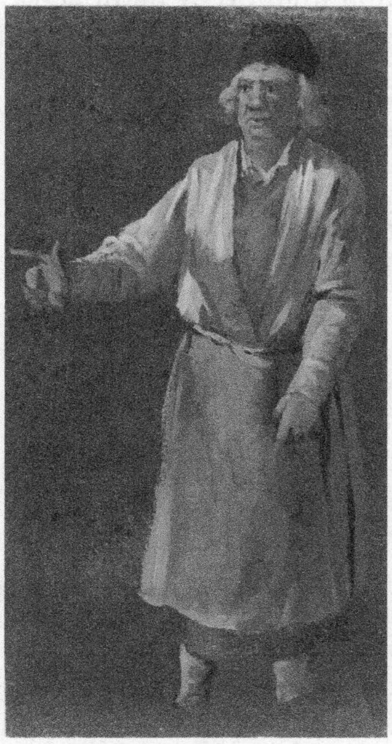

These heavily soiled aprons became somewhat of a badge of honor: the less clean the apron, the more successful the surgeon—or so onlookers thought. To make matters worse, these aprons were typically never washed.

During the Black Plague, doctors wore a type of full body armor to battle this **pestilence**. Their attire resembled the illustration on page 164: a leather hat; a mask that covered the entire head; a beak that held pungent herbs or spices to purify the bad air that circulated around the sick patient; a full-length, heavy robe covered in wax; leather breeches underneath the robe; and leather gloves and boots to protect the hands and feet. The doctor also carried a stick to keep others at a distance from him.

Many centuries would pass before physicians began to wear any type of specialized garment when treating patients. In 1884, Gustav Neuber, a German surgeon, embraced Lister's theories about the importance of antisepsis, pioneering the modern operating room and the use of aseptic garb by surgeons. Neuber was the first doctor to require his staff to wear sterilized caps, gowns, and shoe covers and to wash their hands frequently with **mercuric chloride**. For the first time, the healthcare community recognized that aseptic hand washing and garbing protected not only physicians but patients as well.

Neuber also required his surgical team to don face masks—crude prototypes of which have been worn by inventors and scientists for hundreds of years. Historical records have demonstrated the use of masks for filtering out "bad air" or gases. These masks were typically made of sap- or wax-cloth, leather, wool, or rubber and covered the whole face and even the entire head. The masks often held potent, protective herbs and spices to purify the surrounding air.

By the advent of the twentieth century, documents concerning the **Spanish Flu pandemic of 1918** reveal that caregivers wore face masks. Building on Lister's research that infection can be transmitted through airborne microorganisms, some healthcare personnel treating victims of the highly contagious disease wore crudely fashioned gauze masks in an attempt to protect themselves from disease. It quickly became apparent that this simple act not only protected the hospital staff but also helped to reduce the rates of infection among patients they treated.

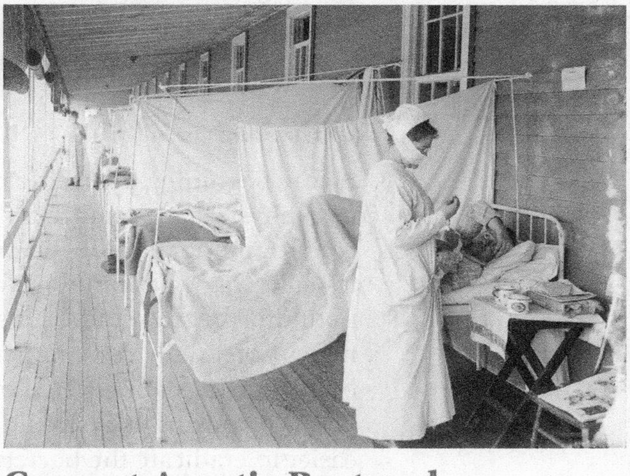

## Current Aseptic Protocol

Garbing in sterile surgical attire became routine practice in the United States by the early 1940s. Wearing this type of sterile garb drastically reduced the incidence of **nosocomial infection** in the hospital setting. Sterile compounding pharmacies took their cue from the medical industry and followed suit by garbing in sterile gowns when they prepared CSPs for patient recipients.

Today, aseptic garbing, hand washing, and gloving are fundamental procedures that pharmacy technicians follow in sterile compounding pharmacies around the world. Critical to patient safety, these procedures are regulated by USP Chapter <797>.

# Part 1: Concepts

Garbing, hand washing, and gloving are important components of aseptic technique. These procedures help avoid the introduction of **pathogens**, or disease-causing microorganisms, while working with sterile compounding products and supplies. Maintaining **asepsis** in product preparation is critical for the hospitalized patients receiving these CSPs. Because these patients are recovering from surgery, injury, or infection, they have compromised immune systems that cannot mount an effective defense against pathogens, putting them at risk for further complications and even death. Thus, in order to minimize the risk of contamination by pathogens, sterile compounding technicians must adhere to strict aseptic technique both in the preparatory steps of garbing, hand washing, and gloving and while performing the sterile compounding procedures.

**POINTER**

Although the aseptic garbing, hand-washing, and gloving procedures presented in Chapter 6 are geared toward the IV technician, USP Chapter <797> regulations state that all personnel who enter the clean room must follow the same preparatory procedures.

Correct garbing, hand washing, and gloving are also important safety measures for those preparing the products: the sterile compounding personnel who need protection from exposure to drugs and hazardous chemicals. In fact, chronic exposure to certain drugs, especially antibiotics, during the sterile compounding process might cause healthcare workers to develop an allergy or immunity to the drugs. Therefore, intravenous (IV) technicians must first understand the USP Chapter <797> guidelines, practice the procedures, and demonstrate mastery of aseptic garbing, hand washing, and gloving to appropriate personnel in order to ensure the safety of patients and of pharmacy and hospital personnel.

## Self-Assessment for Compliance

Before beginning the sterile compounding process, IV technicians must assess their own physical appearance for any violations that could compromise the sterile compounding procedure. For example, as a technician, you must not wear cosmetics, hair spray, perfume, artificial nails, or nail polish while performing sterile compounding because these substances can flake and compromise the aseptic environment, potentially contaminating the CSPs. You must remove any jewelry, including body piercings not covered by a gown and mask, because these items can harbor microorganisms. You should also keep your fingernails closely trimmed to make it easier to eradicate the **bacteria** under the nails. Finally, any technicians who have weeping sores, sunburn, rash, or respiratory infection should not work in the clean room until these conditions have improved.

## Use of Personal Protective Equipment

Next, sterile compounding personnel begin the process of donning **personal protective equipment (PPE)**. These items minimize the risk of contamination of the sterile compounding area and the CSPs. In addition to donning PPE, IV technicians also perform an aseptic hand washing, a hand-washing procedure that is more stringent than basic hand washing.

***Aseptic Garbing*** IV technicians prepare to work in the clean room by donning shoe covers, a hair cover, and a face mask. If appropriate, personnel may also put on a beard cover. Wearing these protective items minimizes the risk of contamination during compounding procedures.

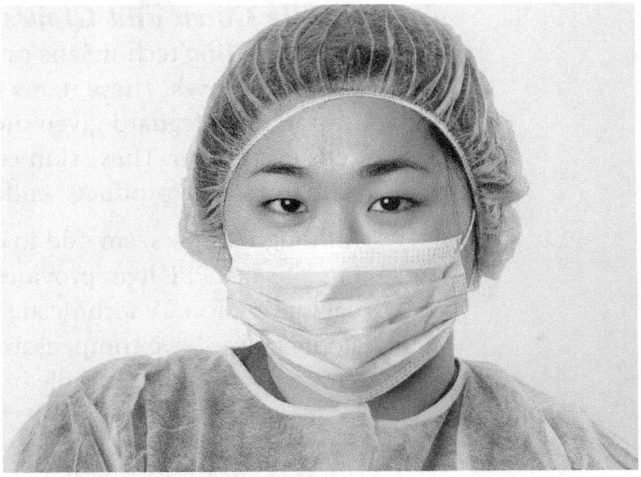
An IV technician wearing aseptic garb.

***Aseptic Hand Washing*** In aseptic hand washing, IV technicians wash their forearms and hands using an appropriate **antimicrobial agent** and following a specific sequence. Special attention should be paid to areas that harbor multiple microorganisms, such as under the fingernails and in the creases of skin. In order to become proficient at aseptic hand washing, technicians need to practice the steps until the process becomes second nature. Learning this process is critical because the most common source of contamination in the preparation of parenteral products is **touch contamination** by a healthcare worker who has not practiced correct aseptic technique in hand washing.

Sterile compounding technicians need to know not only the aseptic hand-washing process but also the circumstances under which the process must be performed or repeated. The following situations require the completion of aseptic hand washing:

- when first entering the sterile compounding area
- when reentering the sterile compounding area
- after eating
- after using the restroom
- after sneezing or coughing
- after a major contamination, such as a needle stick or a drug spill with a volume greater than 5 mL
- after the hands touch any item that is obviously contaminated, such as the floor, the waste receptacle or sharps container, or a visibly soiled item

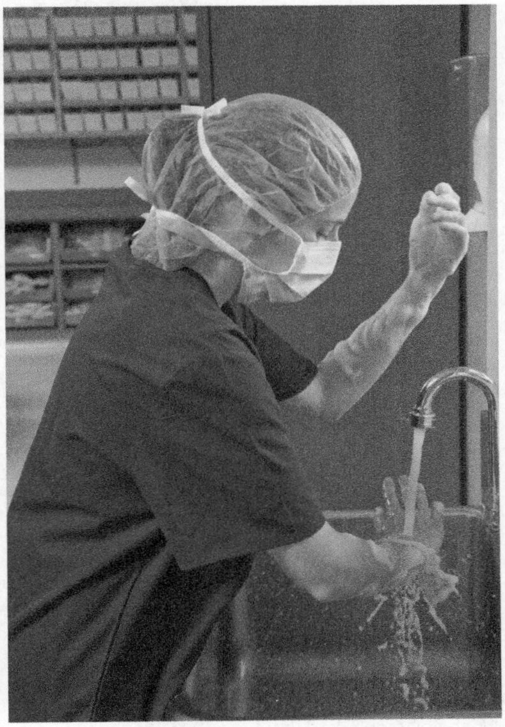
Sterile compounding technician performing a complete aseptic hand-washing procedure.

In certain situations, sterile compounding personnel may cleanse their hands or gloves with sterile, foamed 70% isopropyl alcohol (IPA). The following scenarios allow the use of this product:

- upon entering the anteroom, prior to donning PPE
- after using a calculator or pen
- after spilling a few drops of liquid on the gloved hand
- when there is potential for minor hand contamination such as after adjusting eyeglasses or handling labels or medication orders

***Sterile Gown and Gloves*** After hand washing has been completed, sterile compounding technicians put on the last two PPE items: a sterile gown and a pair of sterile gloves. These items minimize skin exposure in the compounding area, an important safeguard given the fact that a human sheds more than one million skin cells every hour. These skin cells harbor multiple organisms that could contaminate the sterile products, endangering patient recipients.

Although it may seem odd to don sterile gloves after completing aseptic hand washing, this last PPE item provides an additional barrier or backup against product contamination. IV technicians who have aseptically cleansed hands placed inside of sterile gloves have compensated for two possible scenarios: First, the ripping or puncturing of gloves by a needle or glass shard; and second, the growth of microorganisms on poorly cleansed hands enclosed in the warm, moist environment of gloves. These microorganisms could then seep through the **micropores** of the gloves, contaminating the CSPs. Either situation could ultimately put the patient recipient at risk for infection, but applying sterile gloves over aseptically washed hands reduces the potential for both.

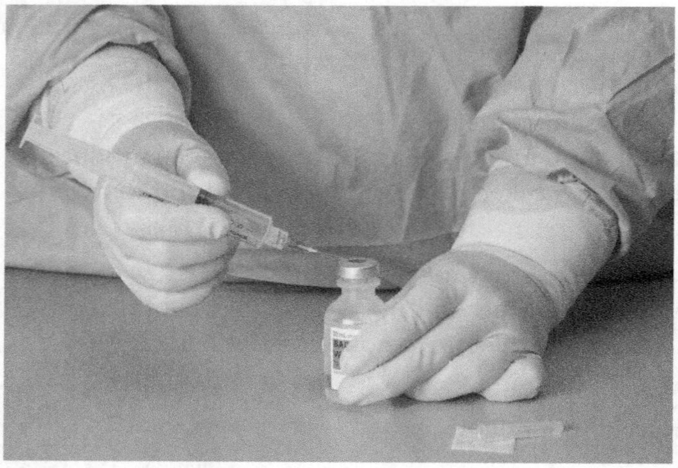

Gloving before the preparation of sterile products provides an additional safeguard to touch contamination.

**BE AWARE**

Eye shields, or goggles, are an optional PPE item. However, they must be worn by sterile compounding personnel who are using harsh disinfectants in the clean room or by those preparing hazardous drugs, such as chemotherapy. Chapter 14: Chemotherapy Products and Procedures provides more information about eye shields.

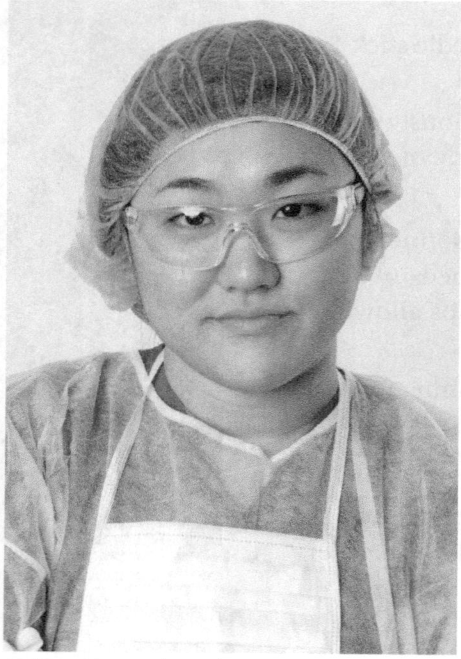

An IV technician dressed in protective, aseptic garb to prevent contamination of a CSP.

# Concepts Self-Check

## Check Your Understanding

*Write your answers on a separate sheet of paper, as modeled in these examples: 1d; 2c; 3b; etc. Check your answers using the Answer Key in Appendix A.*

**1.** What is the most common source of microbial contamination in CSPs?

a. poor hand washing
b. torn gloves
c. circulating air
d. soiled shoe covers

**2.** Which of the following situations requires a complete aseptic hand washing?

a. entering the sterile compounding area after your lunch break
b. being cut by a broken ampule
c. spilling 10 mL of IV penicillin on your hand
d. all of the above

**3.** Which of the following situations warrants hand cleansing with sterile, foamed 70% IPA?

a. before donning PPE
b. after adjusting eyeglasses
c. after handling a CSP label
d. all of the above

**4.** Why is it important that sterile compounding personnel don sterile gloves before preparing products?

a. to protect long fingernails
b. to provide added protection against pathogen transmission
c. to avoid any potential drug interaction with nail polish
d. to protect wrist and hand jewelry from corrosive chemicals

**5.** Which of these physical conditions precludes IV technicians from working in a sterile compounding facility?

a. gastric reflux
b. cardiac arrhythmia
c. osteoarthritis
d. weeping sores

## Apply Your Knowledge

*On a separate sheet of paper, write your answers to the questions posed in the paragraph below. Use complete sentences and take time to create a thorough and thoughtful response. Check your answers against the Answer Key in Appendix A.*

In Part 1 of this chapter, you learned that touch contamination is the most common source of contamination in the preparation of CSPs. With that in mind, consider the following scenario:

> You happen to notice that a co-worker inadvertently touched the faucet with one hand while performing an aseptic hand washing. It appears that he is unaware of the contamination and continues on with the procedure.

What is the most appropriate course of action for you to take? Would you take a different course of action if it appeared as though he *did* notice the break in technique but continued with the procedure anyhow? Why or why not?

# Part 2: Training

*Before performing this lab, review the Sterile Compounding Area Procedures listed on pages 162–163 at the end of the Unit 2 opener, and preview the accompanying process validation checklist in Appendix D.*

## Understand the Resources and Supplies

USP Chapter <797> prescribes special requirements for aseptic garbing, hand washing, and gloving. This chapter and the corresponding lab provide resources and supplies that are in alignment with the directives set forth in USP Chapter <797>.

### Essential Supplies

Most sterile compounding procedures require the same essential supply items to be available for use in both the anteroom and the clean room. For the anteroom, these supplies include aseptic foot and head garb, such as disposable shoe covers, a hair cover, a face mask, and a beard cover (if appropriate)—as well as an approved hand-cleansing agent. Clean room supplies include sterile, foamed 70% IPA and sterile gloves.

***Foot and Head Garb*** Personnel who work in the sterile compounding room must don appropriate footwear for safety and comfort. IV technicians should wear close-toed shoes because of the potential for injury by needles or broken glass. Clean, well-fitting walking or running shoes are a safe option and can provide technicians with the comfort and increased stamina they need for standing for hours in front of the laminar airflow hood. Sterile compounders also need to place disposable shoe covers over their shoes to keep dirt and other substances from contaminating the clean room floor. These shoe covers are removed and thrown away upon leaving the anteroom.

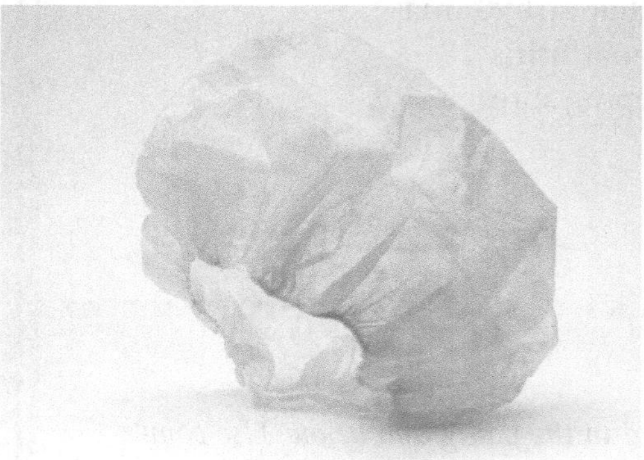

Disposable bouffant-style head cover.

Personnel in the sterile compounding area must also wear hair covers. The options for hair covers include disposable caps and washable caps in surgical or bouffant styles. In general, surgical caps tie behind the head, and bouffant caps have a band of elastic that secure them to the head. Disposable bouffant-style caps are the most common type of hair cover for pharmacy personnel, who must remove and throw them away upon leaving the sterile compounding lab. Washable caps are available in both surgical and bouffant styles and must be cleaned in the hospital laundry after each use. No matter which style IV technicians choose, the most important consideration is that the selected hair cover completely covers all of the hair.

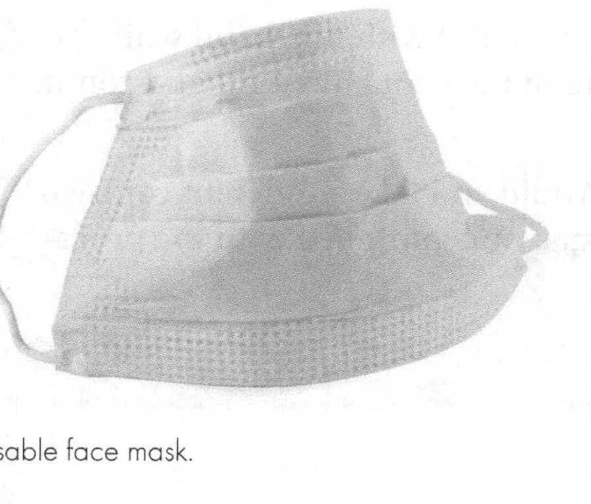

Disposable face mask.

Lastly, pharmacy personnel wear face masks to catch the bacteria held in the liquid droplets and **aerosols** that emanate from the mouth and nose. Masks may have ties or elastic to secure them to the face, and most masks are made from paper or another nonwoven material and are discarded after each use. IV technicians with facial hair should also wear beard covers, which are similar to face masks but cover all visible facial hair, including beards, moustaches, and sideburns.

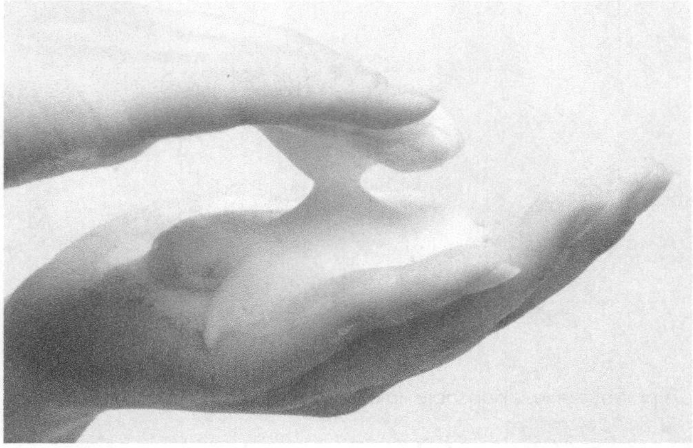

Hand cleansing.

***Hand Cleansers*** Several cleansing agents are available for aseptic hand washing in the sterile compounding environment. Each commonly used type of hand cleanser has benefits and well-defined uses, and compounding facilities choose the types that suit them. To help prevent the formation of microbes that are resistant to a specific cleansing agent, facilities should occasionally change their type of hand cleanser.

- **Chloroxylenol** is an effective, common cleansing agent appropriate for aseptic hand washing.
- **Chlorhexidine gluconate** is also a common and appropriate cleansing agent for aseptic hand washing.
- **Isopropyl alcohol (IPA)** rinses, gels, or foams are frequently used prior to donning PPE, and between aseptic hand-washing procedures when there is minor hand contamination from handling labels or medication orders or adjusting eyeglasses. Whenever they touch anything that is potentially contaminated, technicians should use this cleansing agent to quickly re-clean the hands or gloves, provided that a complete aseptic hand washing has already been performed.
- **Iodophors** (such as **povidone-iodine**) have very effective antimicrobial properties, but they irritate the skin. Thus, sterile compounding technicians typically use this cleansing agent only if nothing else is available.
- **Triclosan**, common in household soaps, is appropriate for general hand washing in other areas of the pharmacy, but not acceptable for aseptic hand washing.

***Scrubs, Gowns, and Gloves*** Keep in mind that the laminar airflow hood generates a certain amount of heat when on. Thus, when dressing to enter the sterile compounding area, layer your attire so that it is both appropriate for the warmth level and comfortable and practical for the tasks at hand. Technicians should don clean scrub uniforms (available in most hospitals or uniform supply stores) that should only be worn when preparing sterile products. If scrubs are not available, preparers should dress in clean, lightweight clothing that is not prone to shedding and that has not been exposed to pet hair.

Sterile compounding technicians must wear, as the outer layer of clothing, either a sterile, lint-free, disposable gown, or a gown that has been freshly laundered and sterilized by the hospital's laundry department. The gown should completely cover the front of the technician, have a secure neck closure, tie in the back, and fit snugly around the wrists.

Technicians should also don sterile, powder-free gloves. Synthetic, nonlatex gloves are available for people with latex allergies. As a general rule, note that size six gloves are small, size seven gloves are medium, and size eight gloves are large. Gloves

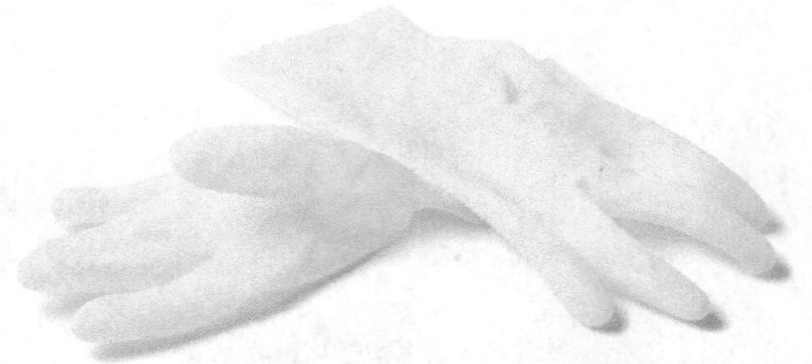

A pair of sterile, disposable, latex gloves.

should be close-fitting to allow for maximum finger dexterity but not so tight that they compromise circulation or cause discomfort. Experiment until you find the size that fits best. Gloves are for one-time use only; you should discard them when leaving the sterile compounding area or anteroom.

## Procedure-Specific Supplies

In addition to the previously listed essential supplies, each sterile compounding procedure requires supply items specific to the procedure being performed. For aseptic hand-washing procedures, a designated sink and hand-washing supplies should be available in the anteroom for use by sterile compounding personnel.

***Designated Sink for Aseptic Hand Washing*** USP Chapter <797> regulations describe the features and location of a sink designated for aseptic hand washing. The sink should be used only for aseptic hand washing by pharmacy personnel who are preparing to enter the sterile compounding room. This specialized and restricted-use sink is designed to minimize splashing and reduce the possibility of contamination during the hand-washing procedure.

The sink must be located in the anteroom or just outside the door of the clean room. It should be deep and have a gooseneck faucet and hot and cold running water. Preferably, foot pedals should be used to turn the water on and off. If a sink with foot pedals is not available, personnel must let the water run throughout the entire scrub and rinse procedure and then turn off the faucet with clean, lint-free paper towels. The sink must be clean and free of any items that might cause splashing, such as sponges or IV bags.

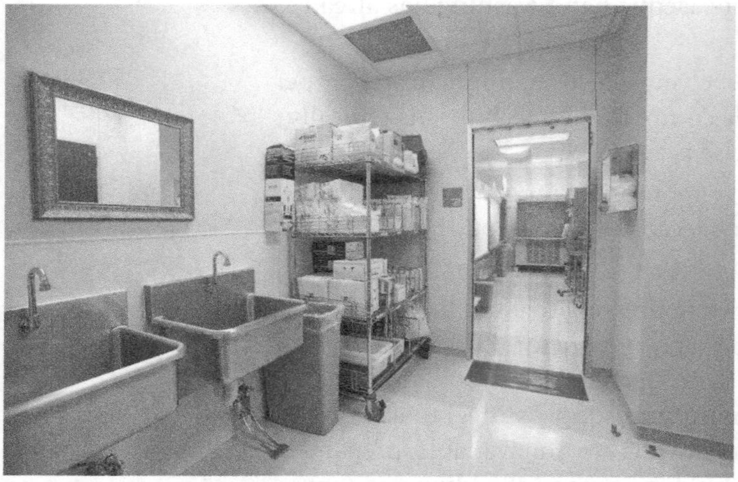

Anteroom sinks with gooseneck faucets and foot pedals.

***Hand-Washing Supplies*** Policies and procedures regarding the use of scrub sponges or scrub brushes in the aseptic hand-washing process vary slightly among sterile compounding facilities. As a sterile compounder, you perform a very **basic aseptic hand washing** by vigorously washing both hands and forearms for at least 30 seconds with an appropriate antimicrobial agent. You must focus extra attention on areas that harbor multiple microorganisms, such as under the fingernails and in the creases of skin, and you must wash your arms up to the elbow. Compared with doing a complete aseptic hand washing, you perform the basic hand-washing procedure more quickly and without using a surgical sponge or brush. However, the two types of hand washing are otherwise the same.

**BE AWARE**

Never use the brush side of a surgical scrub tool to cleanse the skin. Doing so may cause skin particles to flake off into the clean environment, resulting in contamination.

Many facilities, especially those that prepare medium-risk CSPs such as total parenteral nutrition solutions and high-risk CSPs such as those compounded from nonsterile ingredients, prefer to perform the hand-washing procedure using a sterile, prepackaged, **surgical scrub sponge/brush** presaturated with an approved antimicrobial soap. The sterile surgical scrub sponge/brush is a very effective tool for ensuring a correct aseptic hand-washing process. Use the sponge side of the tool to cleanse the skin; use the brush side to scrub under the fingernails and around the nail cuticles. Perform the rinse procedures so that soapy water runs off toward the elbow. This arm position helps to maintain the cleanliness of the fingertips, which will come in direct contact with the CSPs. Dry the hands and forearms with aseptic, lint-free, disposable towels or an aseptic hand dryer. The towel container must be designed so it does not compromise the cleanliness or integrity of the towels.

# Preview the Lab Procedure

*The following material provides a brief overview of the lab procedure that you will perform. First, read the* Preview the Lab Procedure *section. Then read each step of the* Procedural Lab *section carefully, visualizing every action. Next, reinforce your understanding of the process by watching the demonstration video. Once you are in the lab, your instructor will demonstrate the procedure, and then you will perform the procedure by following the steps in the* Procedural Lab *section. Practice the lab procedure multiple times. After sufficient practice, you will complete the lab procedure for process validation by your instructor.*

**POINTER**

Sterile compounding personnel must comply with certain restrictions when working in the anteroom and clean room areas. These restrictions include no gum chewing, horseplay, or food or drink in both the anteroom and clean room, and no hair spray, perfume, makeup, artificial or polished nails, or jewelry in the sterile compounding environment.

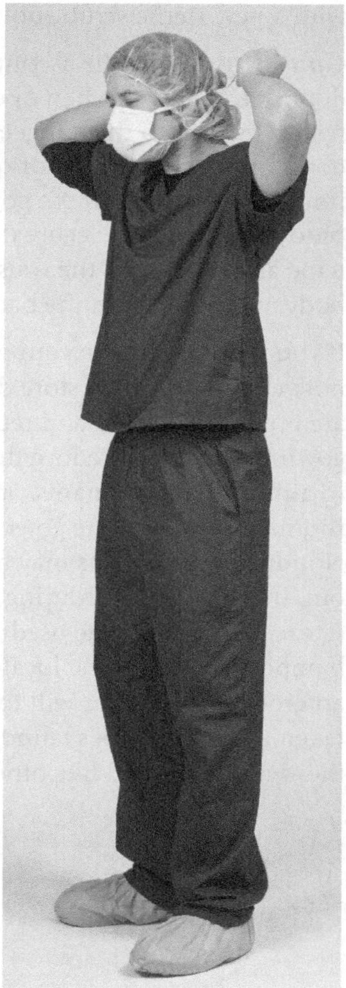

IV technician donning a face mask.

## Anteroom Preparatory Procedures

You perform the preparatory steps of garbing, hand washing, and gloving in the anteroom before entering the sterile product preparation area. The entire process begins with the dirtiest or most contaminated item, the shoes, and ends with the donning of gloves. Because hands and gloves come in direct contact with the sterile product, they must be the cleanest area.

***Garbing*** When you enter the anteroom, you first remove any outer garments that you are wearing, such as a coat, sweater, jacket, or hat. If you are not already wearing appropriate lab attire, you change into a clean scrub uniform, or other lightweight clothing. Next, cleanse your hands with sterile, foamed 70% IPA. Although not mandated by USP Chapter <797>, it is considered best practice to cleanse the hands with sterile, foamed 70% IPA prior to donning PPE, and again after donning shoe and hair covers.

**POINTER**

Sterile compounding technicians with long hair may find it helpful to put hair in a ponytail or otherwise tie it back before putting on hair covers. These individuals should also make sure that during the procedures all of their hair remains inside of the cap.

Next, you put on a clean pair of shoe covers. Once your shoe covers are in place, reapply sterile, foamed 70% IPA to your hands and put a hair cover on your head, making sure that all hair is tucked under the cap.

Once the shoe covers and hair cover are in place, reapply sterile, foamed 70% IPA to your hands and position a face mask over the nose and mouth. The face mask should cover the entire face, from below the chin to the bridge of the nose. If you position the top tie of the mask above the ears, the mask won't slip down on your face. Men with visible facial hair should also wear a beard cover.

**USP Chapter <797>**

Correct aseptic hand-washing technique requires sterile compounding personnel to alternate between the left and right hand, moving from the fingers up toward the elbows.

***Aseptic Hand Washing*** Once you are appropriately garbed, proceed to the sink for aseptic hand washing. Because fingertips directly contact the sterile product, aseptic hand washing is designed to move dirt from the fingertips toward the elbows. Thus, the hand-washing procedure repeatedly alternates between the hands and gradually works toward the elbows. The average acceptable aseptic hand washing takes a minimum of 30 seconds, but a careful and thorough job requires 2–4 minutes.

The surgical scrub sponge/brush is for one-time use only and should be thrown away immediately after use. Exercise caution not to contaminate the fingers, hands, arms, or the scrub sponge/brush at any time by inadvertently touching the sink or faucet. Should this happen, you must repeat the entire hand-washing procedure with a new sterile scrub sponge/brush.

**USP Chapter <797>**

Do not apply lotion to your hands after completing the hand-washing procedure. Doing so causes hand contamination.

***Gowning*** After the aseptic hand washing, you don a clean gown. When opening the gown or removing it from the hanger, be sure that the gown does not touch the floor or other surface at any time. You should pull the gown up the arms and onto the shoulders. Secure the neck closure at the nape and then wrap the waist ties around your body and tie them in the back.

If you need to remove your gown and your shift is not yet over, you may store disposable gowns that are not visibly soiled and reuse them. Turn the gown inside out to reduce the chance of exposure to airborne contaminants, and store it in the anteroom. Throw away the gown at the end of the shift. Nondisposable gowns may also be hung up, inside out, in the anteroom during the shift. At the end of each shift, place the used gowns in the laundry hamper that should be located just outside the anteroom. The gowns will then be picked up and taken to the hospital's laundry department where they will be washed like other sterile linens.

**USP Chapter <797>**

Gowns that are kept in the anteroom while technicians are away from the sterile compounding area must not touch the floor or come into contact with any potential contaminants.

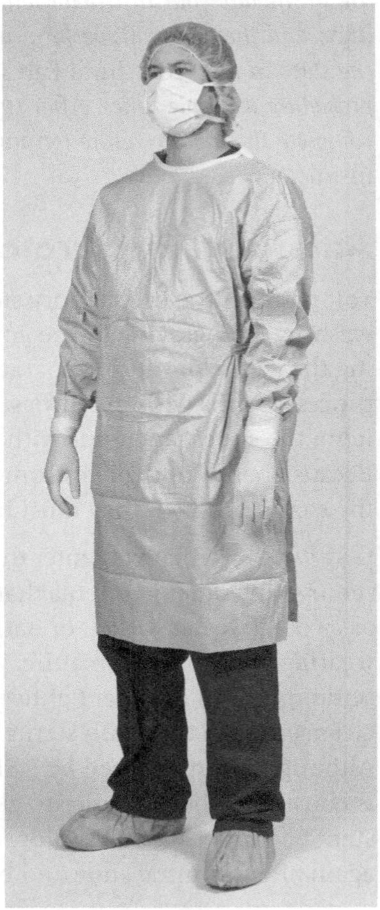

A fully gowned and gloved IV technician.

***Sterile Gloving*** The last part of the garbing, hand-washing, and gloving procedures involves the donning of sterile, powder-free gloves. In most cases, this procedure will be performed immediately upon entering the clean room. However, to facilitate training during this procedural lab, you will don sterile gloves while in the anteroom. First, you cleanse the hands with a small amount of sterile, foamed 70% IPA. Next, you open the outer packet of the gloves to reveal the inner, sterile packet containing the gloves. You then unwrap the sterile packet carefully so that the gloves do not come into contact with any nonsterile surface. You then carefully pull each glove onto the hand and over the wrist cuff of the gown, until it is firmly seated on the forearm, just above the cuff. This placement ensures that the gloves will not slip down below the gown's cuffs.

Gloves may be re-cleaned with sterile, foamed 70% IPA as needed, provided that they are fully intact and have not experienced major contamination. Inspect the gloves regularly throughout the shift. Immediately replace gloves when you notice a hole or tear. Sterile gloves are for one-time use and must be disposed of immediately upon leaving the sterile compounding area.

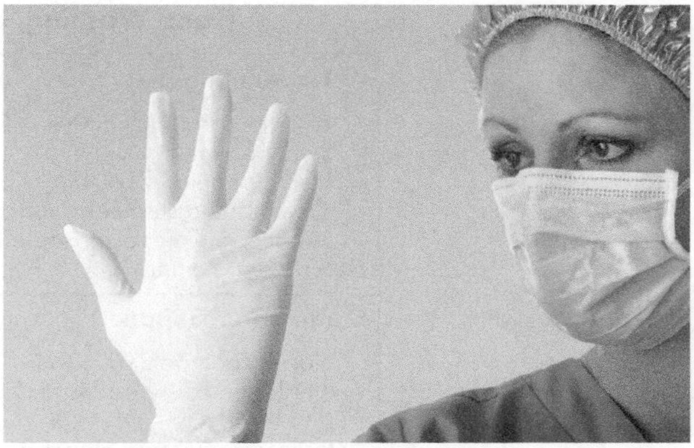
IV technician inspecting a glove for holes or tears.

## Removal of PPE Items

Upon completion of sterile compounding procedures and prior to leaving the anteroom, sterile compounding personnel must correctly remove the PPE items worn. Remove PPE items in the reverse order from how they were donned, starting with glove removal and ending with shoe covers.

# Watch the Demonstration Video

*Watch the Chapter 6 Demonstration Video, which shows the step-by-step aseptic garbing, hand-washing, and gloving procedures.*

Training Videos DVD

# Procedural Lab

*This lab walks you through the step-by-step actions that you must follow for aseptic garbing, hand washing, and gloving. Take your time. Work through each step methodically and with close attention to detail.*

## Supplies

### *Essential Supplies*

To complete the Unit 2 procedural labs, you will need to ensure that various essential anteroom and clean room supplies such as those listed in Table 6.1 are available for your use.

**Table 6.1 Essential Anteroom and Clean Room Supplies for Aseptic Garbing, Hand Washing, and Gloving**

| |
|---|
| **Anteroom Supplies** |
| aseptic garb, including shoe covers, hair cover, face mask, and beard cover (if appropriate)<br>sterile gown<br>sterile, foamed 70% IPA<br>presaturated surgical scrub sponge/brush<br>aseptic, lint-free, disposable towels<br>waste container |
| **Clean Room Supplies** |
| sterile, foamed 70% IPA<br>sterile, powder-free gloves* |
| *Sterile, powder-free gloves are usually donned in the clean room; however, for the purposes of the Chapter 6 procedural lab, they will be donned in the anteroom. |

**POINTER**

To keep the mask from riding up and into your field of vision, shape it over the bridge of the nose by gently pinching the thin aluminum strip woven into the top of the mask.

**BE AWARE**

Do not allow the surgical scrub sponge/brush to come into contact with any surface while you are removing it from the packet. If you accidentally drop the sponge/brush in the sink while hand washing, discard it, open a new sponge/brush packet, and restart the hand-washing procedure from the beginning.

## Procedure

### *Garbing*

1. Remove any outer garments and jewelry.
2. Cleanse your hands with sterile, foamed 70% IPA. Hold a can of foamed alcohol so that the tip is pointed down into the palm of the opposite hand. Press against the tip with the index finger of the hand holding the can, releasing into the palm a small amount of alcohol, approximately the size of a quarter or a golf ball. Rub your hands together making sure that the alcohol coats the palms, the backs of the hands, and each finger. Allow the alcohol to evaporate.

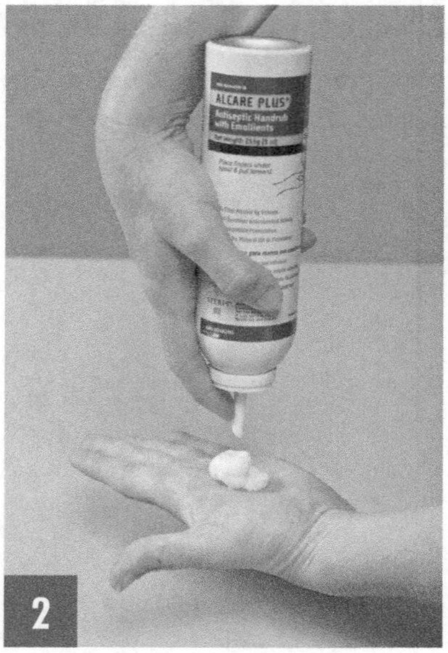

2

3. Don shoe covers, one at a time. Slip the longer end over the toe of the shoe. Pull the cover around the bottom of the shoe and onto the heel. The cover should completely envelop the shoe.

4. Reapply sterile, foamed 70% IPA to your hands and allow it to dry.
5. Put on the hair cover. Gather or tie back loose hair and place the bouffant-style cap over your head so that most of the hair is at the back. Position the back elastic against the back of your neck. Pull the front over your head until the elastic is against your forehead. Tuck any loose hair under the cover. All hair must be covered.
6. Reapply sterile, foamed 70% IPA to your hands and allow it to dry.
7. Don a face mask. Place the top of the mask on the bridge of the nose. Tie the upper ties behind the head, just above your ears. Tie the lower ties behind the neck. Position the mask securely over the nose, mouth, and chin. If you have facial hair, don a beard cover as well.

### *Aseptic Hand Washing*

8. Proceed to the sink and prepare for aseptic hand washing. Before opening the surgical scrub sponge/brush, squeeze the packet several times to activate the soapsuds. Then open the packet, remove the sterile sponge/brush, and hold it in your dominant hand. Use your other hand to dispose of the wrapper in the waste container. Press the foot pedals to begin the flow of water. Allow the water to run until it is warm.
9. Wet your hands and arms. Still holding the scrub sponge/brush, use the nail pick (found loosely embedded in the sponge side of the tool) to clean under each of your fingernails. When you have finished, dispose of the pick in the waste container.
10. Apply a *small amount* of water to the scrub sponge/brush. Squeeze the scrub sponge/brush with a gentle pumping motion and use only a small amount of water. This technique helps to prevent too much soap from being wasted down the drain. Squeeze and dampen as needed so that you have a good soapy lather throughout the entire procedure.
11. Using the *brush side* of the tool, scrub under the fingernail of the thumb of the left hand. Move to the other fingernails, one by one, in order from thumb to pinkie. Repeat the scrubbing process on the fingernails of the right hand.
12. Using the *sponge side* of the tool, clean each of the four surfaces (top, side, bottom, side) of the thumb of the left hand. Clean the webbing between the thumb and forefinger. Next, clean all four surfaces of the forefinger. Continue cleaning the remaining fingers of the left hand sequentially, cleaning the webbing in between each finger before moving on to the next finger. Repeat the cleaning pattern on the thumb and fingers of the right hand.
13. After cleaning the thumb and fingers of the left hand and the right hand, return to the left hand and clean the left palm with the sponge. Then clean the right palm.
14. After cleaning the palm of the right hand, return to cleaning the left hand and clean the back of the hand with the sponge. Then clean the back of the right hand with the sponge.

**POINTER**

Whether you are left-handed or right-handed, you initially perform the aseptic hand-washing procedure in exactly the same order as your classmates. After you have mastered the technique, your instructor may allow you to change order by scrubbing your dominant hand first.

**USP Chapter <797>**

After cleaning the palm of a hand, do not go back and clean the fingers again. USP Chapter <797> guidelines stipulate that the cleaning process should not be reversed.

15. Next, clean the left forearm, moving gradually, and in a circular pattern, around and around the arm, proceeding from the wrist up to the elbow. Then clean the right forearm using the same technique.

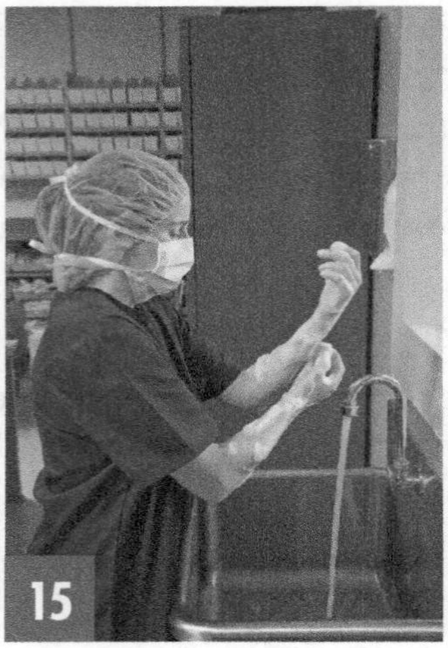


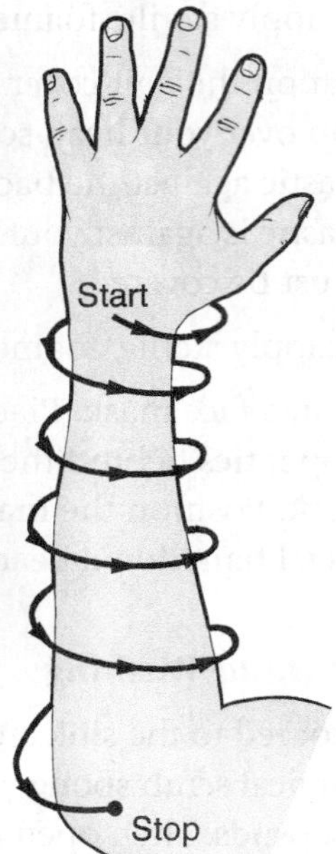


With your fingers pointing up, begin washing at the wrist and work around the forearm in a circular pattern ending at the elbow.

USP <797>

Avoid shaking your hands into the sink to dislodge water. Doing so causes water to run down toward your fingertips, thereby contaminating them.

16. Having completed the cleaning process, you now dispose of the scrub sponge/brush without touching the waste container or its contents.

17. Press the foot pedals on the sink so that you have a nice flow of warm water. Rinse the left hand and forearm, holding your arm with fingertips pointing up so you rinse the fingers first and the water runs down toward the elbow. Then rinse the right hand and forearm. If the sink does not have a foot pedal, turn the faucet on and allow it to run throughout the entire procedure.

**BE AWARE**

Do not touch the sink or faucet at any time during the rinsing procedure. Keep your fingers pointing upward throughout the entire rinse. Do not allow the water to run down toward your fingertips because this action compromises the aseptic nature of the procedure.

18. Using an aseptic, lint-free, paper towel, dry both hands, and then dry the forearms, moving toward the elbow. Keep your fingers pointing up throughout the drying procedure. When finished drying, dispose of the paper towel in the waste container.

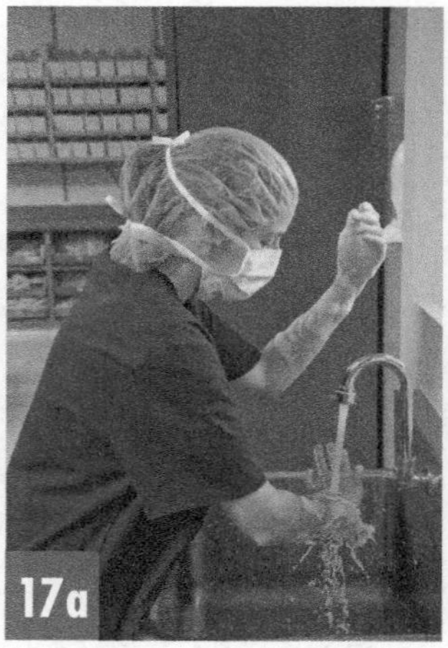


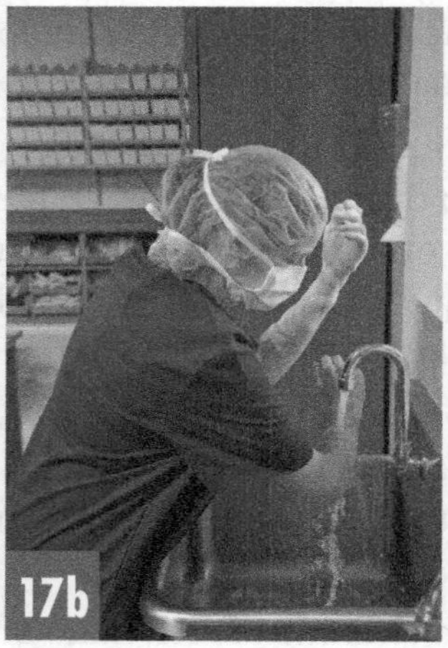


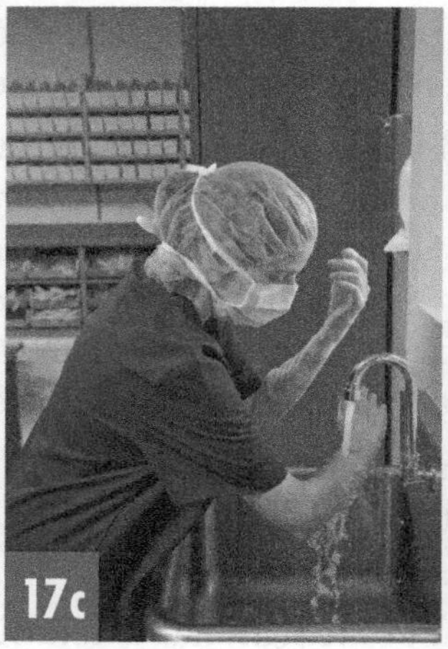


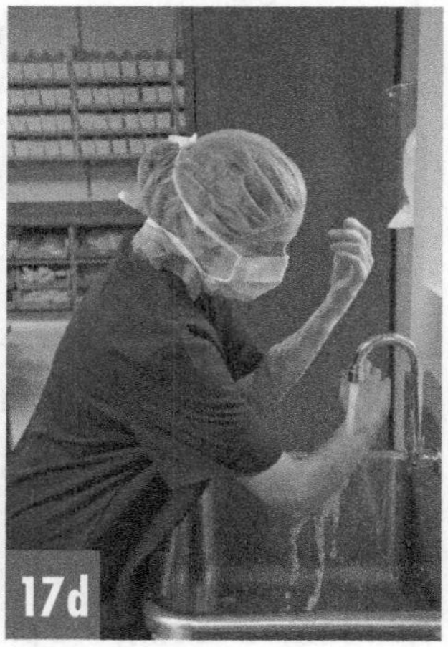

### *Gowning and Gloving*

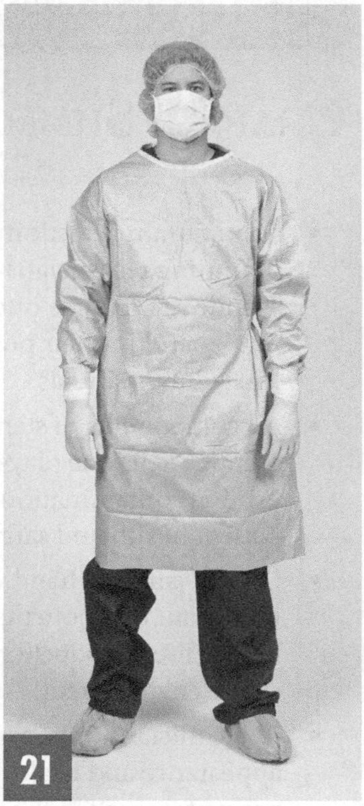

21

**19.** Carefully open the package containing the sterile gown. Don the gown, making sure it does not touch a contaminated surface, such as the floor or a work surface. Insert one arm into the open sleeve and then pull it up onto the shoulder. Insert the other arm into the other sleeve and pull the gown up to the neck. Secure the neck closure of the gown at the nape. Wrap the waist ties around your body and tie them in back.

**20.** Sterilize your hands with sterile, foamed 70% IPA.

**21.** Open the outer wrapper of a packet of sterile gloves. Place the inner packet on a clean surface, such as a table or countertop that has been recently cleaned with sterile 70% IPA. Open the inner glove packet. Do not touch the fingertips of the glove at any time during the donning process. Note that the gloves are labeled "left" and "right." Place the glove on the left hand by grasping the inner part of the cuff (it will be folded over for easy access) with the right hand and carefully pulling the glove onto the left hand, up to the wrist, and over the cuff of the gown. Repeat the gloving process with the other hand.

### *Removal of PPE upon Leaving Anteroom*

**22.** Remove one glove by grasping the cuff and pulling it down and off the hand. The glove should now be inside out. Continue holding this glove in the hand that remains gloved. Grasp the cuff of the glove on the other hand and pull it off of the hand. One glove is now inside the other glove. Dispose of this glove bundle in a standard waste container.

**23.** Untie the strings of the gown and then remove the gown by pulling it off at the shoulders. As you pull it toward the fingers, the gown turns inside out. Make sure that the gown never touches the floor or any other potentially contaminated surface. At the end of your shift, throw away your disposable gown or place your reusable gown in a designated laundry hamper outside the anteroom. Reusable gowns will be picked up and taken to the hospital's laundry facility for cleaning.

**24.** Remove your face mask, hair cover, and shoe covers, in that order. Discard them in a standard waste container.

**POINTER**

After removing PPE, wash your hands with soap and water before leaving the anteroom. Hand cleansing will remove any residue from the compounding process that may have inadvertently transferred onto your hands.

**POINTER**

You may reuse your gown throughout your shift, provided that it is not obviously contaminated or visibly soiled. While you are on break, hang the gown, inside out, in the anteroom area that is designated for gown storage.

# Process Validation by Instructor

*Your instructor will use the process validation checklist provided in Appendix D to evaluate your technique for this lab. In order to receive ACPE certification, and prior to making CSPs for patient use, you must correctly perform each component of the lab procedure. Review the Chapter 6 lab and thoroughly practice each of the steps prior to your evaluation.*

# Part 3: Assessment

## Chapter Summary

- To maintain infection control, sterile compounding technicians must follow the strict aseptic procedures outlined in USP Chapter <797> and in their pharmacies' Policy & Procedure manuals.
- All components of sterile compounding and aseptic technique play an important role in preventing contamination of the CSP, thus ensuring patient health and safety.
- Correct garbing, hand washing, and gloving are important components of aseptic technique and reduce the introduction of pathogens into the sterile environment.
- IV technicians must assess their own physical appearance and health condition prior to preparing for work in the clean room.
- Donning PPE items such as shoe covers, a hair or beard cover, a face mask, a sterile gown, and gloves is required for sterile compounding personnel.
- Correct removal, storage, and disposal of used PPE items also help to maintain aseptic technique protocol.
- Sterile compounding requires aseptic hand washing with an antimicrobial agent.
- The correct order of preparation for sterile compounding work is donning shoe covers, a hair cover, a face mask, and a beard cover (if appropriate). These garbing procedures are following by an aseptic hand washing and then by donning a sterile gown and sterile gloves.
- Food, drink, gum chewing, and horseplay are prohibited in the sterile compounding area.
- Sterile, foamed 70% IPA should be used prior to garbing as well as upon minor contamination (such as adjusting eyeglasses) during sterile compounding procedures.
- A complete aseptic hand washing must be performed prior to donning a sterile gown and upon any major contamination (such as a needle stick or large spill).
- A complete aseptic hand washing should take a minimum of 30 seconds but usually takes between 2–4 minutes.

## Key Terms

**aerosols** small liquid or solid particles that are temporarily suspended in air or in another gaseous medium

**amulet** a small, decorative object, often worn around the neck, that is used to bring good luck or protection to the wearer

**antimicrobial agent** a cleansing product that is designed to either slow the growth of, or kill, microbes and bacteria

**asepsis** a state or condition in which the sterile compounding area and the CSP remain free from pathogenic microorganisms

**autoclave** a device that uses heat and/or steam to sterilize inanimate objects such as surgical instruments, sterile linens, and certain high-risk CSPs

**bacteria** single-celled microorganisms that may contaminate the CSP and lead to a serious infection in the patient recipient

**basic aseptic hand washing** a type of hand washing that lasts approximately 30 seconds, using an antimicrobial soap but no scrub/sponge tool; may be performed after minor glove contamination (such as after using a calculator) but is most often done after removing sterile garb just prior to exiting the anteroom

**Black Plague** a devastating pandemic thought to be spread by the fleas on rats; estimated to have killed 50 percent of Europe's population in the mid-fourteenth century; also known as the Black Death

**carbolic acid** an organic compound that was frequently used in early disinfection practices

**chlorhexidine gluconate** an antimicrobial agent that is widely effective against contaminants that may be encountered in sterile compounding; commonly used in the surgical scrub sponge/brush products utilized in aseptic hand washing

**chloroxylenol** a chlorine-based phenol derivative that is used as an antiseptic cleansing agent in pharmacy and presurgical hand washing

**compounded sterile preparations (CSPs)** the mixing of one or more sterile products using aseptic technique

**contagion** any transmittable infectious agent or contagious disease

**cross contamination** the spread of microorganisms, pathogens, or disease from person to person, or room to room, due to poor hand-washing or disinfection practices

**elixir** an orally administered pharmaceutical compound that is comprised of one or more medications dissolved or suspended in liquid; a liquid medication, often with an alcohol component, that is administered orally

**fomite** an inanimate object such as clothing or bedding that is capable of spreading disease

**garbing** the process of donning aseptic shoe covers, a hair cover, a face mask, and a sterile gown and gloves in preparation for working in the clean room

**germ theory** the theory that all diseases are caused by microorganisms, and that these germs can be transmitted among humans

**infection control** standard practices, including hand washing, surface disinfection, and garbing, that are designed to reduce the likelihood of nosocomial infections in the healthcare setting

**iodophors** anti-infective, antimicrobial agents used for presurgical cleansing

**isopropyl alcohol (IPA)** a cleaning agent commonly used to clean and prepare surfaces in the sterile compounding environment

**latex medical glove** a type of glove used by sterile compounding personnel and other healthcare workers to prevent the spread of disease and protect both the patient and the worker

**mercuric chloride** a mercury derivative used in the eighteenth century as a surface and hand disinfectant

**microorganism** a microscopic living organism such as a bacterium, fungus, or virus

**micropores** microscopic holes inherent in manufactured membranes, such as those used to create gloves

**nosocomial infection** a hospital-acquired infection; any infection that a patient acquires as a result of treatment in a healthcare facility

**pathogen** a disease-causing microorganism

**personal protective equipment (PPE)** specialized clothing and equipment worn by sterile compounding personnel to protect them from hazardous chemicals and to protect the CSP from contaminants

**pestilence** a deadly disease epidemic such as the Plague

**povidone-iodine** an anti-infective, antimicrobial agent used for presurgical cleansing

**Spanish Flu pandemic of 1918** an influenza pandemic, believed to have originated in China, that killed approximately 40 million people worldwide; a virulent strain of influenza whose name was attributed to a particularly high mortality rate in Spain

**strigil** a small, curved tool used to scrape dirt from the body during personal hygiene rituals

**surgical scrub sponge/brush** a dual-sided tool that is typically presaturated with chlorhexadine or another similar anti-infective solution and used in aseptic and presurgical hand washing

**touch contamination** transmission of contaminants through the touching of nonsterile surfaces or a break in aseptic technique; the most common and potentially dangerous form of CSP contamination

**triclosan** a cleansing agent present in many household soaps

## Check the Basics

*On a separate sheet of paper, write your answers as modeled in these examples:* 1d; 2c; 3b; *etc.*

**1.** What should you do if you accidentally drop the sterile scrub sponge/brush in the sink while hand washing?

a. Pick up the scrub sponge/brush and resume hand washing per lab protocol.
b. Pick up the scrub sponge/brush, rinse it off, and resume hand washing.
c. Discard the dropped scrub sponge/brush, open a new scrub sponge/brush packet, and begin the hand-washing procedure again.
d. Discard the dropped scrub sponge/brush, open a new scrub sponge/brush packet, and resume scrubbing wherever you left off.

**2.** Which statement most accurately describes the rinsing procedure?

a. The water should run off toward the fingertips.
b. The water should run off toward the elbow.
c. The water should run off toward the elbow, and then the hands should be shaken into the sink to remove excess water.
d. It makes no difference how you rinse your hands since they are already clean.

**3.** How long should it take to complete a correct aseptic hand washing?

a. a minimum of 30 seconds and up to 4 minutes
b. exactly 30 seconds
c. a minimum of 2 minutes
d. at least 10 minutes

**4.** What should you do if your hand accidentally touches the sink or faucet during the aseptic hand-washing procedure?

a. Rinse your hand with water and continue the hand-washing procedure from the point where you left off.
b. Repeat the entire procedure with a new, sterile scrub sponge/brush.
c. Provided that the sink and faucet have been cleaned recently, do not do anything.
d. Spray alcohol on your hands and start over with the same scrub sponge/brush.

**5.** Which statement is accurate regarding the use of a sterile scrub sponge/brush?

a. A sterile scrub sponge/brush should never be used for aseptic hand washing.
b. The brush side of the sterile scrub sponge/brush should be used during the entire hand-washing procedure.
c. The brush side of the sterile scrub sponge/brush should be used to clean the fingernails; the sponge side of the sterile scrub should be used to cleanse the skin.
d. The sponge side of the sterile scrub sponge/brush should be used during the entire hand-washing procedure.

**6.** Which of the following items may be reused if it is not visibly soiled and it remains in the sterile compounding area or anteroom?

a. gown
b. gown and shoe covers
c. gown and hair cover
d. gown, hair cover, shoe covers, and face mask

**7.** What is the correct order of preparation for sterile compounding?

a. shoe covers, hair cover, face mask, hand washing, gown, gloves
b. gown, shoe covers, face mask, hand washing, gloves, hair cover
c. hand washing, gloves, gown, shoe covers, hair cover, face mask
d. shoe covers, hair cover, gown, face mask, hand washing, gloves

**8.** Which type of gloves is most appropriate for use in compounding sterile products?

a. powdered gloves that must be washed before entering the clean room
b. powder-free gloves that must be washed before entering the clean room
c. sterile, powder-free gloves
d. sterile, powdered gloves

9. What is the correct order of cleansing the fingers and hands during an aseptic hand washing?
   a. palm, fingers, and nail scrub of the left hand—followed by the right hand
   b. nail scrub, fingers, and palm of the left hand—followed by the right hand
   c. fingers, palm, and nail scrub of the right hand—followed by the left hand
   d. nail scrub, palm, and fingers of the right hand—followed by the left hand

10. Which is the correct method for cleansing the forearms during an aseptic hand washing?
    a. Scrub in an up-and-down motion, gradually working around the arm and toward the elbow.
    b. Scrub in a back-and-forth motion, gradually working around the arm and toward the elbow.
    c. Scrub in a circular motion, gradually working around the arm and toward the elbow.
    d. none of the above

## Make Connections

*On a separate sheet of paper, write your answers to the following three questions, using complete sentences and making sure your answers are thorough and thoughtful. Note that the third question requires Internet access.*

1. Process validation involves the instructor's observation, critique, and grading of the IV technician's aseptic technique. In what ways might the process validation experience benefit the technician?

2. What rationale might you offer for using a sterile, antimicrobial, presaturated scrub sponge/brush while performing aseptic hand washing rather than washing your hands without a sponge/brush?

3. Access the website for the Centers for Disease Control and Prevention (CDC). In the search bar, type *Hand Hygiene Basics* to obtain general hand hygiene information for healthcare personnel. In what ways does this basic hand hygiene information differ from aseptic hand washing?

## Meet the Challenge

***Scenario*** This "illuminating" activity will give you the opportunity to see how well you perform an aseptic hand washing.

***Challenge*** Your instructor has a handout that tests your ability to correctly perform an aseptic hand-washing procedure. To meet this challenge, ask your instructor for the handout and work with a partner or small group to complete the activity.

### ADDITIONAL RESOURCES

*Go to the Paradigm Internet Resources Center at* www.paradigmcollege.net/sterilecomp *to access live links related to these Chapter 6 topics:*

+ USP Chapter <797> standards for sterile compounding
+ CDC guidelines on hand washing and prevention of infection

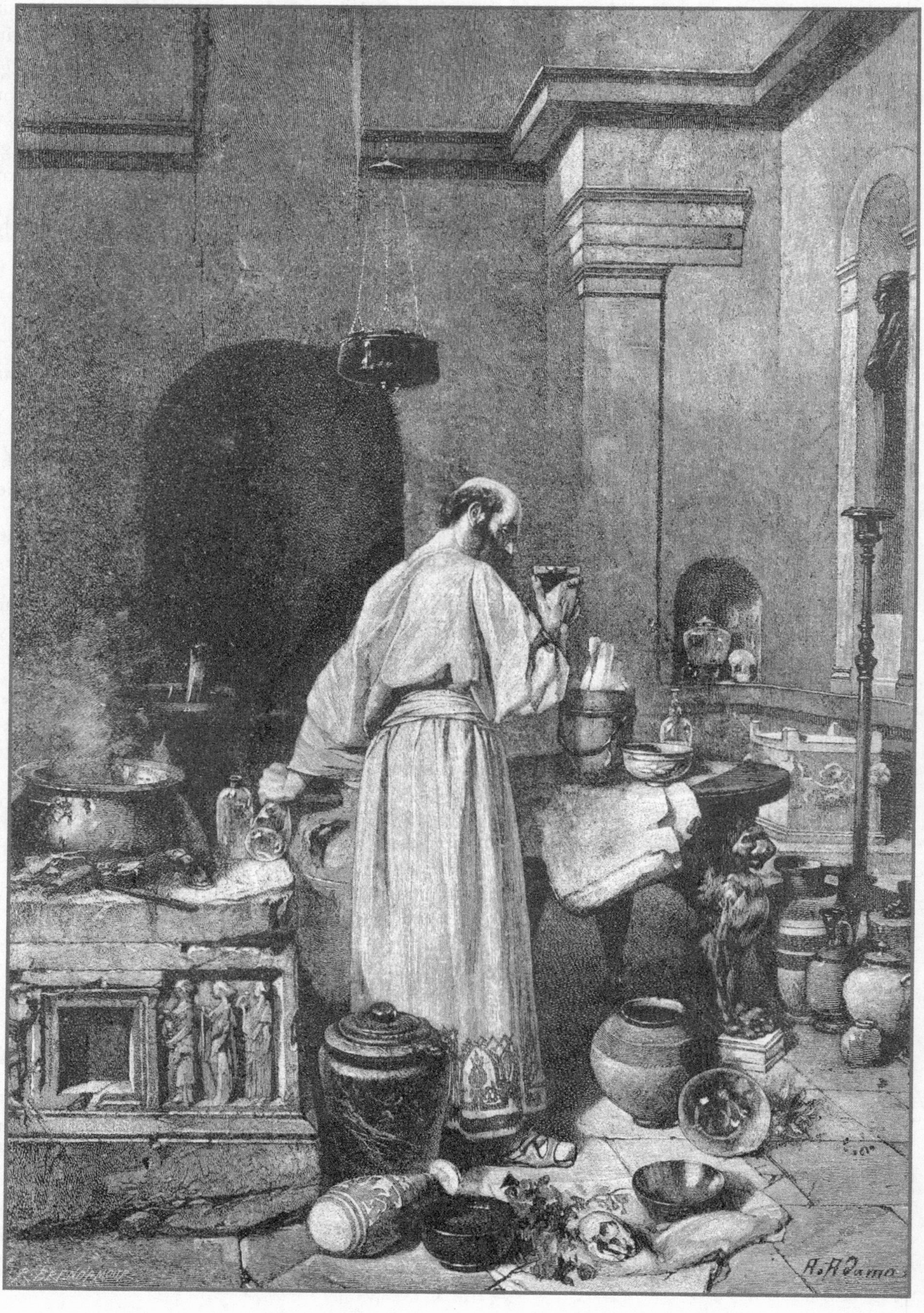

# Chapter 7

# Cleaning the Horizontal Laminar Airflow Hood

## Learning Objectives

- Gain an awareness of early cleanliness methods and disinfection practices.
- Understand the rationale for using a hood when preparing sterile products.
- Describe the components of the horizontal laminar airflow hood.
- Explain the proper methods for cleaning the horizontal laminar airflow hood.
- Demonstrate excellent technique in the cleaning of the horizontal laminar airflow hood.

As you learned in Chapter 6, the process of germ transmission was not fully understood prior to the nineteenth century. However, archaeological evidence from the sites of early civilizations, such as Mesopotamia, shows that these cultures did implement certain cleanliness and **disinfection** practices. In fact, ancient Egyptian cultures, guided by their religious doctrines, were fastidious about personal cleanliness. Their notion that cleanliness was next to godliness stemmed from their belief that illness or disease was the mortal punishment from the gods for unholy behavior. Therefore, participating in cleanliness rituals cleansed not only the body but the soul.

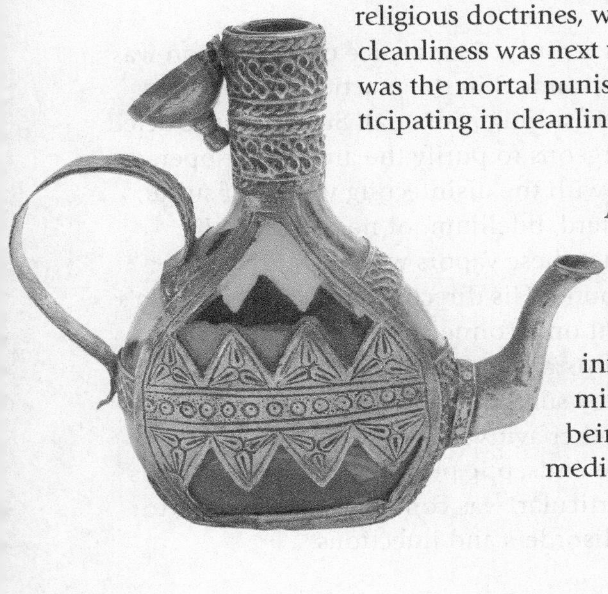

### Ancient Uses of Essential Oils

As part of their bathing rituals, Egyptian citizens applied **essential oils**—such as cedarwood, myrrh, cinnamon bark, thyme, clove, palm, eucalyptus, and fir—to ward off infection. Essential oils were thought to cleanse the body, mind, and spirit of toxins, thereby restoring health and well-being. This early healing practice spawned a form of alternative medicine still used today: **aromatherapy**.

Although these early cleansing practices were limited in effectiveness, they did provide some degree of protection against illness and infection. Recognizing the protective factors, or **antiseptic** properties, of these oils, ancient Egyptians began to soak bandages in these liquids and apply the poultices to wounds. They also introduced essential oils, as well as vinegar (an organic acid), into body cavities during the embalming process to cleanse the bodies before they laid the cadavers in the sunlight for drying. Their discoveries of the disinfectant properties of acids and drying have been applied for centuries in medical practice.

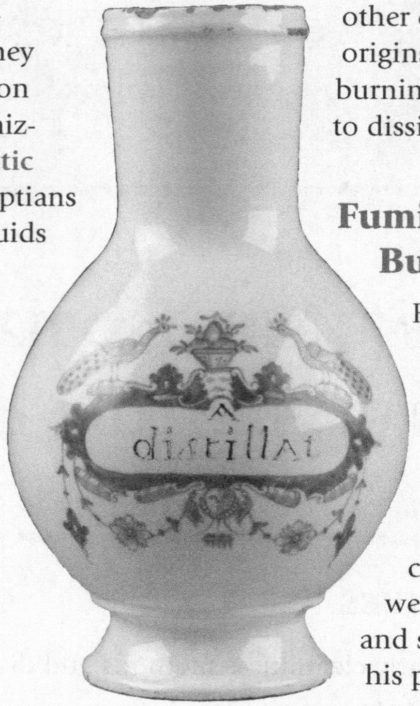


## Early Disinfection Practices

In addition to using plants and tree resins, Egyptians found that several metallic and nonmetallic elements had antiseptic properties as well. They used copper vessels to hold their drinking water, mercury compounds in their mummification processes, and sulfur to fumigate the dwellings of the diseased and dying. In fact, mercury and sulfur are considered to be two of the oldest disinfectants. Mercury was used among primitive cultures to treat wounds; the use of sulfur can be traced back to Book XII of *The Odyssey* by Greek poet Homer, recorded in 800 BCE. In the epic poem, the main character Odysseus orders that his house be fumigated with sulfur after he discovers that his enemies had occupied his house during his long absence. His intention was to purify his dwelling from their evil spirits. Aside from these early disinfectants, two other disinfection practices had their origins in ancient civilizations: burial and burning. Both practices were implemented to dissipate evil spirits and contagion.

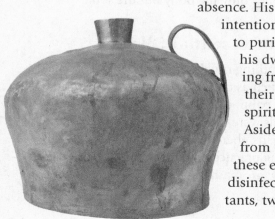

## Fumigation and Burning Methods

Early Greek and Roman practitioners, such as Hippocrates and Galen, approached illness and disease from a more scientific standpoint than the Egyptians did. Hippocrates dismissed the idea that illness and disease were spiritual curses, believing instead that they were the result of the patient's lifestyle and surrounding environment. Like his predecessors, Hippocrates recommended the practice of **fumigation** as a disinfectant, encouraging his fellow citizens to burn herbs in the street to purify the air and ward off disease. He also used herbs (balsam, in particular), the distillate of wine, boiling water, and acetum or vinegar to cleanse wounds. In fact, the potent antibacterial properties of the acid in vinegar continued to be used in the treatment of wounds up through the nineteenth century. Hippocrates' successor, Galen, reportedly boiled his surgical instruments before tending to the wounds of soldiers, revealing a rudimentary knowledge of the effects of **heat sterilization** on bacteria and viruses.

By the first century, the practice of fumigation was a standard protocol in the practice of **ayurvedic medicine**. East Indian shaman Sushruta instructed ancient surgeons to purify the air of their operating rooms with the disinfecting vapors of sulfur, white mustard, bdellium, or neem leaves. He believed that these vapors would sterilize the surgical wound. His directive indicated Sushruta's keen insight on a connection between **airborne contaminants** and infection, a notion that was confirmed by subsequent generations. Sushruta, as well as other ayurvedic practitioners, also recognized the antiseptic properties of heavy metals. Zinc, in particular, was commonly prescribed to treat skin disorders and infections.

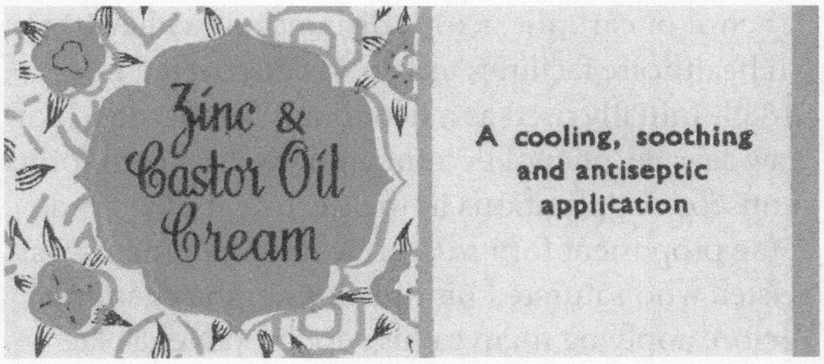


The disinfectant practices of fumigation and burning continued into the Middle Ages, a time of epidemic plagues and untold deaths. Those citizens who succumbed to various forms of plagues had their homes fumigated with sulfur and their clothing incinerated in attempts to halt the spreading of the disease. Ironically, personal hygiene was discouraged at this time for it was thought that hot water would open the skin's pores, allowing disease to creep within the body and reside. The deadly combination of poor personal hygiene, unsanitary disposal of waste, and crowded living conditions contributed to the spread of disease.

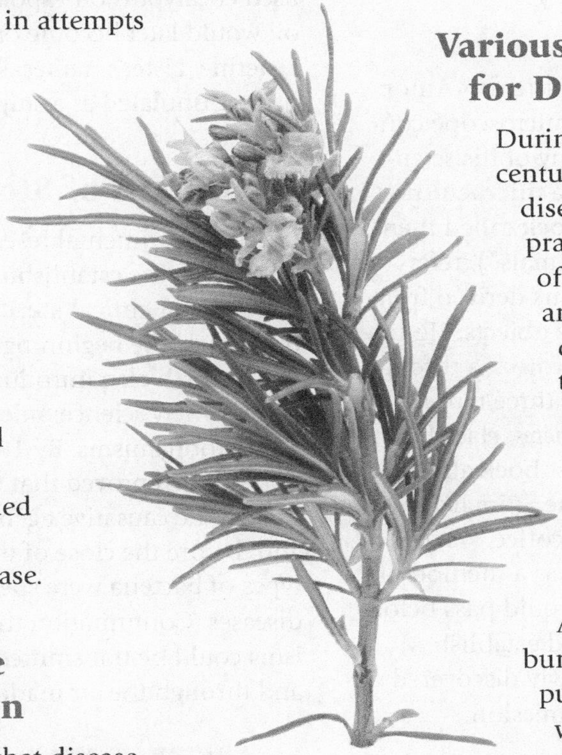

## Seminaria and the Spread of Infection

It wasn't until the 1500s that disease transmission was clearly understood. Italian physician Girolamo Fracastoro (also known as Hieronymus Fracastorius) proposed a theory that infectious diseases could be transmitted by three means: direct contact with an infected person, indirect contact with **fomites** (clothing or objects belonging to the infected person), or airborne transmission. In his book *On Contagion, Contagious Diseases, and Their Treatment*, published in 1546, Fracastoro claimed that invisible particles, or **seminaria**, created by the atmosphere were responsible for the spread of infection among populations. These seminaria were specific to individual diseases, could replicate themselves, and affected the balance of the body's humors. Fracastoro concluded that these seminaria were emitted in the noxious fumes of decaying organic matter, or **miasmas**, from diseased cadavers. Still, it would be another 300 years before scientists would prove the existence of these seminaria (later named **microbes**) and refine an understanding of their origin and role in disease transmission.

## Various Remedies for Disease Transmission

During the sixteenth and seventeenth centuries, with limited knowledge of disease transmission, healthcare practitioners recommended a variety of substances to disinfect objects and purify the air. Some of these disinfectants hearkened back to traditional herbal remedies. Lavender, for example, was considered to be a protectant against infection. As a result, glovemakers began to perfume their gloves with lavender to halt the spread of cholera. Another herb, rosemary, was burned to fumigate hospitals and purify the air. Acids such as vinegar, wine, and, surprisingly, urine were used as antiseptics for dressing wounds; **alkalis** such as soda and lime were used to disinfect surfaces such as public drinking fountains and dwellings of both citizens and animals. None of these remedies, however, could counteract the effects of poor sanitation and hygiene on the transmission of disease.

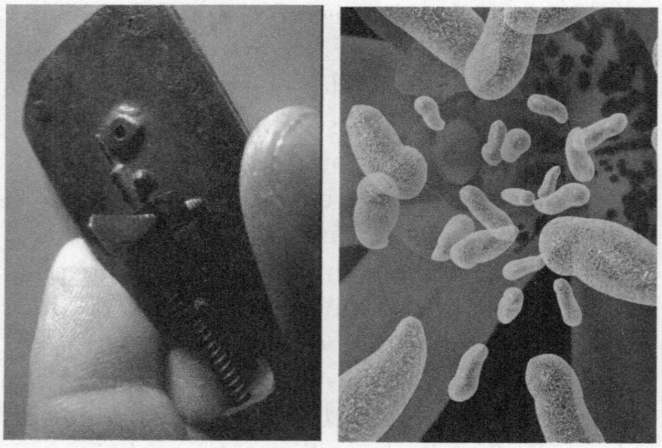

## Leeuwenhoek's Discovery of a Microculture

In the seventeenth century, Dutch scientist Anton van Leeuwenhoek's hand-crafted microscope confirmed what was suspected by many of his scientific predecessors: the presence of a **microculture** of cells and organisms. Leeuwenhoek called them "animalcules" (meaning "little animals"), referring to the idea that these organisms derived from animate life rather than inanimate objects. He carefully observed the movement of **protozoa** through his crude lenses and described the three types of **bacteria** as *cocci, bacilli,* and *spirochetes*, classification terms still used today. Leeuwenhoek also made the serendipitous discovery that the animalcules "could not endure the heat of my coffee," laying the foundation for the use of heat as a method of disinfection. Two hundred years would pass before British surgeon Joseph Lister would establish the relationship between these newly discovered microorganisms and disease transmission.

## Chemical Disinfectants and Infection Control

By the eighteenth and nineteenth centuries, advances in chemistry provided chemical forms of disinfectants. The discovery of **chlorine** in 1774 and **hypochlorites** in 1789 led to their use in the nineteenth century to treat infectious waste before disposal. These substances also served as disinfecting agents in hospital rooms. Another chemical, **iodine**, was introduced in 1811 as a cure for goiter, but its antiseptic properties made it a commonly used wound treatment for soldiers during the Civil War.

**Phenol** or **carbolic acid**, a disinfectant widely used in healthcare facilities today, was discovered in 1834. Initially used as a deodorant for the stench of raw sewage, phenol became more well-known for its antiseptic applications in the treatment of wounds. One proponent for its use in wound treatments was Lister, who saturated his dressings in the chemical before applying them to his surgical patients. He also employed a pump to mist the operative area with the acid. As a result, Lister observed a significant reduction in the mortality rate of his patients. Lister also understood the importance of disinfecting the room air of the operative environment. He used eucalyptus oil vapors as a fumigant. Eucalyptus oil would later become one of the key ingredients in Listerine, Lister's namesake product that was originally formulated as a surgical disinfectant.

## Institution of Sterile Practices

Lister's experimental research on disease transmission led to the establishment of sterile practices, including **chemical sterilization** of surgical instruments and the beginnings of **infection control**. His research also introduced the healthcare field to a brand-new science: **microbiology**, or the study of microorganisms. By 1876, German physician Robert Koch proved that these microorganisms were indeed the causative agents of infectious disease and, before the close of the nineteenth century, 20 types of bacteria were specifically linked to certain diseases. Confirmation that these microorganisms could be transmitted through direct contact and through the air made healthcare practitioners

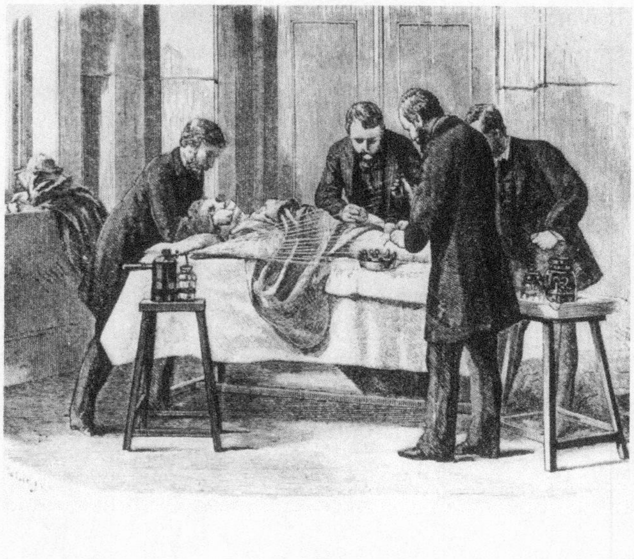

recognize the importance of creating a sterile environment for surgical procedures. Consequently, German surgeon Ernst von Bergmann was the first physician to use an **autoclave** to sterilize his surgical instruments using steam rather than chemicals. This **steam sterilization** method effectively reduced mortality rates among his surgical patients.

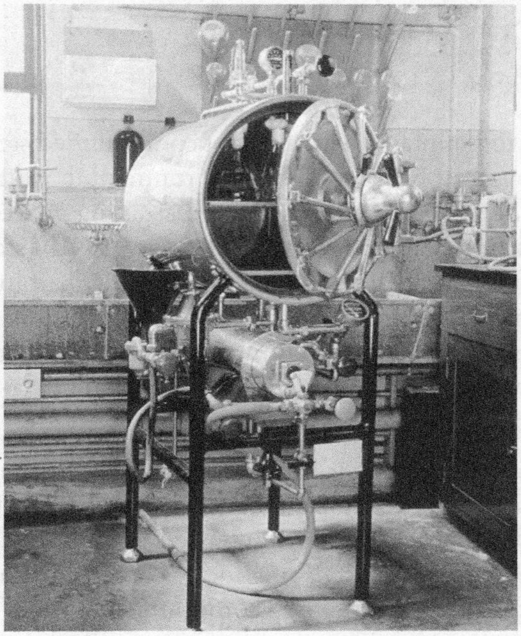

Another important advancement in aseptic hospital protocol at the end of the nineteenth century involved the use of alcohol (ethanol), one of the oldest medicinal treatments that can be traced back to primitive cultures. Alcohol already had a long history as a wound antiseptic, but it wasn't until 1888 that German doctor and professor Paul Fürbringer recognized the benefits of using alcohol to disinfect the hands before a medical procedure. Prior to this discovery, carbolic acid had been used as a skin disinfectant; however, its application had the detrimental side effect of damaging the skin's underlying tissues. It would take several microbiologists many years to determine the exact concentration and time exposure needed to kill microorganisms on the skin, however. Today, alcohol is still being used to disinfect gloves and various other compounding and supply items used during sterile compounding procedures.

## Modern Applications of Disinfectants

In the twentieth century, the use of disinfectants was driven by public health concerns. **Hydrogen peroxide**, a chemical originally used as a deodorizer, saw new use as a disinfectant of drinking water, as did chlorine, a chemical that was also used as a disinfectant in the food industry. **Ammonia compounds** and **cresol solutions** became widely used in both residences and healthcare facilities as a surface disinfectant. Even soaps for personal hygiene advertised their disinfectant properties, their manufacturers promising consumers increased protection against infectious diseases, a major public health concern at the turn of the century. Surprisingly, these disinfectant soaps contained carbolic acid, a powerful surface disinfectant that was later determined to be a poison and, in its undiluted form, potentially fatal on contact.

The latter half of the twentieth century saw an increased use of manufactured disinfectants containing harsh chemicals. This prevalent practice came to the attention of the Environmental Protection Agency (EPA), whose members voiced their concerns about the potential environmental and health risks of these disinfectant products. Consequently, the EPA required that all surface disinfectants be registered and classified with the agency, a practice that continues today.

In current sterile compounding practices, sterile 70% **isopropyl alcohol (IPA)** is the disinfectant of choice for hood-cleaning procedures. This disinfectant is used in combination with an aseptic wipe and has been shown to kill or inhibit the growth of microorganisms on the surface of the hood. It is the responsibility of all sterile compounding personnel to understand the use of disinfectants in the hood-cleaning procedure and their role in maintaining the highest safety standards for the compounding of sterile preparations.

CRUDE CARBOLIC ACID
POISON! CAUTION!
ANTIDOTE.—Dilute Alcohol or Whiskey and albuminous substances, Milk, White of Eggs, etc.
STAR DRUG STORE
510 & 512-23RD STREET,
GALVESTON, TEX.

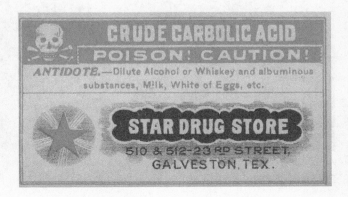

# Part 1: Concepts

In order to maintain the sterility of compounded sterile preparations (CSPs), special attention must be given to the environment in which the CSP is prepared. Chapter 2 details the setup, characteristics, and cleaning of the anteroom and clean room, as well as the different types of hoods that are used in sterile compounding. Chapter 6 describes the proper aseptic hand-washing and garbing procedures that must be performed. Strict adherence to the aseptic protocols addressed in these chapters provides a safe, contaminant-free environment for the compounding of sterile products. A breach anywhere in these procedures may result in contamination that, if left unchecked, could taint multiple CSPs and endanger the lives of many patient recipients.

In addition to adhering to strict aseptic protocol in anteroom and clean room procedures, pharmacy technicians must ensure that the interior of the laminar airflow hood, where sterile compounding takes place, also remains free of contaminants. The aseptic environment of the hood is accomplished through several means: the aseptic technique of the sterile compounder while working in the hood, the movement of HEPA-filtered air as it blows across the work surface, and the correct cleaning and disinfection of the hood.

Proper cleaning of the hood (in this case, the **horizontal laminar airflow hood**) is vital to maintaining the sterility of CSPs. The intravenous (IV) technician must have a thorough knowledge of the hood-cleaning process, from the preparatory steps that are performed in the anteroom to the documentation that must be completed at the end of the procedure. In addition, the technician must be able to consistently demonstrate excellent technique for cleaning the hood. Detailed guidelines on all aspects of the hood-cleaning process can be found in USP Chapter <797>.

## Anteroom Preparation

Although the laminar airflow hood is located in the clean room, preparation for the hood-cleaning process begins in the **anteroom**. (To review the characteristics and setup of the anteroom and clean room, see Chapter 2.) In the anteroom, the IV technician gathers the required hood-cleaning supplies—including lint-free, aseptic hood-cleaning wipes; sterile water; and sterile 70% IPA—and cleans the exterior surfaces of the supply containers with a presaturated aseptic cleaning wipe. These steps must be completed before transporting the supplies into the clean room. Once the supplies are ready, the sterile compounder dons aseptic garb and performs an aseptic hand washing before donning a sterile gown. (Detailed information on how to perform aseptic hand washing, garbing, and gloving can be found in Chapter 6.)

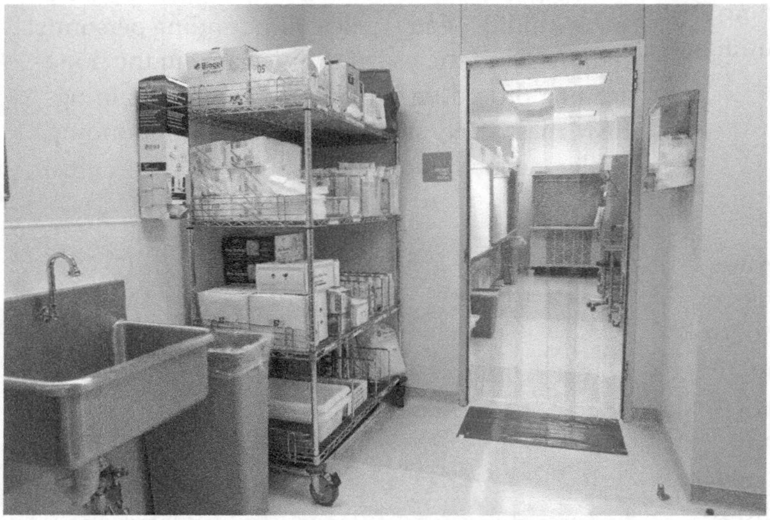

Anteroom used for sterile compounding preparatory procedures, including garbing and aseptic hand washing.

## Clean Room Equipment

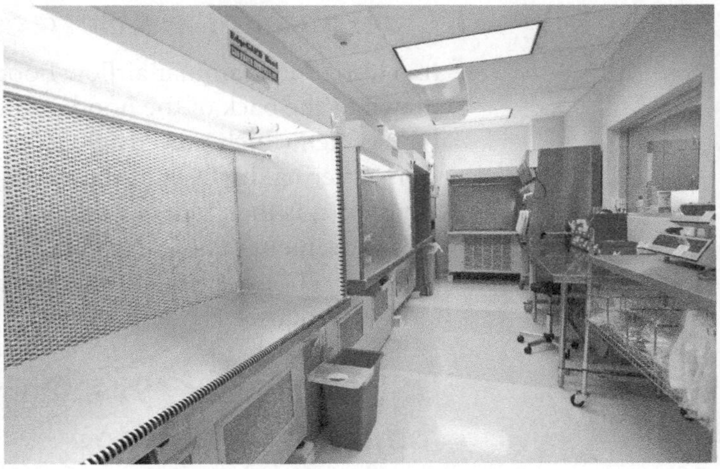

Horizontal laminar airflow hood within the clean room.

Within the clean room is the central piece of equipment used in sterile compounding: the laminar airflow hood. This hood maintains the Class 5 ISO environment necessary for the preparation of CSPs. The number of hoods in the clean room is determined by the volume of CSPs that the lab produces; therefore, there may be one or several horizontal laminar airflow hoods within the clean room, as well as a barrier isolator hood. The vertical laminar airflow hoods used in the preparation of chemotherapy or nuclear medicine are housed in their own separate, negative-pressure room.

## Components of the Horizontal Laminar Airflow Hood

The horizontal laminar airflow hood, sometimes referred to as the cabinet or workbench, is a surgical steel framework with an interior illuminated by overhead lights. The components of the hood work in tandem to maintain a controlled air environment through continuous air filtration. This constant movement of filtered air prevents contaminants from entering and tainting the sterile compounding process. Important components of the hood include the work surface, blower, prefilter, and HEPA filter.

***Work Surface*** The work surface is the stainless-steel surface upon which all sterile compounding procedures take place. Supply items are placed on the work surface within the direct compounding area (DCA), thus allowing HEPA-filtered air to bathe the critical sites of the supply items used to make the CSP.

***Blower*** The blower, or fan, is sealed within the rear of the cabinet and is not readily visible. The blower draws the room air through the prefilter and then pushes it through the HEPA filter and across the work surface of the hood. This air movement operates at a specific and constant velocity, which creates the Class 5 ISO environment. During the hood recertification process, this airflow velocity is measured to verify that the proper air environment is being maintained.

***Prefilter*** The prefilter, located in the front or top of the hood, prevents large particles of dust, hair, and other debris from entering the hood. Like other industrial filters, the prefilter must be replaced on a regular basis. According to USP Chapter <797> guidelines, replacement should occur every 30 days, and these filter changes must be documented. (Refer to Chapter 2 for guidelines on the prefilter checklist and recertification procedures.)

***HEPA Filter*** The HEPA filter, located at the back of the hood, behind a protective grill, traps most microbial contaminants, viruses, fungi, bacteria, and other pollutants, many of which are invisible to the naked eye. The HEPA filter is a permanent filter. It must be recertified by an independent hood/HEPA filter certification company every six months or every time the hood is moved. If the HEPA filter is worn or damaged such that the airflow coming through the filter no longer meets USP Chapter <797> standards, the filter will not pass the recertification process and the entire hood will need to be replaced. Records must be kept to document whenever the HEPA filter is recertified.

## Operation of the Horizontal Hood

In a horizontal laminar airflow hood, room air is pulled through the prefilter and drawn to the back of the hood. A blower then pushes the prefiltered air through the HEPA filter, which prevents 99.97% of all airborne particles of 0.5 micron or larger from entering the DCA of the hood. The HEPA-filtered air, which is now virtually sterile, is then blown horizontally across the work surface toward the worker. This movement of air creates an aseptic work area for the sterile compounding of products. (To understand the components and operation of the horizontal laminar airflow hood, see Figure 7.1 below.)

## USP Chapter <797> Guidelines for Cleaning the Horizontal Hood

USP Chapter <797> cites specific guidelines for the preparation and cleaning of the horizontal laminar airflow hood. This protocol states:

- the minimum timetable for hood cleaning (at the beginning of every shift, before every **batch compounding** session, and every 30 minutes during continuous sterile compounding)
- any circumstances that dictate repeated cleaning of the hood (after any spills, when surface contamination is known or suspected)
- the aseptic garbing, hand-washing, and gloving procedures that must be performed by the worker prior to the hood cleaning
- the supplies that must be used for the hood-cleaning procedure, including lint-free, aseptic hood-cleaning wipes; sterile water; and sterile 70% IPA
- the specific order of the hood-cleaning procedure
- the required documentation of the hood-cleaning process

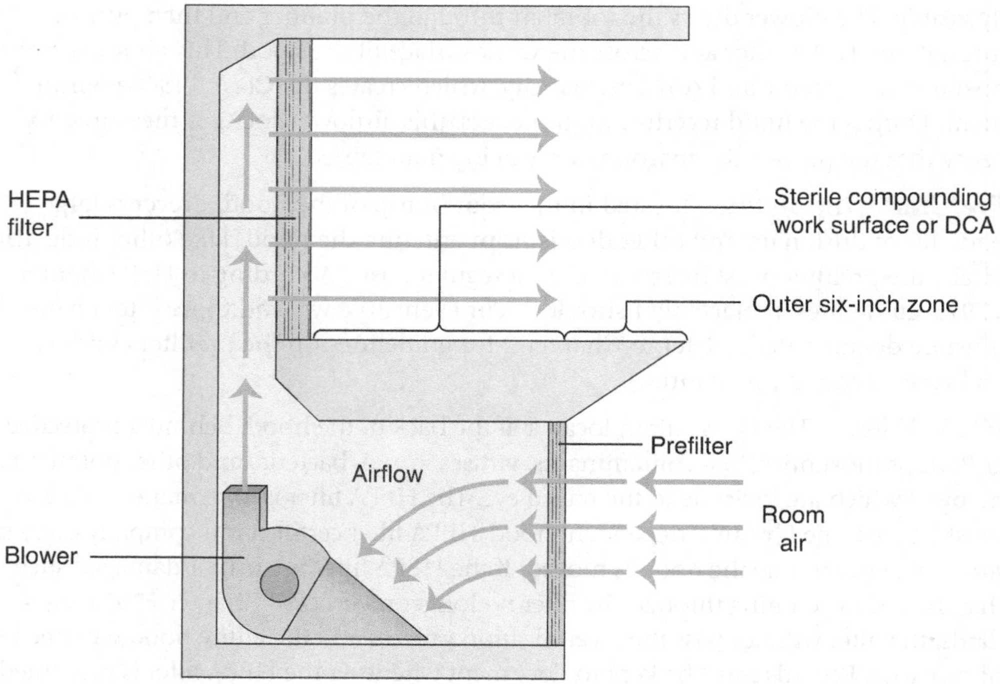


**FIGURE 7.1**

**Cross Section of Horizontal Laminar Airflow Hood (Side View)**

Room air is drawn into the cabinet through the prefilter and then through the blower, which forces the air upward, through the HEPA filter, and horizontally across the work surface toward the worker.

# Concepts Self-Check

## Check Your Understanding

*Write your answers on a separate sheet of paper, as modeled in these examples:* 1d; 2c; 3b; *etc. Check your answers using the Answer Key in Appendix A.*

**1.** Evidence of disinfection practices dates back as far as which time period?

a. ancient Mesopotamia
b. the Middle Ages
c. the eighteenth century
d. the nineteenth century

**2.** Who is credited with discovering the three types of bacteria—cocci, bacilli, and spirochetes?

a. Galen
b. Fracastoro
c. Leeuwenhoek
d. Lister

**3.** Which of the following scientists invented a type of disinfectant that is still in use today?

a. Galen
b. Fracastoro
c. Leeuwenhoek
d. Lister

**4.** Which of the following factors influence sterile compounding procedures?

a. setup, characteristics, and cleaning of the anteroom and clean room
b. HEPA-filtered air and proper disinfection of the hood
c. aseptic technique during sterile compounding procedures
d. all of the above

**5.** Which of the following statements regarding hood filters is true?

a. The prefilter must be changed every 30 days or whenever the cabinet is moved.
b. The HEPA filter must be changed every 30 days.
c. The HEPA filter must be changed every 30 days, and the prefilter must be recertified every six months or whenever the cabinet is moved.
d. The prefilter must be changed every 30 days, and the HEPA filter must be recertified every six months or whenever the cabinet is moved.

## Apply Your Knowledge

*On a separate sheet of paper, write your answer to the question posed in the paragraph below. Use complete sentences and take time to create a thorough and thoughtful response. Check your answer against the Answer Key in Appendix A.*

In Part 1 of this chapter, you learned that USP Chapter <797> has established guidelines for how often and under what circumstances a detailed hood-cleaning procedure must be performed. With that in mind, what do these strict regulations indicate about the importance of hood cleaning to patient health and safety?

# Part 2: Training

*Before performing this lab, review the Sterile Compounding Area Procedures listed on pages 162–163 at the end of the Unit 2 opener, and preview the accompanying process validation checklist in Appendix D.*

## Understand the Resources and Supplies

USP Chapter <797> prescribes special requirements for cleaning the horizontal laminar airflow hood. This chapter and the corresponding lab provide resources and supplies that are in alignment with the directives set forth in USP Chapter <797>.

### Essential Supplies

Most sterile compounding procedures require the same essential supply items to be available for use in both the anteroom and the clean room. For the anteroom, these supplies include a pen; a permanent, felt-tip marker; sterile, foamed 70% IPA; aseptic garb, such as shoe covers, hair cover, face mask, and a beard cover (if appropriate); and sterile garb such as a sterile gown. Other essential items include supplies needed for aseptic hand washing, such as an acceptable cleansing agent (for example, chlorhexadine gluconate) and aseptic, lint-free, disposable towels or an aseptic hand dryer. For the clean room, essential supplies include sterile, foamed 70% IPA; sterile, powder-free gloves; a waste container; a sharps container; and a laminar airflow hood (in this case, a horizontal laminar airflow hood).

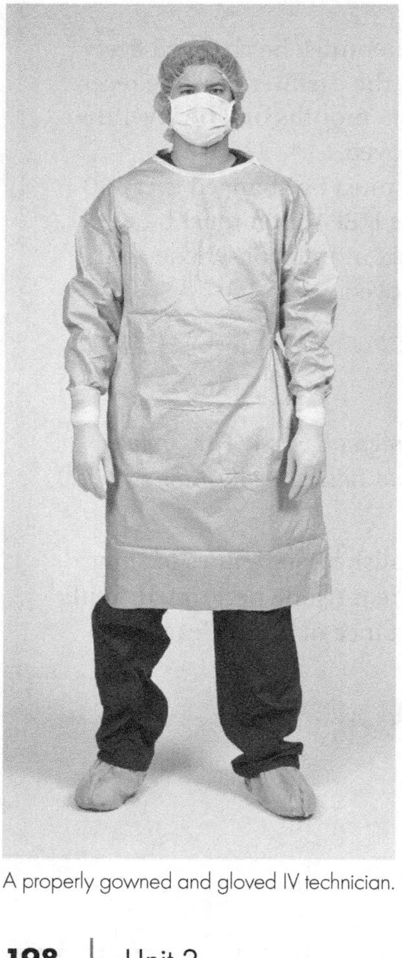

A properly gowned and gloved IV technician.

### Procedure-Specific Supplies

In addition to the previously listed essential supplies, each sterile compounding procedure requires supply items specific to the procedure being performed. The type, number, and amount of procedure-specific supply items are determined by the IV technician prior to the procedure.

***Hood-Cleaning Supplies*** The proper cleaning and disinfection of the hood requires the use of appropriate disinfecting agents and related supplies; the execution of the correct, aseptic cleaning process; and the diligent completion of hood-cleaning documentation. Therefore, a familiarity with the supply items and their specific handling requirements is essential to this sterile compounding procedure.

PRESATURATED CLEANING WIPES To avoid the introduction of contaminants into the clean room, the entire exterior surface of each supply item must be wiped down with presaturated cleaning wipes. The items should then be allowed to dry before being taken into the clean room.

LINT-FREE, ASEPTIC HOOD-CLEANING WIPES The hood must be cleaned with lint-free, nonshedding, **aseptic wipes**. If this type of hood-cleaning wipe is not available, **sterile gauze** is an acceptable substitute. The wipes should be kept inside a container to maintain their aseptic quality, and the container should be stored in the anteroom. Wipes, as well as other cleaning supplies, should be brought into the clean room just prior to their use. If large wipes (4-ply, 8×8 inch) are used to clean the hood, bring 10–12 wipes into the clean room. This quantity is sufficient to clean each section of the hood. If sterile gauze pads (4×4 inch) are used to clean the hood, bring approximately a four-inch stack to clean the entire hood. Sterile compounding personnel must use a new wipe, or approximately 1/10 of the stack of gauze, to clean each section of the hood. Because the six-inch edge of the hood is an area where the HEPA-filtered air mixes with room air, it is considered contaminated. Therefore, as each wipe is brought to the outer edge of the hood, it becomes contaminated and must be thrown away.

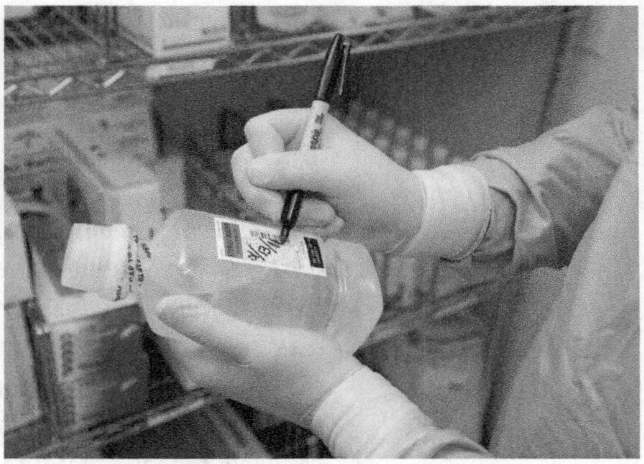

IV technician recording the opening date and time on a bottle.

**Sterile Water** To begin the hood-cleaning process, sterile water is used to remove the **sticky compounding residue** that is insoluble to IPA, the primary agent used to disinfect the hood. The sterile water should be supplied in a 250-mL (or larger) pour bottle that can be recapped to keep the water from becoming contaminated between hood cleanings. Once the bottle is opened, the sterile water should be poured onto the aseptic wipes and then used to wipe down the hood surfaces. When the task is completed, the IV technician should record the opening date and time on the bottle's label. This documentation is important because sterile water contains no preservatives; therefore, any remaining fluid in the bottle must be disposed of after 24 hours.

**Sterile 70% IPA** Sterile 70% IPA is used as the primary **hood-cleaning disinfectant** because it kills or inhibits the growth of microorganisms. The alcohol should be supplied in a 473-mL (or larger) pour bottle that can be recapped to keep the alcohol from becoming contaminated between hood cleanings. Once the bottle is opened, the alcohol should be poured onto the aseptic wipes and then used to wipe down the hood surfaces. When the task is completed, the IV technician should record the opening date and time on the bottle's label. This documentation ensures that any remaining fluid in the bottle is discarded after 24 hours, thus preventing microbial contamination of the product.

**Hood-Cleaning Documentation** The hood-cleaning checklist (see Figure 7.2) is kept in the anteroom inside of a plastic sheet protector, or some other easily wiped container. The checklist is an official document that may be reviewed by regulatory and compliance organizations such as the State Board of Pharmacy or the Joint Commission (formerly the Joint Commission on Accreditation of Health-Care Organizations or JCAHO). The IV technician will clean the hood many times within the course of a work shift. It is his or her responsibility to fill out the **hood-cleaning checklist** whenever the hood-cleaning procedure is performed. Hood-cleaning checklists typically contain the date, time,

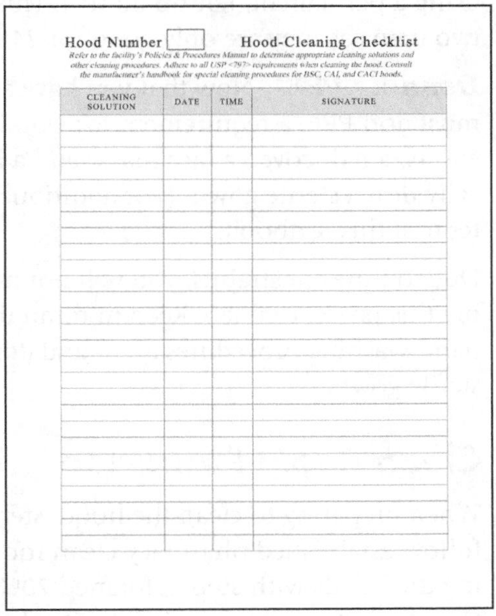

Hood Number ☐ Hood-Cleaning Checklist

*Refer to the facility's Policies & Procedures Manual to determine appropriate cleaning solutions and other cleaning procedures. Adhere to all USP <797> requirements when cleaning the hood. Consult the manufacturer's handbook for special cleaning procedures for BSC, CAI, and CACI hoods.*

| CLEANING SOLUTION | DATE | TIME | SIGNATURE |
|---|---|---|---|

**FIGURE 7.2**

**Sample of a Hood-Cleaning Checklist**

and IV technician's name or initials. If there is more than one hood located in the clean room, a separate hood-cleaning checklist should be maintained for each hood.

# Preview the Lab Procedure

*The following material provides a brief overview of the lab procedure that you will perform. First, read the* Preview the Lab Procedure *section. Then read each step of the* Procedural Lab *carefully, visualizing every action. Next, reinforce your understanding of the process by watching the demonstration video. Once you are in the lab, your instructor will demonstrate the procedure, and then you will perform the procedure by following the steps in the* Procedural Lab *section. Practice the lab procedure multiple times. After sufficient practice, you will complete the lab procedure for process validation by your instructor.*

***Note:*** *This procedural lab requires the use of a basic, open-sided, horizontal laminar airflow hood. For pharmacies that do not have this type of hood, IV technicians should consult the* Instruction Guide *provided by the hood's manufacturer or their facility's P&P manual to determine which procedures may need to be adjusted to suit their hood.*

**POINTER**
Sterile compounding personnel must comply with certain restrictions when working in the anteroom and clean room areas. These restrictions include no gum chewing, horseplay, or food or drink in both the anteroom and clean room, and no hair spray, perfume, makeup, artificial or polished nails, or jewelry in the sterile compounding environment.

## Anteroom Preparatory Procedures

Prior to entering the clean room, you need to complete several preparatory steps in the anteroom, a transition area that provides a space for implementing the standard pharmacy protocols discussed in Chapter 3 and Chapter 6.

***Gathering and Cleaning of Supplies*** First, you must gather the supplies that you need for the hood-cleaning procedure: lint-free, aseptic cleaning wipes; sterile water; and sterile 70% IPA. You also need to gather sterile, foamed 70% IPA, which you apply to your hands before donning sterile gloves in the clean room. The outside of the containers of alcohol and water must be sprayed with a suitable cleansing agent or wiped down with presaturated cleaning wipes prior to entering the clean room in order to remove dust or other contaminants. If you are opening new bottles of sterile water or sterile 70% IPA, you must write the date and time on the bottles using a permanent, felt-tip marker. This date determines the expiration date of these two items as they are only good for 24 hours after opening.

***Donning PPE*** Now that you have assembled your hood-cleaning supplies, you must don PPE, a requirement for working in the clean room. Put on aseptic shoe covers, a hair cover, a face mask, and a beard cover (if appropriate). Lastly, aseptically don a sterile gown. (For additional assistance in aseptic garbing, refer to Chapter 6 of this textbook.)

Due to time constraints, you will not perform aseptic hand-washing procedures during this procedural lab. Keep in mind that, in sterile compounding practice, aseptic hand-washing procedures are mandatory and must be performed prior to donning a sterile gown.

## Clean Room Preparatory Procedures

When preparing to clean the hood, sterile compounding personnel must diligently follow established pharmacy clean room protocols. These protocols include cleansing the hands with sterile, foamed 70% IPA and donning sterile gloves. (For additional assistance in donning sterile gloves, refer to Chapter 6 of this textbook.)

Once these preparatory procedures have been completed, the hood-cleaning process may begin.

***Arranging Supplies in the Hood*** Upon entering the clean room, place half of the four-inch stack of aseptic wipes onto the hood's work surface. The wipes should be placed at least six inches inside of the hood because the outer six-inch edge of the work surface is exposed to potentially contaminated room air. Place the remaining stack of wipes, along with the sterile, foamed 70% IPA and the bottles of sterile water and sterile 70% IPA, onto a clean table or shelf within the clean room. Avoid placing anything, such as the sharps or waste containers, in front of the prefilter; these items could obstruct the airflow into the cabinet.

**POINTER**

The power to the hood runs continuously. If for any reason the hood is turned off, turn on the hood and allow it to run for 30 minutes prior to cleaning.

**BE AWARE**

Take care to never touch the HEPA filter or allow fluid or aspirate to come into contact with the filter as these actions may cause irreparable damage.

## Hood-Cleaning Procedure

With the supply items arranged on the hood, you are ready to begin the hood-cleaning procedure. Pour a small amount of sterile water onto the wipes located within the hood. The amount of water should be enough to lightly saturate each of the wipes, but not so much that it pools on the hood's work surface. Once the wipes are lightly saturated, recap the sterile water bottle and return it to the table. Remember that you must use a new wipe for each section of the hood-cleaning procedure because the wipe becomes contaminated when it reaches the outer edge of the hood.

**POINTER**

The HEPA filter is typically never cleaned. Provided that care is taken not to damage this filter, it can provide acceptable airflow volume for many years.

Pick up the first wipe from the top of the stack. If the hood contains a hang bar and hooks, clean them first. Then clean the ceiling of the hood using overlapping *side-to-side* strokes and moving from the inside of the hood (closest to the HEPA filter) to the outer edge of the hood. Next, clean one side of the hood using overlapping *down-and-up* strokes and moving from the inside of the hood to the outside edge of the hood. This is followed by cleaning the other side of the hood in a similar manner (see Figure 7.3 on the following page).

Finally, select a new, water-saturated aseptic wipe and clean the work surface of the hood using overlapping, *side-to-side* strokes and moving from the inside of the hood to the outer edge of the hood. Cleaning strokes should always overlap so that no surface is left unclean (see Figure 7.4 on the following page).

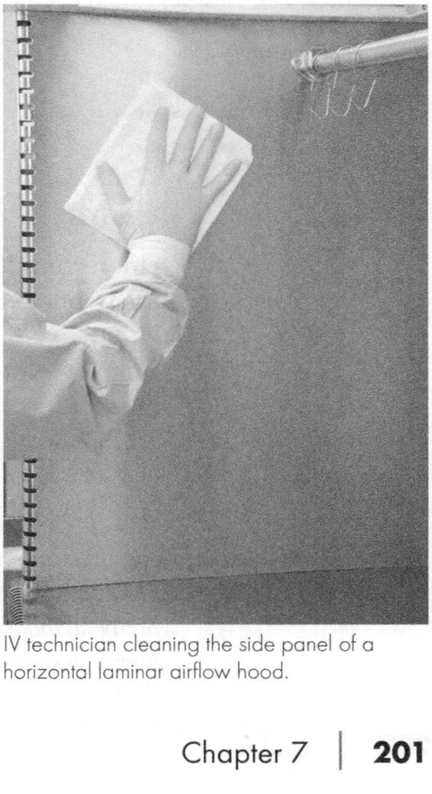

IV technician cleaning the side panel of a horizontal laminar airflow hood.

Cleaning strokes should sweep from one edge of the hood to the other in a single motion. Avoid using short, staccato, back-and-forth strokes as they create **turbulence** in the sterile airflow and may cause you to miss small portions of the hood during the cleaning procedure. The final cleaning stroke for each section (ceiling, sides, and work surface) should wipe down the outer front edge of the cabinet. Refer to the Chapter 7 demonstration video for this part of the step-by-step procedure.

Once the initial hood cleaning has been completed using the sterile water, you must repeat the process using the sterile 70% IPA. Pick up the second stack of cleaning wipes and place them into the hood. Pour a small amount of sterile 70% IPA onto the wipes. The amount of alcohol should be enough to lightly saturate each of the wipes, but not so much that it pools on the hood's work surface. Recap the alcohol bottle and return it to the table. Complete the entire cleaning procedure using the same order and method as you did with the sterile water.

FIGURE 7.3

**Horizontal Laminar Airflow Hood: Proper Cleaning of Side Panels**
Cleaning of side panels starts at the interior upper corner (designated as a red "X"), near the HEPA filter, and proceeds in sweeping, overlapping, down-and-up motions that move toward the outer edge of the hood.

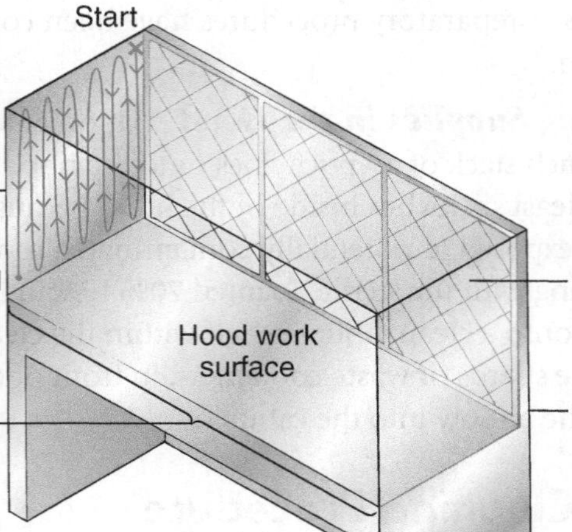


FIGURE 7.4

**Horizontal Laminar Airflow Hood: Proper Cleaning of Work Surface**
Cleaning of work surface starts at the interior, back corner (designated as a red "X"), near the HEPA filter, and proceeds in sweeping, overlapping, side-to-side motions that move toward the outer edge of the hood.

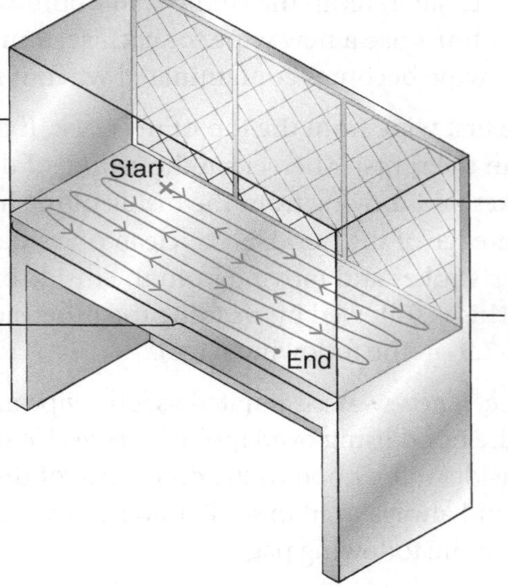


## Completing the Checklist and Removing PPE

Upon completion of the hood-cleaning procedure, return to the anteroom. Complete the hood-cleaning checklist by recording the date, time, and your name or initials as required. Then remove your PPE in the opposite order in which you put them on. (See Chapter 6 for step-by-step instructions on how to aseptically remove your PPE.)

# Watch the Demonstration Video

*Watch the Chapter 7 Demonstration Video, which shows the step-by-step aseptic procedures for cleaning the horizontal laminar airflow hood. For the purposes of the Chapter 7 Demonstration Video, aseptic hand washing will not be demonstrated. Refer to the Chapter 6 video for a demonstration of aseptic hand-washing procedures.*

Training Videos DVD

# Procedural Lab

*This lab walks you through the step-by-step actions that you must follow to properly clean the horizontal laminar airflow hood. Take your time. Work through each step methodically and with close attention to detail.*

***Note:*** *For the purposes of this procedural lab, you will not perform aseptic hand-washing procedures unless directed to do so by your instructor. Should your instructor ask you to perform these procedures, refer to Chapter 6 for instructions on aseptic hand washing.*

***Note:*** *For steps 1–3, please refer to Chapter 3 for gathering and cleaning of supplies. For steps 4–7, refer to Chapter 6 for a reminder of the step-by step procedures that are required for aseptic garbing. Steps 1–7 and steps 20–21 should be performed in the anteroom. Steps 8–19 should be performed in the clean room.*

## Supplies

### *Essential Supplies*

To complete the Unit 2 procedural labs, you will need to ensure that various essential anteroom and clean room supplies such as those listed in Table 7.1 are available for your use.

**Table 7.1 Essential Anteroom and Clean Room Supplies for Sterile Compounding**

| Anteroom Supplies |
|---|
| pen |
| permanent, felt-tip marker |
| aseptic garb, including shoe covers, hair cover, face mask, and beard cover (if appropriate) |
| sterile gown |
| presaturated, aseptic cleaning wipes |
| sterile, foamed 70% IPA |
| waste container |
| hood-cleaning checklist |
| **Clean Room Supplies** |
| sterile, foamed 70% IPA |
| sterile, powder-free gloves |
| aseptic, lint-free hood-cleaning wipes |
| sterile water in a pour bottle |
| sterile 70% IPA in a pour bottle |
| waste container |
| horizontal laminar airflow hood |

## Procedure

### *Gathering Supplies and Documenting Usage*

1. Prior to entering the clean room, you must gather all of the supplies that you need for the preparation and cleaning of the hood: sterile, foamed 70% IPA; sterile, powder-free gloves; one pour bottle of sterile water; one pour bottle of sterile 70% IPA; and approximately 10–12 large, aseptic, lint-free hood-cleaning wipes. If hood-cleaning wipes are not available, you may use an approximately four-inch stack of sterile, 4×4-inch gauze pads.

**BE AWARE**

Avoiding air turbulence in the clean room is important to maintaining a controlled air environment for sterile compounding. Therefore, gather your supplies before entering the clean room to avoid the airflow disruptions that occur when entering and exiting the clean room.

2. Use a permanent, felt-tip marker to write the date and time on the bottles of sterile water and sterile alcohol. Remember that these bottles must be disposed of after 24 hours.
3. Spray or wipe the entire surface of both bottles with presaturated, aseptic cleaning wipes. Allow the alcohol to air-dry thoroughly.

**POINTER**

During aseptic garbing, best practice is to reapply sterile, foamed 70% IPA to your hands after donning shoe covers and again after donning a hair cover.

### *Garbing*

4. Don shoe covers.
5. Put on a hair cover.
6. Don a face mask and beard cover (if appropriate).

### *Gowning*

7. Don a sterile gown.

   *Note:* For the purposes of this training lab, you will skip the mandatory aseptic hand-washing procedure.

### *Entering the Clean Room and Gloving*

8. Bring the sterile, powder-free gloves; aseptic, lint-free hood-cleaning wipes; sterile, foamed 70% IPA; and the pour bottles of sterile water and sterile alcohol with you into the clean room. Place half of the stack of wipes onto the hood's work surface, at least six inches inside of the hood. Place the remaining stack of wipes, foamed alcohol, and pour bottles of water and alcohol onto a clean shelf or table inside of the clean room.
9. Sterilize your hands using sterile, foamed 70% IPA. Allow your hands to dry.
10. Don sterile, powder-free gloves.

**BE AWARE**

Never let fluid come into contact with the HEPA filter. This action may impair the filter and irreparably damage the hood.

### *Cleaning the Horizontal Laminar Airflow Hood*

11. Remove any extraneous items, such as unused vials, from the hood. These items may be temporarily placed onto a shelf or table inside of the clean room, returned to the refrigerator if appropriate, or thrown away if beyond their 24-hour expiration date.
12. Unscrew the top from the sterile water bottle while holding it at least six inches inside of the hood. This will help to ensure that the contents of the bottle remain free of contaminants. Pour enough water onto the hood-cleaning wipes so that all of the wipes are lightly saturated. The wipes should be wet enough to leave a streak when wiped on the hood surface, but not so wet as to leave pools of water, drip or run down the sides of the hood, or leak into the HEPA filter.
13. Recap the sterile water bottle inside the hood's DCA. Place the bottle of sterile water on a shelf or table within the clean room.
14. Take the top one-fifth of the stack of saturated hood-cleaning wipes into your dominant hand. If the hood contains a hang bar and hooks, clean them first. After cleaning the hang bar and hooks, place the used wipe into the waste container.

**BE AWARE**

Hood-cleaning supplies such as sterile, foamed 70% IPA; sterile water; and sterile 70% IPA in a pour bottle may remain on a shelf or table within the clean room to be used for up to 24 hours from the time they were opened. After that time, they should be discarded to prevent microbial contamination of the supplies and, consequently, contamination of the hood from their use.

15. Pick up a new one-fifth of the stack of cleaning wipes and, beginning at the inside back corner of the ceiling of the hood, clean the hood ceiling using overlapping *side-to-side* motions. Gradually move from the area closest to the HEPA filter to the outside edge of the hood ceiling. When you reach the outside edge of the hood ceiling, wipe down the front edge of the hood ceiling and then throw the wipe into the waste container that is kept near the hood.
16. Pick up the next one-fifth of the water-saturated stack of wipes. Beginning with the interior upper corner of one side panel of the hood, clean the side panel using overlapping strokes in a *down-and-up* motion. Gradually move from the area closest to the HEPA filter to the outside edge of the hood's side panel. When you reach the outside edge of the hood's side panel, wipe down the front edge of the side panel, then throw away the wipe.

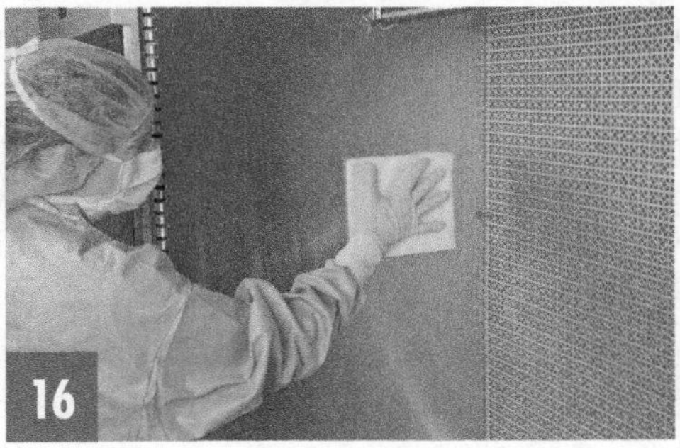
16

17. Pick up the next one-fifth of the water-saturated stack of wipes and repeat step 16 on the other side panel.
18. Take the remaining one-fifth of the water-saturated wipes and clean the work surface. Start in the back corner of the hood, closest to the HEPA filter. Clean in a *side-to-side* motion using overlapping strokes and gradually moving to the outer edge of the hood's work surface. When you reach the outside edge of the work surface, wipe down the front edge of the work surface and then throw away the wipe.

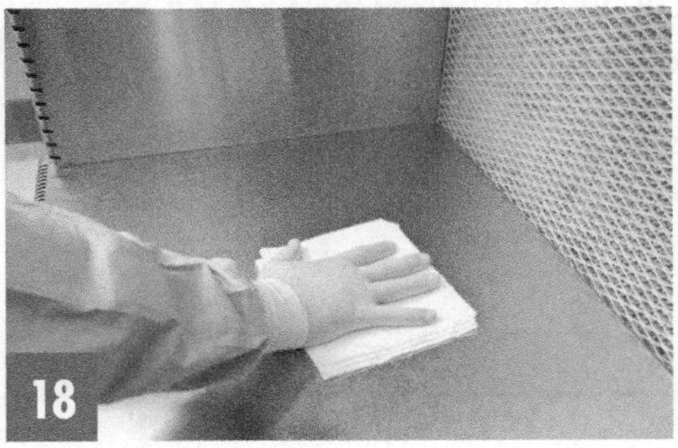
18

19. Repeat steps 12–18 of the procedure using the remaining stack of aseptic wipes saturated with sterile 70% IPA.

***Removing PPE***

20. Return to the anteroom and record the date, time, and your name or initials on the hood-cleaning checklist.
21. Remove and dispose of your gloves and aseptic garb according to established guidelines.

**POINTER**

If the placement of the hang bar and hooks are such that you cannot clean the hood's ceiling without touching them, you are advised to clean the ceiling first, followed by the hang bar and hooks. This will avoid potential contamination that may be created by inadvertently touching the clean hang bar or hooks during the cleaning of the hood's ceiling.

**BE AWARE**

Do not reuse a wipe once it has come to the outer edge of the hood—it is now contaminated. Throw it away and get a clean wipe.

**POINTER**

Remember to use a *down-and-up* motion when cleaning the side panels of the hood and a *side-to-side* motion when cleaning the hood's ceiling and work surface. Be sure that each stroke overlaps the previous stroke slightly as you move from the innermost part of the hood to the outer edge.

# Process Validation by Instructor

*Your instructor will use the process validation checklist provided in Appendix D to evaluate your technique for this lab. In order to receive ACPE certification, and prior to making CSPs for patient use, you must correctly perform each component of the lab procedure. Review the Chapter 7 lab and thoroughly practice each of the steps prior to your evaluation.*

# Part 3: Assessment

## Chapter Summary

- Proper cleaning and disinfection of the hood is necessary for maintaining high safety standards in the preparation of CSPs.
- The primary components of the horizontal laminar airflow hood include the work surface, blower, prefilter, and HEPA filter.
- In the anteroom, sterile compounding personnel must gather hood-cleaning supplies and wipe them down with alcohol.
- Also in the anteroom, sterile compounding personnel must don aseptic garb, perform aseptic hand washing, and put on a sterile gown.
- Immediately upon entering the clean room, sterile compounding personnel must apply sterile, foamed 70% IPA to their hands and then don sterile gloves.
- IV technicians should use aseptic, lint-free wipes or sterile gauze for hood cleaning.
- Sterile water is used for the initial cleaning of the hood because it dissolves sticky residue that may be insoluble in alcohol. Sterile, 70% IPA is used for the final hood cleaning because it kills or inhibits the growth of microorganisms.
- During the hood-cleaning process, IV technicians should exercise care so that liquid does not come in contact with the HEPA filter.
- Hood cleaning should be performed in the following order: hang bar and hooks, ceiling, side, opposite side, work surface.
- The ceiling and work surface of the hood should be cleaned in overlapping, side-to-side strokes, and the sides of the hood should be cleaned in overlapping, down-and-up strokes. The cleaning process should start in the area closest to the HEPA filter and move toward the edge of the hood.
- The IV technician must record the date and time of every hood cleaning, along with his or her initials, on the hood-cleaning checklist.

## Key Terms

**airborne contaminant** any microbial contaminant (such as a bacterium or a virus) or particle (such as dust) that may be spread by air, potentially transmitting illness or disease or causing contamination to the hood or CSP

**alkali** an alkaline substance, often found in the ashes of various plants, that was once used as a disinfectant

**ammonia compound** an ammonia-based solution that is used for surface disinfection

**anteroom** a room or area, immediately before the clean room, in which sterile compounding supplies are staged; an area with a ≥ ISO Class 8 environment

**antiseptic** an agent capable of reducing or preventing infection

**aromatherapy** a therapy or treatment that uses the oil or essence of various plants and herbs

**aseptic wipe** contaminant-free wipe used to clean the hood

**autoclave** an apparatus that uses superheated steam under high pressure to sterilize supplies

**ayurvedic medicine** a form of alternative medicine native to India

**bacteria** organisms capable of producing disease

**batch compounding** the creation of multiple doses of a uniform strength of a drug during a single compounding period; a large number of products prepared during a single sterile compounding session

**blower** a hood component that draws the room air through the prefilter and then pushes it through the HEPA filter and across the work surface

**cabinet** the framework that houses all components of the laminar airflow hood such as the prefilter, blower, HEPA filter, and work surface; also known as a hood, primary engineering control (PEC), or laminar airflow workbench (LAFW)

**chemical sterilization** a method of surface sterilization used on objects or equipment; the process of using an agent—such as alcohol, bleach, or ammonia—to kill microorganisms

**chlorine** a corrosive chemical that is used as a surface disinfectant or germicidal agent

**clean room** a room in which the concentration of airborne particles is minimized by the use of HEPA filtration systems and aseptic technique; an area with a ≥ ISO Class 7 environment

**creosol solution** a liquid derivative of wood or coal tar that was once used as a disinfectant

**disinfection** the act of cleaning or decontaminating an object to prevent infection

**essential oils** a variety of plant or herbal oils that are used in alternative medicine therapies

**fomite** any inanimate object, such as clothing or bedding, that is capable of transferring germs from one person to another

**fumigation** a process that uses fumes to kill microorganisms or disinfect a room or building

**fungi** organisms that produce spores capable of contaminating a CSP

**heat sterilization** the process of using heat to destroy microorganisms, thereby sterilizing the object or solution

**HEPA filter** a filter that effectively removes particulates, from the air, greatly reducing airborne contamination; high-efficiency particulate airflow filter

**hood-cleaning checklist** a preprinted sheet or form on which IV technicians record the date and time of each hood cleaning, along with their name or initials

**hood-cleaning disinfectant** a solution, such as sterile 70% IPA, used to clean the hood

**horizontal laminar airflow hood** a type of hood in which sterile products are prepared and in which HEPA-filtered air blows horizontally across the work surface toward the worker; components of the hood include the hang bar, hooks, ceiling, walls, and work surface

**hydrogen peroxide** a solution that is used as a skin disinfectant

**hypochlorite** a chemical compound such as sodium hypochlorite (bleach) that is used as a surface disinfectant

**infection control** procedures designed to reduce or prevent nosocomial infection

**iodine** a tincture used as a topical antiseptic

**isopropyl alcohol (IPA)** a liquid often used for cleaning and disinfection within the sterile compounding environment

**miasmas** harmful fumes from decaying organic matter

**microbe** a microscopic organism capable of transmitting disease

**microbiology** the scientific study of microscopic organisms

**microculture** a microscopic culture of cells or organisms

**phenol (carbolic acid)** a type of surface disinfectant that is widely used in many healthcare settings

**prefilter** a filter located in the front or top of the hood that prevents large particles of dust, hair, and other debris from entering the hood

**protozoa** a single-celled organism that feeds on organic compounds and is capable of movement

**seminaria** an early term used to describe microbes and the process of disease transmission

**steam sterilization** a method of sterilization used for certain types of equipment or supplies

**sterile gauze** wipes made of medical-grade gauze that are free of lint and other contaminants and are used to clean the hood

**sticky compounding residue** a buildup of compounding materials—such as dextrose, sodium, or various drugs—that adheres to the hood's work surface

**turbulence** air that is not uniform in its direction and/or velocity; turbulent air is present along the outer six-inch edge of the hood, behind CSP supply items in the hood, at the threshold between the positive-pressure clean room and the relatively negative pressure of the anteroom, and around the IV technician as he or she moves about the clean room during compounding procedures

**work surface** the stainless steel surface upon which all sterile compounding procedures take place

## Check the Basics

*On a separate sheet of paper, write your answers as modeled in these examples: 1d; 2c; 3b; etc.*

1. What is the correct order of garbing?
   a. hair cover, shoe covers, face mask, gown, gloves
   b. shoe covers, hair cover, face mask, gown, gloves
   c. shoe covers, hair cover, face mask, gloves, gown
   d. shoe covers, face mask, hair cover, gown, gloves

2. In the anteroom, supplies such as sterile water in a pour bottle should be cleaned by:
   a. wiping with sterile water
   b. spraying with sterile water
   c. spraying or wiping with sterile 90% IPA
   d. spraying or wiping with sterile 70% IPA

3. Which products can be used when cleaning the horizontal laminar airflow hood?
   a. aseptic, lint-free wipes or sterile gauze pads
   b. aseptic, lint-free paper towels or sterile gauze pads
   c. regular paper towels or sterile gauze pads
   d. lint-free wipes or lint-free gauze pads

4. Preservative-free products should be disposed of no longer than how long after opening?
   a. immediately after cleaning the hood
   b. at the end of the shift
   c. after 24 hours
   d. after one week

5. Why is sterile water used as a preliminary hood-cleaning agent?
   a. It sterilizes the hood.
   b. It removes residue insoluble to alcohol.
   c. It removes alcohol residue on the hood.
   d. It removes dust on the hood's surface.

6. Which of the following is the most appropriate agent for primary hood cleaning?
   a. sterile water
   b. foamed alcohol
   c. IPA
   d. sterile 70% IPA

7. How should the hood-cleaning wipes be moistened?
   a. Pour enough fluid so that it heavily saturates the wipes and pools onto the hood's surface.
   b. Lightly saturate the wipes so that they leave streaks when drawn across the hood's surface.
   c. Pour the fluid directly onto the hood's surface and then spread the liquid with the wipes.
   d. Heavily saturate the wipes so that they thoroughly clean the HEPA filter during hood cleaning.

8. What is the proper order for cleaning the horizontal laminar airflow hood?
   a. hang bar and hooks, ceiling, side, opposite side, work surface
   b. ceiling, hang bar and hooks, side, HEPA filter, work surface
   c. work surface, side, opposite side, ceiling, hang bar and hooks
   d. HEPA filter, hang bar and hooks, ceiling, side, work surface

9. The correct method for cleaning the work surface of the hood is:
   a. from back to front using overlapping strokes
   b. from back to front using short, staccato strokes
   c. from side to side using overlapping strokes and moving from the outside of the hood toward the HEPA filter
   d. from side to side using overlapping strokes and moving from the inside of the hood toward the outside edge of the hood

10. What task must be performed after the hood-cleaning procedure?
    a. aseptic hand washing
    b. disposal of any extraneous items in the hood
    c. completion of the hood-cleaning checklist
    d. all of the above

# Make Connections

*On a separate sheet of paper, write your answers to the following three questions, using complete sentences and making sure your answers are thorough and thoughtful. Note that the third question requires Internet access.*

1. You are required to clean the hood every 30 minutes during continuous compounding periods. What does this requirement indicate about continuous compounding periods?
2. What is the rationale for performing some of the hood-cleaning strokes in a side-to-side motion and others in a down-and-up motion?
3. Do an Internet search for Section 1330.670 Compounded Sterile Preparation Standards, taken from the Joint Committee on Administrative Rules – Administrative Code. This is a listing of some of the standards for sterile product preparation as defined by the state of Illinois. Read Section C, Numbers 1 and 2, and then answer the following questions:
   A. According to this document, what is the requirement for hood/HEPA filter recertification?
   B. How does the Illinois requirement for hood/HEPA filter recertification differ from the recertification requirement stated in USP Chapter <797>?
   C. What factors would you consider when determining whether you would follow state or federal guidelines?

# Meet the Challenge

***Scenario*** This "sullied" activity will give you the opportunity to identify any breaks in technique when cleaning the hood.

***Challenge*** Your instructor has a handout outlining the supplies and procedures for an activity centered around the hood-cleaning process. This procedure tests your understanding of the correct technique that must be used for a proper disinfection of the work surface of the hood. To meet this challenge, ask your instructor for the handout and work with a partner or a small group to complete the activity.

## Additional Resources

*Go to the Paradigm Internet Resources Center at* www.paradigmcollege.net/sterilecomp *to access live links related to these Chapter 7 topics:*

- USP Chapter <797>
- *USP <797> Guidebook*
- Section 1330.670 Compounded Sterile Preparation Standards, taken from the Joint Committee on Administrative Rules – Administrative Code, Illinois State Board of Pharmacy

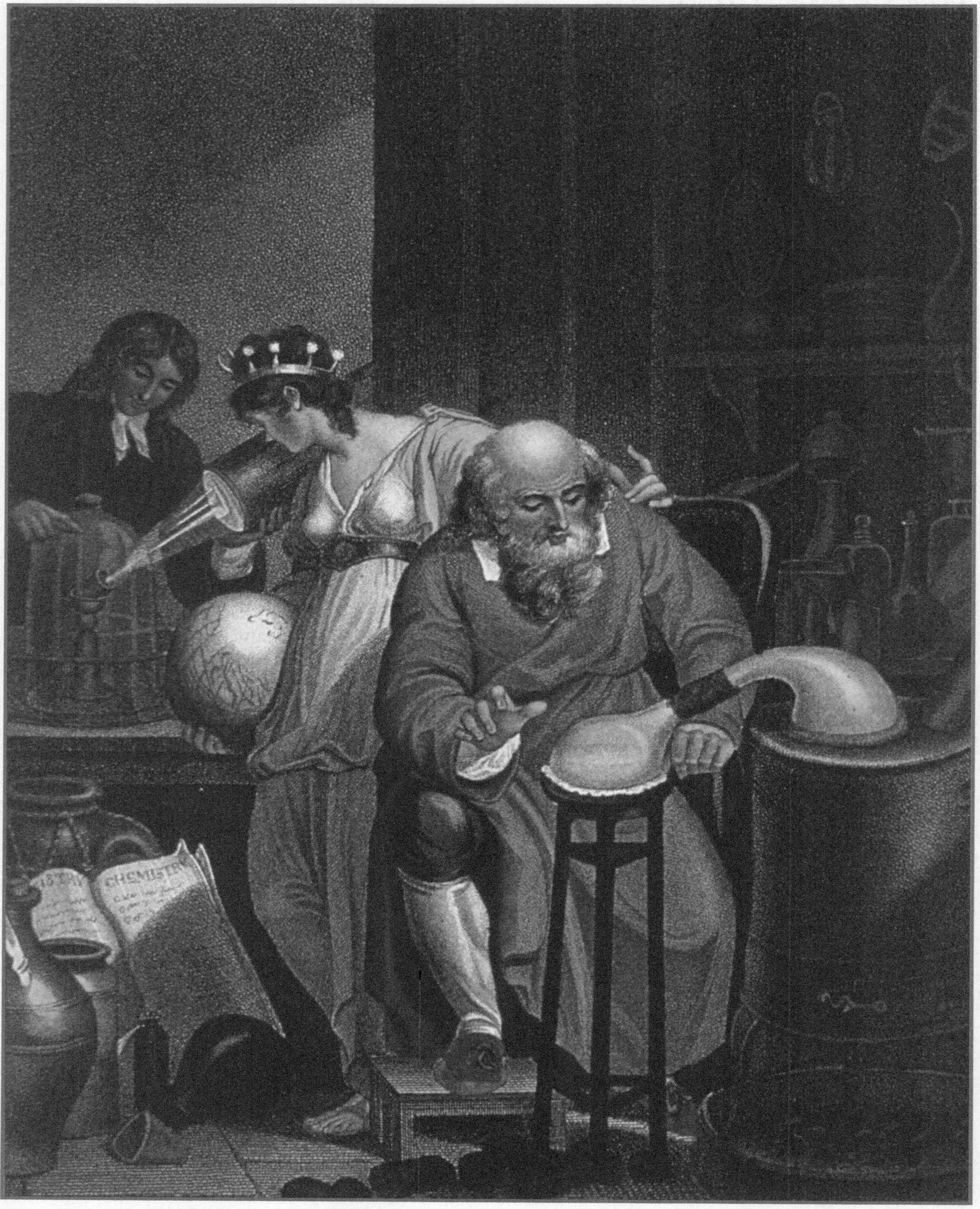
CHEMISTRY

# Large-Volume Parenteral Preparations

## Learning Objectives

- Gain an awareness of the historical roots of large-volume parenteral preparations.
- Understand the physiology of fluid balance and the chemical properties of parenteral products.
- Identify the risks associated with parenteral administration.
- Describe the components and critical sites of various large-volume parenteral preparation supply items.
- Identify the USP Chapter <797> procedures that must be performed prior to compounding large-volume parenteral preparations.
- Demonstrate correct aseptic technique in preparing large-volume parenteral products.

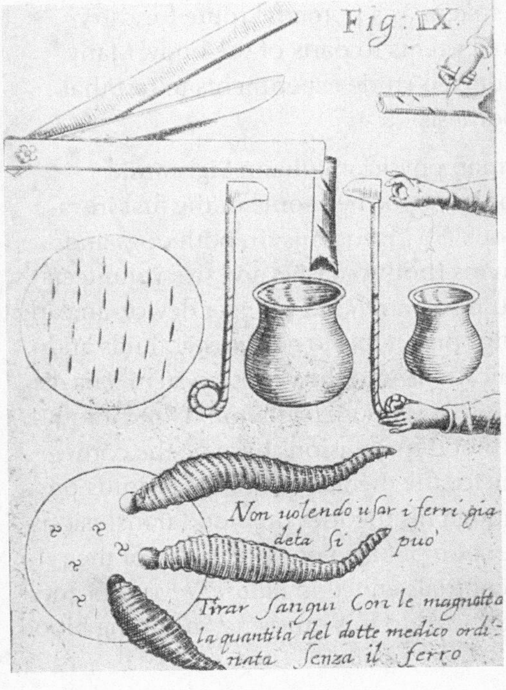

Fig: IX
Non uolendo usar i ferri gia deta si puo'
Tirar Sangui Con le magnotta la quantita del dotte medico ordinata Senza il ferro


Since the age of Hippocrates, medical practitioners have understood fluid balance in the human body to be of vital importance. Before the nineteenth century, the cause of an illness was usually attributed to an imbalance in one of the four **humors**: blood, phlegm, black bile, and yellow bile. Physicians would determine which humor was causing the condition and then prescribe a therapeutic regimen—including diet, rest or physical activity, and herbal remedies—to counteract that imbalance. Other, more extreme practices included bloodletting, purging, diuresis, or irrigation. For example, doctors would prescribe the ingestion of potent herbal concoctions to purge a patient's excess bile or would let a patient's excess blood by using a crude syringe-like device, called a **clyster**, or by applying **leeches**. These healing practices focused on the *withdrawal or extraction* of bodily fluids to restore equilibrium and good health. Many centuries would pass before the medical community recognized the healthful benefits of the *infusion* or *injection* of fluids to restore or maintain good health.

## Discovery of the Circulatory System

Early practitioners recognized that the most important of the four humors was blood, for it was the vital force of life. Galen was the first medical practitioner to study the circulatory system and establish the differences between arterial and venous blood. He believed that arterial blood originated in the heart and venous blood originated in the liver. He also believed that these two circulatory systems operated independently of each other, assisted by invisible pores in the heart through which blood and air combined to form spirit. For many centuries, Galen's theories on blood circulation were accepted by physicians, though they were gradually refined over the years.

In the tenth century, Persian physician and philosopher Avicenna became the first to correctly explain the pulse as the alternating expansion and contraction of the heart, though he did not fully understand the heart's structure or the passageways of circulation. His definitive work *Al-Qanun fi al-Tibb* (*The Canon of Medicine*) became the standard textbook for several medical universities during this period. *The Canon of Medicine* was also the first book to establish principles regarding the testing of medications, thus laying the foundation for the study of clinical pharmacology.

In 1242, Syrian physician Ibn al-Nafis discovered pulmonary circulation and correctly described the functions of the pulse. Unlike Galen, Ibn al-Nafis knew that blood traveled from the right ventricle to the left ventricle through the lungs, and not through a porous connection between the two ventricles.

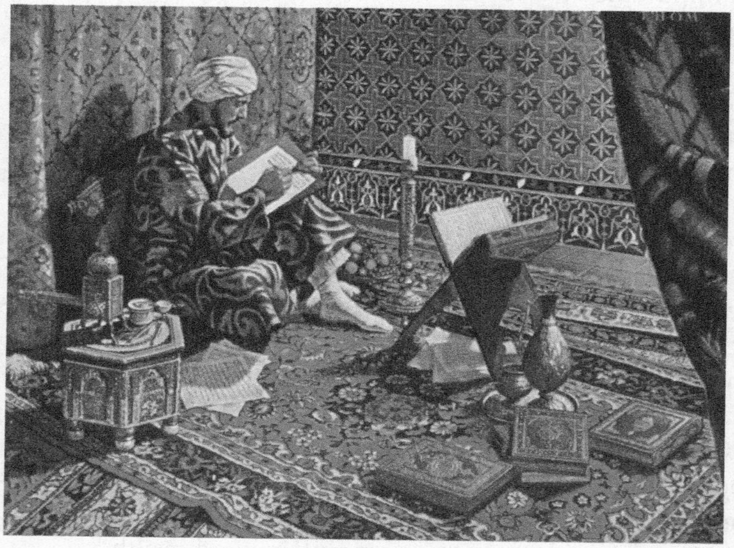

His rudimentary research of coronary and capillary circulations played a critical role in understanding the physiology of the circulatory system.

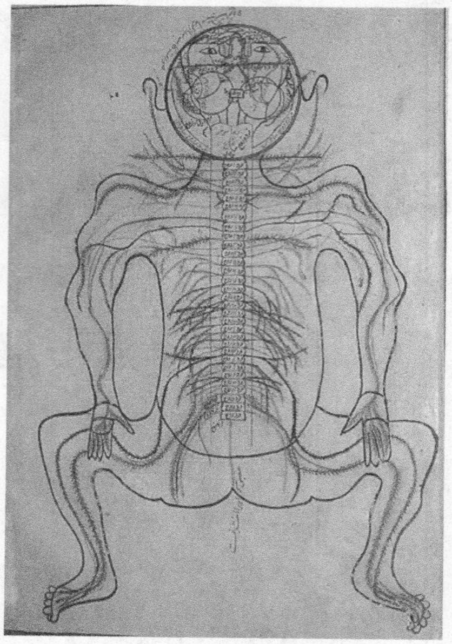

In 1616, English physician and anatomist William Harvey firmly disproved Galen's theories by discovering the continuous, circular flow of blood. This discovery led to the understanding that the human body has a single circulatory system, with the heart serving as the central pump for blood flow. It would take 35 more years for Italian doctor Marcello Malpighi to discover capillaries, the crucial link between arteries and veins, thus proving Ibn al-Nafis's theory posed 400 years earlier.

## Circulation as a Treatment Route

With this newfound understanding of human anatomy, physicians and scientists began to see the circulatory system as a potential route for carrying medicinal agents to parts of the body. Many conducted crude experiments to test that hypothesis.

German physician Johann Sigismund Elsholtz performed some of the first intravenous (IV) infusions on both dogs and humans (both cadavers and live volunteers). He used a barrel-and-plunger device, an early syringe prototype, to administer fluids and medications into the venous system. His discussion of venous circulation, IV techniques, and blood transfusions became the cornerstone for the therapeutic use of IV infusions. Although his theories on blood transfusions were soon put into practice, many of the patient trials ended in failure. Several factors contributed to this outcome, including blood

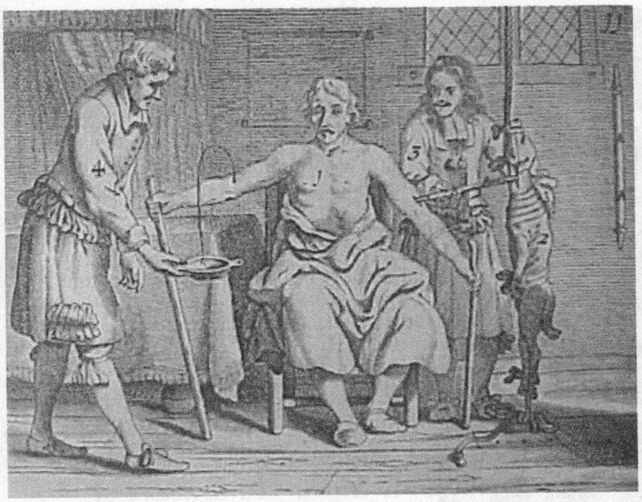

incompatibility (using animal blood for human transfusions) and coagulability. As a result, blood transfusions were outlawed in 1668 and remained illegal for another 150 years. It was not until 1829 that British physiologist James Blundell performed the first successful transfusion and proved that only human blood was safe for the procedure.

## Origins of Fluid Replacement

An Indian blue cholera pandemic in Europe and Asia in 1831–1832 led to a major breakthrough in the use of IV therapy. Cholera—like the destructive plague, typhus, and dysentery—provoked severe fluid loss and dehydration. Previous treatment for this disease included patient ingestion of "curative" substances such as opium, magnesia, cayenne pepper, brandy, copper sulphate, and hydrocyanic acid; the use of purgatives such as rhubarb root, croton oil, and turpentine; and the obligatory practice of bloodletting—all methods that robbed the afflicted of their few precious remaining fluids. Public confusion and anger over the varying treatments and subsequent poor results led to a mistrust of medical practitioners and widespread refusal of experimental treatment options.

At the start of the cholera pandemic, Irish physician William Brooke O'Shaughnessy began to experiment with fluid replacement therapy by injecting dogs with saline solution. He based his work on the research of British physician William Stevens, who had successfully treated patients suffering from tropical fevers with oral salt solutions. O'Shaughnessy injected "two to three drachms of muriate of soda and two scruples of the subcarbonate of soda in six pints of water" using a tube attached to a syringe. He found that the treatment had no ill effects on the animals and suggested that physicians try this therapy on cholera victims to replenish their associated fluid loss. Relying on O'Shaughnessy's research, Scottish physician Thomas Latta injected multiple doses of saline solution into the veins of 15 dying patients, one ounce at a time, in a desperate attempt to revive them. To his surprise, five patients improved upon injection with the solution.

## Experiments with Large-Volume Infusions

Although the majority of Latta's initial patients would die, prominent members of the medical community considered the results favorable in light of the highly advanced stages of illness at which the patients were treated. Latta's pioneering work in IV infusion therapy laid the groundwork for others to experiment with the formulation of large-volume IV infusions by including different solution additives (sodium, carbonate, chloride, potassium) and varying their concentrations. In fact, British physician Sydney Ringer used Latta's findings in his own frog-heart research. Ringer discovered that adding a small amount of potassium to a sodium chloride solution extended the heart's function. From Ringer's experiments came the lactated Ringer's solution that is still used in IV therapy today.

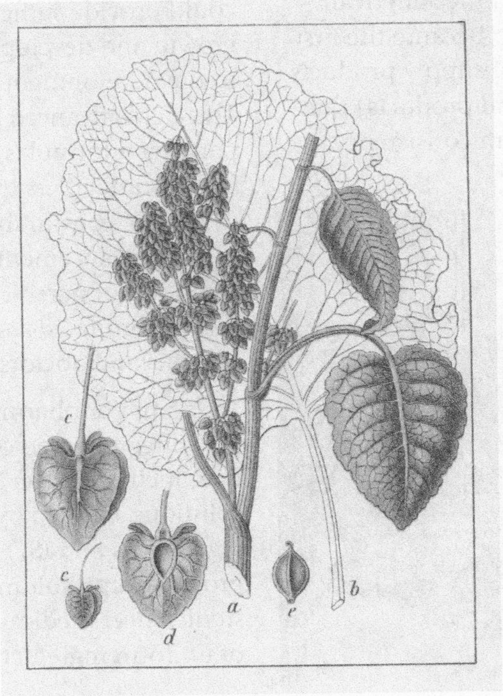


Nineteenth-century German surgeon Albert Landerer was another individual to build on Latta's work, becoming the first physician to successfully provide a large-volume parenteral infusion to a patient with **hypovolemia**, a state of decreased volume of circulating blood. He also used his saline solution, combined with cinnamic acid from Peruvian balsam, to treat **phthisis**. Although Landerer's treatment was not a reliable cure, it restored patients' weight and energy with surprising success, effectively stopping further lung and other organ degeneration.

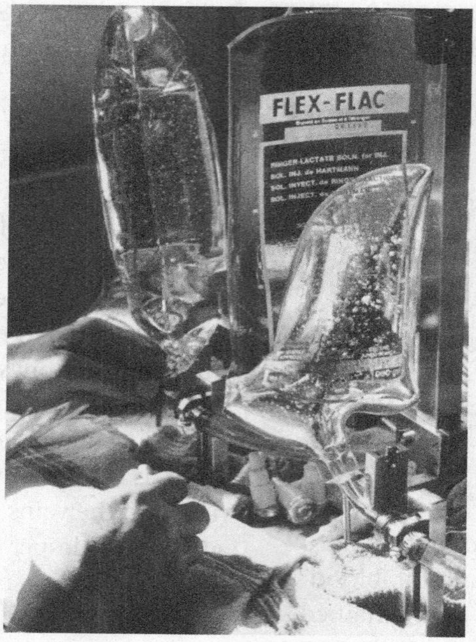


In 1931, two Iowa physicians, Dr. Ralph Falk and Dr. Donald Baxter, formed the Don Baxter Intravenous Products Company. More than 50 years later, the American Hospital Supply Company would merge with the Baxter Company to become the world's largest manufacturer of large-volume parenteral solutions and a number of other hospital supply products.

Over the remainder of the twentieth century, several advances were made in IV infusion therapy, including an expansion of treatment options and a refinement of IV supplies and administration techniques.

## Innovations in IV Therapy

By the beginning of the twentieth century, physicians used large-volume parenteral infusions (mainly water and sodium chloride solutions) only in cases of dire necessity, despite Landerer's recommendation for their use as an early-stage treatment for hypovolemia. Mortality rates among patients who received infusion therapy were high, partly due to poor-quality ingredients and contaminated supplies. But as the demand for high-quality IV solutions grew, the need for a source of mass-produced IV base solutions uniformly prepared to **medical-grade quality standards** became apparent.

In 1922, Foster G. McGaw created the American Hospital Supply Company, which became the first company to manufacture hospital supply products (including large-volume parenteral products) that were high quality and of a uniform consistency.

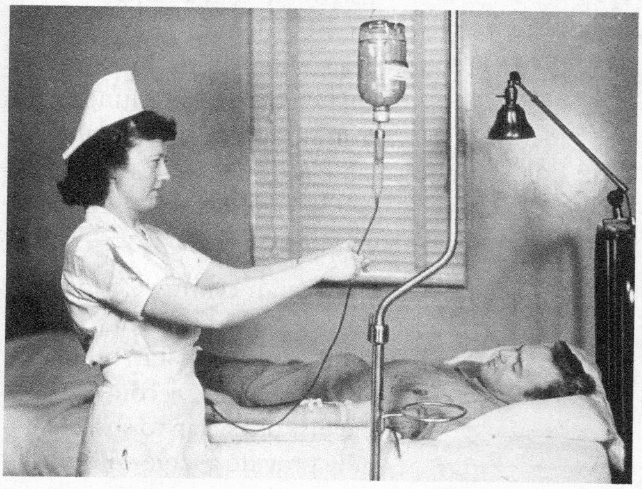

One important innovation was the introduction of the **slow-drip IV administration method** by English physicians Hugh Leslie Marriot and Alan Kekwick in 1935. This method enabled a continuous and consistent introduction of fluids without the constant presence of doctors or IV nurses. This technology increased the number of patients who could be treated and reduced the possibility of human error in the administration of fluids. Thirty years later, a team at the University of Pennsylvania's Department of Surgical Research showed that IV therapy could provide sufficient nutrients to support normal growth and development in juvenile beagles, leading to the development of **total parenteral nutrition**. This field advanced rapidly with improvements in parenteral formulas and technology such as **winged infusion needles**, **tunneled catheters**, and **flexible, plastic IV bags** in the 1970s. Scientific and technological advancements like these continue to fuel the evolution of parenteral administration, a method that encountered sometimes violent opposition from patients and doctors less than 200 years ago.

Today, major pharmaceutical manufacturing companies offer a myriad of pharmaceutical supply products, including over 200 large-volume parenteral base solutions. Guided by Food and Drug Administration regulations and ISO standards, such companies mass produce large-volume parenteral solutions that are sterile, meet medical-grade quality standards, and are of uniform ingredient strength and purity.

# Part 1: Concepts

In hospital pharmacy settings, IV technicians are largely responsible for preparing **parenteral solutions** for patient administration. Parenteral solutions are medications administered by any route other than through the alimentary canal (digestive tract). Injectable parenteral medications are administered to patients who are unable to swallow or whose digestive systems preclude the use of oral medications. Commonly ordered by physicians or other healthcare personnel, parenteral solutions maintain or correct the **fluid status** of patients whose conditions disrupt their bodies' innate fluid balance. To understand the use of parenteral preparations, sterile compounding personnel must understand the physiology of fluid balance.

> **POINTER**
> The word *parenteral* comes from the Greek roots *para*, meaning "beside," and *enteron*, meaning "intestine." Therefore, a parenteral preparation refers to a product that bypasses—or goes "beside" rather than through—the gastrointestinal tract.

## Physiology of Fluid Balance

Water is a critical element of the human body, composing approximately 70% of the body's weight. Water is primarily found *within* the cells of the body, or **intracellular spaces**, but it also can be found in the spaces *between* the cells, or **interstitial spaces**, and in the spaces *outside* the cells, or **extracellular spaces**. Water is also a component of blood vessels, where it is found in the **intravascular spaces**.

Maintaining the proper level of fluid and electrolytes within the body, called **homeostasis**, is essential for human life. Fluid enters the body through the normal processes of drinking and eating and exits the body through the processes of perspiration, respiration, urination, and bowel evacuation (see Figure 8.1 on the following page). When certain conditions affect normal fluid intake and output levels—such as an inability to swallow, vomiting, diarrhea, excessive urination, excessive sweating, or blood loss—patients may be at risk for **dehydration**. Dehydration occurs when the amount of water entering the body is less than the amount of water leaving the body. Because an extreme loss of fluid may lead to kidney failure, cardiac arrest, or death, patients must be rehydrated with fluids as quickly as possible. The quickest method of rehydration is through the injection of parenteral solutions into the blood supply. For this reason, the vast majority of compounded sterile preparations (CSPs) prepared by IV technicians are large-volume parenteral products.

## Properties of Parenteral Products

Because parenteral products are administered directly into a patient's blood supply, these solutions must have certain **chemical properties** or *characteristics* that render them safe for patient administration. Most IV base solutions are manufactured to meet these safety characteristics. Still, IV technicians should have a basic understanding of the chemical properties of parenteral solutions to better understand the sterile compounding process. Some characteristics include pH value, osmolarity, osmolality, and tonicity, as well as the compatibility of CSP additives. This chapter provides a broad introduction to the properties of parenteral products. Chapters 13 and 14 of this textbook provide more detailed information about the chemical properties, administration risks, and special compounding procedures associated with CSPs that do not have a neutral pH value, as well as CSPs that are not isotonic or isoosmotic.

FIGURE 8.1

**Daily Fluid Balance**

Regulation mechanisms such as thirst and urine output help the body maintain proper fluid balance. The yellow box at the right provides an example of the average daily intake and loss of fluid for an adult.

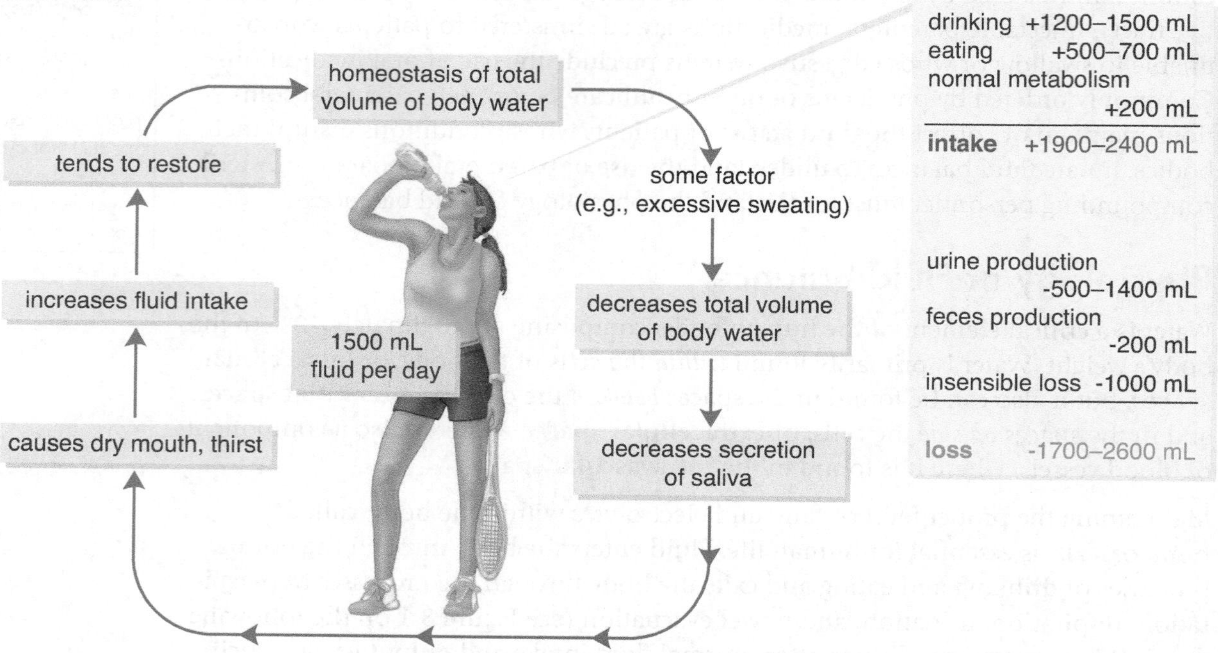


***pH Value*** IV preparations must have chemical properties that do not damage blood vessels. To achieve this effect, IV solutions must possess characteristics similar to human blood serum. The degree of **alkalinity** or **acidity** of a solution is referred to as its **pH value** and is measured on a scale from 0 to 14. A pH of 0 is extremely acidic, whereas a pH of 14 is extremely alkaline (basic). Any solution with a pH of less than 7.0 is considered to be acidic. Any solution with a pH greater than 7.0 is considered to be alkaline. A solution with a pH of 7.0 is considered to be **neutral**.

Human blood plasma has a pH of 7.4, which is slightly alkaline. The pH of blood plasma must be maintained for optimal health. Because an IV solution is administered directly into the patient's bloodstream, the solution must have a pH that does not significantly alter blood pH. Therefore, parenteral solutions are generally neutral to slightly acidic in nature. IV fluids with a pH value of less than 3.5 or greater than 7.5 may damage blood vessels or cause a disruption of normal cell function. Standard IV base solutions—such as dextrose 5% in water ($D_5W$), lactated Ringer's (LR), and normal saline (NS)—have pH values ranging from 3.5 to 6.2. In some instances, these ≠ neutral solutions can cause a burning or stinging sensation when injected into a patient's vein. This problem may be compounded when the CSP contains an acidic electrolyte such as potassium chloride. Some facilities inject a **buffer solution**, such as sterile sodium bicarbonate, into the CSP to neutralize the pH and prevent patient discomfort.

***Osmolarity and Osmolality*** Two other chemical properties of CSPs are osmolarity and osmolality. **Osmolarity** is a measure of the number of **milliosmoles** of **solute** per liter of solution (mOsm/L). With regard to CSPs, osmolarity refers to the osmotic pressure applied by a solution across a cell wall. **Osmotic pressure** is the pressure required to maintain equilibrium within the cells. **Osmolality** is a measure of the number of milliosmoles of solute per kilogram of solvent (mOsm/kg). As it pertains to CSPs, osmolality refers to the number of ions or molecules in a solution. Osmolarity and osmolality affect the flow of fluid into and out of cells within the body. To maintain optimal health, the cells should be maintained in a state of **equilibrium**. Therefore, CSPs must be neither **hyperosmotic** nor **hypoosmotic**. This state of equilibrium is called **isoosmotic**, meaning that the solution has relatively the same number of dissolved particles and the same osmotic pressure as human blood plasma.

***Tonicity*** **Tonicity** refers to the way that cells or tissues respond to surrounding fluid (see Figure 8.2 below). Cells within the human body have a semipermeable membrane through which fluid and solutes move in and around. Based on the movement of fluid and solutes, the tonicity of a solution can be classified as hypertonic, hypotonic, or isotonic. A **hypertonic** solution contains a greater number of dissolved particles than human blood plasma. If cells are subjected to a hypertonic solution, water will be drawn out of the cells, causing the cells to shrivel. A **hypotonic** solution contains fewer dissolved particles than human blood plasma. If cells are subjected to a hypotonic solution, water will be drawn into the cells, causing

**POINTER**

Although the terms *osmolarity* and *tonicity* are often used interchangeably, these chemical properties are distinct. Osmolarity is an absolute measure of the movement of fluid and solutes through a cell membrane, whereas tonicity is a relative measure of the movement of fluid and solutes through a cell membrane.

FIGURE 8.2

**Tonicity Effects on Cells in Solution**

Body cells can be bathed with isotonic solution without a net change between intracellular and extracellular concentrations.

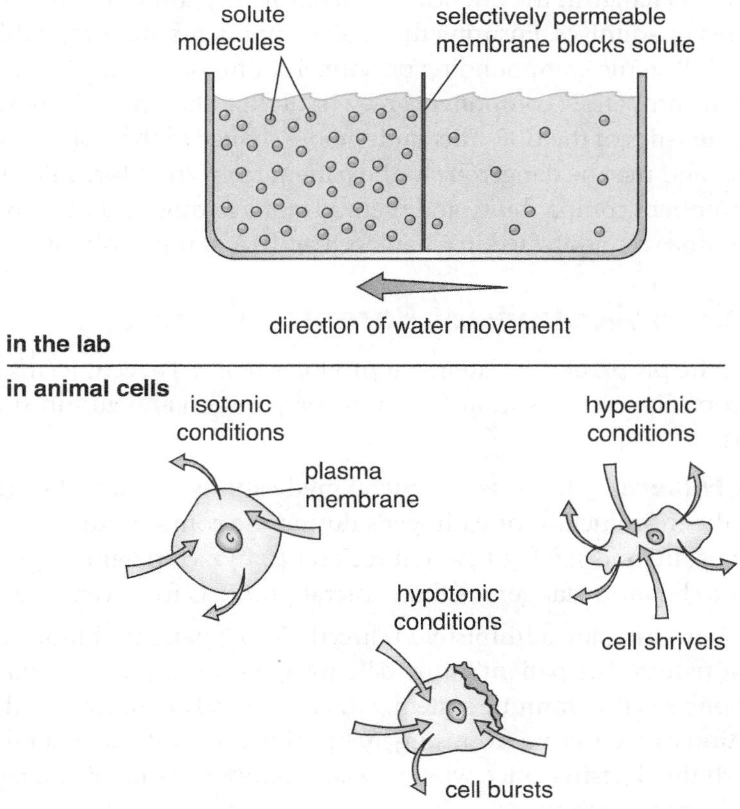

the cells to swell. Both situations are potentially damaging to the cells and may be harmful to a patient. In addition to causing ulceration or other damage to the blood vessel or surrounding tissue, the administration of solutions that are either hypertonic or hypotonic could lead to cardiovascular collapse or overload, resulting in serious injury or death. In contrast, an **isotonic** solution contains a number of dissolved particles equivalent to human blood plasma. The most commonly prescribed CSPs are either isotonic, slightly hypertonic, or slightly hypotonic.

Some conditions require treatment with a parenteral solution that is either hypertonic or hypotonic. For instance, a total parenteral nutrition (TPN) preparation is a type of hypertonic large-volume parenteral (LVP) solution administered to patients needing long-term IV nutrition. If a TPN solution were to be administered through a peripheral vein, the hypertonic solution would cause the destruction or collapse of the smaller, peripheral vein. Therefore, TPNs and other hypertonic solutions are generally administered into larger veins such as the **subclavian vein** or the **superior vena cava**. These larger veins have significantly more blood flowing through them and can more easily accommodate the hypertonic solution.

Unlike hypertonic solutions, hypotonic solutions, such as 0.225% sodium chloride (¼ NS), are rarely administered to patients. Occasionally, critical care patients who are experiencing **diuresis** are treated with these solutions to replace the high volume of fluid output without significantly increasing **plasma sodium concentration** ($P_{Na}$). These patients must be monitored closely to ensure that they do not develop a potentially life-threatening electrolyte imbalance such as **hyponatremia**.

***Compatibility*** With regard to CSPs, **compatibility** may be defined as the ability to combine two or more base components or additives within a solution, without creating a resultant change in the physical or chemical properties of any of the solution components or additives. Ensuring that CSP components are compatible is the responsibility of all sterile compounding personnel. Compounding a CSP comprised of one or more incompatible components may result in a change to the physical or chemical characteristics of the CSP. This undesirable change to the CSP is called an **incompatibility** and may be dangerous to the patient recipient. More information about CSP component compatibility and methods for avoiding and identifying potential incompatibilities are addressed in Chapters 9 and 13 of this textbook.

## Potential Complications of Parenteral Therapy

Understanding the properties of parenteral products makes IV technicians aware of the potential complications associated with the preparation and administration of these solutions.

***Preparation Hazards*** Because parenteral medications circulate through the blood supply, the introduction of pathogens during the compounding process can jeopardize the health and safety of patient recipients. In fact, parenteral medications are considered to be more dangerous than enteral products for several reasons:

- Parenteral products are administered directly into a patient's blood supply, organs, or tissues. The patient's only defense against any potential pathogens in these products is the immune system, which is already compromised by fighting infection or recovering from surgery or injury. In contrast, enteral products go through the digestive tract, where an abundance of flora defend against many pathogenic organisms.

- Parenteral solutions injected into the bloodstream have little or no chance of reversal if a medication error (incorrect drug or dosage) is made. By contrast, some enteral medications can be reversed with the administration of ipecac or activated charcoal, if necessary.
- Parenteral administration introduces 100% of the drug into the bloodstream, whereas enteral medications are broken down in the digestive tract, which allows only a portion of the drug to reach the patient's blood supply.

***Administration Hazards*** In addition to the risks involved in the preparation of the product, the administration of parenteral therapy involves potential complications that may lead to injury or, possibly, death for patient recipients. Therefore, *all* patients receiving parenteral fluids should be monitored for **nosocomial infection**, **extravasation**, **tissuing**, **phlebitis**, **cellulitis**, **embolism**, **allergic reaction** (including **anaphylaxis**), **Stevens-Johnson syndrome**, and **nephrotoxicity**. To manage these complications, healthcare practitioners use various techniques, including the use of access points, to administer LVPs. **Access points** are the specific areas of the body where an IV needle, catheter, or lock is placed. These points are determined by the medical conditions of the patients or the type of CSP being administered.

The most common access point is through a **peripheral vein**, into which a nurse inserts a needle, a **catheter**, or **cannula**, which is attached to IV tubing. This type of IV line is known as a **peripheral IV line** is most often used for a patient who requires short-term treatment (usually 72 hours or less) with IV fluids. Patients who require long-term treatment may need a **PICC line**, in which a sheath is inserted through a peripheral vein and then, using the guidance of an ultrasound and various x-rays, is threaded through the vein until the catheter is situated in the superior vena cava or the right atrium. The PICC line remains in place until the treatment regimen is complete. Other IV access points include the subclavian vein, superior vena cava, or femoral vein. These access points are reached through the use of various access devices such as the **central line**, **Hickman line**, **Broviac line**, and various **implantable ports**. These access points, their access mechanisms, and the medical conditions that might necessitate their use, are discussed in Chapters 12–14 of this textbook.

***Adherence to USP Chapter <797> Guidelines*** In light of these potential complications, IV technicians must adhere to strict aseptic technique when preparing parenteral medications, and healthcare personnel must be vigilant during their administration to patients. Chapters 8–14 of this textbook align with the directives set forth in USP Chapter <797> regarding the importance of proper aseptic technique in the preparation of different types of parenteral products. This chapter begins with a discussion of the most commonly prepared LVP solutions.

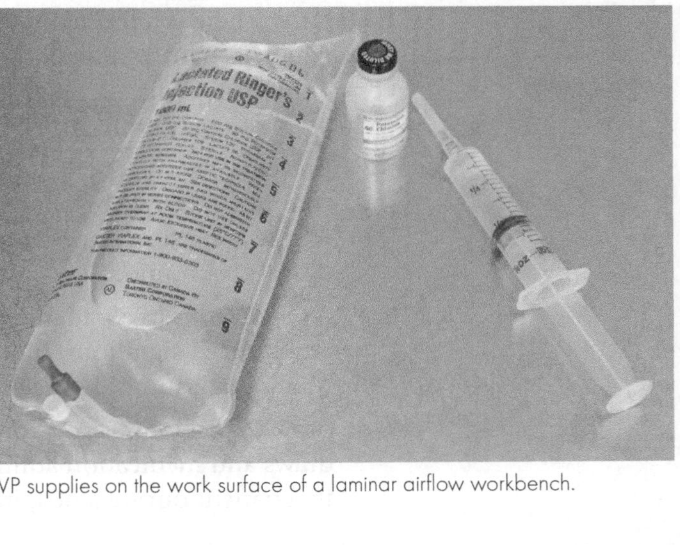

LVP supplies on the work surface of a laminar airflow workbench.

## LVP Preparations

**Large-volume parenteral (LVP) preparations**—or, simply, **LVPs**—are sterile solutions of 250 mL or greater that are administered parenterally.

Because most inpatients receive an LVP during their hospital stay, many of the procedures you perform as a sterile compounding technician involve the aseptic preparation of these products for IV administration. These large-volume IV solutions are frequently referred to as "main" IV lines for they provide fluids directly into patients' veins.

The most common LVPs are IV solutions compounded from a standard solution or **base solution** such as 0.9% sodium chloride (also known as NS), dextrose 5% in water ($D_5W$), dextrose 5% in normal saline ($D_5NS$), and LR solution. The most common volumes for LVPs are 250 mL, 500 mL, and 1000 mL. These IV solutions can be administered as either a continuous infusion or a drip.

**Common IV Base Solutions and Their Abbreviations:**

- Dextrose 5% in water ($D_5W$ or D5W)
- Dextrose 5% in 0.225% sodium chloride ($D_5$ ¼ NS or D5 ¼NS)
- Dextrose 5% in 0.33% sodium chloride ($D_5$ ⅓ NS or D5 ⅓NS)
- Dextrose 5% in 0.45% sodium chloride ($D_5$ ½ NS or D5 ½NS)
- Dextrose 5% in 0.9% sodium chloride ($D_5$ NS or D5 NS)
- 0.9% sodium chloride (NS)
- Lactated Ringer's (LR or RL)
- Dextrose 5% in lactated Ringer's ($D_5$ LR or $D_5$ RL, or D5 LR or D5 RL)

***Continuous Infusion*** A **continuous infusion**—also called a **maintenance infusion**, **replacement infusion**, or **hydration infusion**—typically consists of a base solution with **additives**. This type of IV solution may be administered at an IV flow rate ranging from 40 mL/hour up to 250 mL/hour, depending on the patient's hydration and electrolyte needs. The most common additives are electrolytes or, occasionally, vitamins to replace a patient's depleted fluid volume or electrolyte stores, such as potassium chloride, sodium chloride, sodium bicarbonate, magnesium sulfate, and multivitamins. There is a limited selection of premade LVPs with additives; therefore, most continuous infusions are prepared by an IV technician. A continuous infusion is used to:

- prevent or correct dehydration and restore electrolyte balance in a patient whose condition impedes adequate fluid consumption
- replace fluids in a patient who has experienced significant blood loss from trauma or a surgical procedure
- provide easy vein access for blood draws and medication administration in a patient during a hospital stay

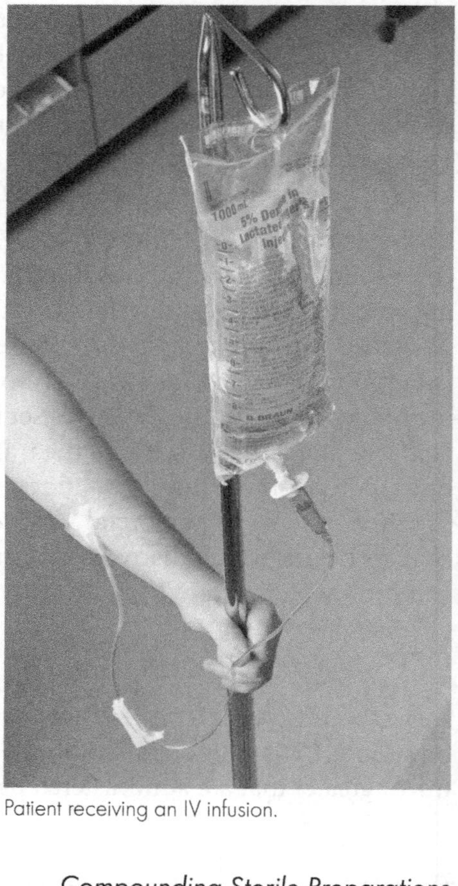

Patient receiving an IV infusion.

***Drip*** A second type of LVP solution is referred to as a **drip**. Unlike continuous infusions, drip solutions are used to continuously deliver an IV medication to treat a specific medical condition. Some common drip solutions are heparin, aminophylline, dopamine, dobutamine, nitroglycerin, nitroprusside, amiodarone, and insulin. The medication is injected into an IV base solution that typically has a volume of either 250 mL or 500 mL. A limited selection of premade drip solutions is available; therefore, most drips are prepared by an IV technician.

In general, drip solutions are infused at a much slower rate than other types of LVP solutions, often 20 mL/hour or less. A physician may order an IV drip to administer a specific dose of medication—for example, an order for the anticoagulant heparin to be administered continuously at an IV rate of 1000 units/hour. Or, a physician may order an IV drip to be "**titrated to effect**." In this instance, a medication such as nitroglycerin is administered at such a rate as to relieve the patient's chest pain. The nurse may increase or decrease the flow rate of the nitroglycerin drip based on the effect the medication has on the patient. Once the patient's medical condition has improved or the desired result has been achieved, the drip is discontinued.

## USP Chapter <797> Guidelines for LVPs

During the preparatory and compounding procedures of LVPs, the IV technician must adhere to the overarching principles set forth in USP Chapter <797>. These guidelines are reinforced in each facility's P&P manual as well. In accordance with these guidelines, sterile compounding personnel must pay strict attention to aseptic technique protocols both in the anteroom and clean room. Any breach in these protocols may result in medication errors, sepsis, or, possibly, death for patient recipients. Therefore, as an IV technician, you bear primary responsibility for the preparation and integrity of the CSPs. With that in mind, only those personnel who have been specially trained, process validated, and certified in aseptic technique and sterile product preparation should be allowed to compound sterile products. Part 2 of this chapter guides you through the discovery and demonstration of proper aseptic technique in LVP preparation.

# Concepts Self-Check

## Check Your Understanding

*Write your answers on a separate sheet of paper, as modeled in these examples:* 1d; 2c; 3b; *etc. Check your answers using the Answer Key in Appendix A.*

**1.** Which of the following was a main reason why consistent, successful treatment with LVP solutions was not widely implemented prior to the 1920s?
   a. tainted solutions and supplies due to nonsterile compounding procedures
   b. absence of guidelines to ensure uniform quality and quantity of LVP ingredients
   c. lack of sources to supply mass-produced, sterile, IV base solutions
   d. all of the above

**2.** Sterile parenterals are most often administered by which route?
   a. oral
   b. topical
   c. intravenous
   d. subcutaneous

**3.** Which of the following physical or chemical characteristics must be considered with regard to CSPs?
   a. pH value
   b. osmolarity, osmolality, and tonicity
   c. compatibility of solution components
   d. all of the above
   e. only *a* and *b*

**4.** Which of the following statements most closely describes the term *continuous infusion*?
   a. an LVP that administers a medication to relieve chest pain
   b. an LVP that administers a medication that is titrated to effect
   c. an LVP that administers a specific dose of a medication
   d. an LVP that administers continuous hydration and electrolytes

**5.** Which of the following items provides guidance for aseptic technique procedures that must be followed during LVP preparation?
   a. the facility's P&P manual, which reinforces the principles set forth in USP Chapter <797>
   b. USP Chapter <797>, which reinforces the guidelines established by the facility's P&P manual
   c. the hood manufacturer's guidebook, which reinforces the guidelines established by the facility's P&P manual
   d. none of the above

## Apply Your Knowledge

*On a separate sheet of paper, write your answers to the questions posed in the paragraph below. Use complete sentences and take time to create a thorough and thoughtful response. Check your answers against the Answer Key in Appendix A.*

In Part 1 of this chapter, you learned that early pioneers in LVP development and administration experienced many setbacks, including a high mortality rate from infections brought on by the use of contaminated solutions and containers. With that in mind, what is the significance of using medical-grade containers and ingredients in the sterile compounding process? What does it indicate about the need for aseptic technique in LVP preparation procedures?

# Part 2: Training

*Before performing this lab, review the Sterile Compounding Area Procedures listed on pages 162–163 at the end of the Unit 2 opener, and preview the accompanying process validation checklist in Appendix D.*

## Understand the Resources and Supplies

USP Chapter <797> prescribes special requirements for the preparation of LVP products. This chapter and the corresponding lab provide resources and supplies that are in alignment with the directives set forth in USP Chapter <797>.

### Essential Supplies

Most sterile compounding procedures require the same essential supply items to be available for use in both the anteroom and the clean room. For the anteroom, these supplies include a standard calculator, aseptic garb, presaturated **aseptic cleaning wipes**, a waste container, and various other compounding supplies such as those needed for aseptic hand washing and hood cleaning. In the clean room, essential supply items include sterile, foamed 70% IPA, sterile gloves, sterile 70% IPA swabs, a sharps container, a waste container, and a laminar airflow hood.

### Procedure-Specific Supplies

In addition to the previously listed essential supplies, each sterile compounding procedure requires supply items specific to the procedure being performed. The type, number, and amount of procedure-specific supply items are determined by an IV technician prior to performing the procedure, based on information provided on the CSP label and the medication additive label. After reading these labels, the IV technician performs one or more calculations that reveal the number and volume of additives needed to prepare the CSP. This information, in turn, dictates the number, size, and types of syringes needed for the procedure.

***LVP Supplies*** The process of compounding LVP preparations involves the manipulation of regular needles and, in particular, vials and IV base solutions. Familiarity with the appearance of these items as well as any specific handling requirements is essential to sterile compounding procedures.

VIALS A **vial** is a sealed, sterile container, made of plastic or glass, that has a rubber top through which an IV technician draws fluid. Vials contain a sterile medication either in a powdered form, which must be dissolved with a liquid **diluent**, or in a liquid form. The most commonly used diluents are sterile water and normal saline. Because a vial is a **closed-system container**, or a container from which air cannot freely flow in or out, an IV technician uses a **milking technique** to easily and safely release the **negative pressure** within a vial. To perform this technique, the IV technician adds **positive pressure** to the closed system by introducing an amount of air to the vial that is equal to, or slightly less than, the volume of liquid to be withdrawn from the vial. The air from the syringe is then injected, a small amount at a time, into the vial, while alternately transferring small volumes of liquid from the vial into the

**FIGURE 8.3**

**Vial and Needle-and-Syringe Unit**

Note the critical areas and the syringe measurement point.

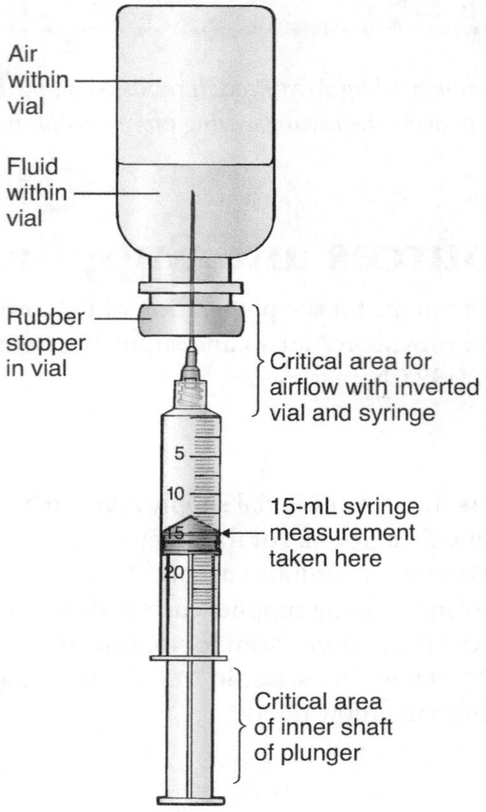


syringe. The syringe measurement is taken where the shoulder of the rubber plunger meets the barrel of the syringe (see Figure 8.3).

Using the milking technique is an important element of working with vials. This technique prevents **aspiration** and other problems associated with negative or positive pressure. The Meet the Challenge activity at the end of this chapter provides more experience with the type of negative and positive pressure situations that you may encounter when preparing LVPs.

When handling a vial, an IV technician must also be careful to avoid coring. **Coring** is an undesired event that occurs when a needle is inserted incorrectly into the rubber stopper atop a solution vial, causing a small bit of the stopper to tear off and contaminate the solution inside the vial. To avoid coring, the IV technician should insert the needle into the vial's rubber top with the bevel of the needle pointing upward and with the needle bending slightly upon contact. If coring does occur, the IV technician must dispose of the contaminated vial and needle-and-syringe unit and repeat the procedure using new supplies.

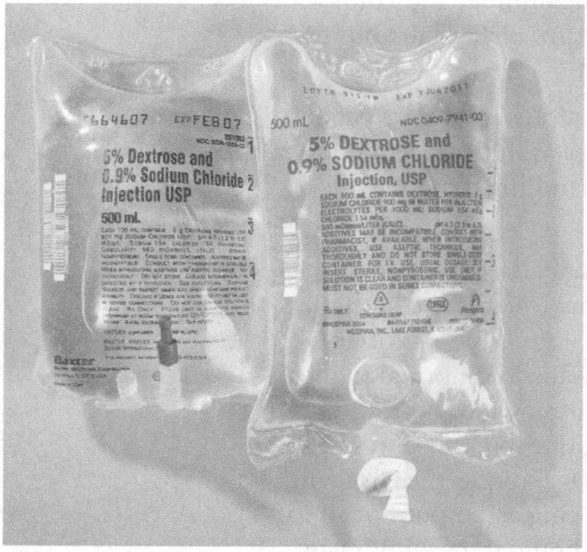


IV bags with a tail injection port (left) and a button injection port (right).

**IV BASE SOLUTIONS** An IV base solution is commonly provided by the manufacturer in an IV bag made of flexible plastic or polyvinyl chloride (PVC). This material allows the bag to expand when fluid is injected into the bag and to contract when fluid is withdrawn from the bag. Therefore, unlike the closed system of a vial, air pressure within the bag can fluctuate, requiring no equalization measures to be taken.

The injection port of the IV bag may be one of two types, depending on the manufacturer: a button or nipple injection port or a tail injection port. The **button or nipple injection port** can be found at the bottom of the IV bag's face, or the bottom front of the IV bag where the manufacturer's printed information is located. The **tail injection port**, the most common type of IV injection port, is located at the very bottom of the IV bag. Recognizing these two different types of ports is important to the placement of the IV bag in the hood. IV technicians must ensure that the bag's position in the hood maintains a proper airflow from the HEPA filter to the injection port, a critical site. The port itself is constructed of a material that is not prone to coring. Consequently, unlike a vial, the needle should be inserted directly into the injection port without regard to the position of the needle bevel and without creating any bend to the needle.

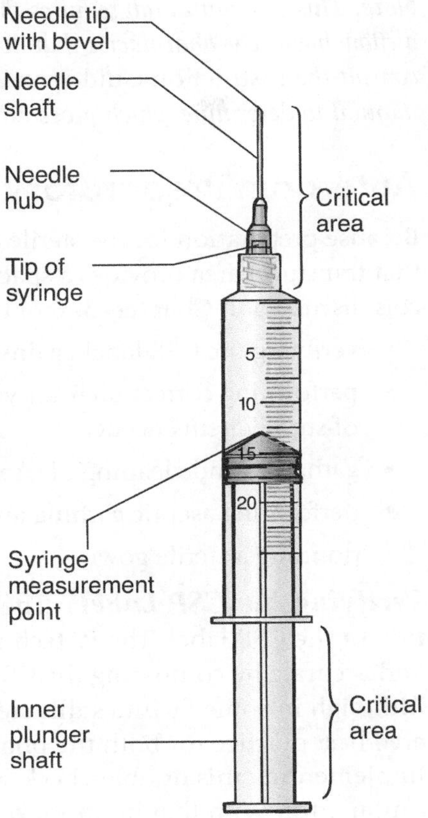


FIGURE 8.4

**Critical Areas of a Needle and Syringe**

## Critical Sites of Essential Supplies and LVP Supplies

Before beginning preparatory procedures in the anteroom or clean room, the IV technician must recall the **critical sites** of the supplies. Identifying the critical site of each supply item will help you to determine the proper procedure for handling the supply item once you have entered the clean room and begin working in the hood.

The critical sites of essential supply items include the opened sterile 70% IPA swabs. The critical sites of the LVP supplies include the needle, syringe tip, and the piston plunger and inner plunger shaft of the syringe (see Figure 8.4). The critical sites of these essential and procedure-specific supply items are supplied by the manufacturer in sterile condition and, therefore, should not be swabbed with IPA prior to use.

The critical sites of the other LVP supplies used for the Chapter 8 procedural lab include the injection port of the IV base solution and the vial top. These critical sites must be swabbed with sterile, 70% IPA prior to needle insertion to decrease the likelihood of contaminating the solution during the injection or withdrawal procedures.

After identifying the critical sites of all supply items, care must be taken not to taint the critical site of any of the supply items through **touch contamination**, **shadowing**, or incorrect placement of the item within the hood. (For additional assistance on the handling of critical sites of sterile compounding supplies, refer to Chapter 3 of this textbook.)

# Preview the Lab Procedure

*The following material provides a brief overview of the lab procedure that you will perform. First, read the* Preview the Lab Procedure *section. Then read each step of the* Procedural Lab *section carefully, visualizing every action. Next, reinforce your understanding of the process by watching the demonstration video. Once you are in the lab, your instructor will demonstrate the procedure, and then you will perform the procedure by following the steps in the* Procedural Lab *section. Practice the lab procedure multiple times. After sufficient practice, you will complete the lab procedure for process validation by your instructor.*

**POINTER**
Sterile compounding personnel must comply with certain restrictions when working in the anteroom and clean room areas. These restrictions include no gum chewing, horse-play, or food or drink in both the anteroom and clean room, and no hair spray, perfume, make-up, artificial or polished nails, or jewelry in the sterile compounding environment.

**POINTER**
Refer to your facility's P&P manual to determine the approved cleaning agent to be used for wiping down the supply items and the transport vehicle.

***Note:*** *This procedural lab requires the use of a basic, open-sided, horizontal laminar airflow hood. For pharmacies that do not have this type of hood, IV technicians should consult the* Instruction Guide *provided by the hood's manufacturer or their facility's P&P manual to determine which procedures may need to be adjusted to suit their hood.*

## Anteroom Preparatory Procedures

Because preparation for the sterile compounding process begins in the anteroom, that transition area provides a space for implementing the standard pharmacy protocols discussed in Chapters 3–6 of this textbook, including:

- verifying the CSP label against the medication order
- performing correct pharmacy calculations to determine type, size, and number of supply items needed
- gathering and cleaning of supplies
- performing aseptic garbing and hand washing
- donning a sterile gown

***Verifying the CSP Label*** The first step in the preparation of an LVP is verification of the CSP label. The IV technician should check that the CSP label is legible and accurate by comparing the CSP label to the physician's medication order. Although in some facilities this step is performed by the pharmacist, it is considered best practice for both the pharmacist and IV technician to perform this task. Implementing this double-check system helps to reduce the likelihood of a medication error. With that in mind, you should compare the medication order to the CSP label to verify that the following items match exactly: the name, room number, and ID number of the patient; the name, strength, and amount or quantity of the drug or additive; the name, concentration, and volume of the base solution; and the designated IV flow rate or administration time. (For additional assistance in reading and understanding medication orders, labels, and common abbreviations, refer to Chapter 4 and Appendix B of this textbook.)

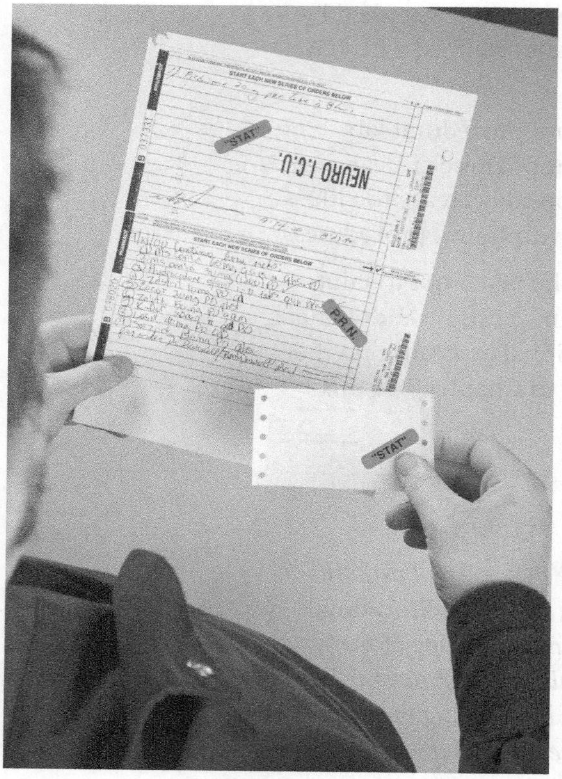

IV technician comparing a CSP label to a medication order.

***Performing Pharmacy Calculations*** Once you have verified the accuracy of the CSP label, you need to determine the type, size, and number of supply items needed for the procedure. Using information gleaned from the CSP label and the label on each medication or additive, calculate the desired volume of each additive or ingredient to be used in the procedure. The **desired volume** is the volume that you must withdraw from the vial to deliver the dose ordered by the physician. (For additional assistance on performing calculations, refer to Chapter 5 of this textbook.)

***Gathering and Cleaning of Supplies*** After performing the calculations, place the CSP label into a small plastic bag, place the medication order into a large plastic bag, and seal both bags. You should then gather the necessary supplies, including an appropriately sized syringe for the desired volume needed, and obtain a **transport vehicle**—such as a stainless-steel cart, a basket, or a tray—to facilitate an easy transfer of supplies into and out of the clean room.

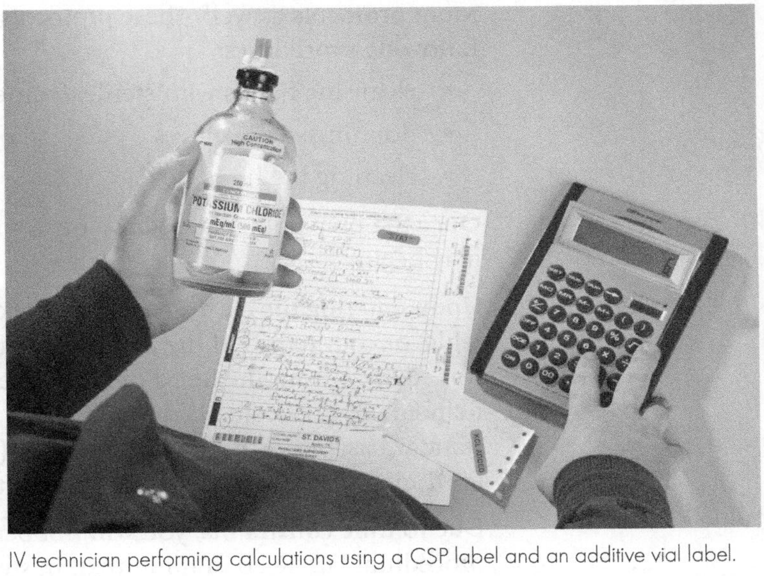

IV technician performing calculations using a CSP label and an additive vial label.

With the supplies and transport vehicle at hand, wipe down or spray the exterior surface of every supply item, as well as the transport vehicle, with an appropriate cleaning agent, such as a commercially available product formulated from methyl, alcohol, IPA, ammonia, hydrogen peroxide, or peracetic acid. Most supplies are provided by the manufacturer as individually wrapped items in a protective outer covering, sometimes called a **dust cover**. The IV technician must wipe the entire exterior surface or dust cover of each supply item individually, taking care that the entire surface comes into contact with the cleaning agent. If using a spray device to clean supply items, the IV technician must be sure to saturate the entire surface of each supply item's exterior cover and allow the supply item to dry completely before transferring it into the clean room. Be sure to also wipe down or spray the exterior surfaces of the plastic bags containing the medication order and CSP label. After cleaning the exterior surface of each supply item, place the item into the transport vehicle. Dispose of used wipes in a waste receptacle in the anteroom.

***Donning PPE*** Now that you have assembled your clean supplies, you must put on personal protective equipment (PPE), a requirement for working in the clean room. Before donning your aseptic garb, be sure that you are wearing close-toed shoes and either a scrub uniform or other approved lightweight, nonshedding clothing. Then put on aseptic shoe covers, a hair cover, a face mask, and, if appropriate, a beard cover. Lastly, don a sterile gown. (For additional assistance in aseptic garbing, refer to Chapter 6 of this textbook.)

Due to time constraints, you will not perform aseptic hand-washing procedures during this procedural lab. Keep in mind that, in sterile compounding practice, aseptic hand-washing procedures are mandatory and must be performed prior to donning a sterile gown.

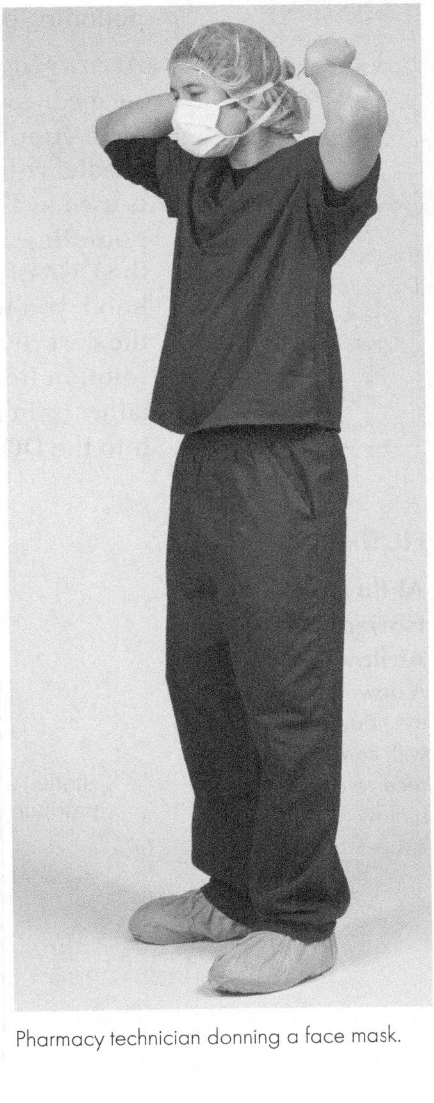
Pharmacy technician donning a face mask.

## Clean Room Preparatory Procedures

When preparing LVPs for patient administration, sterile compounding personnel must diligently follow established pharmacy clean room protocols as well. These protocols, discussed in Chapters 6 and 7, include the following procedures:

- cleansing hands with sterile, foamed 70% IPA
- donning sterile gloves
- cleaning the hood

Once the preparatory steps have been completed, LVP compounding procedures may begin.

Upon entering the clean room, place the transport basket or tray onto a clean shelf, table, or countertop. If the transport vehicle used is a cart, wheel it so that it is positioned away from the hood prefilter. Cleanse your hands and forearms with sterile, foamed 70% IPA and allow them to dry thoroughly. Don sterile gloves according to standard aseptic technique procedures. (For additional assistance on the procedure for donning sterile gloves, refer to Chapter 6 of this textbook.)

Due to time constraints, you will not perform hood-cleaning procedures during this procedural lab. Keep in mind that, in sterile compounding practice, hood-cleaning procedures are mandatory and must be performed prior to beginning sterile compounding procedures and at intervals prescribed by USP Chapter <797>.

**POINTER**

Some sterile compounding personnel prefer to dispose of waste as it is generated. Others prefer to create a waste or discard pile within the outer six-inch edge of the hood. If you use a discard pile, be sure to place the waste so that it does not mix with supply items or interfere in any way with CSP preparation.

***Arranging and Preparing Supplies in the Hood*** Once the hood has been cleaned, you must transfer the clean supplies from the transport vehicle or clean countertop to certain areas of the hood. Place small supply items, such as the vial, needle, syringe, and alcohol swabs, in the outer **six-inch zone** of the hood, which is used as a staging area prior to bringing the supplies into the hood's **direct compounding area (DCA)**. Set large supply items such as the IV base solution into the DCA of the hood (see Figure 8.5). Before placing the IV base solution in the hood, you need to remove the IV bag's dust cover. To do so, locate the **tear line** on the dust cover and rip open the outer package along this line. Remove the IV base solution from the dust cover and discard the cover into an appropriate waste container or in a **discard pile** located in the outer six-inch zone. Then place the IV bag into the DCA of the hood, or at least six inches *inside* the hood. Be sure to position

**FIGURE 8.5**

**Airflow in a Horizontal Laminar Airflow Workbench**

A downward view onto the hood's work surface with items placed to receive uninterrupted airflow.

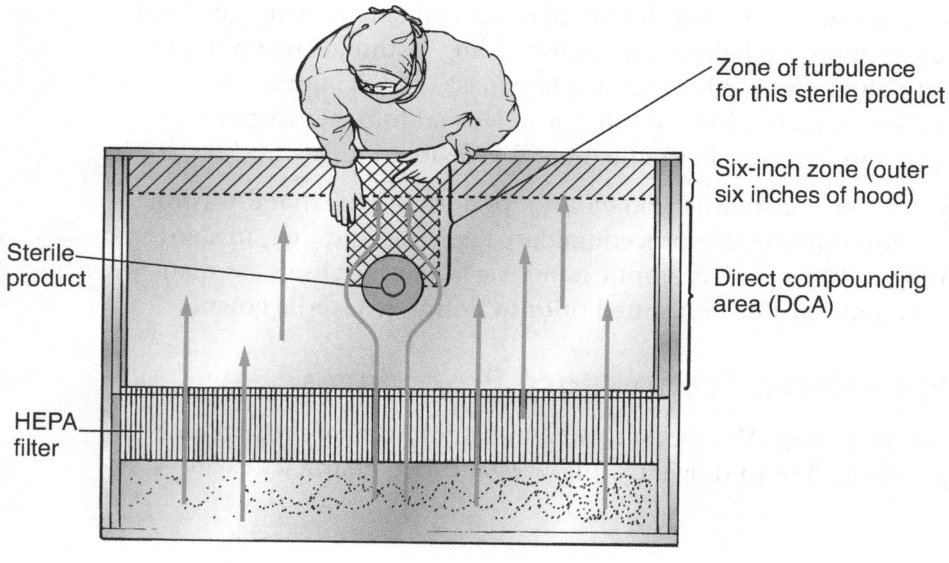

the injection port of the IV bag (in this case, a tail injection port) so that it receives uninterrupted airflow from the HEPA filter.

## LVP Compounding Procedure

With the small supply items arranged in the outer six-inch zone and the large supply items placed in the DCA, you are ready to begin the LVP compounding procedure. Remember that as you bring each small supply item into the DCA, it should be placed so that its critical site(s) receives a continuous airflow from the HEPA filter at the back of the hood. Also, be sure that the syringe and uncapped needle are handled in such a way as to avoid touch contamination and shadowing of the syringe tip and the needle hub. (For additional information on the hood's components and airflow movement, refer to Chapter 2 of this textbook.)

**POINTER**

Avoid repeatedly or vigorously rubbing the swab over a critical area as this action may cause fibers from the swab to adhere to the critical area, thereby contaminating it.

Keeping the critical sites in mind, start the procedure by bringing the vial into the DCA. Remove the **flip-top cap**, placing the cap into the discard pile. Position the vial top so that it receives uninterrupted airflow from the HEPA filter. Pick up an alcohol swab, move it into an area of the DCA so that it receives uninterrupted airflow from the HEPA filter, and carefully tear open the package. Place the empty swab package into the discard pile. Then swab the top of the vial and place the used swab into the discard pile.

**USP Chapter <797>**

Because manufacturers supply the syringe tip and all parts of the needle in sterile form, you must not swab them with IPA. Doing so may contaminate these critical sites.

Next, bring the syringe into the DCA and carefully remove the outer wrapper of the syringe without touching or shadowing the syringe tip. Grasp the barrel of the syringe and avoid placing the syringe onto the hood's work surface as this will contaminate it. Place the syringe wrapper into the discard pile. If there is a cap on the tip of the syringe, carefully remove it and place it into the discard pile. Without touching or shadowing the syringe tip, position the syringe in your hand to allow adequate airflow to the syringe tip and then open the needle and hold it by its cap. Be sure to avoid touching or shadowing the needle hub. Using a twisting motion, attach the capped needle hub to the Luer-lock on the syringe tip. Temporarily place the needle-and-syringe unit onto the hood's work surface within the DCA.

Next, open a new alcohol swab and place it on the hood's work surface, within the DCA. Pick up the syringe and pull down on the flat knob of the syringe plunger to draw a volume of air into the syringe that is equal to the desired volume of the additive. This desired volume was determined by your earlier mathematical calculation. Holding the syringe by the barrel, carefully remove the needle cap and place it onto the alcohol swab. Because most sterile compounding procedures require the IV technician to recap the needle, placing it onto an alcohol swab helps to maintain the needle cap's sterility.

Grasp the barrel of the syringe between your thumb and forefinger, as you would a pencil or dart, and rotate the barrel so that the needle bevel is pointed upward toward the ceiling. Brace the vial against the hood's work surface and place the needle tip, bevel up, onto the vial top. Insert the needle into the vial using a slight upward rotation of the wrist. Keep the tip of the needle in contact with the vial's rubber top at all times to help avoid coring. There should be a very slight bend to the needle as it penetrates the vial top (see Figure 8.6 on the following page).

Invert the vial using a clockwise motion. Inject air into the vial using the milking technique, thereby creating positive pressure that forces a volume of fluid from the

**FIGURE 8.6**

**Correct Needle Insertion into a Vial**
Note the slight bend of the needle during the insertion.

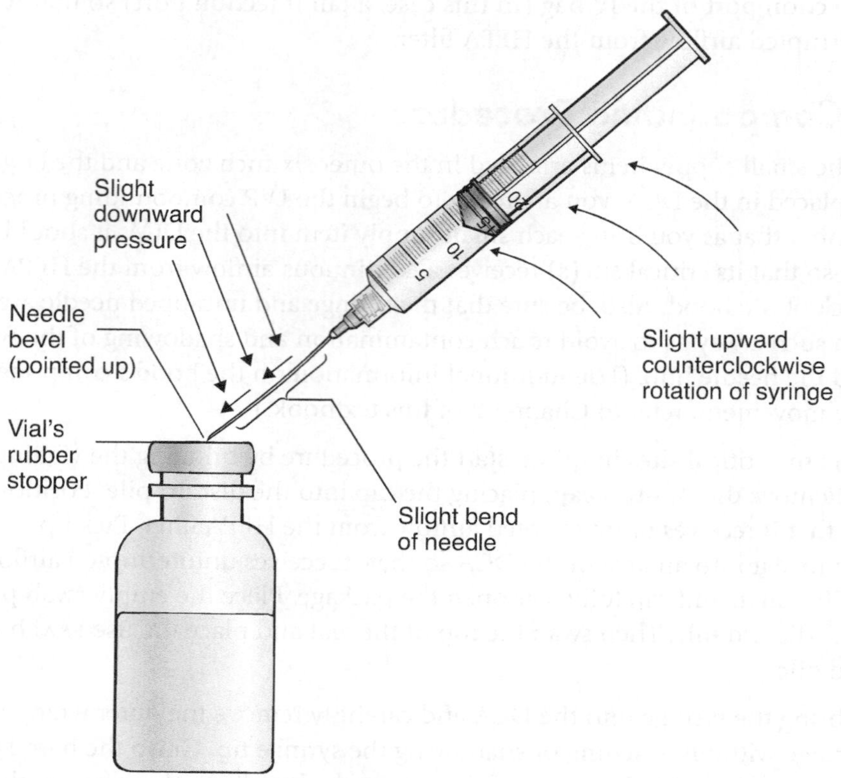


**POINTER**

The extra fluid volume that you have drawn up for this procedure allows you to easily remove any bubbles without having to withdraw additional fluid to meet the required final dose volume.

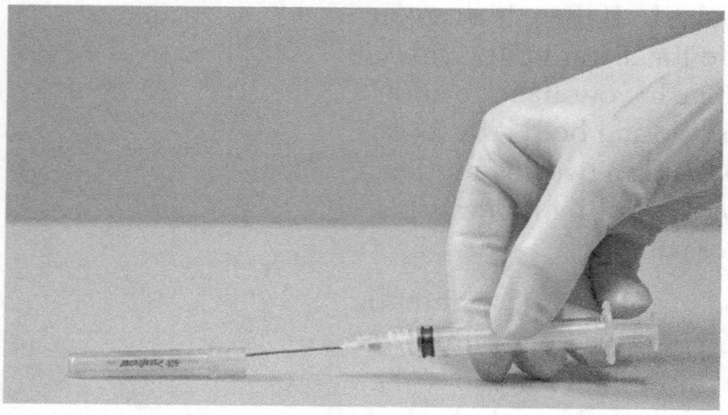
Scoop method of recapping a needle.

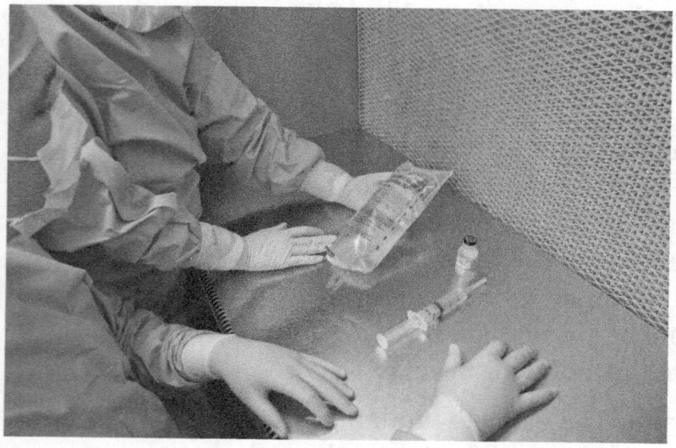
Pharmacist checking the CSP ingredients prepared by an IV technician.

vial into the syringe. Repeat this procedure until you have withdrawn a volume of fluid from the vial into the syringe that equals approximately 1 mL more than the desired dose volume. Without removing the syringe from the vial, brace the syringe against your palm, and tap the barrel of the syringe to force air bubbles upward toward the needle. Once all of the air bubbles from the syringe have gathered at the tip of the syringe, push up on the flat knob to expel the air and any extra fluid back into the vial, until the desired volume (determined by your earlier calculations) of bubble-free fluid remains in the syringe.

Return the vial, with syringe attached, to the hood's work surface using a counterclockwise motion. Grasp the syringe at the barrel and carefully pull the syringe, with needle attached, from the vial. Carefully recap the needle, using the **scoop method**. The scoop method involves the technician placing the tip of the needle into the cap that is lying on an IPA swab on the hood's work surface. The IV technician uses the needle-and-syringe unit to scoop the needle cap onto the needle. This method helps prevent an inadvertent needle stick but also increases the potential for contamination of the needle-and-syringe unit due to the needle accidently touching the hood's work surface.

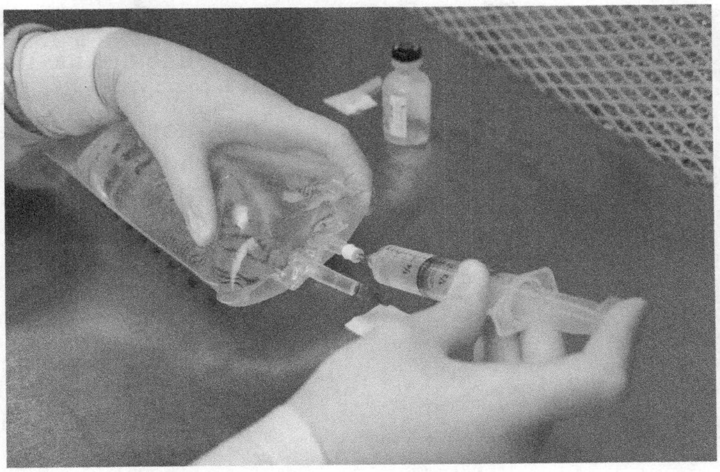

Injection of an additive into an LVP.

Arrange the vial, the filled and capped syringe, and the IV bag within the DCA to await a **verification check** by a pharmacist or your instructor. The IV bag should be placed on the hood, face up, so the pharmacist or instructor can easily read the preprinted information on the face of the bag without having to touch or reposition it. The vial should be placed to the immediate right of the IV bag, and the syringe should be placed to the immediate right of the vial. Turn the vial and syringe so that the checking pharmacist or instructor can easily read the vial label and syringe volume without having to touch or reposition either the vial or syringe. Place the medication order and CSP label, both in their plastic bags, in front of the CSP ingredients, in the outer six-inch zone of the hood. Be sure to avoid the area where you have located the discard pile.

Next, ask for a verification check by the checking pharmacist or your instructor. Make sure that the CSP components are positioned so that their readings can be quickly and easily observed without manipulation by the checkers. To do so, you may need to temporarily adjust the positions of the items, which may interrupt airflow to a critical site. If that happens, be sure to wipe the affected critical site with a new alcohol swab prior to injection. Once the instructor has verified that you have drawn up the correct desired volume of the additive, reposition the IV bag so that the tail injection port receives uninterrupted airflow. Bring a new alcohol swab into the DCA, position it so that the package receives uninterrupted airflow from the HEPA filter, and carefully tear open the package. Place the empty swab package into the discard pile. Swab the tail injection port of the IV bag, and then place the used alcohol swab onto the hood's work surface, directly under the injection port.

Remove the needle cap and place it onto the alcohol swab that you previously used to rest the cap. Grasp the syringe at the barrel, holding it as you would a dart. Then, with your other hand, stabilize the tail injection port of the IV bag. While maintaining a clear airflow to the area where the injection port and needle come into contact, carefully insert the needle into the injection port of the IV bag. The needle should be inserted straight into the injection port without regard to the position of the needle bevel. Caution should be taken to avoid puncturing the sidewall of the injection port during needle insertion.

**POINTER**

Some facilities prefer that the IV technician inject the additive into the IV or IV piggyback bag prior to the final verification check. In this case, the IV technician would inject the additive, remove the recapped needle from the empty additive syringe, and pull the plunger back to replicate the volume of the additive that was injected. The IV technician would then place the empty syringe and empty vial next to the CSP, which is subsequently checked by a pharmacist. Refer to your facility's P&P manual to determine the procedures for a pharmacist verification check.

**POINTER**

Although not a mandatory procedure, placing the used alcohol swab under the tail injection port is considered to be a best practice procedure. Performing this step provides two potential benefits: First, the alcohol swab will absorb any fluid that may drip from the injection port during injection; second, the alcohol swab acts as a buffer between the contaminated hood surface and the tail injection port, which tends to curl downward. Therefore, the alcohol swab helps maintain the sterility of the CSP.

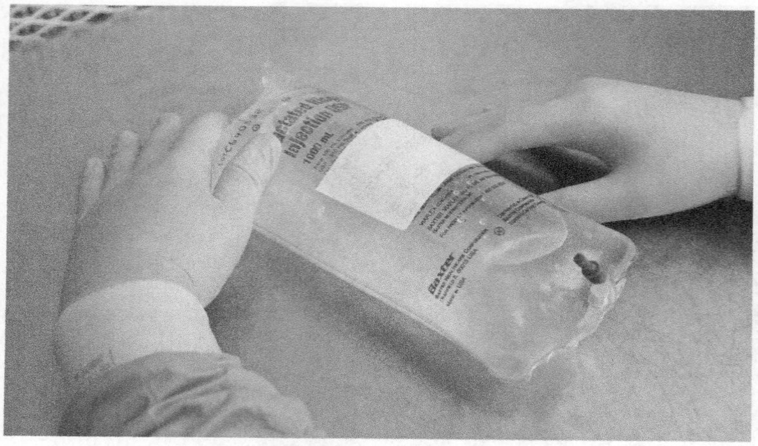


Labeling the CSP.

Once the needle is completely inserted into the injection port, push up on the flat knob of the plunger to inject the medication (in this case, potassium chloride) into the IV bag. Take care not to touch or shadow the injection port or needle at any time during the procedure.

Grasping the syringe only at the barrel, remove the syringe with attached needle from the IV bag. To avoid an inadvertent needle stick, do not recap the needle. Immediately place the syringe with attached needle into the sharps container.

Hold the IV bag up toward the light and squeeze it, examining the bag for leaks, **precipitates**, or evidence of incompatibility. If you observe any of these signs, you must dispose of the CSP and repeat the entire compounding procedure. (Refer to your facility's P&P manual for guidance on correct CSP disposal.) Provided the bag is free of these problems, label the CSP by affixing the adhesive label backing to the face of the IV bag so that it does not come into contact with the injection port or obscure the graduation markings on the IV bag. Then affix an IVA seal over the injection port of the bag.

**BE AWARE**

If you encounter resistance during needle insertion, the needle may have entered the tail injection port at a slight angle and be encountering resistance from the harder, outer plastic sidewall that covers the exterior surface of the tail. If so, immediately remove and reinsert the needle, ensuring it is inserted straight into the port.

Finally, dispose of the waste from the discard pile, as well as the needle cap and the used alcohol swabs, into the waste container. Place the CSP and the vial into the transport vehicle and return these supplies to the anteroom. Once there, use the felt-tip marker to record the opening date, time, and your initials on the vial and store the vial in the refrigerator or some other designated area. If you performed an aseptic hood-cleaning procedure for this lab, complete the required hood-cleaning log sheet. Then remove PPE using proper aseptic technique. (For additional assistance on the aseptic removal of PPE, refer to Chapter 6 of this textbook.)

**POINTER**

IVA seals are not used in all facilities. These seals are a preferred, but not required, supply item. Refer to your facility's P&P manual to determine whether IVA seals are part of your compounding procedures.

# Watch the Demonstration Video

*Watch the Chapter 8 Demonstration Video, which shows the step-by-step aseptic procedures for compounding LVPs. For the purposes of the Chapter 8 Demonstration Video, neither aseptic hand washing nor hood cleaning is demonstrated. Refer to the Chapter 6 video for a demonstration of aseptic hand-washing procedures, and to the Chapter 7 video for a demonstration of correct hood-cleaning procedures.*

Training Videos DVD

# Procedural Lab

*This lab walks you through the step-by-step actions that you must follow to compound LVPs using aseptic technique. Take your time. Work through each step methodically and with close attention to detail.*

***Note:** For the purposes of this procedural lab, you will not perform aseptic hand-washing and hood-cleaning procedures unless directed to do so by your instructor. Should your instructor ask you to perform these procedures, refer to Chapter 6 for instructions on aseptic hand washing and to Chapter 7 for directions on correct hood cleaning.*

***Note:** For steps 1–3, please refer to Chapter 4 for a reminder of the step-by-step procedures required for medication order and CSP label verification. For steps 4 and 5, please refer to Chapter 5 for assistance in performing calculations. For steps 6–10, refer to Chapter 3 for a reminder of the process for cleaning supplies. For steps 11–14, refer to Chapter 6 for step-by-step aseptic garbing, hand-washing, and gloving procedures. You should perform steps 1–14 and steps 48–49 in the anteroom. You should perform steps 15–47 in the clean room.*

## Supplies

### *Essential Supplies*

To complete the Unit 2 procedural labs, you will need to ensure that various essential anteroom and clean room supplies such as those listed in Table 8.1 are available for your use.

**Table 8.1 Essential Anteroom and Clean Room Supplies for Sterile Compounding**

| Anteroom Supplies |
|---|
| medication order and CSP label<br>calculator<br>pen<br>permanent, felt-tip marker<br>plastic bags (small and large)<br>aseptic garb, including shoe covers, hair cover, face mask, and beard cover (if appropriate)<br>sterile gown<br>presaturated, aseptic cleaning wipes<br>sterile, foamed 70% IPA<br>waste container<br>transport vehicle (optional) |
| **Clean Room Supplies** |
| sterile, foamed 70% IPA<br>sterile, powder-free gloves<br>sterile 70% IPA swabs, individually packaged × 3<br>sharps container<br>waste container<br>laminar airflow hood |

### *Procedure-Specific Supplies*

In addition to the supplies listed in Table 8.1, gather the following items specific to the Chapter 8 LVP procedural lab:

- regular needle (nonfilter, nonvented needle, either 18 or 19 gauge)
- potassium chloride 2 mEq/mL; 20-mL vial size (or larger)

- 20-mL Luer-lock syringe
- 1000 mL of LR solution in an IV bag with a tail injection port
- IVA seals (optional)

## Procedure

### *Verifying the Label(s)*

1. Review the CSP label to verify that the patient's name, room number, and ID number match the information contained on the medication order. To help you with this task, compare the CSP label (see Figure 8.7) to the medication order and patient ID label (see Figure 8.8).

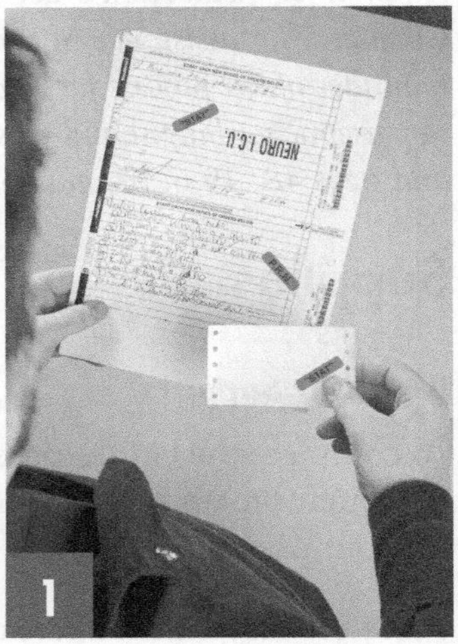


**FIGURE 8.7**
**CSP Label for Potassium Chloride**

****Large-Volume Parenteral****
Memorial Hospital

**Pt. Name:** Will Van Ingen **Room:** Neuro ICU
**Pt. ID#:** 8873662 **Rx#:** 74521

**Potassium Chloride 30 mEq**
**Lactated Ringer's 1000 mL**
**Rate: 40 mL/hr**

Expires ______
RPh ______
Tech ______

Keep refrigerated – warm to room temperature before use.

2. Check the CSP label to verify that the additive name (in this case, potassium chloride) and dosage match what is on the medication order.
3. Scan the CSP label to verify that the base solution name (in this case, LR solution), strength, and volume, as well as the IV flow rate, match what is on the medication order.

### *Calculating Desired Volume*

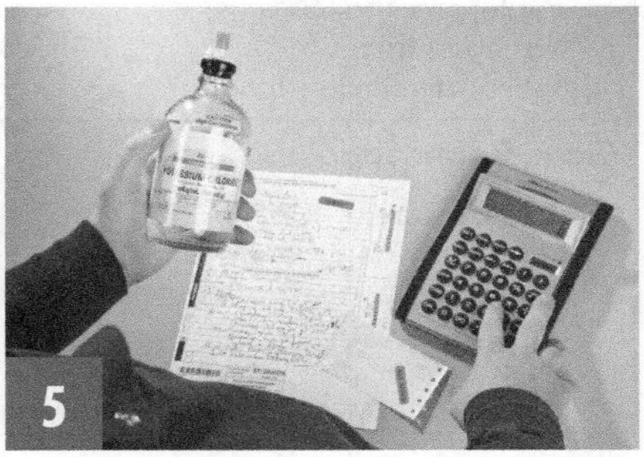


4. Read the label on the potassium chloride vial to determine the concentration of the potassium chloride solution.
5. Perform the calculations based on the information provided on the potassium chloride label. Provided that the label indicates that potassium chloride has a concentration of 2 mEq/mL, use the following formula to calculate the dose:

$$\frac{2\text{ mEq}}{1\text{ mL}} = \frac{30\text{ mEq}}{x\text{ mL}}$$

*Cross-multiply, then divide to solve for $x$ the desired dosage volume. (For additional assistance, refer to Chapter 5 for step-by-step dosage calculation procedures.)

**FIGURE 8.8**

**Daily Order**

**ID#:** 8873662
**Name:** Will Van Ingen
**DOB:** 4/21/83
**Room:** Neuro ICU
**Dr.:** Petra Nicolaissen

**MEMORIAL HOSPITAL**
**PHYSICIAN'S MEDICATION ORDER**

BEAR DOWN ON HARD SURFACE WITH BALLPOINT PEN

GENERIC EQUIVALENT IS AUTHORIZED UNLESS CHECKED IN THIS COLUMN

ALLERGY OR SENSITIVITY TO PCN, EES

NONE KNOWN ☐ SIGNED:

DIAGNOSIS

COMPLETED OR DISCONTINUED

| DATE | TIME | ORDERS | PHYSICIAN'S SIG. | NAME | DATE | TIME |
|---|---|---|---|---|---|---|
| | | Height 5' 9" Weight 152 lbs | | | | |
| 7/27/2013 | | Start IV of LR w/30 mEq of KCl @ 40 mL/hr | | | | |
| | | | Petra Nicolaissen, MD | | | |

"STAT"

PHARMACY COPY

### *Gathering and Cleaning Supplies*

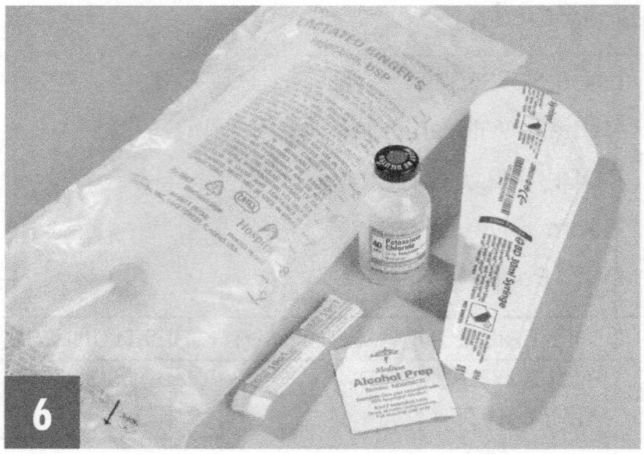

6. Place the medication order into the large plastic bag and the CSP label into the small plastic bag. Gather all supply items listed in the Supplies section of the procedural lab.
7. Open the package of aseptic cleaning wipes. Remove one or, if necessary, more wipes, and thoroughly wipe down the entire transport vehicle.
8. Place the used wipes into the waste receptacle.
9. Remove a new aseptic cleaning wipe and wipe down the exterior surface of the IV bag's dust cover. Place the cleaned IV bag into the transport vehicle. Place the used wipe into the waste receptacle.
10. Repeat the cleaning procedure outlined in step 9 with each of the remaining supply items.

**POINTER**

During aseptic garbing, best practice is to reapply sterile, foamed 70% IPA to your hands after donning shoe covers and again after donning a hair cover.

### *Garbing*

11. Don shoe covers.
12. Put on a hair cover.
13. Don a face mask and beard cover (if appropriate).

    *Note:* For the purposes of this training lab, you will skip the mandatory aseptic hand-washing procedure.
14. Don a sterile gown.
15. Bring all supply items, including an unopened package of sterile gloves, into the clean room.
16. Place the transport vehicle onto a clean surface or countertop within the clean room. If a cart is used, position it so that it does not interrupt airflow into the hood prefilter.
17. Apply sterile, foamed 70% IPA to your hands. Allow them to air-dry and then don sterile gloves.

    *Note:* For the purposes of this training lab, you will skip the mandatory hood-cleaning procedure.

### *Compounding the LVP Solution*

**18.** Tear open the dust cover and remove the IV bag of LR solution. Place the bag into the DCA of the hood and the dust cover into the waste receptacle. Place small supply items, such as the needle, vial, syringe, and alcohol swabs into the outer six-inch zone of the hood.

**19.** Remove the plastic, flip-top cap from the potassium chloride vial by holding the vial in your hand and forcing the cap upward with your thumb or forefinger. Remove the cap from the vial's rubber top and place the plastic cap into the discard pile. Place the vial into the DCA so that it receives uninterrupted airflow from the HEPA filter.

**20.** Tear open a sterile, 70% IPA swab while holding it within the DCA. Swab the vial top by holding the vial between the thumb and forefinger of your dominant hand, and then rubbing the swab once or twice across the vial's rubber top. Place the used swab and the empty swab package into the discard pile.

**21.** Remove the 20-mL syringe from its outer wrap. If necessary, remove the cap from the hub of the syringe. Place the syringe outer wrap and cap into the discard pile in the outer six-inch zone of the hood.

**22.** Tear open a new, sterile, 70% IPA swab while holding it within the DCA. Place the swab onto the hood's work surface so that it receives uninterrupted airflow from the HEPA filter. Place the empty swab package into the discard pile.

**23.** Without touching or shadowing the syringe tip, grasp the barrel of the syringe in your dominant hand, keeping the syringe's position within the DCA. Be sure that the syringe tip receives uninterrupted airflow from the HEPA filter.

**24.** While carefully holding the barrel of the syringe in your dominant hand, carefully peel apart the needle package, using the fingers of both hands. Take care not to touch or shadow the needle hub at any time. Using a twisting motion, gently screw the needle hub onto the syringe tip.

**25.** Hold the capped syringe in your nondominant hand. Use your dominant hand to pull down on the flat knob of the plunger to draw approximately 15 mL of air into the syringe.

**26.** Using your dominant hand, grasp the syringe at the barrel. Hold it as you would a dart. Hold the syringe steadily and use your nondominant hand to remove the needle cap by pulling it carefully but firmly off of the needle. Place the needle cap on top of the alcohol swab on the hood's work surface.

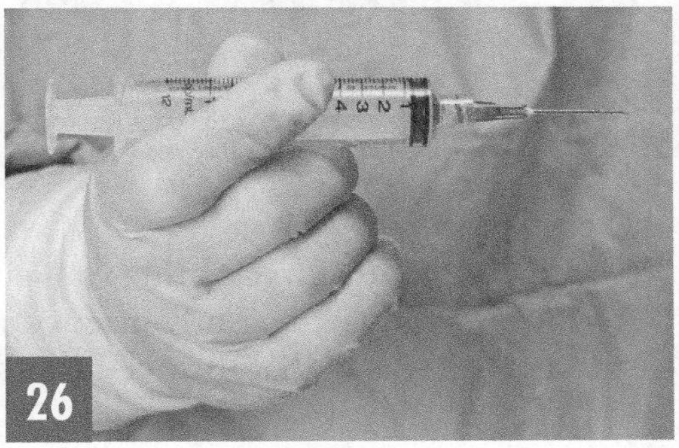


**USP Chapter <797>**

If you inadvertently touch or shadow the needle or syringe tip, immediately place the contaminated items into the sharps container, gather new supply items, and repeat the compounding procedure using new sterile supplies.

**POINTER**

Take care to hold the vial and syringe so that the airflow to the critical area—the area from the tip of the syringe to the neck of the vial, including the entire needle and the vial's rubber top—remains unobstructed.

**27.** Use your fingers to rotate the barrel of the syringe so that the bevel of the needle is pointed up toward the ceiling.

**28.** Using your nondominant hand, brace the potassium chloride vial against the hood's work surface. Lay the tip of the needle, bevel up, onto the center of the vial's rubber top.

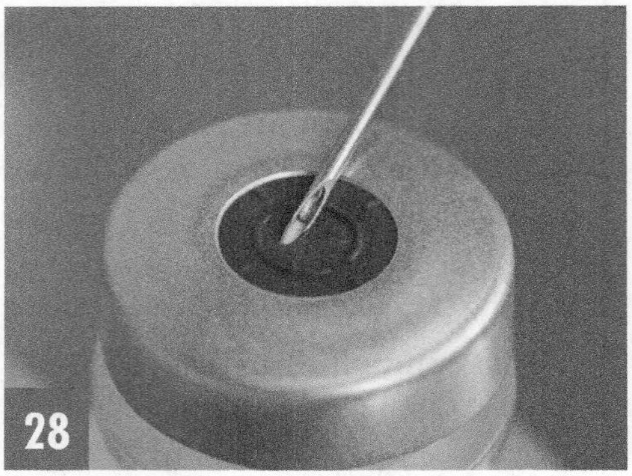
28

**29.** Insert the needle into the vial using a slight upward rotation of the wrist (rotating in a counterclockwise direction if you are right-handed, and in the opposite direction if you are left-handed). Keep the tip of the needle in contact with the vial's rubber top at all times. There should be a slight, almost imperceptible, bend to the needle as it enters the vial.

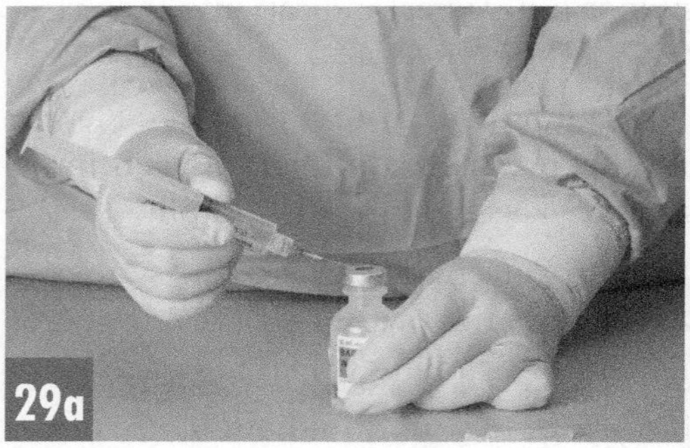
29a

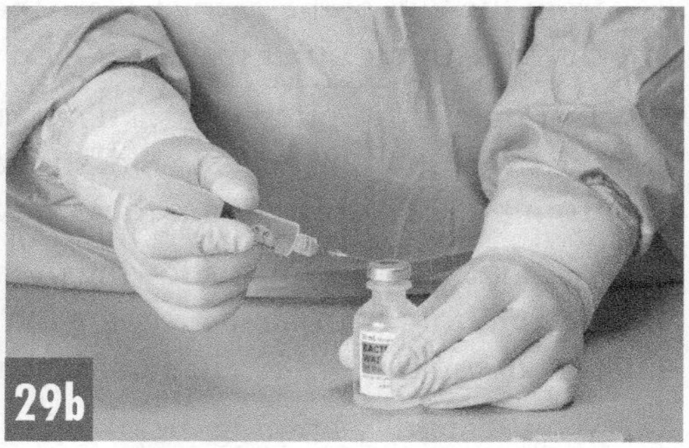
29b

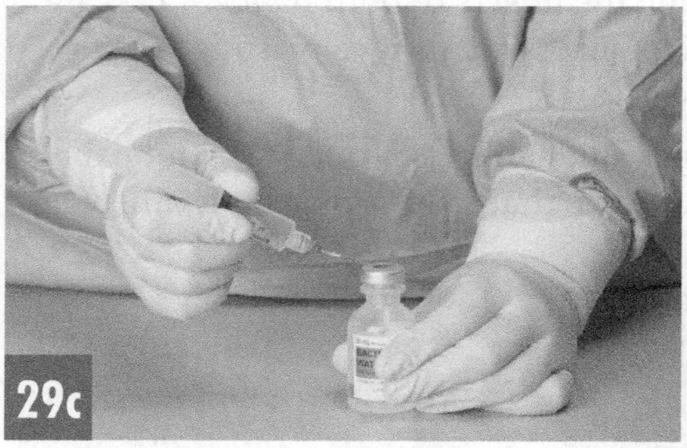
29c

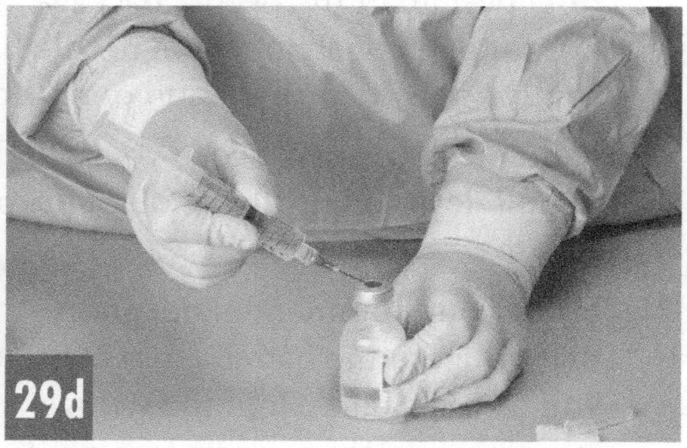
29d

**30.** Hold the potassium chloride vial with your nondominant hand and the syringe, with needle firmly inserted into the vial, with your dominant hand. Invert the vial so that the needle-and-syringe unit is now below the vial.

31. Use the thumb of your dominant hand to gradually push up on the flat knob of the plunger to inject a small amount of air (approximately 5 mL) into the potassium chloride vial, creating a slight positive pressure within the vial. Release the plunger and allow fluid to flow into the syringe. Repeat this milking process until you have a minimum of 16 mL of potassium chloride solution in the syringe.

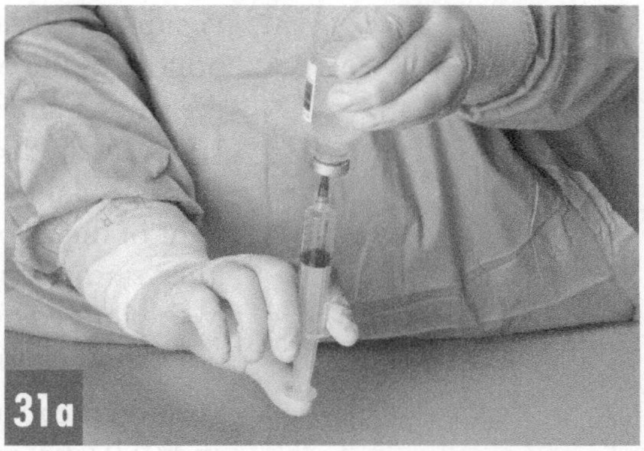

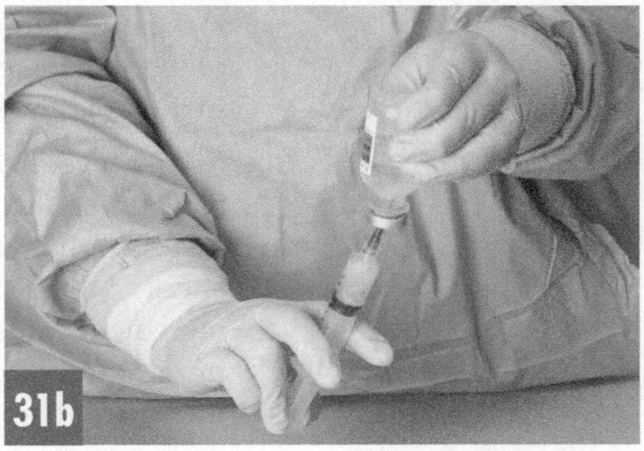

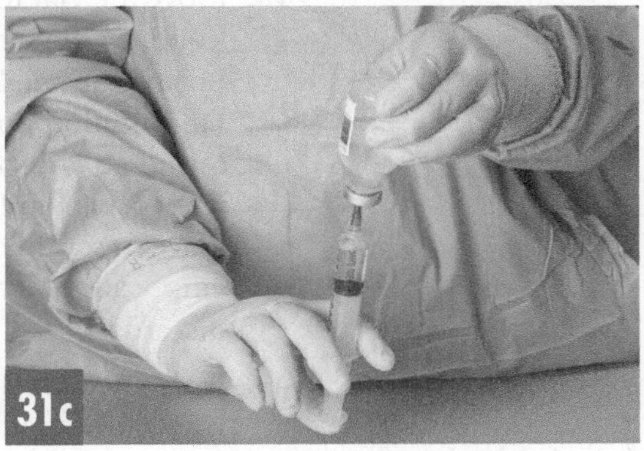

32. While ensuring that the needle remains entirely within the vial, hold the vial between the thumb and forefinger of your nondominant hand, allowing the barrel of the syringe to rest against the palm of that hand. Be sure to position your nondominant hand in a manner that continues to allow airflow to the critical site. Then, using your dominant hand, tap the barrel of the syringe with your fingers to force air bubbles within the fluid up toward the tip of the syringe. You must take care to perform this action in such a way that you do not bring your dominant hand between the critical site and the HEPA filter at any time.
33. Push up on the flat knob of the plunger with the thumb of your dominant hand to expel the air bubbles that have gathered near the tip of the syringe, along with any extra fluid, including the extra 1 mL of fluid that was drawn up to facilitate bubble removal.
34. Verify that the syringe now contains the desired amount of medication (for this dose, the desired volume is 15 mL).
35. While keeping the needle firmly inserted in the vial, return the vial and syringe to the original starting position, with the upright vial braced against the hood's work surface and the dominant hand grasping the barrel of the inverted syringe. Slowly remove the needle-and-syringe unit from the medication vial. Remember to avoid touching the plunger or flat knob of the syringe at any time while removing the needle-and-syringe unit from the vial.
36. Carefully recap the needle and place the capped needle-and-syringe unit onto the hood's work surface, within the DCA.

37. Position the IV bag so that the bottom of the bag faces toward the worker and away from the HEPA filter. Place the potassium chloride vial to the immediate right of the IV bag. Place the filled syringe with capped needle to the immediate right of the potassium chloride vial.

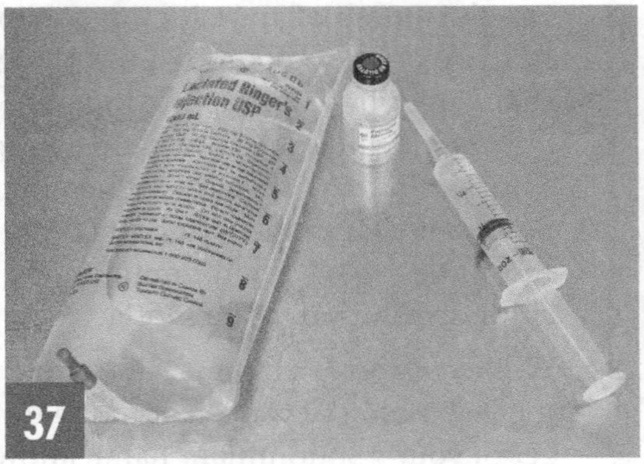

37

38. Position the medication order and CSP label in the outer six-inch zone, immediately in front of the CSP ingredients. *Note:* The medication order and CSP label must remain in their plastic bags until compounding procedures are complete.

**USP Chapter <797>**

Some IV technicians prefer to hang the IV bag from the hood's hang bar throughout the procedure. While this is too time-consuming for most facilities, it is acceptable provided that airflow from the HEPA filter to the IV bag's injection port is not interrupted at any time.

39. Ask for a verification check by your instructor. Once your instructor has completed the check of the CSP ingredients, the ingredients must be repositioned prior to injecting the medication into the IV bag.

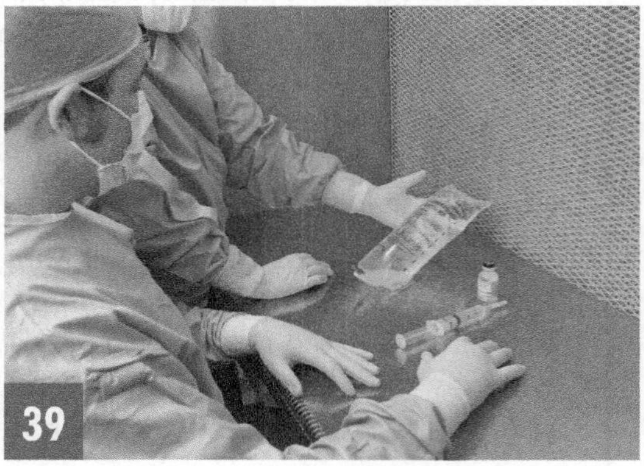
39

40. Move the vial to the side of the hood, away from the IV bag. Reposition the IV bag so that the tail injection port receives uninterrupted airflow from the HEPA filter. Open an IV swab within the DCA and swab the injection port of the bag. Place the swab on the work surface directly under the injection port. Place the empty swab package into the discard pile.

**POINTER**

When inserting a needle into the injection port of an IV bag, it is not necessary to consider the direction of the bevel. The needle should be inserted straight into the bag without angle and without bending the needle.

41. Hold the barrel of the syringe in your dominant hand. Remove the cap of the needle and place the needle cap onto the alcohol swab you placed on the hood's work surface in step 22.

42. Hold the injection port steady with your nondominant hand, taking care to avoid shadowing or touching the injection port.

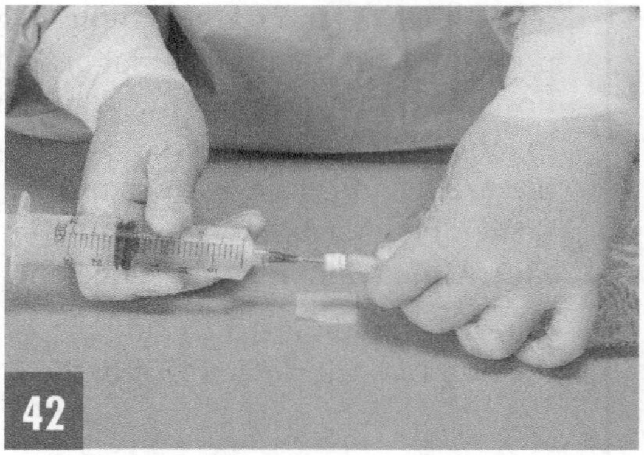
42

43. Inject the medication into the bag by pressing on the flat knob of the plunger with the thumb or forefinger of the dominant hand.

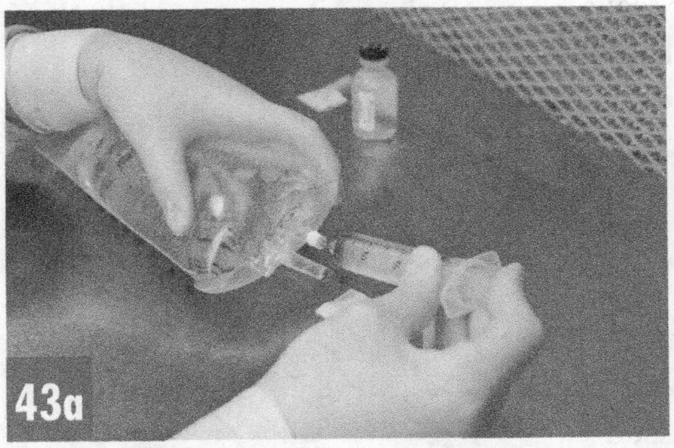


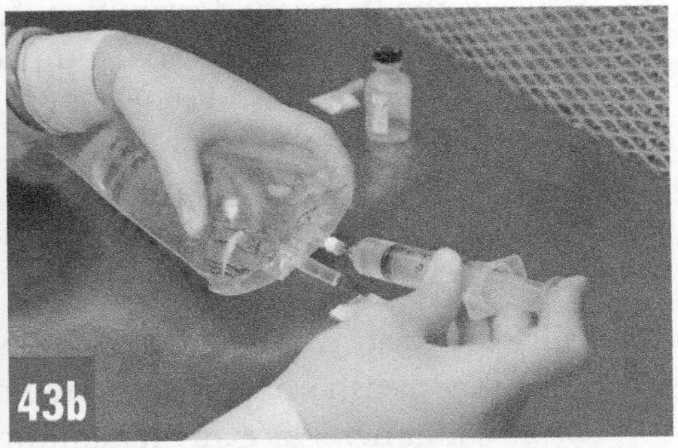


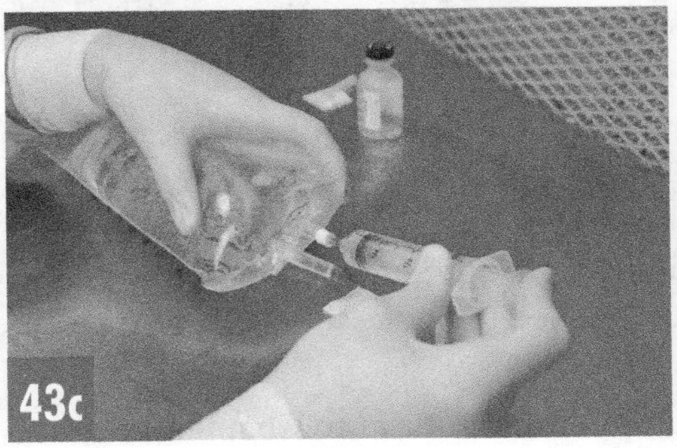


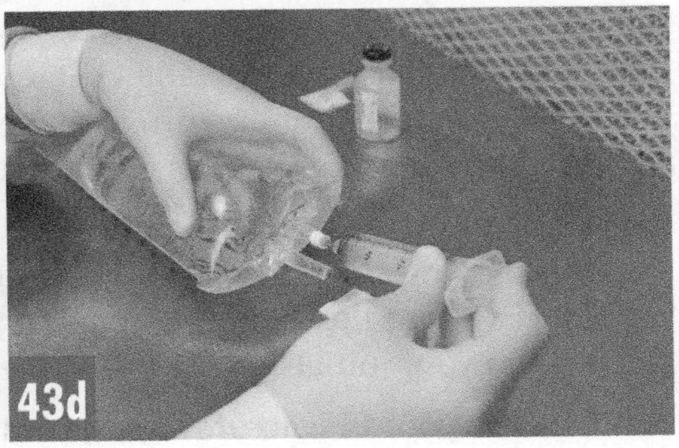


44. Holding only the barrel of the syringe, carefully remove the needle-and-syringe unit from the IV bag.

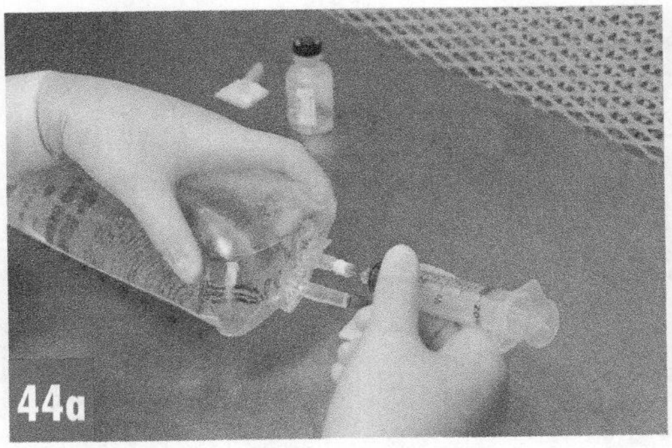


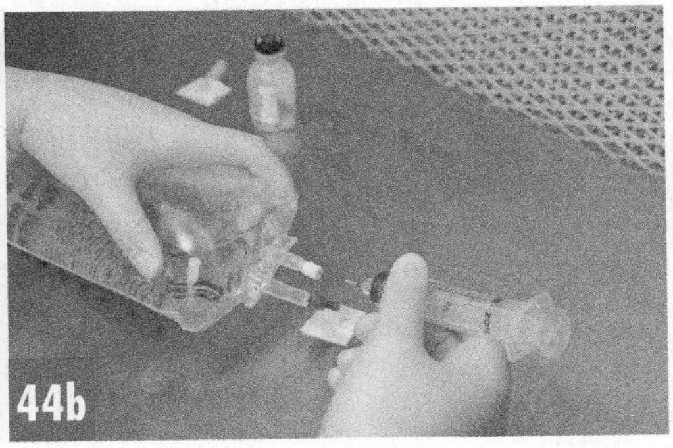


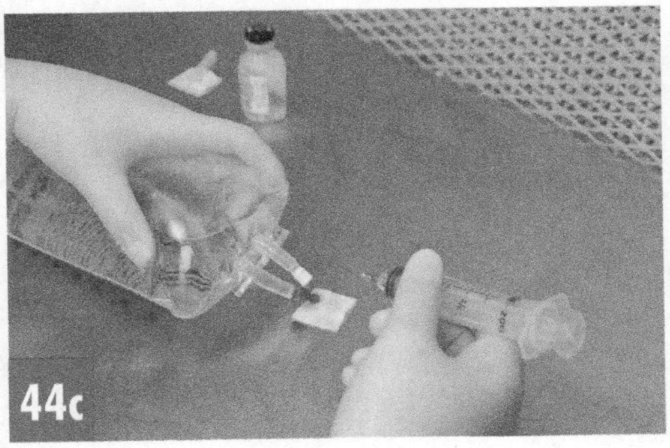

**POINTER**

Although some IV technicians prefer to recap the needle upon completion of the compounding procedure, it is considered best practice to place the needle-and-syringe unit into the sharps container *without* recapping the needle. That way, technicians can avoid inadvertent needle sticks.

**45.** Place the needle-and-syringe unit into the sharps container.

**46.** Squeeze the IV bag and examine it for leaks, precipitates, or evidence of incompatibility. Cover the injection port with an IVA seal. Remove the CSP label from the plastic bag and affix the label to the IV bag.

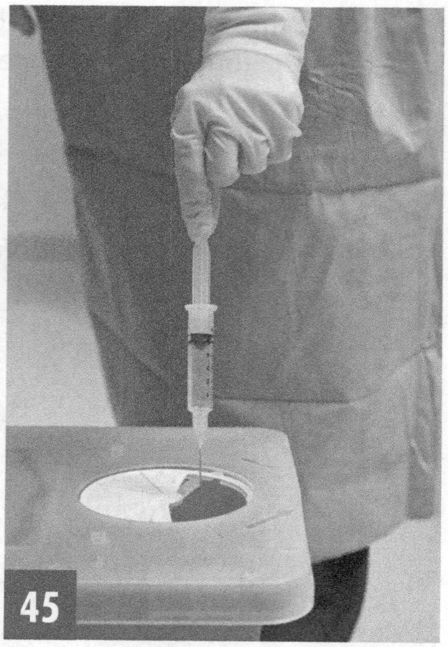

45

### *Cleaning Up After the Procedure*

**47.** Place the waste from the discard pile and any other nonsharps waste into the regular waste container. Place any remaining used swabs and the needle cap into the waste container. Place the vial and CSP into the transport vehicle and return the items to the anteroom to complete the compounding procedure.

**48.** Once in the anteroom, record your initials in the proper location on the CSP label. Record the date and time that you opened the potassium chloride vial as well as your initials on the vial's label.

**49.** Remove your PPE according to standard procedures. Refer to Chapter 6 for step-by-step PPE removal procedures. Return any unused supply items to their proper locations in the anteroom.

**50.** Ask for a final check from your instructor.

**POINTER**

Facilities vary with regard to where the CSP label should be positioned on the IV or IV piggyback bag. Some facilities prefer the label affixed to the back of the bag, so that none of the manufacturer's information is obscured. Others prefer the label on the front, so that the CSP and IV base solution information is visible on the same side. Refer to your facility's P&P manual to determine the proper procedure for affixing CSP labels.

# Process Validation by Instructor

*Your instructor will use the process validation checklist provided in Appendix D to evaluate your technique for this lab. In order to receive ACPE certification, and prior to making CSPs for patient use, you must correctly perform each component of the lab procedure. Review the Chapter 8 lab and thoroughly practice each of the steps prior to your evaluation.*

# Part 3: Assessment

## Chapter Summary

- Early practitioners theorized that illness and disease stemmed from an imbalance in one or more of the body's humors.
- The discovery of the circulatory system led physicians and scientists to the possibility of its use as a potential route for medicinal agents.
- Dr. Thomas Latta's work with cholera patients was the impetus for further investigation into the healing potential of IV fluids.
- Dr. Albert Landerer was the first person to successfully treat patients with LVP infusions.
- Mass production of IV base solutions led to more quality-control measures for ingredients and containers.
- IV infusion therapy became more refined with the creation of innovative supplies and equipment that could treat more patients with less chance of human error.
- LVP solutions, commonly called IV fluids, are required for most hospital inpatients.
- Most LVPs are maintenance infusions that provide hydration and/or electrolytes.
- Drip solutions are used to continuously deliver an IV medication to treat a specific medical condition.
- In addition to the risk of patient infection, IV therapy comes with other potential complications including extravasation, tissuing, phlebitis, cellulitis, and embolism.
- Patients requiring long-term IV therapy may receive it through various IV access points such as a peripheral, subclavian, or femoral vein, or through the superior vena cava. These veins are accessed through a PICC line, central line, Hickman line, Broviac line, or various implantable ports.
- The most common access point is through a peripheral vein.
- Anteroom procedures include CSP label verification, dosage calculations, gathering and exterior cleaning of supply items, garbing, aseptic hand washing, and donning a sterile gown.
- Initial clean room procedures include applying sterile, foamed 70% IPA to your hands, donning sterile gloves, and cleaning the hood.
- Small supply items may be staged within the outer six-inch zone of the hood.
- The dust cover of the IV bag should be removed, and the bag should then be placed within the DCA.
- The critical sites of supply items used in LVP preparation include the needle, the syringe tip and plunger, the vial top, IPA swabs, and the injection port of the IV bag.
- The syringe tip and plunger, as well as the entire needle (except the needle cap), should never be touched or shadowed and must always be maintained within the DCA. These critical sites should also never be swabbed with alcohol.
- The vial's rubber top and IV injection port should be maintained in the DCA, must be swabbed with a sterile 70% IPA swab, and must never be touched or shadowed after the site has been swabbed.
- The syringe should be held by the barrel as you would a dart, with the needle bevel pointing up.
- Proper insertion of the needle into the vial will help to avoid coring, an undesired event that causes a small bit of the rubber stopper to tear off and contaminate the solution inside the vial.
- Coring may result in potential harm to the patient recipient of the CSP.
- The IV technician should inject an amount of air into the vial that is equal to, or slightly less than, the amount of fluid to be withdrawn. This technique, called the milking technique, creates positive pressure within the vial and therefore assists with fluid withdrawal.

- After preparing the CSP ingredients, the IV technician should arrange the supply items on the hood's work surface for a verification check by a pharmacist or instructor.
- Upon completion of the verification check, the CSP ingredients and other supply items must be rearranged within the DCA so that the injection port of the IV bag and the needle-and-syringe unit receive uninterrupted airflow from the HEPA filter.
- The injection port of an IV bag must be cleaned with an IPA swab prior to needle insertion.
- When injecting into a tail injection port, the IV technician must exercise care to avoid rupturing the sidewall of the injection port with an improperly inserted needle.
- Used needles and syringes should be disposed of in a sharps container.
- Other waste items should be discarded in a regular waste receptacle.
- At the completion of the compounding procedure, the IV technician should return any extra supply items and the transport vehicle to the anteroom; document the date, time, and his or her initials on the label of the vial; record his or her initials and the date on the label of the CSP; and remove PPE according to standard procedures.

## Key Terms

**access point** the area where an IV needle, catheter, or lock is placed for access to a patient's vein

**acidity** one of the chemical properties of a parenteral solution; any solution with a pH less than 7.0 is considered to be acidic

**additive** a medication or electrolyte that is injected into a large-volume or small-volume parenteral solution for administration to a patient; a drug that is injected into an IV solution

**alkalinity** one of the chemical properties of a parenteral solution; any solution with a pH greater than 7.0 is considered to be alkaline

**allergic reaction** a disorder of hypersensitivity to a normally harmless substance, resulting in various symptoms of the nose, eyes, ears, skin, airways, and digestive system

**anaphylaxis** a potentially life-threatening allergic reaction

**aseptic cleaning wipes** presaturated cleaning wipes used to wipe down the exterior surfaces of supply items prior to bringing them into the anteroom

**aspiration** a fine mist or aerosolized powder that may be expelled inadvertently into the hood during sterile compounding procedures; an undesired consequence of incorrect aseptic technique

**base solution** a sterile solution to which additives may be injected prior to IV administration

**Broviac line** IV access gained through the use of a tunneled central venous catheter; may also be called a Broviac catheter

**buffer solution** a solution, such as sodium bicarbonate, that is sometimes injected into a CSP to neutralize the CSP's acidity and, therefore, prevent discomfort in a patient recipient

**button or nipple injection port** a type of injection port located on the face of certain IV base solution bags

**cannula** a small, sterile tube or needle that may be used to gain or maintain access to a patient's vein or artery for delivery of IV fluids or medications; may contain a sharp trocar for creating an entrance point into the vein; see also *catheter*

**capillaries** small blood vessels that connect arteries and veins

**catheter** a small, sterile tube or needle that may be used to gain or maintain access to a patient's vein or artery for delivery of IV fluids or medications; see also *cannula*

**cellulitis** inflammation or infection of the tissues beneath the skin

**central line** IV access through a central venous catheter placed into a large vein in the neck

**chemical property** the chemical nature of a parenteral solution—specifically, the solution's pH value, tonicity, osmolarity, osmolality, and compatibility; may also be called a characteristic

**circulatory system** the system by which blood is moved throughout the body; may also be called the cardiovascular system

**clinical pharmacology** the study of the effects of drugs on the human body

**closed-system container** a type of sterile container; a sealed, noncollapsible container, such as a vial; the type of container in which air pressure must be equalized prior to the withdrawal of fluid

**clyster** an ancient, syringe-like device used to remove bodily fluids such as pus or blood

**compatibility** the ability to combine two or more base components or additives within a solution without creating a resultant change in the physical or chemical properties of any of the solution components or additives

**continuous infusion** an IV infusion that is administered continuously in order to rehydrate or manage the electrolyte needs of a patient; see also *maintenance infusion*, *replacement infusion*, and *hydration infusion*

**coring** a small piece of rubber that is torn from the vial top and unintentionally ends up in the sterile solution; an inadvertent event caused by incorrect needle insertion into a vial

**critical site** part of a supply item that includes any fluid pathway surface or fluid pathway opening at risk for contamination by touch or airflow interruption

**dehydration** a condition of diminished fluid volume; excessive loss of body fluids

**desired volume** the volume of a medication or an additive that must be drawn up to provide a specific dosage

**diluent** a fluid, typically sterile water or normal saline, used to dissolve or reconstitute a drug in powdered form or to dilute a liquid medication to a lesser concentration

**direct compounding area (DCA)** within a hood, the area that is closest to the hood's HEPA filter, receives uninterrupted airflow, and is the location where sterile compounding procedures are performed; the area that extends from the hood's HEPA filter out to where the innermost part of the six-inch zone begins; may also be called first air

**discard pile** a small pile, kept in the outer six-inch zone of the hood, where used supply items or supply wrappers may be gathered until being placed into the waste receptacle at the completion of sterile compounding procedures

**diuresis** excessive excretion of urine

**drip** an IV infusion that is used to deliver a continuous dose of a medication such as heparin or nitroglycerin

**dust cover** the outer packaging of a sterile supply item

**embolism** any solid, liquid, or gaseous mass floating within a vein that may become lodged in an artery causing blockage of blood flow

**equilibrium** a condition of balance or homeostasis

**extracellular space** the space outside each living cell

**extravasation** a condition of fluid leaking from the vein into surrounding tissue; a potential undesired result of some IV therapies

**flexible, plastic IV bag** a sterile, flexible container used for IV base solutions; a type of container that expands and contracts; a PVC IV bag

**flip-top cap** the removable, hard-plastic cap that covers the vial's rubber top

**fluid status** the condition or level of hydration in the body

**Hickman line** IV access through a catheter tunneled between two large veins, one in the neck and one in the chest wall; often used for chemotherapy administration; may also be called a Hickman catheter

**homeostasis** a condition of balance or stability; the body's ability for physiological regulation

**humors** a medieval medical theory, often credited to Hippocrates, that believed optimal health may be attained only when the four elemental body fluids (blood, phlegm, black bile, and yellow bile) were in perfect balance

**hydration infusion** a type of LVP infusion used to continuously administer IV fluid

**hyperosmotic** a solution that has a higher osmotic pressure than human blood serum

**hypertonic** a solution that has a higher number of dissolved particles than human blood serum

**hyponatremia** a condition of abnormally low blood sodium

**hypoosmotic** a solution that has a lower osmotic pressure than human blood serum

**hypotonic** a solution that has a lower number of dissolved particles than human blood serum

**hypovolemia** a condition of low blood volume due to blood loss or dehydration

**implantable port** a type of IV line that is placed completely inside the body, usually in the neck or chest; also known as a PORT-A-CATH, or GROSHONG catheter

**incompatibility** a sign that two or more solutions or ingredients within a solution are not suitable for use in combination, evidenced by the presence of precipitates, crystallized particles, flakes, or a darkening or coloring of a compounded solution

**interstitial space** the fluid-filled space that surrounds each living cell

**intracellular space** the space within each living cell

**intravascular space** the space within a blood vessel

**intravenous (IV) infusion** an LVP that is administered into a vein

**isoosmotic** a solution that has an osmotic pressure equal to human blood serum

**isotonic** a solution that has the same number of dissolved particles as human blood serum

**lactated Ringer's (LR) solution** a type of LVP solution; often used as a base solution for CSPs

**large-volume parenteral (LVP) preparation** an IV fluid of more than 250 mL that may contain medications, nutrients, or electrolytes; may also be referred to as, simply, an LVP

**leech** a type of bloodsucking worm used in ancient medicine to purge the body of excess blood; sterilized leeches are used in modern medicine to remove excess swelling around severed limbs or appendages that have been reattached

**maintenance infusion** a type of continuous IV infusion in which a LVP base solution provides the primary, ongoing source of hydration for a patient; often used to deliver continuous infusion of fluids and electrolytes such as potassium, sodium, and dextrose

**medical-grade quality standards** a product that meets ISO or USP established criteria for medical use; having been prepared within an ISO Class 5 environment

**milking technique** a process, used to dilute a powdered drug or withdraw a liquid drug, in which positive air pressure is used to equalize pressure within a vial; technique allows for greater ease in withdrawal of fluid from the vial

**milliosmoles** molecular weight equal to 1/1000th of an osmole

**negative pressure** the pressure within a container, such as a vial or an empty evacuated container, that is less than the air pressure outside of the container

**nephrotoxicity** a condition of kidney damage resulting from certain drugs or drug doses

**neutral** a solution that has a pH value of 7.0

**nosocomial infection** an infection acquired while in a hospital; often drug-resistant and difficult to treat

**osmolality** a count of the number of particles in a solution

**osmolarity** the concentration of osmotically active particles in a solution

**osmotic pressure** the pressure that must be applied to a solution to prevent the flow of water across a cell

**parenteral solution** a solution that is administered parenterally; a sterile solution, such as an LVP solution, that is administered into a vein

**peripheral IV line** an IV tubing, line, or lock that is placed into a patient's peripheral vein; an IV access point within the patient's arm or leg

**peripheral vein** a vein located in the arms, hands, legs, or feet; a vein outside of the chest, abdomen or head

**phlebitis** inflammation of a vein

**phthisis** a Greek term meaning "to waste away"; used to refer to tuberculosis or other diseases characterized by severe weight loss and muscle wasting

**pH value** a measurement of the acidity or alkalinity of a solution

**PICC line** peripherally inserted central catheter; inserted into a peripheral vein and then advanced internally into increasingly larger veins; allows for long-term IV therapy

**plasma sodium concentration ($P_{Na}$)** the concentration of sodium as measured in blood plasma

**positive pressure** a procedure in which air or fluid is injected into a vial, thereby creating positive air pressure within the vial, which assists with the withdrawal of fluid from the vial when using the milking technique

**precipitate** any particulate matter formed as a result of incompatibility; an undesired solid or semi-solid substance within an IV solution

**pulmonary circulation** the process by which blood and oxygen are circulated through the body

**replacement infusion** a continuous, infusion used to replace fluids and electrolytes; a method of relieving dehydration by administering IV fluids

**saline solution** water mixed with salt; a crude type of IV solution

**scoop method** a safe method of recapping the needle attached to a filled syringe; the filled needle-and-syringe unit are used to scoop the cap onto the needle

**shadowing** contamination caused by an interruption of airflow from the hood's HEPA filter to the critical site of any supply item

**six-inch zone** the outermost edge of the hood, closest to the worker and farthest from airflow origin at the HEPA filter; a poor environment for preparing sterile products because it receives lower velocity airflow than do areas closer to the HEPA filter

**slow-drip IV administration method** an early method of safely administering IV fluids

**solute** a dissolved substance

**Stevens-Johnson syndrome** a rare condition in which the skin blisters and may slough off; caused by an immune system disorder or an adverse reaction to medication

**subclavian vein** one of a pair of veins, located in the chest, through which blood flows from the arms to the heart; a common access point for administration of certain hypertonic, acidic, or hyperosmolar solutions

**superior vena cava** the large vein that returns blood from the head and upper body to the heart

**tail injection port** a type of injection port located at the very bottom of certain types of LVP and IV piggyback (IVPB) base solution bags

**tear line** a small perforation on the dust cover of some supply items that indicates the location or direction in which the cover should be torn for removal from the supply item

**tissuing** leakage of IV fluid into surrounding tissue; may cause swelling or other undesired effects

**"titrated to effect"** a type of continuously administered LVP in which the IV flow rate is adjusted to run faster or slower, depending on the patient's response to the medication (e.g., decreasing a nitroglycerin drip rate as a patient's chest pain subsides)

**tonicity** the number of dissolved particles in a solution

**total parenteral nutrition** an advanced sterile compound that intravenously provides the patient with a 24-hour supply of all the fluids, proteins, amino acids, calories, vitamins, minerals, and nutrients needed for life; an IV preparation for the patient who has long-term nutritional needs but cannot receive oral feedings

**touch contamination** contamination caused when the critical site of a supply item is touched by the preparer's finger, hand, the hood's work surface, or any nonsterile item; the most common and dangerous form of contamination of CSPs

**transport vehicle** a container, such as a cart, basket, or bucket, used to bring supply items from the anteroom into the clean room

**tunneled catheter** a type of surgically implanted catheter or port

**verification check** the process performed by the pharmacist or instructor just prior to injection of the parenteral medication into a reservoir such as an IV bag or IVPB; second check that includes verifying the CSP label, medication order, diluent, drug dosage volume, and base solution

**vial** a container for sterile liquid or powdered medication

**winged infusion needle** a type of catheter used to administer IV solutions; also called a butterfly needle or butterfly catheter

## Check the Basics

*On a separate sheet of paper, write your answers as modeled in these examples:* 1d; 2c; 3b; *etc.*

1. Within the sterile compounding environment, what is the primary use for aseptic, presaturated cleaning wipes?
   a. wiping the critical site of the vial
   b. wiping down the hood prior to compounding procedures
   c. wiping the critical site of the IV bag
   d. wiping down supply items prior to entering the clean room

2. Upon entering the clean room, where should the IV technician place the transport vehicle?
   a. within the DCA of the hood
   b. within the outer six-inch zone of the hood
   c. in front of the prefilter
   d. none of the above

3. Where should small supply items such as needles and swabs be kept during sterile compounding procedures?
   a. within the DCA of the hood
   b. within the outer six-inch zone of the hood
   c. on a clean surface or countertop within the clean room, but outside of the hood
   d. none of the above

4. Where should a large item, such as an IV bag that has been removed from its dust cover, be kept during sterile compounding procedures?
   a. within the DCA of the hood
   b. within the outer six-inch zone of the hood
   c. on a clean surface or countertop within the clean room, but outside of the hood
   d. none of the above

5. Which of the following groups of supply components lists *all* of the critical sites that must not be touched or shadowed during LVP preparation?
   a. the needle cap, alcohol swab packet, vial cap, and syringe package
   b. the needle package, syringe, vial, and alcohol swab
   c. the needle, syringe tip, vial top, and injection port
   d. the needle, syringe, alcohol swab, and IV bag

6. Which of the following describes the proper method of holding a syringe when inserting the needle-and-syringe unit into a vial?
   a. Using your dominant hand, hold the syringe barrel like a dart, with the needle bevel pointing up.
   b. Using your nondominant hand, hold the syringe barrel like a dart, with the needle bevel pointing up.
   c. Using your dominant hand, hold the syringe barrel like a dart, with the needle bevel pointing down.
   d. Using your nondominant hand, hold the syringe barrel like a dart, with the needle bevel pointing down.

7. Based on the desired volume that you determined by dosage calculation, what is the most appropriate syringe size for drawing up the potassium chloride dose?
   a. 10 mL
   b. 20 mL
   c. 30 mL
   d. 60 mL

8. Which of the following critical sites should *never* be cleaned with an alcohol swab?
   a. the injection port and vial top
   b. the vial top and needle cap
   c. the needle and syringe tip
   d. the flat knob and flip-top cap

9. Which critical site(s) must be cleaned with an alcohol swab prior to injection during LVP preparation?
   a. the vial top
   b. the IV bag injection port
   c. neither *a* or *b*
   d. both *a* and *b*

10. What is the proper method of needle insertion into the port of an IV bag?
    a. The needle should be bevel up and slightly bent to prevent coring.
    b. The needle should be bevel down and slightly bent to prevent coring.
    c. The needle should be inserted straight into the port without bending and without regard for the position of the bevel.
    d. none of the above

## Make Connections

*On a separate sheet of paper, write your answers to the following three questions, using complete sentences and making sure your answers are thorough and thoughtful. Note that the third question requires Internet access.*

1. Considering what you have learned about aseptic technique and the importance of maintaining the sterility of CSPs, what action would you take if you noticed that there were particles floating within the final CSP container?

2. What is the rationale for creating positive pressure within a vial prior to withdrawing fluid from the vial?

3. Use any Internet search engine to access the National Library of Medicine website. Once there, perform a search for the term *peripheral IV*. Read at least one of the available articles on this subject. What does the information that you read indicate about peripheral IV solutions?

## Meet the Challenge

***Scenario*** This "pressurized" activity will give you the opportunity to experiment with positive and negative air pressure within a vial.

***Challenge*** Your instructor has a handout outlining the supplies and steps for an activity centered around positive and negative pressure changes. This procedure takes your understanding of how those pressures operate in a vial to a deeper level. To meet this challenge, ask your instructor for the handout and give it a try, either as an individual, in small groups, or as a class.

### ADDITIONAL RESOURCES

*Go to the Paradigm Internet Resources Center at* www.paradigmcollege.net/sterilecomp *to access live links related to these Chapter 8 topics:*

- Medical resources for research on diseases, conditions, medications, and treatments
- Citations for medical and biomedical literature

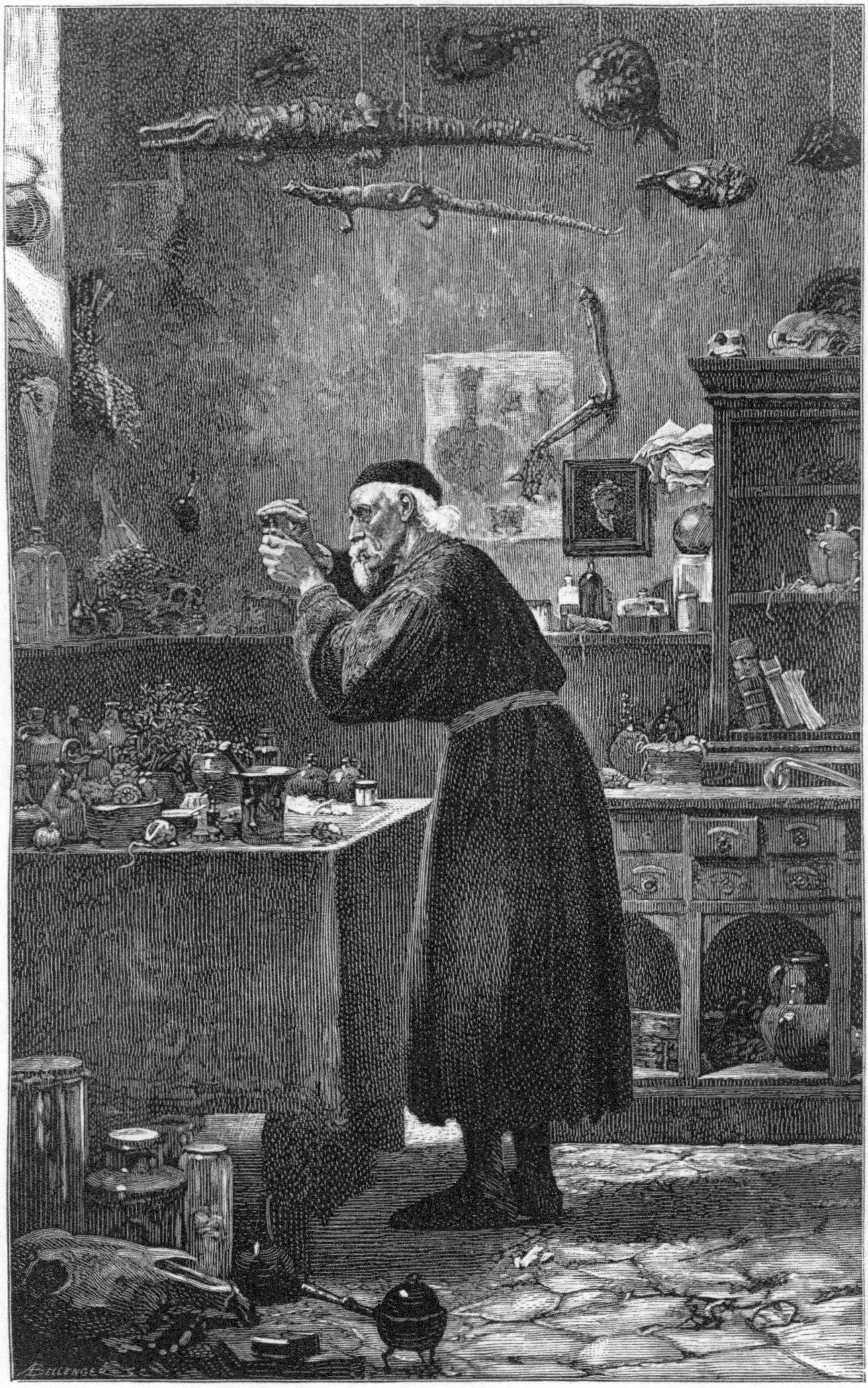

THE APOTHECARY.

Chapter 9

# Small-Volume Parenteral Preparations

## Learning Objectives

- Recognize the origins of small-volume parenteral preparations—in particular, antibiotics.
- Understand the USP Chapter <797> procedures that must be performed prior to sterile compounding procedures.
- Identify the critical sites of various small-volume parenteral preparation supply items, and describe compounding situations in which certain supply items should be used.
- Discover the USP Chapter <797> procedures that must be performed during small-volume parenteral preparation.
- Demonstrate effective technique in the preparation of two small-volume compounded sterile preparations.

Small-volume parenteral (SVP) preparations—antibiotics, in particular—came to the forefront of the pharmaceutical industry in the twentieth century. These powerful antimicrobial drugs have made a lasting impact on society by eliminating many infectious diseases that had long plagued humankind. Yet long before the discovery of pathogenic microorganisms such as fungi and bacteria, and the role they play in the transmission of disease, early civilizations recognized the antimicrobial properties of certain plants, metallic elements, and other substances in the treatment of illness and disease.

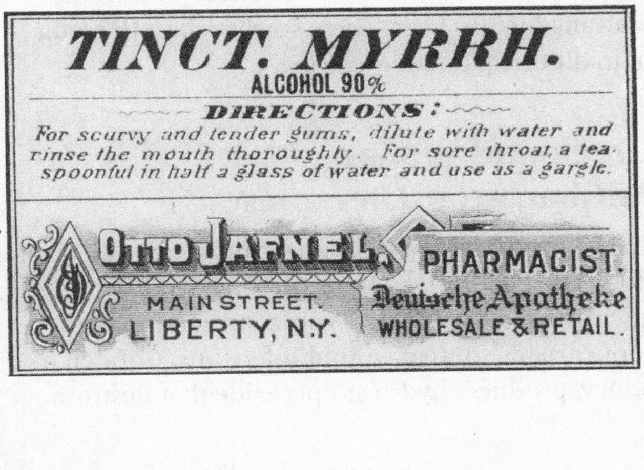


## Early Use of Antibacterial Substances in Egypt and China

Ancient Egyptian medical practitioners recognized the antibacterial and healing properties of resins such as frankincense and myrrh, and metals like copper and mercury. They also possessed an understanding of the connection between mold and antibacterial activity, an insight proven true by Alexander Fleming hundreds of years later. Their discovery of this relationship is evident in a prescription recorded in the Ebers

Papyrus, an ancient document of Egyptian pharmacology from 1535 BCE. This prescription states that if a "wound rots . . . then bind on it spoiled barley bread." Egyptians also utilized plants such as onions, garlic, and radishes in their healing practices. In fact, scientists would eventually discover that garlic contains allicin and radishes contain raphanin, two antibacterial substances that have recently been extracted and studied for antibacterial research.

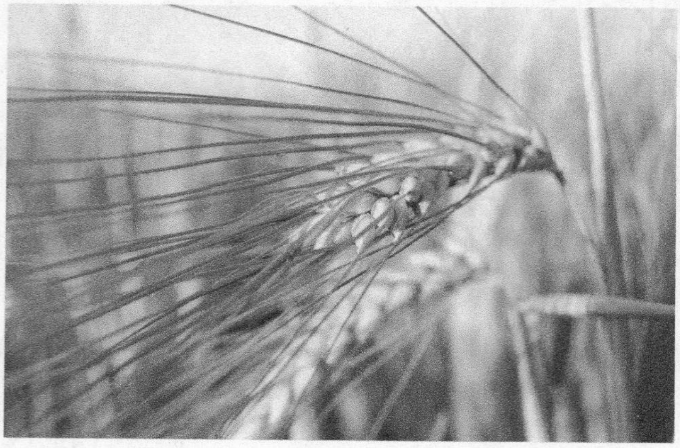

Another substance that early Egyptian healers frequently used to treat infections was honey, which was compounded with lard or copper and used as a poultice for wounds. These ancient physicians had no knowledge of the properties of honey but observed that the substance was an effective remedy for skin infections. No fewer than 147 prescriptions recorded in the Ebers Papyrus mention honey as a main ingredient in a remedy. Honey became a mainstay anti-infective treatment for thousands of years until the emergence of antibiotics at the beginning of the twentieth century—making it one of the oldest antibacterials known to humans. Indeed, scientists have proven that honey has both antibacterial and antifungal properties that effectively destroy microorganisms through the enzymatic production of hydrogen peroxide and the osmolar process of cellular dehydration.

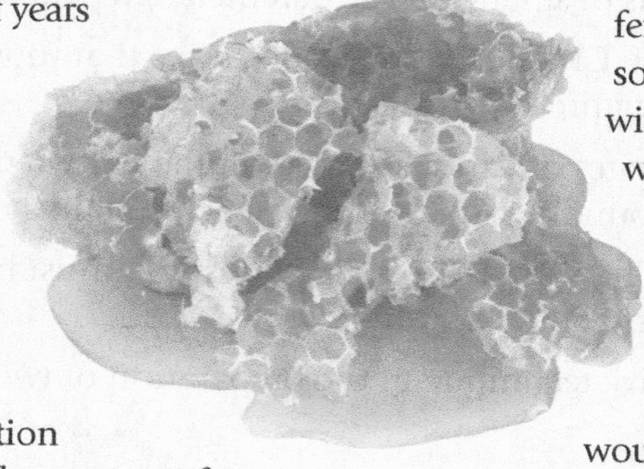

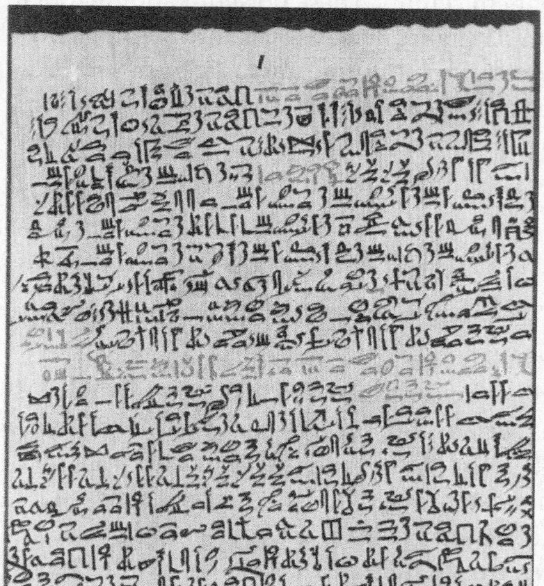

One of the most astonishing discoveries regarding the use of antibiotics in ancient cultures was the appearance of tetracycline residue (a common modern antibiotic) in the bones of Sudanese-Nubian mummies that date back to the fourth century. These early inhabitants most likely ingested fermented grain (in both liquid and solid forms) that was contaminated with *Streptomyces*. Although they were certainly unaware of the antibacterial properties of this substance, what these people did recognize was the association between fermented grain and improved health. Ironically, it would be more than a thousand years before scientists produced the synthetic drug tetracycline, a widely used antibiotic today.

Like their Egyptian counterparts, Chinese practitioners also understood the effects of mold on bacteria. Silk scrolls discovered by archaeologists in tombs at Mawangdui, China, reveal a prescription for the application of moldy soybean curds to heal wound infections and boils. This prescription dates back to the Han dynasty (206 BCE to 25 CE) and is one of 283 prescriptions included on 14 scrolls known as the Mawangdui Silk Texts. These scrolls reflect the roots of traditional Eastern medicine.

## Greek and Roman Antibacterial Therapies

The ancient Greek and Roman empires also understood the healthful benefits of honey and frequently used the substance in combination with copper oxide to treat wound infections. Copper, like honey, produces hydrogen peroxide that destroys

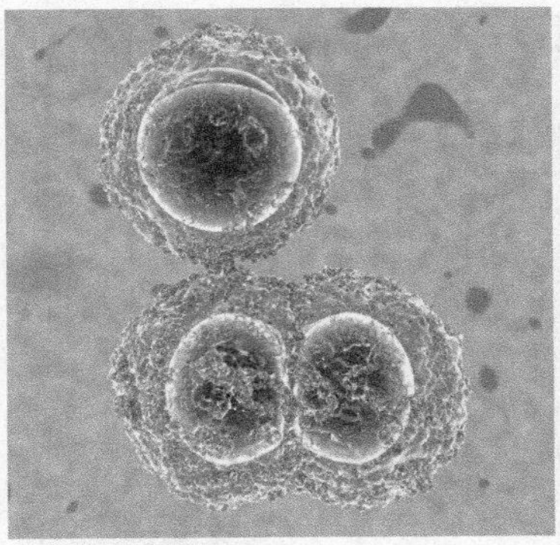

the cell walls of microorganisms—a discovery that wouldn't be confirmed for many centuries. Copper was widely used among European, African, and Asian civilizations as a standard therapy for skin, neurological, and infectious disorders. In recent times, copper has been proven to have both antibacterial and antifungal properties, and its alloy has been shown to be highly effective in killing methicillin-resistant *Staphylococcus aureus* (MRSA) on surfaces.

In addition to copper, the Greeks and Romans also used another metallic element, silver, for its antibacterial properties. These early citizens would store liquids in silver containers to keep them fresh and pure. The practice of using silver for dinnerware and tableware continued for centuries, long before the medical community proved that silver could destroy disease-producing pathogens. Prior to the introduction of antibiotics in the twentieth century, colloidal silver was also used in medicine, particularly in the treatment of burns and as an anti-infective ophthalmic medication for newborns' eyes. Recently, scientists have discovered that colloidal silver can destroy more than 650 disease-causing microorganisms, making this element a potential source for future antibiotics.

## Other Natural Antibiotics Used to Treat Infections

Throughout these early civilizations and well into the Renaissance period, various cultures continued to use plants, herbs, and tree resins to counteract infectious disease. Thyme, usnea (also known as old man's beard), goldenseal, chamomile, and garlic were frequently used as natural antibiotics. To battle the scourge of malaria, a common affliction in Europe in the 1600s, the bark of the cinchona tree was used to produce a powder for ingestion. Although the cinchona tree is native to South America, the seeds of the tree were carried to the European continent by settlers who observed their use in Native American medicines. The tree's bark contained quinine, a substance that effectively killed the malaria-causing protozoa. Quinine was used for centuries to treat malaria and is considered the predecessor of the synthetic antibiotic chloroquinine.

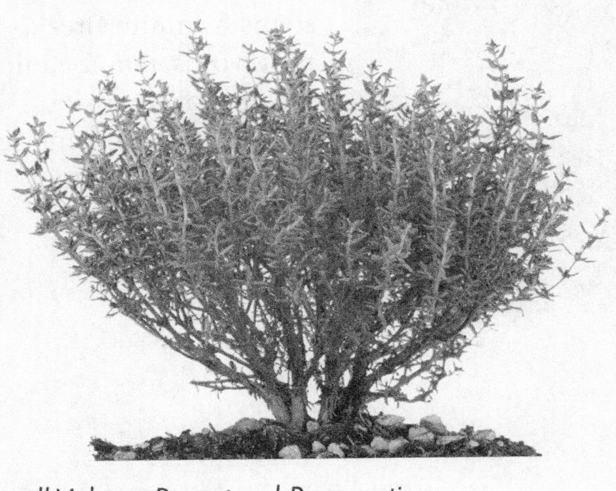

In the 1670s, Dutch scientist Anton van Leeuwenhoek identified bacteria through his hand-crafted microscope—a discovery that laid the foundation for the study of microbiology and germ transmission. Two hundred years later, Joseph Lister proposed his germ theory, which established microorganisms as the causative agents for disease. As Lister's theory was gradually accepted by healthcare practitioners, scientists, physicians, and chemists around the world began to experiment with the use of harmless bacteria to counteract the growth of harmful, disease-causing bacteria. Much of the work of these early pioneers centered on finding a treatment for bacterial infections that often killed people who, if not for contracting an opportunistic infection, would have easily recovered from their otherwise minor initial injuries or illnesses. Two antibacterial agents, pyocyanase and salvarsan, were

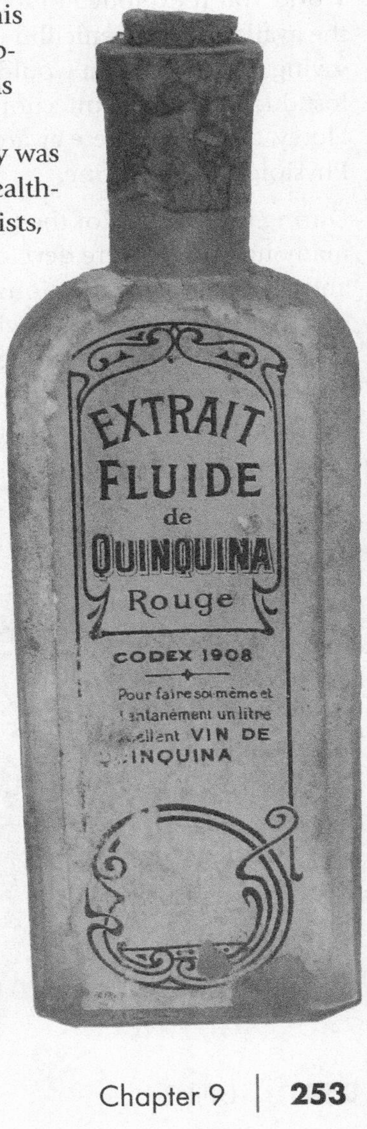

created to combat infectious disease, but both drugs proved to be toxic to patients. Consequently, scientists continued to search for a drug that would successfully kill or inhibit bacterial growth *without* harming the human body.

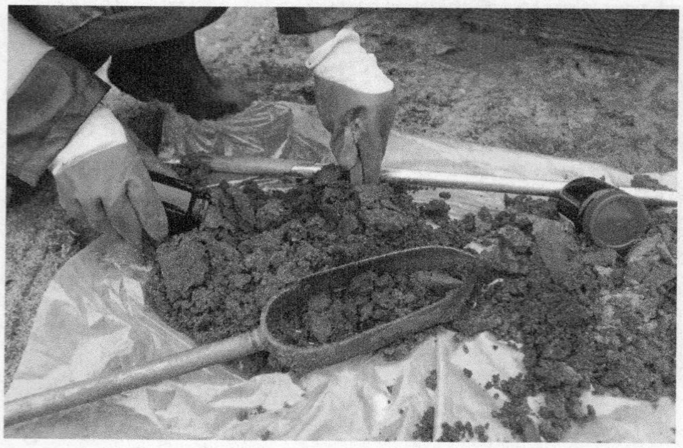

## The Rise of Synthetic Antibiotics

In 1928, Scottish biologist Alexander Fleming discovered that a mold that had inadvertently contaminated an unattended **Petri dish** had destroyed the bacteria *Staphylococcus aureus* that had been growing on the dish. Fleming knew that this serendipitous discovery, an extract of the mold *Penicillium*, held the promise of becoming an antibacterial **wonder drug**. However, it was not until more than a decade later that two scientists at Oxford University, Howard Florey and Ernst Chain, used new chemical techniques to transform Fleming's discovery into the antibacterial drug **penicillin**. As World War II exploded onto the pages of history, the availability of penicillin played a major role in saving many lives that would have otherwise been lost due to bacterial infections. In 1945, Fleming, Florey, and Chain were awarded the Nobel Prize in Physiology or Medicine.

During the last half of the twentieth century, many new drugs were developed to treat bacterial and other types of infections. In 1935, German biochemist Gerhard Domagk, who worked for Bayer Laboratories, developed the first **sulfonamide** by testing the synthetic red dye Prontosil. Domagk was so confident in the results he obtained from clinical trials that he used Prontosil in his own daughter, who had developed a streptococcal infection from a needle that was accidentally embedded in her wrist. Thankfully, his daughter made a complete recovery.

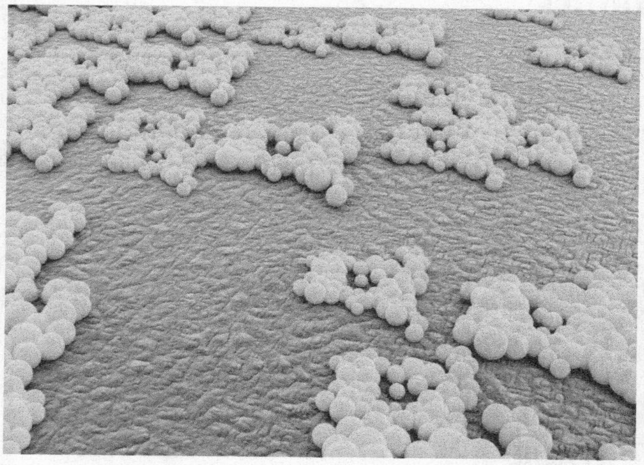

In 1939, Filipino scientist Abelardo Aguilar sent a soil sample to his employer, the Eli Lilly Company. Company scientists were able to use this sample to isolate the antibacterial substance **erythromycin** from a strain of *Streptomyces erythreus*. Several Eli Lilly scientists who worked on the project received acclaim for the discovery of this antibacterial medicine; however, Aguilar was never officially recognized for his contribution to what would become the lifesaving drug erythromycin.

Another important discovery in antibiotics occurred in 1944. American microbiologist Selman Waxman led a team of researchers from Rutgers University in the discovery and development of **streptomycin**, which was isolated from a soil sample containing the antibacterial substance *Streptomyces griseus*. In 1952, Waxman was awarded the Nobel Prize for Medicine for his discovery of streptomycin which, at that time, was the only effective treatment for tuberculosis. Waxman is also credited with introducing the term *antibiotic*, which he used to describe a class of substances that could kill or inhibit the growth of bacteria. The word stems from the Greek root words *anti*, meaning "against or opposite," and *biotikos*, meaning "of life." Therefore, antibiotic literally means "against life."

## Emergence of SVP Preparations

The second half of the twentieth century saw a dramatic rise in the development of drugs used to treat infections and illnesses. At the time, antibiotic drugs were primarily administered via two routes: oral and intramuscular (IM) injections. Both of these routes had potential side effects. Oral medications were not well-tolerated by patients whose digestive systems precluded their use or by patients who had difficulty swallowing. IM injections carried the potential risk of **tissue necrosis** or other injury. Consequently, it became evident to healthcare practitioners that a method for delivering medications directly into the patient's bloodstream was necessary.

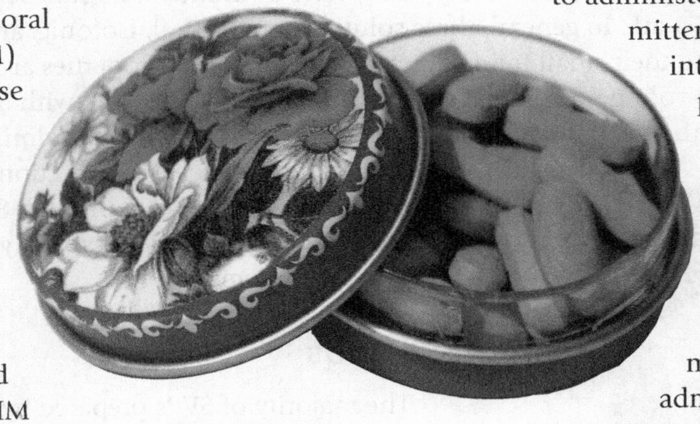

In addition to addressing patient side effects, there were several other compelling reasons to create a new delivery method for antibiotics. Some newly developed drugs required direct administration into the bloodstream to achieve their full **mechanism of action**. Still other drugs were either of too large a volume, required further dilution prior to administration, or were too **caustic** to be delivered by IM or direct intravenous push (IVP) routes into the patient's vein.

In response to the need for an IV delivery method, manufacturers of large-volume parenteral preparations, such as Abbott Labs and Baxter Pharmaceuticals, created a new SVP delivery vehicle called an **intravenous piggyback (IVPB)**. An IVPB is a way to administer an SVP medication intermittently, through an existing intravenous (IV) line, into a patient's vein.

Today, many pharmaceutical companies provide the components needed to perform the sterile compounding of SVP products. Some SVP medications—such as those administered by the subcutaneous (Sub-Q), IM, and IVP routes—are often supplied by the manufacturer in a form that is ready to administer. The nurse simply draws up the injection and administers it to the patient. However, the majority of SVPs are administered by IVPB and, therefore, require sterile compounding. Consequently, this chapter provides the background information, aseptic technique protocol, and specific procedures to be used in the creation of these products.

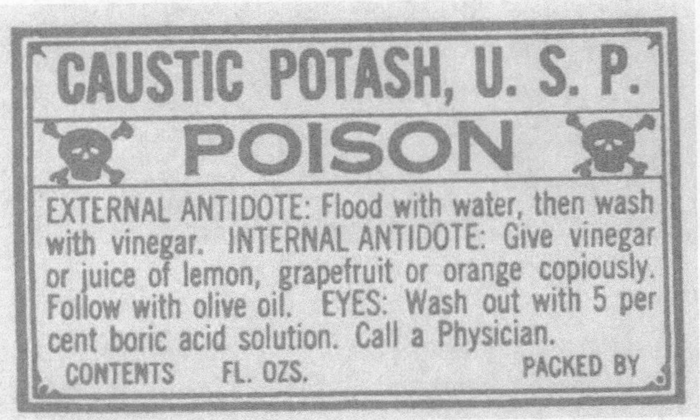
CAUSTIC POTASH, U. S. P.
POISON
EXTERNAL ANTIDOTE: Flood with water, then wash with vinegar. INTERNAL ANTIDOTE: Give vinegar or juice of lemon, grapefruit or orange copiously. Follow with olive oil. EYES: Wash out with 5 per cent boric acid solution. Call a Physician.
CONTENTS FL. OZS.
PACKED BY

# Part 1: Concepts

**Small-volume parenteral (SVP) preparations**—known simply as SVPs—are sterile solutions that typically have a volume of 25 mL, 50 mL, 100 mL, 150 mL, or 250 mL. In general, these solutions are neutral, isotonic, and isosmotic; however, due to their small fluid volumes, their chemical properties are not as significant as large-volume parenteral (LVP) preparations. Most SVPs with a volume ranging from 25 mL to 250 mL are administered by the IVPB route of administration. Some SVPs may be administered by injection. These SVPs are administered parenterally through Sub-Q, IVP, IM, or intrathecal (IT) routes and typically have a much smaller volume than most IVPBs.

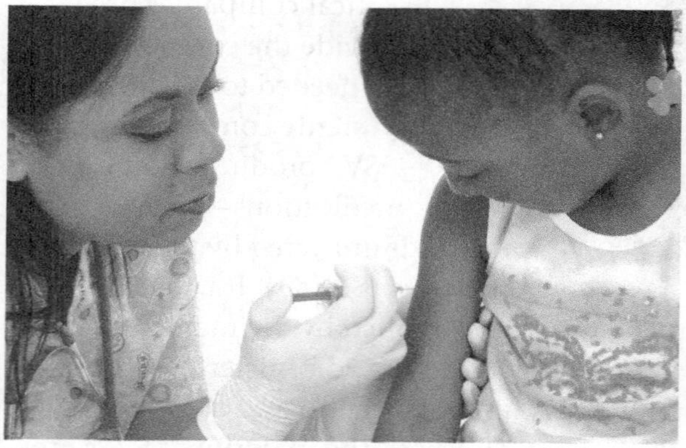

Nurse administering an IM injection.

## IVPBs

The majority of SVPs prepared by sterile compounding personnel are IV piggybacks, or IVPBs. An IVPB is comprised of a small volume of a base solution and a medication. The **standard IV base solution** may be a sterile fluid such as dextrose 5% in water ($D_5W$), normal saline (NS), half normal saline (½ NS), or sterile water. The medication may be an antibiotic, an antibacterial, or any number of drugs that must be diluted. Unlike an LVP that is given for hydration or the **continuous infusion** of medication, an IVPB is used solely for the intermittent IV administration of medication according to a dosing schedule specified by a prescriber. This **intermittent infusion** is accomplished by piggybacking the SVP through the tubing containing a patient's primary IV solution.

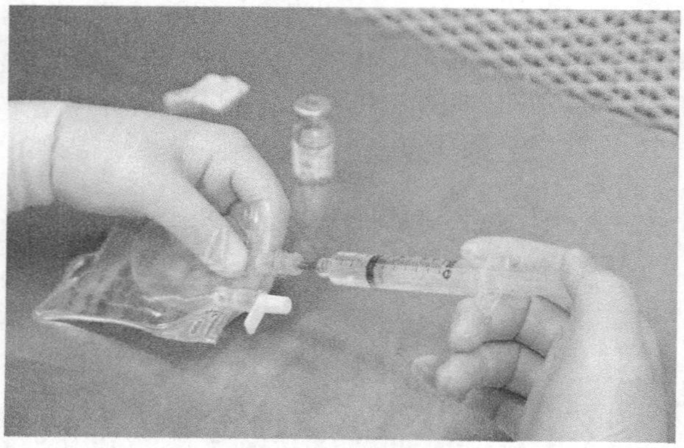

IV technician preparing an IVPB medication.

A limited number of IVPBs are supplied as premixed, shelf-stable, or frozen products. Other types of IVPBs are available in vial and bag systems such as Add-A-Vial, MINI-BAG Plus, or ADD-Vantage. However, the majority of ordered IVPBs must be compounded by an IV technician.

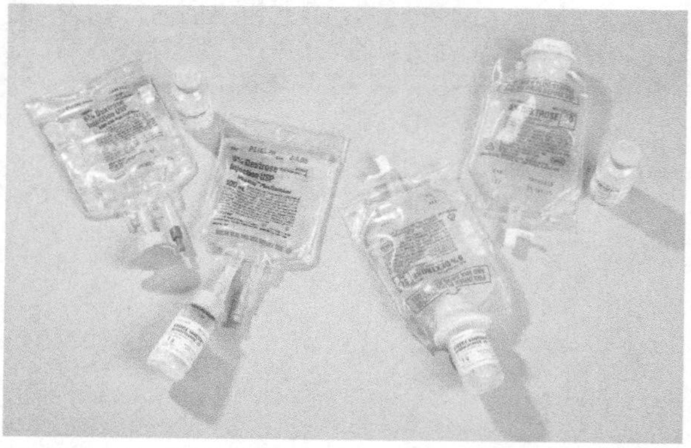

MINI-BAG Plus (left) and ADD-Vantage (right) IVPBs.

## Compounding of IVPBs

The compounding of IVPBs begins with the medication order. When writing a medication order for an IVPB, a prescriber typically indicates the medication name, dose, and **dosing interval** or schedule, without specifying the base solution or volume. Upon the order's arrival in the pharmacy, the pharmacist then assumes the responsibility of determining the appropriate IVPB base solution for that medication and dosage. To make this decision, the pharmacist reads the drug's package insert or consults a helpful resource such as the *Handbook on Injectable Drugs* or Micromedex, an online drug database. The pharmacist considers several factors when choosing the most appropriate IVPB base solution and volume, including:

- the compatibility of the medication with the base solution
- the length of time over which the IVPB is to be administered
- the kidney function and hydration status of the patient recipient
- the minimum or maximum concentration required for safe administration of the drug

Some pharmacy computer programs automatically select the most appropriate IVPB base solution and volume for the medication and print this information onto the compounded sterile preparation (CSP) label at the time of order entry.

IV technicians prepare many different types of IVPBs during the course of a standard eight-hour shift. Some of these IVPBs may include medications such as $H_2$ antagonist drugs (famotidine or ranitidine) or, occasionally, highly concentrated potassium chloride to provide emergency treatment for a patient with hypokalemia. However, most IVPBs prepared by IV technicians are antibiotic preparations.

***Antibiotic Preparations*** Antibiotics are antimicrobial medicines used to treat a variety of infections caused by certain types of **microorganisms**, such as fungi, protozoa, or bacteria. Antibiotics are *not* effective in the treatment of viruses. The terms **antibiotic drugs** and **antibacterial drugs** are sometimes used interchangeably. However, these two classes of drugs have one important distinction: Whereas antibiotics are used to treat multiple types of microorganisms, antibacterial drugs are only used to treat infections caused by bacteria.

Antibiotics are among the most commonly prescribed parenteral medications because most patient recipients either have an existing infection or are at risk for a nosocomial infection. Consequently, these medications are frequently compounded by IV technicians. Antibiotics are prescribed based on their effectiveness in treating a certain type of microorganism. Most bacterial microorganisms are said to be either **gram-positive** or **gram-negative organisms**. In essence, gram-positive bacteria have thicker cell walls than gram-negative bacteria. Patients requiring IVPB antibiotic therapy often undergo blood testing (known as a culture and sensitivity test) to determine which **pathogenic organism** is causing the infection and—if the microorganism is a type of bacteria—whether the organism is gram-positive or gram-negative. The microorganism is exposed to several antibiotics in the laboratory to determine the effectiveness of each drug. The antibiotic that provides the most effective treatment for that specific organism is then ordered by the prescriber.

A number of different classes of antibiotics are commonly used in sterile compounding. Each class of antibiotics targets the infected cell in a different way. For example, some antibiotics inhibit bacterial cell growth by preventing formation of the cell wall. Other antibiotics work by blocking the cell's ability to produce the protein it needs for survival. Still others kill bacteria by inhibiting DNA function within the cell. (See Table 9.1 on the following page for a list of commonly prescribed IVPB antibiotics.)

Table 9.1 **Commonly Prescribed IVPB Antibiotics**

| Antibiotic Class | Examples | Used to Treat |
|---|---|---|
| Aminoglycosides | amikacin, gentamicin, streptomycin, tobramycin | gram-positive bacterial infections<br>gram-negative bacterial infections |
| Carbapenems | imipenem | gram-positive bacterial infections<br>gram-negative bacterial infections |
| Cephalosporins | cefazolin, cefepime, cefotaxime, cefotetan, cefoxitin, ceftazidime, ceftriaxone, cefuroxime | gram-positive bacterial infections<br>gram-negative bacterial infections |
| Chloramphenicol | chloramphenicol | gram-positive bacterial infections<br>gram-negative bacterial infections |
| Glycopeptides | vancomycin | gram-positive bacterial infections |
| Lincomycins | clindamycin | gram-positive bacterial infections<br>gram-negative bacterial infections |
| Macrolides | azithromycin, erythromycin | gram-positive bacterial infections<br>some gram-negative bacteria infections |
| Monobactams | aztreonam | gram-negative bacterial infections |
| Nitroimidazoles | metronidazole | some bacterial infections<br>protozoal infections |
| Oxazolidinones | linezolid, posizolid | poly-resistant gram-positive infections |
| Penicillins | ampicillin, nafcillin, oxacillin, penicillin G, piperacillin, ticarcillin, Timentin (ticarcillin disodium and clavulanate potassium), Unasyn (ampicillin and sulbactam), Zosyn (piperacillin and tazobactam) | gram-positive bacterial infections |
| Polyenes | amphotericin B, nystatin | fungal infections, amoebic infections |
| Polypeptides | bacitracin, polymyxin B | gram-positive bacterial infections<br>gram-negative bacterial infections |
| Quinolones | ciprofloxacin, levofloxacin, moxifloxacin | gram-negative bacterial infections |
| Rifamycins | rifampin | gram-positive bacterial infections |
| Sulfonamides | trimethoprim/sulfamethoxazole | gram-positive bacterial infections<br>gram-negative bacterial infections |
| Tetracyclines | doxycycline, minocycline | gram-positive bacterial infections<br>gram-negative bacterial infections |

## Administration of IVPBs

IVPBs are administered over a short period, usually 15 minutes, 20 minutes, 30 minutes, or 60 minutes. However, these medications can be given over as short as a 10-minute duration or as long as a 24-hour duration. Most IVPBs are administered by piggybacking them through a patient's primary IV line. Occasionally, an IVPB medication is administered to a patient who does not have a primary IV line. In this situation, the IVPB is administered through secondary IV tubing, directly into the patient's vein, via a temporary injection port. This type of injection port—called a **heparin lock**, **saline lock**, or, simply, a *lock*—is attached to a flexible needle that is maintained in the patient's vein. In either case, the IVPB medication is discontinued once the patient's medical condition has improved.

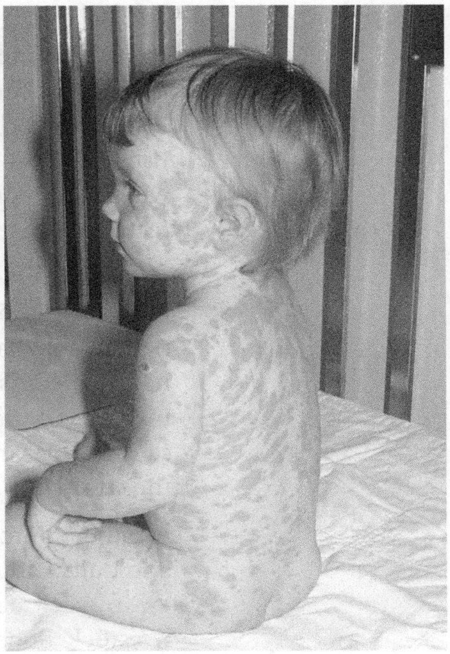

The reaction from Stevens-Johnson syndrome starts as a diffuse red rash that, if left untreated, spreads deeper, causing the dermis to slough off.

## Potential Complications of Parenteral Therapy

The administration of parenteral medications involves certain potential complications that may lead to injury or, possibly, death for patient recipients. Therefore, all patients receiving parenteral therapy should be monitored for the following complications:

- nosocomial infection
- allergic reaction (including anaphylaxis)
- phlebitis
- tissuing
- embolism
- extravasation
- cellulitis
- Stevens-Johnson syndrome
- nephrotoxicity

Other complications are specific to certain types of CSPs, and to varying degrees. For antibiotic SVPs, there is an increased likelihood for **allergic reactions**, including **anaphylaxis**; **Stevens-Johnson syndrome**; and **nephrotoxicity**. Patients receiving these sterile products should be monitored closely for these complications.

***Incompatibility Issues*** In addition to these risks, IVPBs, due to their administration setup, have the potential for **incompatibility** issues with other IVPB or IVP medications. For example, if two incompatible medications are administered through the same IV tubing, a **precipitate** could form, clogging the IV tubing and potentially causing injury to the patient. For this reason, the primary IV tubing or the lock (for patients without a primary IV line) must be flushed after the IVPB medication has been administered. If the patient is receiving a primary IV solution, the **flush** is performed by lowering the empty IVPB bag with secondary tubing attached to a height that allows gravity to force the primary IV solution to back up into the secondary tubing line. Once the primary IV solution has backed up into the IVPB, the IVPB should then be temporarily raised to a height above the primary IV solution. This action will flush any remaining medication out of the secondary IVPB tubing and into the patient's vein. For patients without a primary IV solution, the lock is usually flushed with a small volume (usually 3, 5, or 10 mL) of either NS solution, or a **heparinized saline solution**.

**USP Chapter <797>**

Facilities may vary with regard to the type and volume of flush solution, as well as the frequency of lock flush procedures. Consult your facility's P&P manual to determine the procedures of lock flushes implemented by the nursing staff.

***Antibiotic-Resistant Bacteria*** IV technicians should be aware of a growing health concern in the use of antibiotic therapy—the development of **antibiotic-resistant bacteria**, or bacteria that are resistant to treatment by most or all of the commercially available antibiotics. These robust and virulent pathogens are known as **superbugs** and, consequently, are very difficult to treat. The evolution of superbugs has been influenced by two factors: the widespread use of antimicrobial disinfectants and the overuse of antibiotics. Both of these situations promote bacterial resistance to antibiotics due to repeated or extended exposure. This exposure allows the bacteria to develop resistance mechanisms, such as changes in the cell wall or the development of enzymes that can destroy the antibiotic.

**Antimicrobial Overuse** In general terms, an **antimicrobial** is a substance or chemical compound capable of killing or inhibiting the growth of microorganisms such as bacteria, fungi, protozoa, or viruses. Antimicrobial agents may be found in many hand soaps, cleansers, and **surface disinfectants**, as well as some medicines. The rise in the use of these products has helped to strengthen various **microbes**, some of which are evolving to the point that standard antimicrobial agents will soon be ineffective against them.

**Antibiotic Overuse** The prevalence of overprescribing antibiotics has also led to the development of antibiotic-resistant bacteria. Often, prescribers yield to a patient's demand for an antibiotic for an illness that may be viral, not bacterial, in nature. Because antibiotics are ineffective against viruses, the end result is simply an increased patient immunity to the prescribed antibiotic. So, when that patient is prescribed the same antibiotic for a bacterial infection, the drug is less effective against the strain of bacteria.

Another source of antibiotic overuse comes from the use of antibiotics in the meat and dairy industries, whose policies allow for the administration of **prophylactic antibiotic treatment** to promote animal growth and to prevent and treat illness in livestock. Subsequent ingestion of the food products obtained from the livestock increases an individual's exposure and may lead to development of resistance to certain antibiotics.

***Superbugs as a Global Health Threat*** Due to the widespread use of antimicrobials and antibiotics, superbugs such as methicillin-resistant *Staphylococcus aureus* (MRSA), carbapenem-resistant *Klebsiella pneumoniae* (CRKP), and New Delhi metallo-beta-lactamase (NDM-1) are on the rise and considered by many scientists to pose a serious threat to global health. To address this concern, the World Health Organization (WHO) used World Health Day (April 7, 2011) to issue an urgent plea to healthcare practitioners to decrease antibiotic-resistant bacteria by promoting correct antibiotic use:

> *The message on this World Health Day is loud and clear. The world is on the brink of losing these miracle cures. The emergence and spread of drug-resistant pathogens has accelerated. More and more essential medicines are failing. The therapeutic arsenal is shrinking. The speed with which these drugs are being lost far outpaces the development of replacement drugs. In fact, the R&D pipeline for new antimicrobials has practically run dry. The implications are equally clear. In the absence of urgent corrective and protective actions, the world is heading towards a post-antibiotic era, in which many common infections will no longer have a cure and, once again, kill unabated.*

## USP Chapter <797> Guidelines for SVPs

During the preparatory and compounding procedures of SVPs, an IV technician must adhere to the overarching principles set forth in USP Chapter <797>. These guidelines are reinforced in each facility's P&P manual as well. In accordance with these guidelines, sterile compounding personnel must pay strict attention to aseptic technique protocols both in the anteroom and clean room. Any breach in these protocols may result in medication errors, sepsis, or, possibly, death for the patient recipients. Therefore, as an IV technician, you bear primary responsibility for the preparation and integrity of the CSPs. With that in mind, only those personnel who have been specially trained, process validated, and certified in aseptic technique and sterile product preparation should be allowed to compound sterile products. Part 2 of this chapter guides you through the discovery and demonstration of proper aseptic technique in SVP preparation.

# Concepts Self-Check

## Check Your Understanding

*Write your answers on a separate sheet of paper, as modeled in these examples: 1d; 2c; 3b; etc. Check your answers using the Answer Key in Appendix A.*

**1.** Who first discovered bacteria?

a. Anton van Leeuwenhoek
b. Louis Pasteur
c. Alexander Fleming
d. Abelardo Aguilar

**2.** What is the name of the bacteria that was first discovered to have been destroyed by an extract of the mold *Penicillium*?

a. penicillin
b. *Staphylococcus aureus*
c. erythromycin
d. *Streptomyces erythreus*

**3.** What is the most common route of administration for a medication requiring intermittent infusion?

a. IVP
b. IT
c. IVPB
d. IM

**4.** Which of the following statements best describes the term *antibiotic*?

a. an antimicrobial agent capable of killing or inhibiting the growth of certain bacteria, fungi, and protozoa
b. an antimicrobial agent capable of killing or inhibiting the growth of certain viruses
c. none of the above
d. both *a* and *b*

**5.** Which of the following was identified by the WHO as posing a serious threat to global health?

a. nosocomial infections
b. antibiotic-resistant viruses
c. drug-resistant pathogens
d. microbial infections

## Apply Your Knowledge

*On a separate sheet of paper, write your answers to the questions posed in the paragraph below. Use complete sentences and take time to create a thorough and thoughtful response. Check your answers against the Answer Key in Appendix A.*

In Part 1 of this chapter, you learned that the WHO's 2011 statement regarding antibiotic-resistant superbugs says that "the therapeutic arsenal is shrinking" and that "[t]he speed with which these drugs are being lost far outpaces the development of replacement drugs." With that in mind, what does the organization's statement indicate about the ability of pathogenic organisms to evolve in response to antibiotic therapy? What does it reveal about the difficulty of developing effective ways to combat these superbugs?

# Part 2: Training

*Before performing this lab, review the Sterile Compounding Area Procedures listed on pages 162–163 at the end of the Unit 2 opener, and preview the accompanying process validation checklist in Appendix D.*

## Understand the Resources and Supplies

USP Chapter <797> prescribes a number of special requirements for the preparation of SVP products. This chapter and the corresponding lab provide resources and supplies that are in alignment with the directives set forth in USP Chapter <797>.

### Essential Supplies

Most sterile compounding procedures require the same essential supply items to be available for use in both the anteroom and the clean room. For the anteroom, these supplies include a medication order and CSP label; a standard calculator; a pen; a permanent felt-tip marker; large and small plastic bags; aseptic garb; a sterile gown; presaturated, aseptic cleaning wipes; sterile, foamed 70% IPA; a waste container; and a transport vehicle (optional). (Various other compounding supplies, such as those needed for aseptic hand washing and hood cleaning, are necessary supplies, but, for the purposes of this lab, are not included on the Essential Supplies list.) In the clean room, essential supply items include sterile, foamed 70% IPA; sterile, powder-free gloves; sterile 70% IPA swabs; a sharps container; a waste container; and a laminar airflow hood.

### Procedure-Specific Supplies

In addition to the previously listed essential supplies, each sterile compounding procedure requires supply items specific to the procedure being performed. The type, number, and amount of procedure-specific supply items are determined by the IV technician prior to performing the procedure, based on information provided on the CSP label and the medication additive label. After reading these labels, the IV technician performs one or more calculations that reveal the number and volume of additives needed to prepare the CSP. This information, in turn, dictates the number, size, and type of syringes needed for the procedure.

***IVPB Supplies*** The process of compounding the IVPB preparations in this procedural lab involves the manipulation of regular needles and—in particular—vials, vented needles, and IVPB base solutions. Familiarity with the appearances of these items as well as any specific handling requirements is essential to sterile compounding procedures.

VIALS Most IVPB compounding procedures require an IV technician to **reconstitute** a powdered antibiotic within a vial. To do so, the technician draws up **diluent** (such as sterile water or NS) from a separate vial and injects that fluid into the vial containing the powdered antibiotic. There are several methods that may be used to complete this procedure, including the use of the **milking technique**, a vented needle, or a repeater pump. Each of these reconstitution methods involves techniques or equipment that reconstitute the powder while simultaneously equalizing the air pressure within the vial. Facilities that prepare multiple, large batches of IVPB medications sometimes use a repeater pump for drug reconstitution. This pump allows for the dilution of multiple vials of powder. (For more information on repeater pumps, refer to Chapter 3 of this textbook.)

Sterile compounding personnel must take several precautions during the reconstitution process. Proper needle insertion technique must be implemented to avoid coring the vial's rubber top. In addition to proper needle insertion, care must be taken to relieve the air pressure within the diluent vial prior to withdrawing fluid from the vial. Using the milking technique helps to equalize the pressure within the vial, allowing an easy withdrawal of fluid. (For assistance in understanding or performing the milking technique for fluid withdrawal, refer to Chapter 8 of this textbook.)

An IV technician may also use the milking technique to relieve air pressure within a vial when reconstituting a powder. This air pressure is created when a liquid is injected into the vial of powder. Once the diluent has been injected into the vial, the needle-and-syringe unit used to inject the diluent should remain inserted in the vial until the powder is completely dissolved. At that time, the liquid within the vial can be withdrawn into the attached syringe. Because **positive pressure** was created within the vial when the diluent was injected, the milking technique can be used to withdraw the dissolved powder from the vial without injecting air. This method of reconstituting a powder within a vial is best used when preparing a single CSP in which the entire contents of a vial are injected into the IVPB to provide the desired dose.

**Vented Needles** In addition to regular needles, some IVPB sterile compounding situations require the use of a **vented needle**. Unlike a regular needle that has a beveled tip, a vented needle has a **razor tip** and is surrounded by a tiny **aluminum needle sheath**. When the sheath is properly situated in the vial's rubber top, air is vented out of the vial through the movable metal band. This unique design allows the injection of the diluent into the vial while simultaneously venting air from the vial. The design of the needle prevents the withdrawal of fluid into the syringe, as well as the injection of fluid into an IV or an IVPB. A vented needle is also useful when consecutively diluting multiple powdered stock drug vials.

This type of needle is used solely to reconstitute a powdered medication within a vial. To perform the reconstitution, an IV technician must first draw up the diluent into a syringe using a regular needle and then remove the regular needle and attach a vented needle to the syringe. Lastly, the IV technician inserts the vented needle directly into the vial's rubber top without any angle or bend to the needle.

**IVPB Base Solutions** An IVPB base solution bag is very similar in design and function to that of an LVP bag. However, unlike an LVP bag, the IVPB base solution bag is only available with a tail injection port. Button injection ports are not used on IVPB bags due to their small size and the potential for accidentally puncturing the back

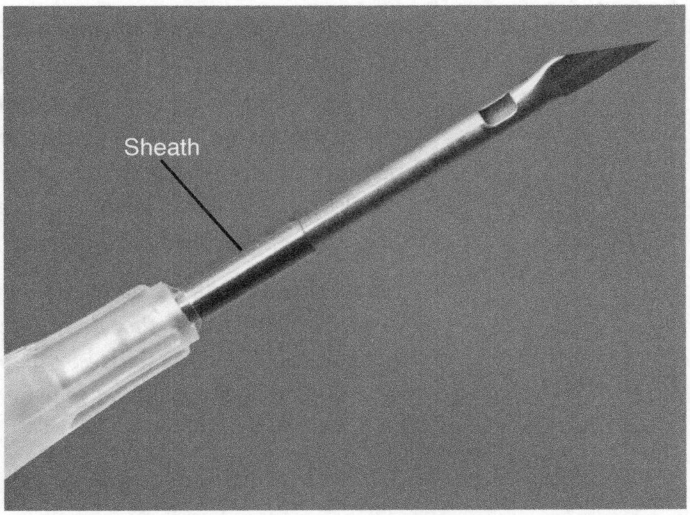


Vented needle; notice the sheath, razor tip, and lack of the type of needle bevel found on a regular needle.

of the bag during injection of the medication. When using an IVPB bag, the needle should be inserted directly into the injection port without regard to the position of the needle bevel, and without creating any bend to the needle, as is done when inserting a needle into a vial. The base solution component of an IVPB is usually either $D_5W$ or NS, with a volume of either 50 mL or 100 mL, depending on which medication is ordered by the prescriber.

## Critical Sites of Essential Supplies and IVPB Supplies

Before beginning preparatory procedures in the anteroom or clean room, the IV technician must recall the critical sites of the supplies. Identifying the critical site of each supply item helps you to determine the proper procedure for handling the supply item once you have entered the clean room and begin working in the hood.

The critical sites of essential supply items include sterile 70% IPA swabs. The critical sites of IVPB supplies include the syringe tip, the piston plunger and inner plunger shaft of the syringe, and the needle. These critical sites are supplied by the manufacturer in sterile form and should, therefore, not be swabbed with alcohol prior to use. In addition to these supplies, this chapter's procedural lab provides instruction in the proper use of a vented needle, a sterile supply item that should never be swabbed with IPA.

The critical sites of the other SVP supplies used for the Chapter 9 procedural lab include the injection port of the IVPB base solution bag and the vial top. These critical sites must be swabbed with sterile 70% IPA prior to needle insertion to decrease the likelihood of contaminating the solution during injection or withdrawal procedures.

After identifying the critical sites of all supply items, care must be taken not to taint the critical site of any supply item through touch contamination, shadowing, or incorrect placement of the item within the hood. (For additional assistance on the handling of critical sites of sterile compounding supplies, refer to Chapter 3 of this textbook.)

**POINTER**

Sterile compounding personnel must comply with certain restrictions when working in the anteroom and clean room areas. These restrictions include no gum chewing, horseplay, or food or drink in both the anteroom and clean room, and no hair spray, perfume, makeup, artificial or polished nails, or jewelry in the sterile compounding environment.

# Preview the Lab Procedure

*The following material provides a brief overview of the lab procedure that you will perform. First, read the* Preview the Lab Procedure *section. Then read each step of the* Procedural Lab *section carefully, visualizing every action. Next, reinforce your understanding of the process by watching the demonstration video. Once you are in the lab, your instructor will demonstrate the procedure, and then you will perform the procedure by following the steps in the* Procedural Lab *section. Practice the lab procedure multiple times. After sufficient practice, you will complete the lab procedure for process validation by your instructor.*

***Note:*** *This procedural lab requires the use of a basic, open-sided, horizontal laminar airflow hood. For pharmacies that do not have this type of hood, IV technicians should consult the* Instruction Guide *provided by the hood's manufacturer or their facility's P&P manual to determine which procedures may need to be adjusted to suit their hood.*

## Anteroom Preparatory Procedures

As you already know, the preparation for the sterile compounding process begins in the anteroom. This transition area provides a space for implementing the standard pharmacy protocols discussed in Chapters 3–6, including:

- verifying the CSP label against the medication order
- performing correct pharmacy calculations to determine type, size, and number of supply items needed
- gathering and cleaning of supplies
- performing aseptic garbing and hand washing
- donning a sterile gown

> **POINTER**
> Refer to your facility's P&P manual to determine the approved cleaning agent to be used for wiping down the supply items and the transport vehicle.

> **POINTER**
> If the powdered drug vial label does not provide the concentrated form strength or the diluent amount, consult the drug's package insert for this information.

***Verifying the CSP Label*** Compare the medication order to the CSP label to verify all information on the CSP label matches the medication order exactly. Then read the CSP label to determine the necessary ingredients for the compounding procedure. Retrieve the ordered **powdered drug** and determine how much diluent must be added to properly reconstitute the drug to its **desired concentration**. The desired concentration is determined by the drug manufacturer and is found on the label of the powdered drug. The label instructs the IV technician to inject a specific amount of a diluent such as sterile water or sterile NS into the powder to provide the desired concentration of the drug in a liquid, injectable form. Once the drug has been reconstituted from its powdered form into its liquid, injectable form, the liquid is now in its **concentrated form**. The concentration listed on the powdered drug vial indicates the strength, or concentration, of the drug as it is in its final, reconstituted form. This ratio of milligrams per milliliter (mg/mL) is called the drug's **final concentration**, or simply, the *concentration*.

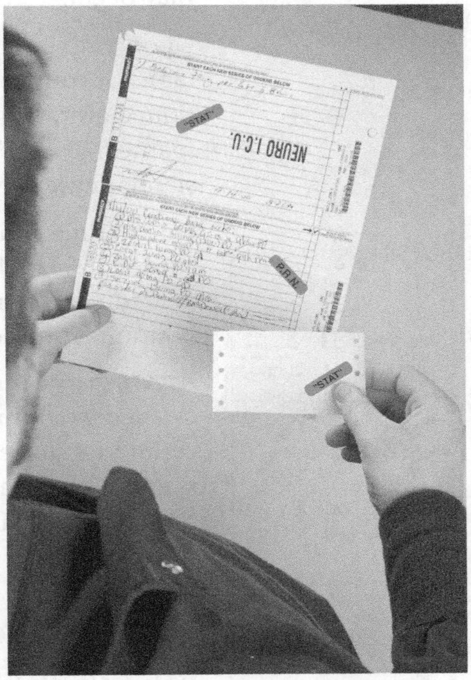

IV technician verifying a medication order with a CSP label.

***Performing Pharmacy Calculations*** Use the CSP label to determine the desired dose ordered by the prescriber. Then use the final concentration given on the label of the powdered drug vial to perform the calculations needed to determine the volume of each ingredient you need to draw up to prepare the CSP.

***Gathering and Cleaning of Supplies*** Once all calculations are complete, you must then gather and wipe down all of the necessary compounding supplies. (For detailed information on the USP Chapter <797>-aligned protocol for this anteroom procedure, refer to the Chapter 8 section titled Gathering and Cleaning of Supplies on page 226.)

***Donning PPE*** Now that you have assembled your clean supplies, you must put on personal protective equipment (PPE), a requirement for working in the clean room. Before donning your aseptic garb, be sure that you are wearing close-toed shoes and either scrub uniforms, or another approved lightweight, nonshedding clothing. Then put on aseptic shoe covers, a hair cover, a face mask, and, if appropriate, a beard cover. Lastly, don a sterile gown.

> **POINTER**
> Whenever you are required to reconstitute a powdered drug vial, you must gather enough needles and syringes for two separate procedures: the drawing up of the appropriate volume of diluent and, subsequently, the appropriate volume of the reconstituted drug.

Due to time constraints, you will not perform aseptic hand-washing procedures during this procedural lab. Keep in mind that, in sterile compounding practice, aseptic hand-washing procedures are mandatory and must be performed prior to donning a sterile gown.

## Clean Room Preparatory Procedures

When preparing SVPs for patient administration, sterile compounding personnel must diligently follow established pharmacy clean room protocols as well. These protocols, discussed in Chapters 6 and 7, include:

- cleansing hands with sterile, foamed 70% IPA
- donning sterile gloves
- cleaning the hood

Once the preparatory steps have been completed, SVP compounding procedures may begin.

Upon entering the clean room, place the transport basket or tray onto a clean shelf, table, or countertop. If the transport vehicle used is a cart, wheel it so that it is positioned away from the hood prefilter. Cleanse your hands and forearms with sterile, foamed 70% IPA and allow them to dry thoroughly. Don sterile gloves according to standard aseptic technique procedures.

**POINTER**

Remember that the discard pile for sterile compounding waste should be kept within the outer six-inch zone of the hood, in an area where the waste does not interfere with compounding procedures or interrupt airflow to the CSP.

Due to time constraints, you will not perform hood-cleaning procedures during this procedural lab. Keep in mind that, in sterile compounding practice, hood-cleaning procedures are mandatory and must be performed prior to beginning sterile compounding procedures and at intervals prescribed by USP Chapter <797>.

***Arranging and Preparing Supplies in the Hood*** Once the hood has been cleaned, you must transfer the clean supplies from the transport vehicle or clean countertop to certain areas of the hood. Place small supply items, such as the needle, syringes, and vials, within the outer six-inch zone of the hood. Remove the dust covers of large supply items, such as the IVPB base solution bag, and place the items into the DCA of the hood. Dispose of the dust covers in the waste container.

## SVP Compounding Procedure, Scenario One: Reconstitution Using the Milking Technique

**USP Chapter <797>**

Take care not to touch or shadow the syringe tip or any portion of the needle, except its cap. If you do, you must place the supply items into the sharps container, gather new supplies, and repeat the procedure from the beginning.

With the small supply items arranged in the outer six-inch zone and the large supply items placed in the DCA, you are ready to begin the SVP compounding procedure. Bring the vial into the DCA of the hood, positioning the vial so that it receives uninterrupted airflow from the high-efficiency particulate airflow (HEPA) filter. Remove the vial's flip-top cap, placing the cap into the discard pile located in the outer six-inch zone. Swab the vial's rubber top with a sterile 70% IPA swab. Place the used swab in the discard pile.

Next, bring the first syringe, which is used to draw up the diluent, into the DCA. Remove the outer wrapper of the syringe and place the wrapper in the discard pile. If the syringe tip has a cap, remove the cap and place it in the discard pile. Without ever placing the uncapped syringe onto the hood surface, grasp the barrel of the syringe, and while holding the syringe in such a way as to maintain uninterrupted airflow from the HEPA filter to the syringe tip, carefully open the *regular* needle.

Grasping only the needle cap, aseptically attach the needle hub by twisting it onto the syringe tip, and temporarily place the syringe-and-needle unit onto the hood surface within the DCA.

Open a new, sterile 70% IPA swab and place it onto the hood surface within the DCA. Pull down on the flat knob of the syringe plunger to draw a volume of air into the syringe equal to the desired volume of the diluent needed. Hold the syringe—with the attached, capped needle—by the barrel. Remove the needle cap and place it onto the alcohol swab.

Grasp the barrel of the empty syringe, as you would a dart, and rotate it so that the needle bevel is pointed upward. Brace the vial against the hood's work surface, and lay the needle tip, bevel up, onto the vial top. Insert the needle into the vial using correct technique to help avoid coring. Invert the vial using a clockwise motion. Gradually inject air into the vial, thereby drawing diluent into the syringe, using the milking technique.

Repeat this procedure until you have withdrawn the appropriate volume of fluid from the diluent vial into the syringe. Without removing the syringe from the vial—and without shadowing the needle, syringe tip, or vial top—brace the syringe against your palm and tap the barrel of the syringe. Utilize proper procedures to eliminate bubbles from the syringe. Verify that you have drawn the desired volume of diluent into the syringe. Use correct technique to remove the needle and syringe from the vial; then carefully recap the needle and place the needle-and-syringe unit onto the hood surface within the DCA. (For detailed information on the USP Chapter <797>-aligned protocol for these clean room procedures, refer to the Chapter 8 section titled LVP Compounding Procedure on page 229.)

**POINTER**

Consult your facility's P&P manual to verify whether a pharmacist needs to check the diluent prior to reconstituting the powdered drug. If so, arrange the diluent vial, filled and capped diluent syringe, and the powdered drug vial on the hood surface for a verification check.

Next, bring the powdered drug vial into the DCA and remove the flip-top cap. Position the vial top within the DCA so that it receives uninterrupted airflow from the HEPA filter. Swab the vial's rubber top with a new, sterile 70% IPA swab, and place the swab on the work surface within the DCA. Remove the needle cap from the diluent syringe, and place the cap onto the alcohol swab. Grasp the barrel of the filled syringe and use correct technique to insert the needle into the powdered drug vial. Gently push down on the syringe flat knob, and use the milking technique to gradually inject diluent into the powdered drug vial, thereby releasing air pressure from the vial into the syringe. Repeat this procedure until all of the diluent from the syringe has been injected into the powdered drug vial, thereby venting the pressure from the vial into the attached syringe.

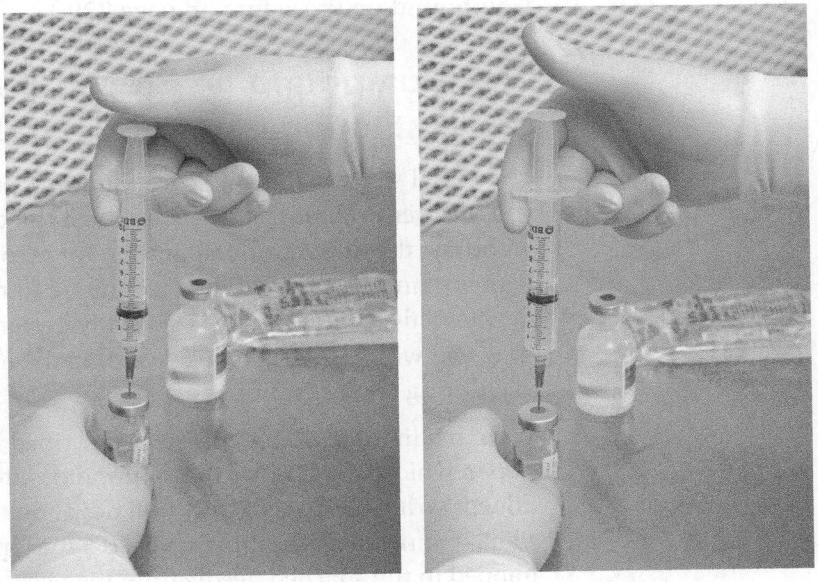
Injection of diluent into a powdered drug vial using the milking technique.

Without removing the syringe from the vial—and without shadowing the critical sites of the needle, syringe, or vial—gently shake the vial and

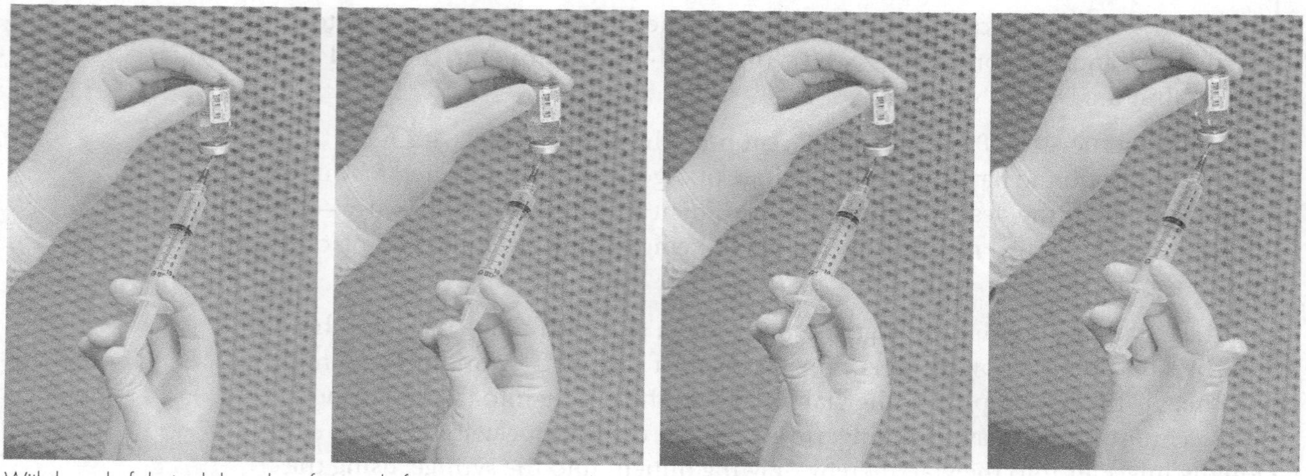

Withdrawal of desired drug dose from vial after reconstitution and venting using the milking technique.

attached needle-and-syringe unit to mix the diluent into the powder. Once the powder is completely dissolved, invert the vial and needle-and-syringe unit (clockwise if you are right-handed; counterclockwise if you are left-handed). Gradually inject the air that was displaced into the syringe back into the attached vial. Use the milking technique to gradually withdraw the reconstituted drug from the vial into the syringe. Utilize the correct procedures to eliminate bubbles from the syringe. Then verify that you have drawn up the desired volume of reconstituted drug into the syringe.

**POINTER**

Consult your facility's P&P manual to determine whether you are permitted to inject the desired concentration of drug into an IVPB base solution bag prior to a verification check. If so, the pharmacist would then check the empty vial, diluent vial, IVPB bag, and empty syringe (drawn back to the representative volume) against the CSP and medication label.

Use proper technique to remove the needle-and-syringe unit from the vial and recap the needle; then place the filled syringe on the hood surface within the DCA. Arrange the supply items and ingredients used in the preparation of the CSP next to the filled syringe to await a verification check by a pharmacist or your instructor. Once the check has been completed, use aseptic technique to inject the medication into the IVPB base solution bag. Properly label the IVPB and affix an IVA seal over the injection port. (For detailed information on the USP Chapter <797>-aligned protocol for these clean room procedures, refer to the Chapter 8 section titled LVP Compounding Procedure on page 229.)

## SVP Compounding Procedure, Scenario Two: Reconstitution Using a Vented Needle

The initial steps in this SVP compounding procedure are similar to the procedure you just performed. The point at which the two procedures diverge occurs once you withdraw the diluent in preparation for reconstitution of the powdered drug vial. Rather than using the milking technique to reconstitute the powder, you use a *vented* needle. This type of needle is specially designed to inject diluent into a powdered drug vial while simultaneously venting the air pressure that builds up inside of the vial during reconstitution.

**POINTER**

A *vented* needle should be used only to inject a diluent into a powdered drug vial. A *regular, nonvented* needle should then be used to withdraw the liquid from the reconstituted drug vial.

With that in mind, follow the steps described in the first procedure, up through the step in which you draw up the appropriate amount of diluent. Then pick up the filled diluent syringe and very gently pull down on the flat knob of the plunger to draw a small volume of air (approximately 0.5 mL) into the syringe. This action pulls any fluid trapped in the attached needle from the needle into the syringe. Carefully remove the entire needle and place it into the sharps container. Using appropriate technique, and without contaminating the syringe or needle, carefully attach a capped vented needle to the syringe tip. Place the syringe with the attached vented needle onto the hood surface within the DCA.

Remove the flip-top cap from the powdered drug vial within the DCA. Swab the vial's rubber top, and place the swab onto the work surface within the DCA. Remove the cap from the vented needle, and place the cap onto the alcohol swab. Grasp the barrel of the filled syringe as you would a dart. Without regard to the position of the bevel, and without any bend to the needle, introduce the vented needle into the vial. Use a direct, downward motion and a gentle stab, ensuring that the sheath of the vented needle is firmly seated in the vial's rubber top.

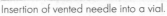

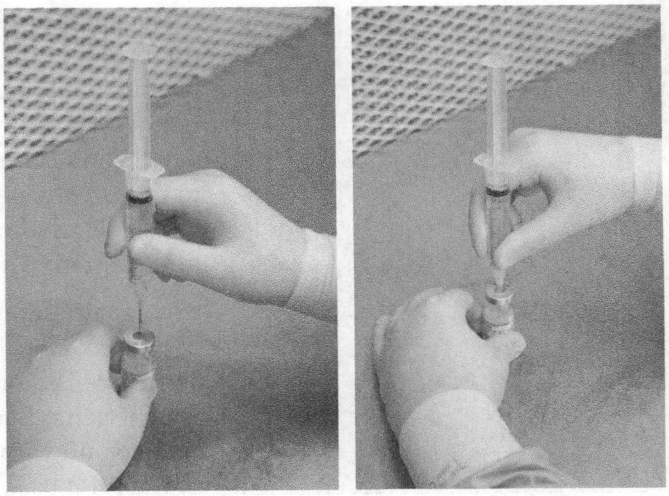
Insertion of vented needle into a vial.

Push down on the flat knob to inject all of the diluent from the syringe into the powdered drug vial (see Figure 9.1). Notice that the vented needle removes the positive pressure typically created when injecting fluid into a vial. This change is evident because the syringe plunger is not forced back toward the preparer, as is the case when positive pressure is created within a vial. As the vented needle vents air out of the vial, the syringe plunger moves easily and completely through the syringe barrel toward the syringe tip during fluid injection.

**USP Chapter <797>**

A few drugs have a chemical property that causes them to break down if shaken. For these drugs, gently swirl the vial to dissolve the powder. As a rule, consult each drug's package insert for any special handling requirements.

Once all of the diluent has been injected into the vial, grasp the barrel of the syringe between your thumb and forefinger and remove the syringe-and-needle unit from the vial.

Place the syringe-and-needle unit immediately into the sharps container. Gently shake the vial to mix the diluent into the powder. Once the powder has been completely reconstituted, prepare a new syringe by aseptically attaching a *regular* needle to the syringe tip.

Without drawing any air into the syringe, use proper technique to insert the needle into the reconstituted drug vial. Invert the reconstituted

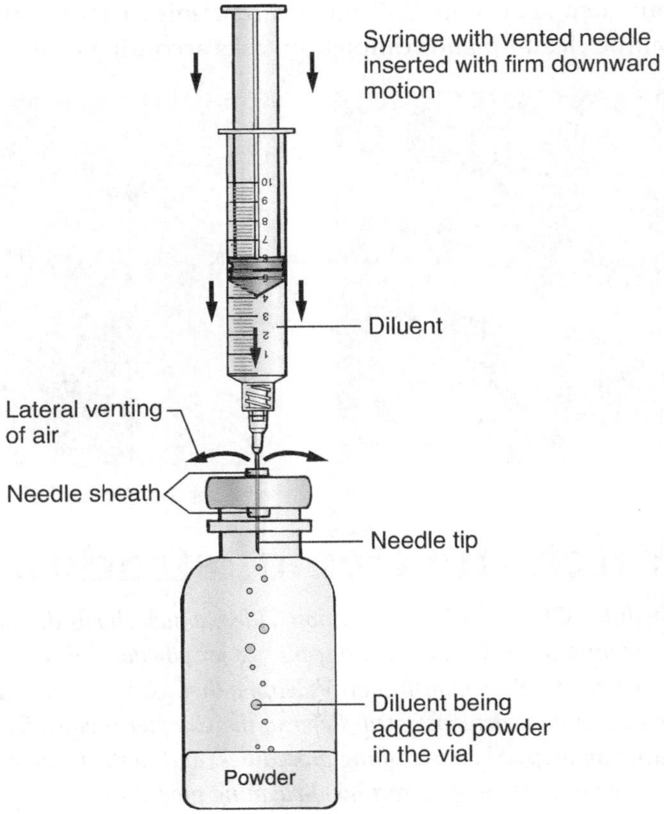


FIGURE 9.1

**Correct Use of a Vented Needle**

Procedure for inserting a vented needle and diluting a powdered drug vial.

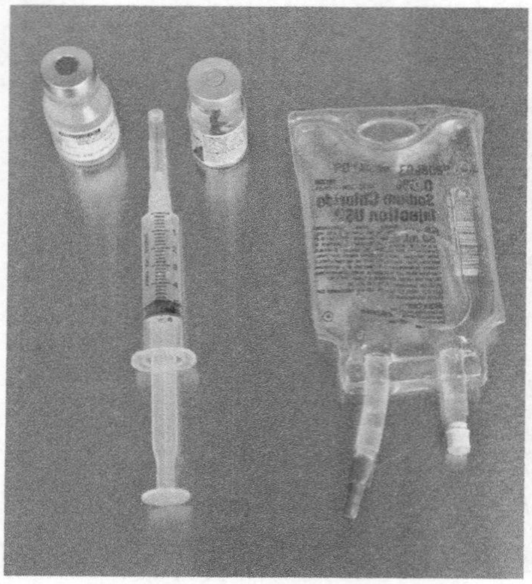


Filled syringe, ampicillin vial, diluent vial, and IVPB on hood awaiting a verification check.

drug vial and, without using the milking technique, pull down on the flat knob of the plunger to draw an appropriate amount of reconstituted drug into the syringe. Use proper aseptic technique to remove bubbles from the syringe, and return the vial with attached needle-and-syringe unit to the work surface. Use proper technique to remove the needle-and-syringe unit from the vial, and recap the needle. Place the filled syringe, with attached regular needle, on the hood surface within the DCA.

Arrange the supply items and ingredients used in the preparation of the second CSP on the hood surface next to the filled syringe to await a verification check by a pharmacist or your instructor. Once the check has been completed, reposition the IVPB and needle-and-syringe unit within the DCA of the hood so that the injection port of the IVPB base solution bag and the entire needle-and-syringe unit receive uninterrupted airflow.

Swab the injection port of the IVPB base solution bag, and then place the swab onto the hood surface, directly under the IVPB injection port. Use aseptic technique to carefully inject the medication into the IVPB, and then remove the needle-and-syringe unit from the IVPB bag. Immediately place the used needle-and-syringe unit into the sharps container.

**POINTER**

IVA seals are not used at all facilities. They are a preferred, but not a required, supply item. Refer to your facility's P&P manual to determine whether IVA seals are required in your facility.

Examine the IVPB for leaks, precipitate, or evidence of incompatibility; if free of these issues, proceed with labeling the CSP by affixing the label to the back of the IVPB bag. Then affix an IVA seal over the injection port of the bag. Place all waste from the discard pile and any nonsharps waste from the work surface into the waste container. Return the CSP and any remaining supply items to the anteroom. Perform routine clean-up and completion tasks according to standard procedures.

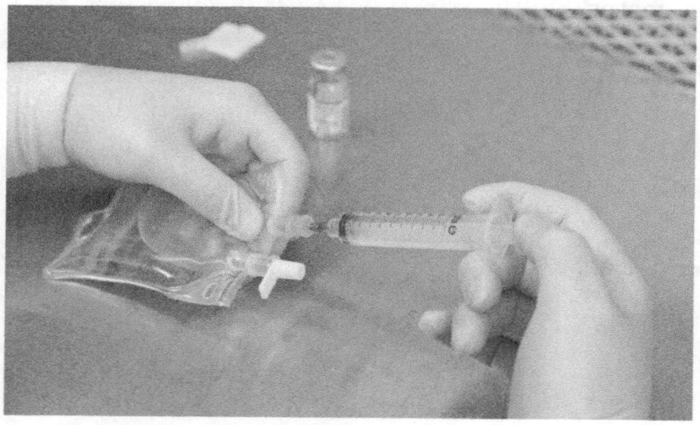

IV technician injecting medication into an IVPB.

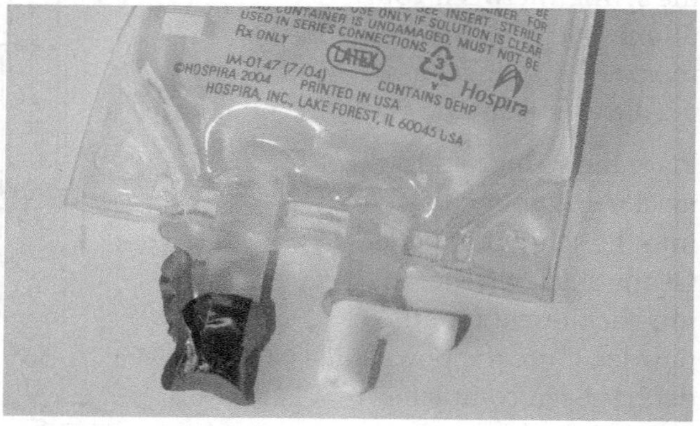


An IVA seal on an IVPB bag.

# Watch the Demonstration Video

*Watch the Chapter 9 Demonstration Video, which shows the step-by-step aseptic procedures for creating SVPs, including two scenarios for powdered drug reconstitution. For the purposes of the Chapter 9 Demonstration Video, neither aseptic hand washing nor hood cleaning is demonstrated. Refer to the Chapter 6 video for a demonstration of aseptic hand-washing procedures, and to the Chapter 7 video for a demonstration of correct hood-cleaning procedures.*

Training Videos DVD

# Procedural Lab

*This lab walks you through the step-by-step actions that you must follow to properly compound two SVP preparations using two reconstitution techniques. Take your time. Work through each step methodically and with close attention to detail.*

**Note:** *For the purposes of this procedural lab, you will not perform aseptic hand-washing or hood-cleaning procedures unless directed to do so by your instructor. Should your instructor ask you to perform these procedures, refer to Chapter 6 for instructions on aseptic hand washing and to Chapter 7 for directions on correct hood cleaning.*

**Note:** *For step 1, please refer to Chapter 4 for a reminder of the step-by-step procedures required for medication order and CSP label verification. For steps 2 and 3, refer to Chapter 5 for pharmacy calculation procedures. For steps 4–8, refer to Chapter 3 for a reminder of the process for gathering and cleaning supplies. For steps 9–15, refer to Chapter 6 for step-by-step aseptic garbing, hand-washing, and gloving procedures. Steps 1–12 and steps 71–73 should be performed in the anteroom. Steps 13–70 should be performed in the clean room.*

## Supplies

### *Essential Supplies*

To complete the Unit 2 procedural labs, you will need to ensure that various essential anteroom and clean room supplies such as those listed in Table 9.2 are available for your use.

**Table 9.2 Essential Anteroom and Clean Room Supplies for Sterile Compounding**

| |
|---|
| **Anteroom Supplies** |
| medication order and CSP label |
| calculator |
| pen |
| permanent, felt-tip marker |
| plastic bags (small and large) |
| aseptic garb, including shoe covers, hair cover, face mask, and beard cover (if appropriate) |
| sterile gown |
| presaturated, aseptic cleaning wipes |
| sterile, foamed 70% IPA |
| waste container |
| transport vehicle (optional) |
| **Clean Room Supplies** |
| sterile, foamed 70% IPA |
| sterile, powder-free gloves |
| sterile 70% IPA swabs, individually packaged × 10 |
| sharps container |
| waste container |
| laminar airflow hood |

### *Procedure-Specific Supplies*

In addition to the supplies listed in Table 9.2, gather the following items specific to the Chapter 9 SVP procedural lab:

- regular needles (nonfilter, nonvented needles, either 18 or 19 gauge) × 3
- ampicillin, 500-mg vial × 2

- sterile water, 10-mL diluent vial × 2
- 10-mL Luer-lock syringes × 3
- 3-mL Luer-lock syringe
- vented needle
- 0.9% sodium chloride, 100-mL IVPB × 2
- IVA seals (optional)

## Procedure

### *Verifying the Label*

1. Review the CSP label to verify that all information on the label matches the medication order. To help you with this task, compare the CSP labels (see Figures 9.2 and 9.3) to the medication order and patient ID label (see Figure 9.5).

**FIGURE 9.2** (left)

**CSP Label for Ampicillin 500 Mg**

**FIGURE 9.3** (right)

**CSP Label for Ampicillin 250 Mg**

****IV Piggyback****
Memorial Hospital
**Pt. Name:** Ogard, Christopher **Room:** 560
**Pt. ID#:** 898372 **Rx#:** 03127

**Ampicillin 500 mg**
**Sodium Chloride 0.9% (NS) 50 mL**
**Rate: over 20 min**

Expires ______
RPh ______
Tech ______

Keep refrigerated – warm to room temperature before use.

****IV Piggyback****
Memorial Hospital
**Pt. Name:** Ogard, Christopher **Room:** 560
**Pt. ID#:** 898372 **Rx#:** 03145

**Ampicillin 250 mg**
**Sodium Chloride 0.9% (NS) 50 mL**
**Rate: over 20 min**

Expires ______
RPh ______
Tech ______

Keep refrigerated – warm to room temperature before use.

### *Calculating Desired Volume*

2. Read the label on one of the ampicillin vials to determine the desired concentration of the drug once it has been reconstituted.

**POINTER**
Most powdered drug vial labels provide reconstitution instructions as well as the resulting, final concentration. Some drug manufacturers, however, provide this information in the package insert instead of on the vial label. Therefore, for the purposes of this procedural lab, reconstitute the powder with 5 mL of sterile water to obtain a concentration of ampicillin 500 mg/5 mL.

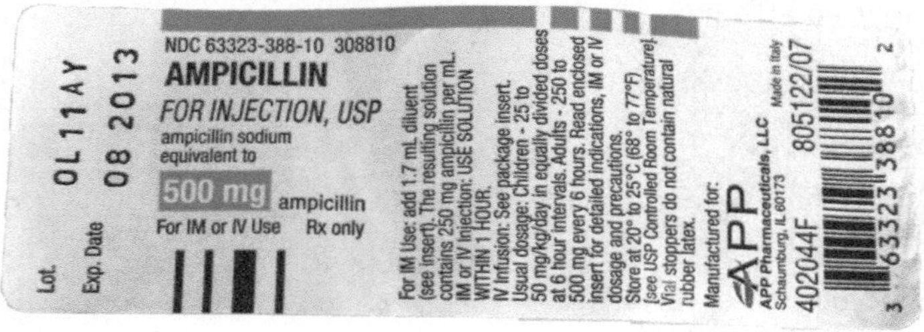


**FIGURE 9.4**
**Medication Label for Ampicillin**

FIGURE 9.5

**Daily Order**

Physicians create daily orders following each patient examination, or to change orders or make new orders.

ID#: 898372
Name: Christopher Ogard
DOB: 9/22/02
Room: 560
Dr.: Llewellyn, Douglas

**MEMORIAL HOSPITAL**
**PHYSICIAN'S MEDICATION ORDER**

BEAR DOWN ON HARD SURFACE WITH BALLPOINT PEN

GENERIC EQUIVALENT IS AUTHORIZED UNLESS CHECKED IN THIS COLUMN

ALLERGY OR SENSITIVITY
TO *Demerol, Sulfa Drugs*
NONE KNOWN ☐ SIGNED:

DIAGNOSIS

| DATE | TIME | ORDERS | PHYSICIAN'S SIG. | | COMPLETED OR DISCONTINUED NAME | DATE | TIME |
|---|---|---|---|---|---|---|---|
| | | *Height 4' 5" Weight 86 lbs* | | | | | |
| | | *C&S, UA, CBC—NOW* | | | | | |
| | | *NPO pre-op* | | | | | |
| | | *Schedule for surgery in AM—* | | | | | |
| | | *obtain consent for open reduction* | | | | | |
| | | *internal Fx—Ⓡ ankle.* | | | | | |
| | | *Give Ampicillin 500 mg IVPB × 1 NOW* | | | | | |
| | | *and Ampicillin 250 mg IVPB × 1 in* | | | | | |
| | | *AM before OR.* | | | | | |
| | | | *Douglas Llewellyn, MD* | | | | |

PHARMACY COPY

**POINTER**
Because you are using the same powdered drug strength and diluent volume for each compounding scenario, the desired concentration is the same for both ampicillin vials.

3. Perform the calculations based on the ampicillin dosage information provided on the CSP label and the ampicillin's final concentration. You must perform a separate calculation for each of the two CSPs that you are required to prepare. Assume that the label indicates that ampicillin, once reconstituted, has a concentration of 500 mg/5 mL. Use the following formula to calculate the dose:

*Scenario One*

$$\frac{500 \text{ mg}}{5 \text{ mL}} = \frac{500 \text{ mg}}{x \text{ mL}}$$

*Scenario Two*

$$\frac{500 \text{ mg}}{5 \text{ mL}} = \frac{250 \text{ mg}}{x \text{ mL}}$$

*Cross-multiply, then divide to solve for $x$ (the desired dosage volume) for each dose. (For additional assistance, refer to Chapter 5 for step-by-step dosage calculation procedures.)

### *Gathering and Cleaning Supplies*

4. Place the medication order into the large plastic bag and each of the CSP labels into separate small plastic bags. Gather all supply items listed in the supply section of the procedural lab.
5. Open the package of aseptic cleaning wipes. Remove one or, if necessary, more wipes, and thoroughly wipe down the entire transport vehicle.
6. Place the used wipes in the waste receptacle.
7. Remove a new aseptic cleaning wipe and wipe down the exterior surface of the IVPB bags' dust covers. Place the cleaned IVPB bags into the transport vehicle. Place the used wipe in the waste receptacle.
8. Repeat the cleaning procedure outlined in step 7 with each of the remaining supply items.

**POINTER**
During aseptic garbing, best practice is to reapply sterile, foamed 70% IPA to your hands after donning shoe covers and again after donning a hair cover.

### *Garbing*

9. Don shoe covers.
10. Put on a hair cover.
11. Don a face mask and beard cover (if appropriate).

    *Note:* For the purposes of this training lab, you will skip the mandatory aseptic hand-washing procedure.
12. Don a sterile gown.
13. Use a transport vehicle to bring all supply items, including an unopened package of sterile, powder-free gloves, into the clean room.
14. Place the transport vehicle onto a clean surface or countertop within the clean room. If a cart is used, position it so that is does not interrupt airflow into the hood prefilter.
15. Apply sterile, foamed 70% IPA to your hands. Allow them to air-dry and then don sterile gloves.

    *Note:* For the purposes of this training lab, you will skip the mandatory hood-cleaning procedure.

### *Compounding the SVP Solution—Scenario One*

16. Tear open the dust cover and remove the first IVPB base solution bag. Place the IVPB bag into the DCA of the hood and the dust cover into the waste receptacle. Place small supply items—such as the needles, syringes, and vials—into the outer six-inch staging area of the hood.
17. Remove the plastic, flip-top cap from one vial of sterile water by holding the vial in your hand and forcing the cap upward with your thumb or forefinger. Place the plastic vial cap in the discard pile. Position the vial within the DCA so that it receives uninterrupted airflow from the HEPA filter.
18. Tear open a sterile, 70% IPA swab while holding it within the DCA. Swab the sterile water vial top by holding the swab between the thumb and forefinger of your dominant hand, and then rubbing it once or twice across the vial's rubber top. Place the used swab onto the hood surface within the DCA, and the empty swab package in the discard pile.
19. Remove one 10-mL syringe from its outer wrap. If necessary, remove the cap from the tip of the syringe. Place the syringe outer wrap and cap in the discard pile in the outer six-inch zone of the hood.
20. Without laying down the uncapped syringe—and without touching or shadowing the syringe tip—hold the barrel of the syringe in your dominant hand, always maintaining your position with the DCA such that the syringe tip receives uninterrupted airflow from the HEPA filter.
21. While holding the barrel of the syringe in your dominant hand—and while keeping the syringe tip pointed toward the HEPA filter—use the fingers of both hands to carefully peel apart the regular needle package. Take care not to touch or shadow the needle hub or syringe tip at any time. Using a twisting motion, gently screw the needle hub onto the syringe tip. Place the needle package in the discard pile.

**POINTER**

The discard pile should contain only nonsharps waste and should be kept in the outer six-inch zone of the hood in an area that does not shadow or disrupt compounding procedures.

**USP Chapter <797>**

If at any time you inadvertently touch or shadow the needle or syringe tip, you must immediately place the contaminated items into the sharps container, gather new supply items, and repeat the compounding procedure.

### *Withdrawing the Correct Diluent Volume Using the Milking Technique*

22. Grasp the empty syringe—with attached, capped needle—in your nondominant hand. Use your dominant hand to pull down on the flat knob of the plunger to draw approximately 5 mL of air into the syringe.
23. Transfer the syringe to your dominant hand, grasping the syringe at the barrel. Hold it as you would a dart. Hold the syringe steadily, and use your nondominant hand to remove the needle cap by pulling it carefully but firmly off of the needle. Place the needle cap, with the open end pointing toward the HEPA filter, on top of the alcohol swab on the hood's work surface.

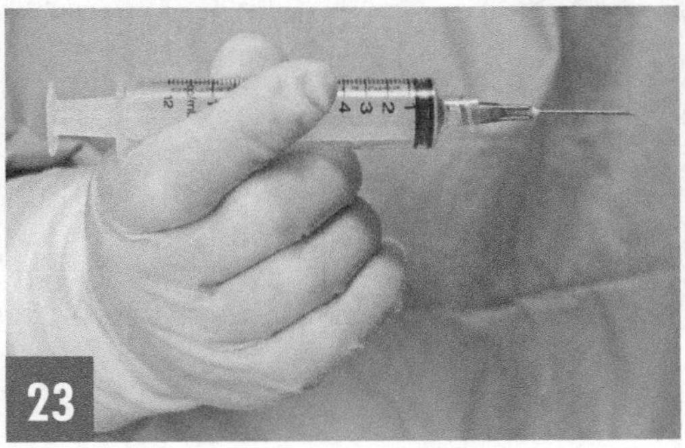


24. Use your fingers to rotate the barrel of the syringe so that the bevel of the needle is pointed up toward the ceiling.

**USP Chapter <797>**

You must never place a needle or syringe on the hood's work surface unless it has an attached needle cap.

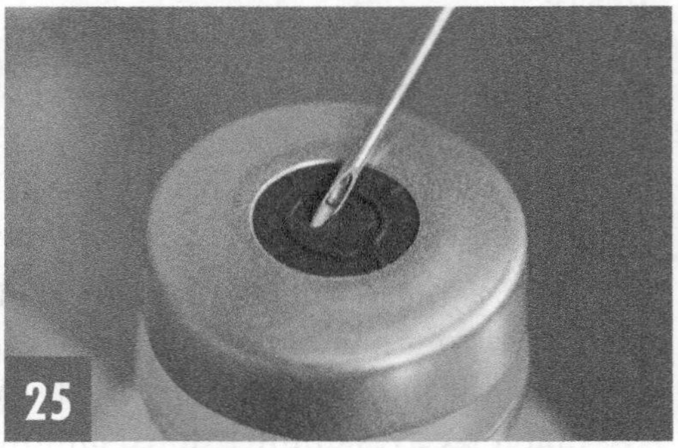


**25.** Using your nondominant hand, brace the sterile water vial against the hood's work surface. Lay the tip of the needle, bevel up, onto the center of the vial's rubber top.

**26.** Insert the needle into the vial using a slight upward rotation of the wrist (rotating in a counterclockwise direction if you are right-handed, and in a clockwise direction if you are left-handed). Keep the tip of the needle in contact with the vial's rubber top at all times. There should be a slight, almost imperceptible, bend to the needle as it enters the vial.

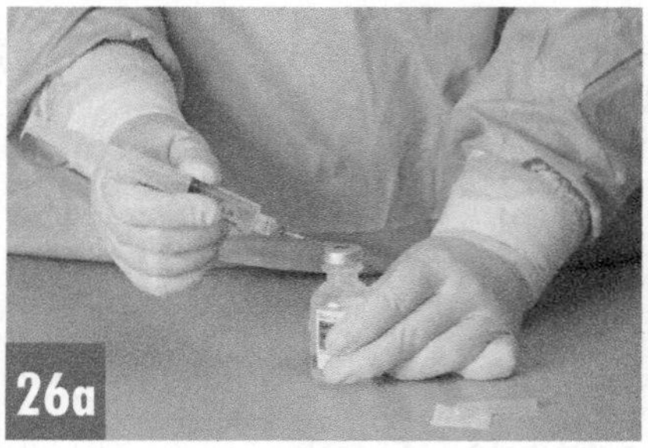


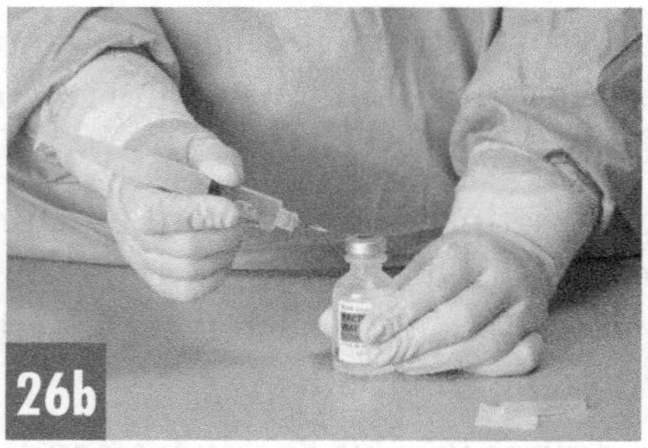


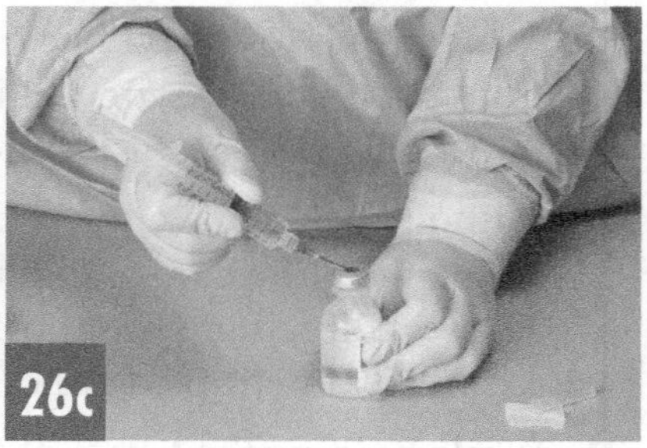


**POINTER**

Take care to hold the vial and syringe so that the airflow to the critical area—the area from the tip of the syringe to the neck of the vial, including the entire needle and the vial's rubber top—remains unobstructed.

**27.** Hold the sterile water vial with your nondominant hand and the syringe, with needle firmly inserted into the vial, with your dominant hand. Invert the vial, using a clockwise motion (a counterclockwise motion if you are left-handed), so that the needle-and-syringe unit is now below the vial.

**28.** Use the thumb of your dominant hand to gradually push up on the flat knob of the plunger to inject a small amount of air (approximately 3 mL) into the sterile water vial, creating a slight positive pressure within the vial. Release the plunger and allow fluid to flow into the syringe. Repeat this milking process until you have a minimum of 5.5 mL of sterile water in the syringe.

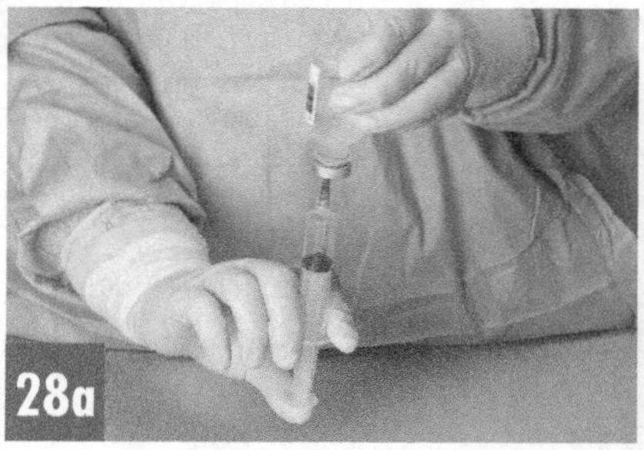


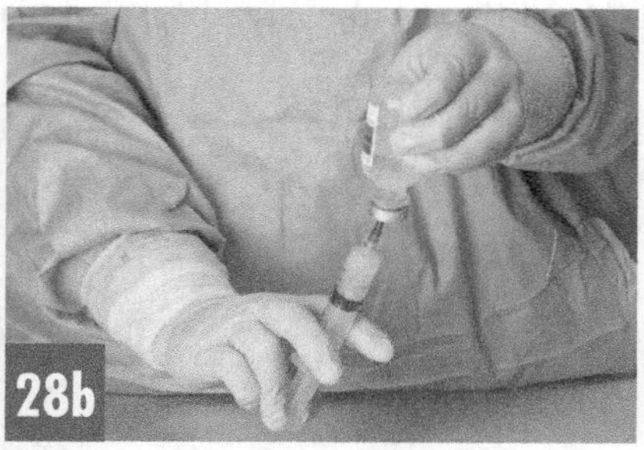


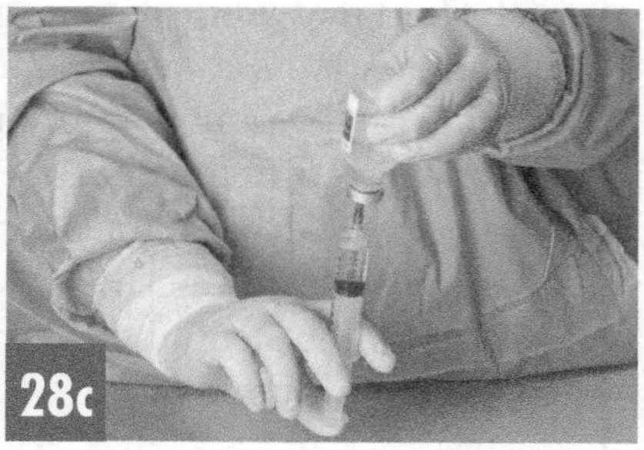

29. While ensuring that the needle remains entirely within the vial, hold the vial between the thumb and forefinger of your nondominant hand, allowing the barrel of the syringe to rest against the palm of that hand. Be sure to position your nondominant hand in a manner that continues to allow airflow to the critical site. Then, using your dominant hand, tap the barrel of the syringe with your fingers to force air bubbles within the fluid up toward the tip of the syringe. You must take care to perform this action in such a way that you do not bring your dominant hand between the critical site and the HEPA filter at any time.
30. Push up on the flat knob of the plunger with the thumb of your dominant hand to expel the air bubbles that have gathered near the tip of the syringe, along with any extra fluid, including the extra 0.5 mL of fluid that was drawn up to facilitate bubble removal.
31. Verify that the syringe now contains the desired amount of diluent. (For the sterile water diluent, the desired volume is 5 mL.)
32. While keeping the needle firmly inserted in the vial, use a counterclockwise rotation (a clockwise rotation if you are left-handed) to return the vial and syringe to the original starting position, with the upright vial braced against the work surface and the dominant hand grasping the barrel of the syringe. Slowly remove the needle-and-syringe unit from the vial of sterile water. Remember to avoid touching the plunger or flat knob of the syringe at any time while removing the needle-and-syringe unit from the vial.
33. Carefully recap the needle and place the capped needle-and-syringe unit, now filled with diluent, onto the work surface within the DCA.

**POINTER**

When using the milking technique to *withdraw* fluid from a vial, the needle-and-syringe unit must remain below the inverted vial. Remember to keep the tip of the needle near the vial's interior neck so that a steady stream of fluid is drawn into the syringe. This precaution helps to avoid drawing excess air into the syringe.

**USP Chapter <797>**

As you hold the vial or brace the syringe against your palm, be sure that your palm faces the HEPA filter. Maintaining this position allows continuous airflow to all critical sites.

### *Reconstituting and Venting a Powdered Drug Vial Using the Milking Technique*

34. Bring a vial of ampicillin into the DCA and remove the vial's flip-top cap. Open a new IPA swab and swab the top of the ampicillin vial. Place the used swab on the hood's work surface, within the DCA. Place the swab wrapper and flip-top cap in the discard pile.
35. Pick up the diluent-filled syringe in your dominant hand, grasping the syringe at the barrel. Hold it as you would a dart. Hold the syringe steadily, and use your nondominant hand to remove the needle cap by pulling it carefully but firmly off of the needle. Place the needle cap, with the open end pointing toward the HEPA filter, on top of the alcohol swab on the hood's work surface.
36. Use your fingers to rotate the barrel of the syringe so that the bevel of the needle is pointed up toward the ceiling.
37. Using your nondominant hand, brace the ampicillin vial against the hood's work surface. Lay the tip of the needle, bevel up, onto the center of the vial's rubber top.

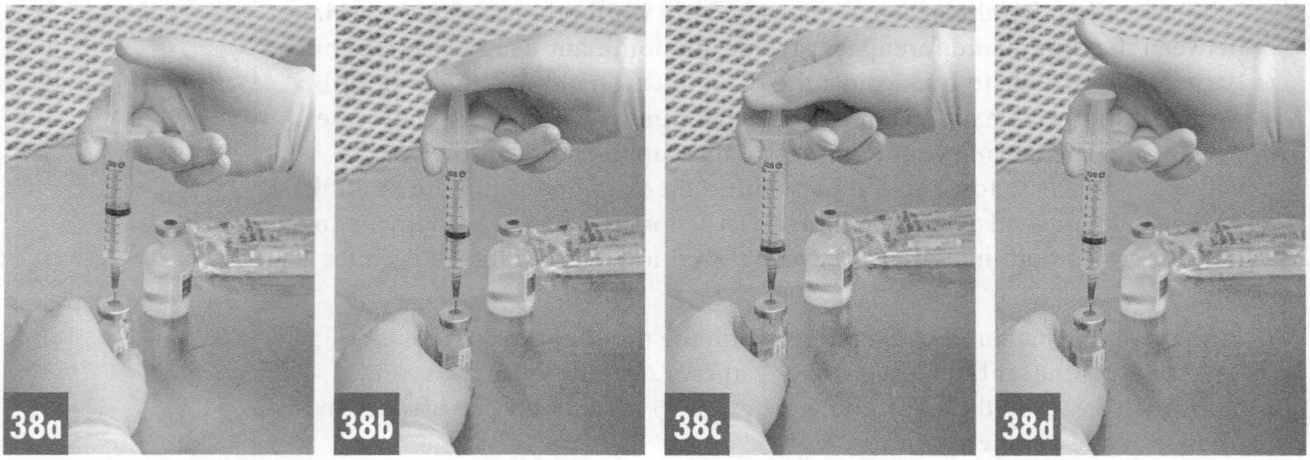


> **POINTER**
> When using the milking technique to *dilute* a powder, brace the vial against the hood surface and keep the tip of the needle near the *interior neck of the vial* to avoid drawing powder from the bottom of the vial into the syringe.

**38.** Stabilize the ampicillin vial against the hood's work surface with your nondominant hand, and maintain the needle-and-syringe unit's position above the vial. Gently push down on the flat knob of the plunger with the thumb of your dominant hand, until you have injected approximately 3 mL of diluent into the ampicillin vial. Release your thumb from the flat knob and allow built-up air pressure to transfer from the ampicillin vial to the syringe. Repeat this milking technique until all of the diluent has been injected into the vial and an equivalent amount of positive air pressure (approximately 5 mL) has transferred into the syringe.

**39.** Hold the vial with your nondominant hand and the syringe barrel with your dominant hand. While keeping the needle inserted completely into the vial, gently shake the syringe and attached vial to mix the diluent and ampicillin powder. Take care not to touch or shadow the critical site of the needle, syringe, or vial at any time.

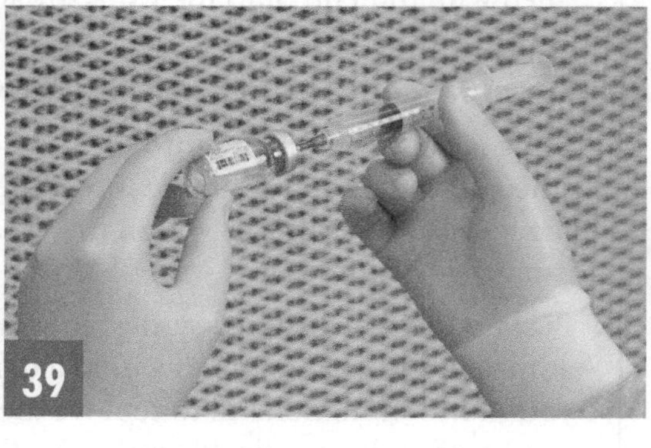


**40.** Repeat steps 27–33 to draw up the correct dose volume of ampicillin—in this case, 5 mL.

**41.** Properly arrange the ampicillin syringe, used ampicillin vial, used diluent vial, and IVPB base solution bag on the work surface of the hood to await a verification check by a pharmacist or your instructor. Position the medication order and CSP label in the outer six-inch zone, immediately in front of the CSP ingredients. *Note:* The medication order and CSP label must remain in their plastic bags until compounding procedures are complete.

**42.** Once the verification check has been completed, rearrange the IVPB bag's injection port and the needle-and-syringe unit within the DCA so that they receive uninterrupted airflow from the HEPA filter.

### *Injecting the Medication into the IVPB Base Solution Bag*

**43.** Open a new IPA swab and swab the injection port of the IVPB bag. Place the swab on the hood's work surface directly under the injection port.

**44.** Grasp the barrel of the ampicillin syringe in your dominant hand, as you would a dart. Remove the cap of the needle and place the needle cap onto the alcohol swab that you placed on the hood's work surface.

**45.** Hold the injection port steady with your nondominant hand, taking care to avoid shadowing or touching the injection port. With your dominant hand, carefully insert the needle straight into the injection port, taking care to avoid puncturing the sidewall of the injection port.

**46.** Inject the medication into the IVPB bag by pressing on the flat knob of the plunger with the thumb or forefinger of your dominant hand.

**47.** Holding only the barrel of the syringe, carefully remove the needle-and-syringe unit from the IVPB bag. Place the needle-and-syringe unit into the sharps container without recapping the needle.

**48.** Squeeze the IVPB bag and examine it for leaks, precipitate, or evidence of incompatibility. If there are no signs of these issues, cover the injection port with an IVA seal. Remove the CSP label for Scenerio One from the plastic bag and affix the label to the IVPB bag.

**49.** Temporarily place the labeled CSP and any used supply items over to the side of the hood, in the outer six-inch zone, while you prepare the CSP for Scenario Two.

### *Compounding the SVP Solution—Scenario Two*

**50.** Repeat steps 17–33 using the second 10-mL syringe and the unused sterile water diluent vial.

**51.** Grasp the filled diluent syringe and hold it so that the capped needle is pointing up. Gently pull the plunger down approximately 0.5 mL. This pulling action draws fluid from the needle into the syringe.

**52.** Unscrew and remove the regular needle and place it into the sharps container.

**53.** Without laying down the uncapped syringe—and without touching or shadowing the syringe tip—hold the barrel of the syringe in your dominant hand, always maintaining your position with the DCA such that the syringe tip receives uninterrupted airflow from the HEPA filter.

**54.** While holding the barrel of the syringe in your dominant hand—and while keeping the syringe tip pointed toward the HEPA filter—use the fingers of both hands to carefully peel apart the vented needle package. Take care not to touch or shadow the syringe tip or vented needle hub at any time. Use a twisting motion to gently screw the vented needle hub onto the syringe tip. Place the vented needle package into the discard pile.

**POINTER**

When inserting a needle into the injection port of an IVPB base solution bag, it is not necessary to consider the direction of the bevel. The needle should be inserted straight into the bag without an angle and without bending the needle.

**USP Chapter <797>**

If precipitates, incompatibility, or leakage are noted, consult with your instructor on how to proceed. In practice, these issues necessitate the disposal of the questionable product and the restart of the compounding procedure with new supplies.

**BE AWARE**

Be sure that you have secured the correct CSP label and that the dosage indicated on the CSP label matches the dosage amount required in Scenario One.

> **POINTER**
> Unlike regular needles, the razor tip of a vented needle does not contain a bevel. The vented needle-and-syringe unit should be inserted into a vial without laying the needle tip onto the vial top, and without any bend to the needle. Apply enough downward pressure when inserting the needle so that the aluminum sheath surrounding the needle is firmly seated into the vial's rubber top. If correctly inserted, the needle itself should be able to move up and down freely while the sheath remains stuck in the vial top.

> **POINTER**
> If a noticeable amount of fluid pools on the vial top during the injection of the diluent, it is likely that you have not fully inserted the needle into the vial top; notify your instructor to receive further guidance.

> **POINTER**
> If the vented needle failed to vent the air out of the vial adequately, it is likely that the syringe was held too close to the vial top. If this situation occurs during the injection of the diluent, notify your instructor for further guidance.

### *Reconstituting and Venting a Powdered Drug Vial Using a Vented Needle*

**55.** Bring the second ampicillin vial into the DCA and remove the vial's flip-top cap. Open a new IPA swab and swab the top of the ampicillin vial. Place the used swab onto the hood's work surface, within the DCA. Place the swab wrapper and flip-top cap in the discard pile.

**56.** Grasping the barrel of the syringe like a dart, remove the cap of the vented needle. Place the vented needle cap onto the IPA swab within the DCA.

**57.** Use your nondominant hand to brace the ampicillin vial against the hood's work surface. With your dominant hand, insert the vented needle directly into the top of the vial with a firm downward motion.

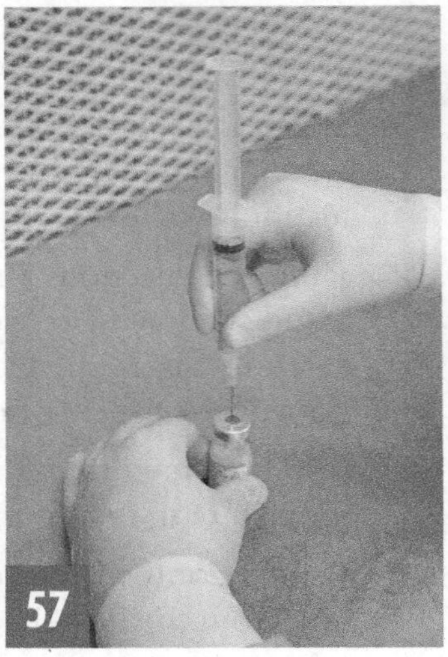
57

**58.** While maintaining the needle in the vial at such a depth that the hub of the needle stays approximately one-eighth inch above the vial's rubber top, inject the diluent into the ampicillin vial.

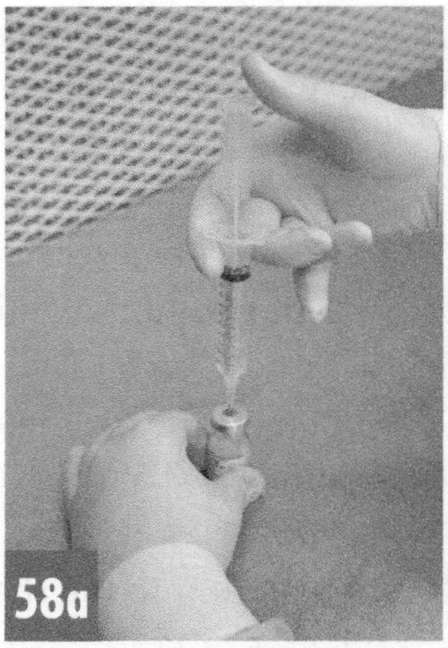
58a

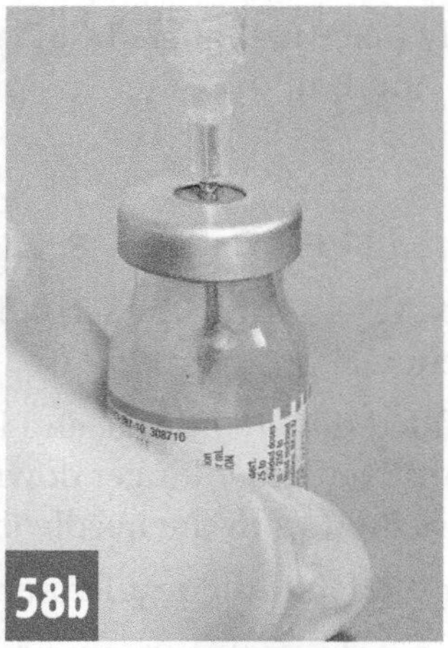
58b

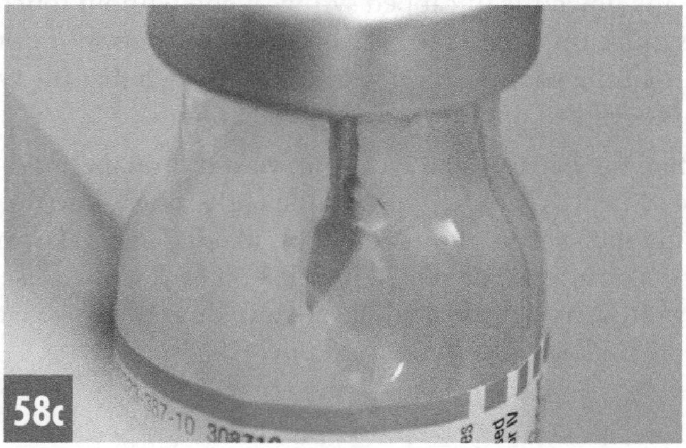
58c

59. Correctly grasp the barrel of the syringe, taking care not to touch the plunger, and remove the needle from the vial. Place the vented needle-and-syringe unit into the sharps container.

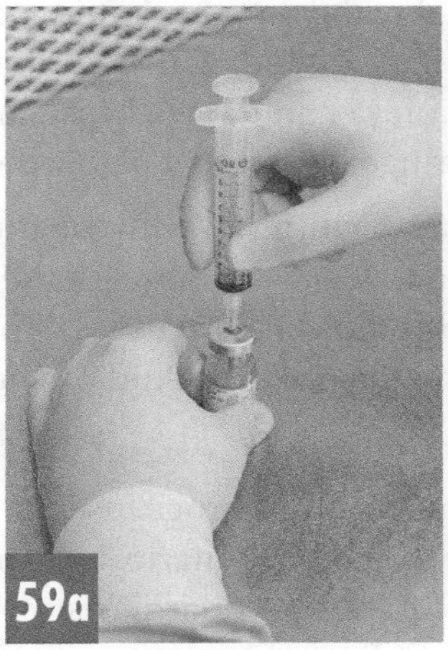
59a

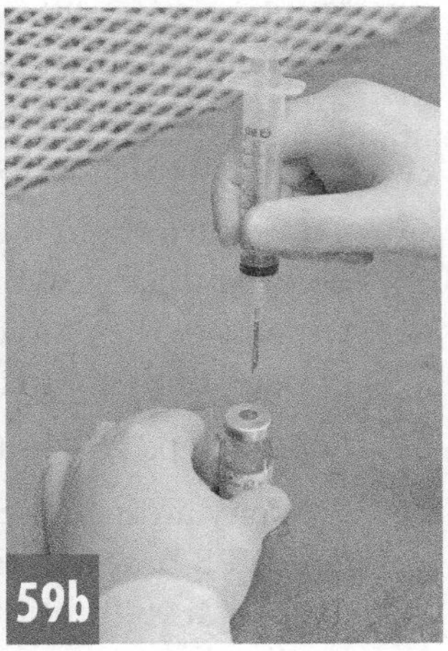
59b

60. Using the 3-mL syringe and a regular needle, repeat steps 18–21 to prepare the regular needle, 3-mL syringe, and diluted ampicillin vial for compounding.

61. Using your dominant hand, grasp the empty 3-mL syringe—with attached regular needle—at the barrel, as you would a dart. Hold the syringe steadily, and with your nondominant hand, remove the needle cap by pulling it carefully but firmly off of the needle. Place the needle cap, with the open end pointing toward the HEPA filter, on top of the alcohol swab on the hood's work surface.

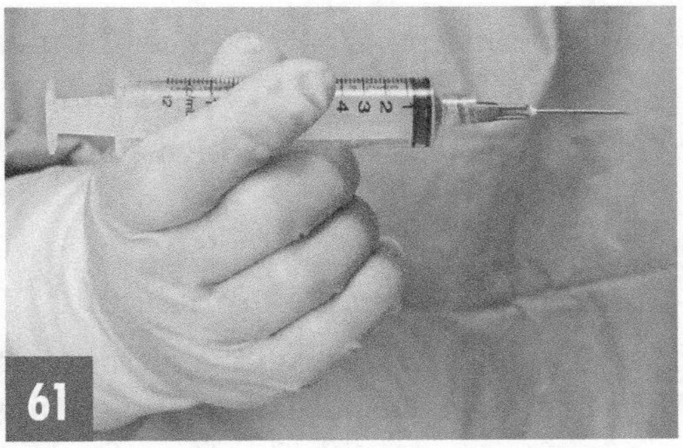
61

62. Use your fingers to rotate the barrel of the syringe so that the bevel of the needle is pointed up toward the ceiling.

63. Using your nondominant hand, brace the diluted ampicillin vial against the hood's work surface. Lay the tip of the needle, bevel up, onto the center of the vial's rubber top.

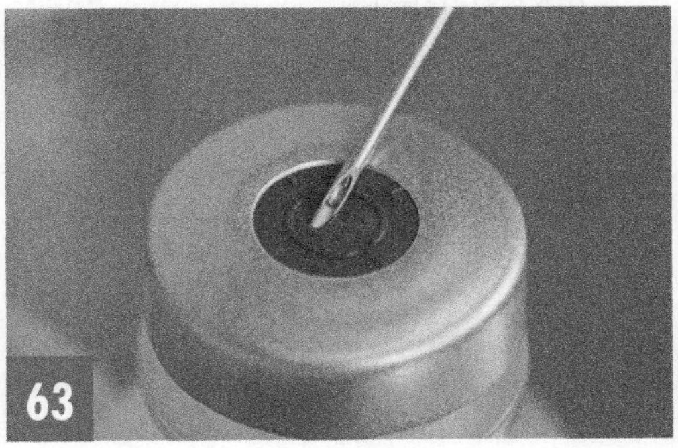
63

64. Insert the needle into the vial using a slight upward rotation of the wrist (rotating in a counterclockwise direction if you are right-handed, and in a clockwise direction if you are left-handed). Keep the tip of the needle in contact with the vial's rubber top at all times. There should be a slight, almost imperceptible bend to the needle as it enters the vial.

**POINTER**

Take care to avoid inserting the regular needle into the hole left in the vial's rubber top by the vented needle, as that may lead to coring. Also, because the vial was previously vented by the vented needle, there is no need to add air to the vial or use the milking technique at this point in the procedure. Injecting air into a vial whose top has been previously punctured by a vented needle may lead to aspiration of fluid from the vial into the DCA.

**POINTER**
Take care to hold the vial and syringe so that the airflow to the critical area—the area from the tip of the syringe to the neck of the vial, including the entire needle and the vial's rubber top—remains unobstructed.

**65.** Hold the ampicillin vial with your nondominant hand and the syringe, with needle firmly inserted into the vial, with your dominant hand. Invert the vial, using a clockwise motion (a counterclockwise motion if you are left-handed), so that the needle-and-syringe unit is now below the vial.

**66.** Continue to hold the ampicillin vial with the thumb and forefinger of your nondominant hand. While holding the barrel of the syringe so that the needle tip remains in the ampicillin fluid within the vial, pull down on the flat knob of the plunger until approximately 3 mL of fluid has been drawn into the syringe.

**67.** Repeat steps 29–33 to draw up exactly 2.5 mL of ampicillin into the syringe.

**68.** Properly arrange the ampicillin syringe, used ampicillin vial, used diluent vial, and IVPB base solution bag for Scenario Two on the work surface of the hood to await a verification check by a pharmacist or your instructor. Position the medication order and CSP label in the outer six-inch zone, immediately in front of the CSP ingredients. *Note:* The medication order and CSP label must remain in their plastic bags until compounding procedures are complete.

**69.** Repeat steps 42–47 to inject the medication into the IVPB bag used for Scenario Two.

**70.** Repeat steps 48–49, which address the inspection and proper labeling of the IVPB bag.

### *Cleaning Up After the Procedures*

**71.** Place the waste from the discard pile and the used vials into the regular waste container. Dispose of any remaining used swabs and needle caps in the waste container as well. Then transfer the labeled CSPs and any remaining supply items from the hood into the transport vehicle and return the vehicle to the anteroom.

**72.** In the anteroom, complete the compounding procedures by using the permanent, felt-tip marker to record your initials in the proper location on both of the CSP labels.

**73.** Remove your PPE according to the standard protocol outlined in Chapter 6. Return any unused supply items to their proper locations.

**74.** Ask for a final verification check from the pharmacist or your instructor.

# Process Validation Checklist

*Your instructor will use the process validation checklist provided in Appendix D to evaluate your technique for this lab. In order to receive ACPE certification, and prior to making CSPs for patient use, you must correctly perform each component of the lab procedure. Review the Chapter 9 lab and thoroughly practice each of the steps prior to your evaluation.*

# Part 3: Assessment

## Chapter Summary

- Antimicrobial substances can be traced back to ancient civilizations of Africa, Asia, and Europe.
- Early cultures had a primitive understanding of the connection between mold and antibacterial activity.
- Scientists experimented with harmless bacteria and its effect on harmful, disease-causing bacteria.
- Alexander Fleming discovered that an extract of the mold *Penicillium* would destroy the bacteria *Staphylococcus aureus*.
- Howard Florey and Ernst Chain first produced the antibacterial medication penicillin, a wonder drug that was mass-produced and went on to save the lives of many individuals in the middle of the twentieth century.
- Abelardo Aguilar discovered a strain of *Streptomyces erythreus* in a soil sample; this bacterium was eventually isolated into the antibacterial substance erythromycin.
- SVP products such as IVPBs were created to safely administer certain medications directly into the bloodstream.
- SVPs, particularly IVPBs, are primarily used to administer IV antibiotic medications.
- IVPBs are intermittent IV infusions of medications diluted in small volumes (ranging from 25 mL to 250 mL) of a base solution such as NS or $D_5W$.
- To reconstitute a powdered drug vial, IV technicians calculate how much diluent must be drawn up for the reconstitution procedure.
- Once the powder has been reconstituted, sterile compounding personnel use the drug's final concentration to perform calculations to determine the drug's dosage volume.
- The milking technique and the use of a vented needle are two primary methods of diluting medication in a powdered drug vial.
- The milking technique is used to aid withdrawal of a liquid from a vial.
- When using the milking technique, an IV technician injects an amount of air (or liquid, if diluting a powder) equal to, or slightly less than, the volume needed to be drawn up. Failure to add enough air to the vial may create a negative pressure environment that will make withdrawal of fluid from the vial difficult. Adding too much air to the vial may create excessive positive pressure within the vial, causing the drug to leak or aspirate into the sterile compounding environment.
- A vented needle is used to relieve air pressure while simultaneously reconstituting a powder within a vial.
- A vented needle is used only for drug reconstitution, never for fluid withdrawal.
- IV technicians should follow the standard aseptic protocol presented in the Sterile Compounding Area Procedures list located at the end of the Unit 2 opener on pages 162–163.

# Key Terms

**allergic reaction** an undesired immune system response to a substance such as an antibiotic; mild allergic reactions include hives and itching; a potentially fatal allergic reaction is called *anaphylaxis* and is characterized by tongue or throat swelling and respiratory distress

**aluminum needle sheath** a small, aluminum ring that encircles the vented needle and is firmly seated into the vial's rubber top, thereby allowing air to vent around the needle and out of the vial

**anaphylaxis** a potentially life-threatening allergic reaction

**antibacterial drug** a drug that is used to kill or inhibit the growth of bacteria

**antibiotic drug** a class of drugs used to treat various bacterial or fungal infections

**antibiotic-resistant bacteria** bacteria that have evolved to the point of being resistant to known antibiotic therapy; a superbug such as MRSA, CRKP, or NDM-1

**antimicrobial** an agent capable of killing or inhibiting the growth of various microorganisms

**caustic** burning, corrosive, or destructive to living tissue; a characteristic of some drugs when injected undiluted directly into muscles or veins

**concentrated form** a sterile, injectable medication that has been reconstituted from a powdered form to a liquid form

**continuous infusion** an LVP solution (with or without additives) administered intravenously to provide hydration and electrolytes; a maintenance or hydration infusion of IV fluids

**desired concentration** a drug manufacturer's predetermined ratio of what a powdered drug's concentration will be after reconstitution

**diluent** an agent used to reconstitute or dissolve a powdered drug so that it may be injected into an IVPB for IV administration

**dosing interval** the prescriber-determined schedule for intermittent administration of a medication; the frequency schedule provided on a medication order that the pharmacy must include on a CSP label; dosing schedule for medication administration

**erythromycin** a broad-spectrum, macrolide antibiotic synthesized from the fungus *Streptomyces erythreus*

**final concentration** a ratio giving the quantity of drug contained in a certain volume of solution; typically stated in milligrams per milliliter (mg/mL); may also be called the drug's *concentration*

**flush** the quantity of NS or other solution used to clear an IV line

**gram-negative organism** a bacterial organism characterized by a thin cell wall; common gram-negative bacteria include *Spirochetes* and *Neisseria*

**gram-positive organism** a bacterial organism characterized by a thick cell wall; common gram-positive bacteria include *Streptococcus, Staphylococcus, Bacillus, Clostridium, Corynebacterium*, and *Listeria*

**heparinized saline solution** a solution comprised of 0.9% sodium chloride with a certain amount of heparin added, such as 10 units/mL; used to flush lock sites or IV lines, thus preventing the formation of blood clots in the heparin lock or IV tubing

**heparin lock** a temporary injection port attached to a flexible needle maintained in the patient's vein; see also *saline lock*

**incompatibility** an undesired situation created when two or more solutions or ingredients separate or develop a precipitate when mixed in the same container such as an IV bag or tubing

**intermittent infusion** the infusion of a parenteral medication, such as an IVPB antibiotic, administered over a short period (10–60 minutes) according to a prescribed time schedule (for example, *q6h, bid, q8h*, etc.)

**intravenous piggyback (IVPB)** a way to administer SVP medications; so named because the medication is usually given on top of, or through, an existing IV line and in addition to the primary IV solution; a method of intermittent infusion

**mechanism of action** the biochemical process by which a drug produces its effect on the body (for instance, by inhibiting an enzyme, activating a certain cellular receptor site, etc.)

**microbe** a microscopic, pathogenic organism such as a bacterium

**microorganism** a microscopic organism

**milking technique** a process of adding a small amount of air or liquid to a vial to create a relatively positive pressure, thus aiding in the withdrawal of fluid from the vial

**nephrotoxicity** a condition of kidney damage resulting from certain drugs or drug doses

**opportunistic infection** an infection that results when a nonpathogenic organism becomes pathogenic due to certain circumstances (such as an impaired immune system)

**pathogenic organism** an organism that causes disease; a bacterium, fungus, virus, or other microscopic organism that causes human disease

**penicillin** any of a large group of antibiotics derived from fungi that belong to the genus *Penicillium*

**Petri dish** a round, shallow, flat-bottomed, straight-sided glass or plastic dish and the similar but slightly larger dish that forms its cover; when filled with a solid growth medium such as agar, it is used to culture microorganisms

**positive pressure** a pressure greater than that of the atmosphere of the surrounding environment; positive pressure within a vial is employed when using the milking technique to withdraw fluid from a vial

**powdered drug** a parenteral drug in powdered form that must be reconstituted before administration

**precipitate** a substance that settles out of a solution in the form of solid particles

**prophylactic antibiotic treatment** antibiotic treatment administered prior to surgery to prevent infection

**razor tip** the type of nonbeveled needle tip found on a vented needle

**reconstitute** to transform a powdered parenteral drug into an injectable liquid through the addition of an appropriate diluent

**saline lock** a flexible needle, cannula, or catheter that provides access to a patient's vein or bloodstream; a place where certain parenteral medications are administered intravenously

**small-volume parenteral (SVP) preparation** a parenteral solution of relatively small volume, usually from 25 to 250 mL; typically administered as an IVPB; lesser-used SVPs such as those administered by IM, Sub-Q, or IVP injection typically range in volume from 0.1 mL to 10 mL

**standard IV base solution** a flexible plastic or polyvinyl chloride bag containing a relatively small volume of solution such as NS, ½ NS, or $D_5W$ and having a tail injection port

***Staphylococcus aureus*** a type of pathogenic, gram-positive bacterial microorganism

**Stevens-Johnson syndrome** rare, often drug-induced, condition in which the skin blisters and may slough off

**streptomycin** a bacteriocidal antibiotic produced by the soil-dwelling bacterium *Streptomyces griseus*

**sulfonamide** a class of antibiotics derived from a sulfur compound

**superbug** a pathogenic organism resistant to known antibiotic treatments; an antibiotic-resistant microorganism such as MRSA, CRKP, and NDM-1

**surface disinfectant** a cleaning agent such as that found in presaturated, aseptic cleaning wipes used in the anteroom; an antimicrobial agent such as soap, or various alcohol, bleach, or peroxide-based surface cleaning agents

**tissue necrosis** the death of living tissue caused by fluid injection or leakage of a caustic, hypertonic, or hyperosmotic IV solution into tissue surrounding the vein

**vented needle** a needle designed to vent (release) air from a vial at the same time liquid is added; may be used instead of the milking technique to add diluent to a powdered drug vial

**wonder drug** a medication that can completely eradicate disease without harming the patient

## CHECK THE BASICS

*On a separate sheet of paper, write your answers as modeled in these examples:* 1d; 2c; 3b; *etc.*

**1.** What is the term commonly used to refer to parenteral medications that must be reconstituted prior to use?

a. powdered drug
b. reconstituted drug
c. diluted drug
d. liquid drug

**2.** In order to reconstitute a powder for parenteral use, an IV technician must determine the amount of diluent needed to provide which of the following?

a. the desired dosage
b. the concentrated formula
c. the desired concentration
d. the diluted form

**3.** The final concentration of a reconstituted drug is often provided on the drug's label using which of the following ratios?

a. mL/mg
b. mg/L
c. mg/mL
d. mg/m²

**4.** In Scenario One, what method is used to create positive pressure within the vial during reconstitution?

a. the venting technique
b. the milking technique
c. the use of a vented needle
d. the use of a vented needle and the milking technique

**5.** Which of the following includes all of the critical sites that must not be touched or shadowed during SVP preparation?

a. the needle cap, alcohol swab packet, vial top, and syringe package
b. the needle package, syringe, vial, and alcohol swab
c. the needle, syringe tip, vial top, and IVPB injection port
d. the needle, syringe, alcohol swab, and IVPB bag

**6.** In Scenario Two, what method is used to vent air pressure from the ampicillin vial during reconstitution?

a. the venting technique
b. the milking technique
c. the use of a vented needle
d. the use of a vented needle and the milking technique

**7.** What is the most appropriate syringe size for drawing up the sterile water diluent volume of 5.5 mL?

a. 3 mL
b. 5 mL
c. 10 mL
d. 20 mL

**8.** What is the most appropriate syringe size for drawing up the volume of ampicillin needed for the CSP in Scenario Two?

a. 3 mL
b. 5 mL
c. 10 mL
d. 20 mL

**9.** Which critical site(s) must be swabbed with alcohol prior to injection during SVP preparation?

a. the vial top
b. the injection port of the IVPB bag
c. neither *a* nor *b*
d. both *a* and *b*

**10.** Prior to labeling the IVPB, an IV technician must check for which of the following issues?

a. leakage from the IVPB bag
b. precipitate formation
c. evidence of incompatibility
d. all of the above

## Make Connections

*On a separate sheet of paper, write your answers to the following three questions, using complete sentences and making sure your answers are thorough and thoughtful. Note that the third question requires Internet access.*

1. The introductory information presented in this chapter discussed the potential danger of bacterial infections. In addition, earlier chapters presented information about the importance of aseptic technique in preventing infection caused by contaminated CSPs. Do you think that bacterial infections could be generated or transmitted by a contaminated CSP? If so, how might that happen?

2. What is the rationale for using different reconstitution and venting methods in different compounding scenarios?

3. Use any Internet search engine to search for *types of bacterial infections*. List at least two types of bacterial infections. Name at least one drug used in the treatment of each of these bacterial infections.

## Meet the Challenge

***Scenario*** This "venting" activity will give you the opportunity to experiment with the use of a vented needle to inject multiple vials from a single syringe.

***Challenge*** Your instructor has a handout outlining the supplies and steps for an activity involving the proper handling of a vented needle. This procedure allows you to experience the benefits and, possibly, the difficulties of using a vented needle during the sterile compounding process. To meet this challenge, ask your instructor for the handout and give it a try, either as an individual, in small groups, or as a class.

### ADDITIONAL RESOURCES

*Go to the Paradigm Internet Resources Center at* www.paradigmcollege.net/sterilecomp *to access live links related to these Chapter 9 topics:*

- Resources for scientific, medical, and biomedical literature
- Information on the prevention of bacteria transmission from the Centers for Disease Control and Prevention
- List of anti-infective pharmaceuticals

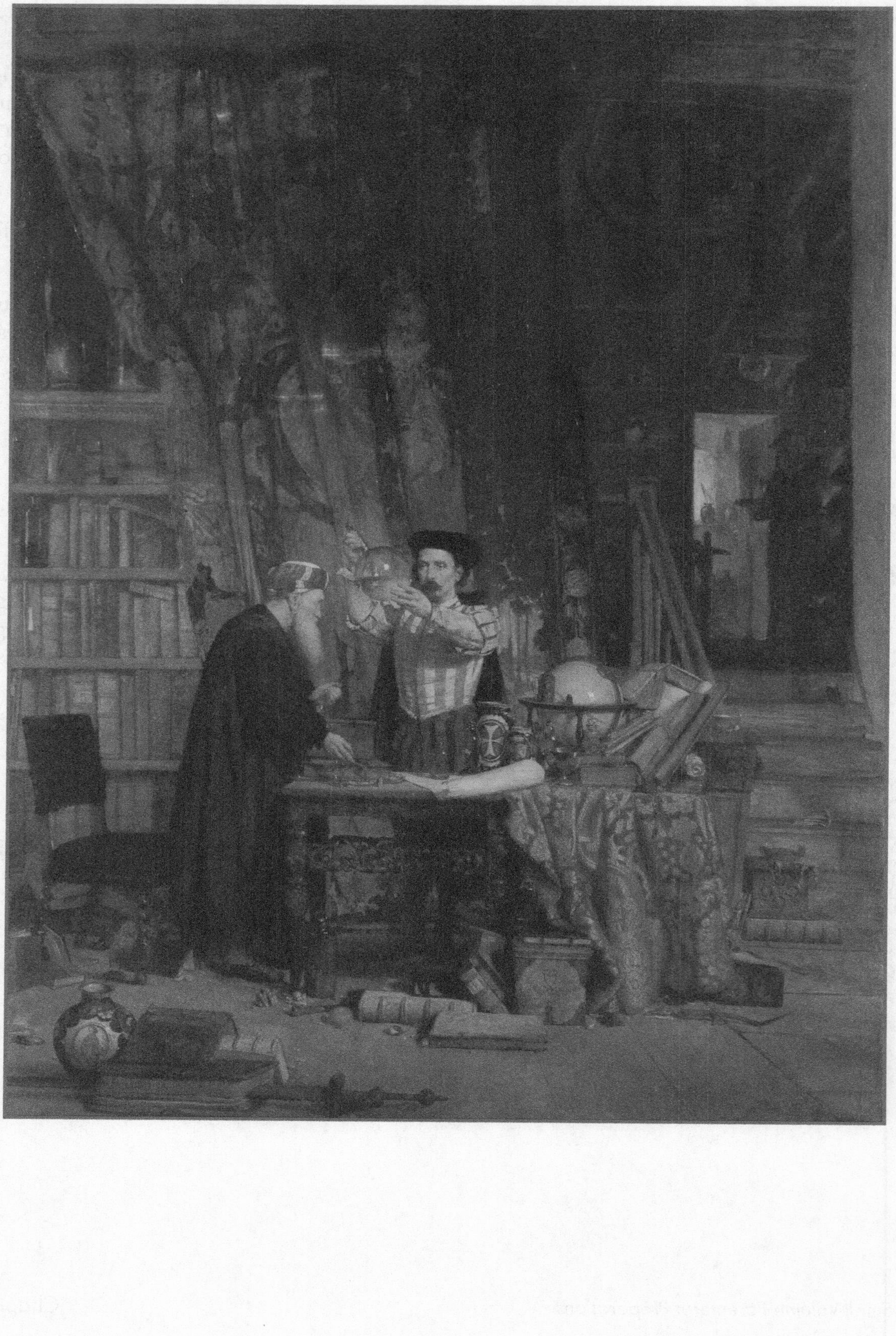

# Chapter 10

# Ampule-Based Preparations

## Learning Objectives

- Gain an awareness of the history of ampules.
- Understand the identifying characteristics of ampules and their purpose in sterile compounding procedures.
- Identify the USP Chapter <797> procedures that must be performed during the compounding of ampule-based preparations.
- Demonstrate excellent aseptic technique in the compounding of ampule-based preparations.
- Recognize the safety issues associated with the opening of ampules.

The **ampule**—sometimes spelled *ampoule* or *ampulla* and commonly referred to as an *amp*—is a small, hermetically sealed container with a distinct, elongated neck. Typically made of glass, ampules are primarily used to store sterile parenteral medications that are incompatible with certain physical and chemical properties of vials. Although modern ampules contain medications commonly used in sterile compounding procedures, these tubular containers have a long and colorful history and, over the centuries, have held fluids more precious than medications.

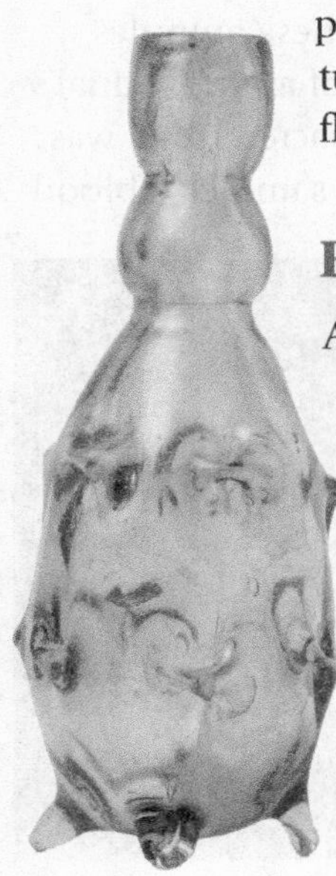

### Early Prototypes of Ampules

Ampules date back to the earliest recorded history, when they were used in various religious ceremonies and burial rituals. The modern ampule possibly evolved from the **tear bottles** (sometimes called *lachrymatories*) of ancient Roman and Middle Eastern societies. These small bottles, found in huge numbers by archaeologists during the excavations of tombs, are believed to have been filled with the tears of mourners, sealed with stone stoppers, and buried with the dead. This ancient rite paid homage to the deceased—the tear bottles symbolizing the love and respect of the mourners. Because the number of tear bottles that accompanied the cadaver indicated the perceived importance of the individual, the wealthy and important members of society may have even hired mourners to attend burial ceremonies for their families and friends. The more passionate grievers who filled the bottles with the most tears would receive the highest compensation from their employers. In fact, the use of tear bottles for moments of grief or mourning has been documented up through the Civil War, when soldiers departing for duty left their wives small ampules that they hoped would be full of tears—symbols of their wives' undying devotion—when they returned. These old tear bottles bear a striking resemblance to the modern tear-shaped ampules used today in the healthcare field.

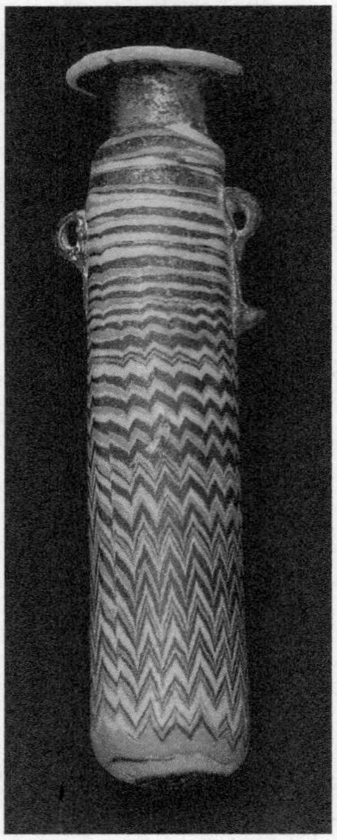

Early cultures used ceremonial ampules for more than just tears. Archaeological expeditions in the Middle East have uncovered ampules containing medicinal oils, perfumes, and cosmetics entombed with ancient pharaohs and other members of the ruling elite. A part of the religious practice of bringing their worldly goods to the underworld, these ampules were filled with the finest substances and sealed tightly to be used in the afterlife. In these early cultures, burial offerings served several purposes for the deceased: They made eternal life similar to the time spent on earth; they provided protection from evil spirits; and they held healing powers for any ailments suffered in the afterlife.

One cosmetic, kohl, was particularly important to Egyptians. This ancient make-up was made by grinding galena, a bluish-gray mineral, and then mixing the powdered residue with soot. Once the process was complete, an individual would use a stick to apply the kohl around the rims of the upper and lower eyelids. Outlining the eyes with this black powder offered the wearer protection from the harsh sun and served as a deterrent to flies—two environmental factors that affected the health of the region's inhabitants. Consequently, kohl was considered to have magical healing powers and was frequently entombed as a personal possession to accompany the body of the deceased into the afterlife. The substance was contained in a kohl flask, similar to the one pictured here, and its characteristic elongated shape was an early prototype of the modern-day ampule.

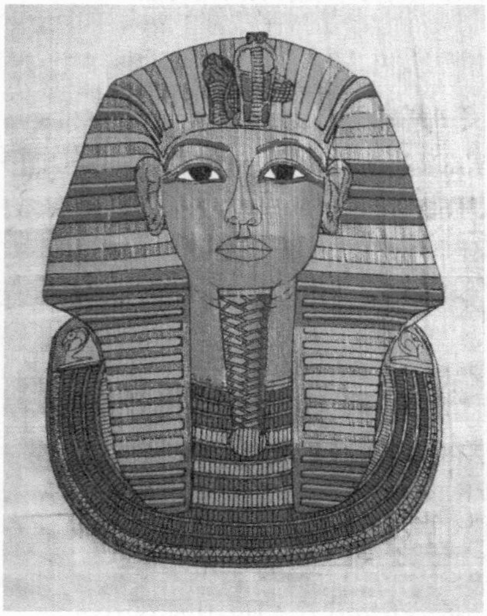

## Ampule Legends

Over the centuries, ampules have housed precious liquids that, according to Eastern Mediterranean legends, offered miracle cures for the ailments of humankind. Ampules containing a substance called red (or pharaonic) mercury have been found in royal Egyptian tombs. According to early Arab medicine and alchemy, this magical substance—a cure for all ailments and an essential ingredient for the transmutation of lesser metals into gold—possessed the physical characteristics of mercury but changed colors and retained a singular form even if spilled. Like the Holy Grail and the Fountain of Youth, this mythical cure inspired many adventurers and thieves to spend their entire lives hunting for this hidden treasure and dreaming of its supernatural rewards.

Similar to Egyptian tombs, Roman catacombs containing the remains of ancient Christians have been found lined with small ampules. These ampules were used to preserve a few drops of an individual's blood after death. Originally, this sacred ritual was performed with holy martyrs—the sample of blood symbolizing their sacrifice to the benefit of humankind. To honor this ancient Roman tradition, citizens of Naples, Italy, annually place an ampule thought to be filled with the dried blood of Saint Januarius (San Gennaro), a fourth-century bishop of Benevento, next to his silver bust likeness

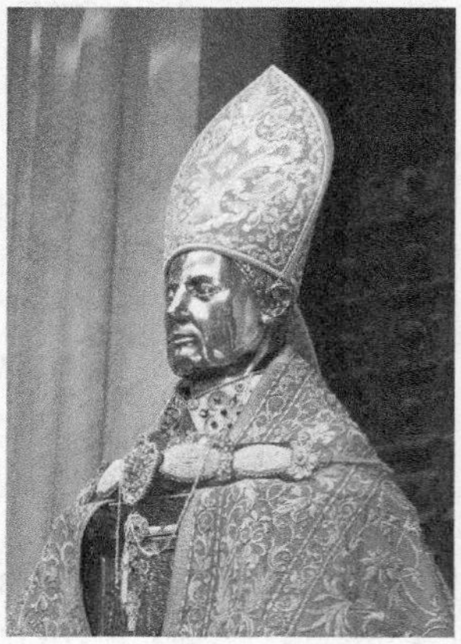

in the Naples Cathedral. This ritual, called the "Blood Miracle of San Gennaro," draws thousands of people who make the pilgrimage to witness the liquefaction of the dried blood in the unopened ampule. The 170-year-old blood miracle remains one of the great mysteries of the world.

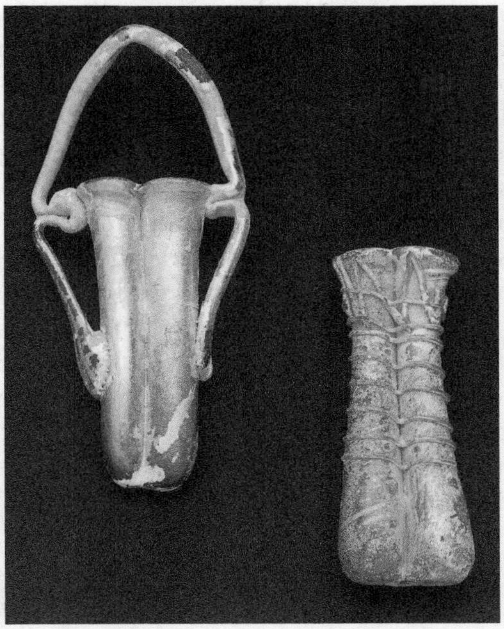

Pilgrims visiting holy sites in the Middle Ages often carried lead or glass ampules to store consecrated oils or other fluids while traveling. Terracotta was also a popular material for the mass production of ampules—such as the ones found at Abu Menas, the ruins of a town and monastery complex in Egypt. This area served as a popular pilgrimage site for Christians between the fourth and seventh centuries who came to see the burial grounds of the famous martyr Menas (often spelled Minas) of Alexandria. Buried in an unknown desert location for hundreds of years, his body was reportedly found after an injured lamb lay on the spot and was healed. Soon the area was renowned for miraculous healing of the hopelessly sick, even attracting the daughter of a ruling emperor, who suffered from severe leprosy. During the night, she had a vision of St. Menas, who informed her of the location of his body. She woke up, completely healed, and told her father about her vision. Consequently, the emperor ordered that the martyr's body be exhumed and a cathedral built upon the sacred ground. The cathedral became the center of a sprawling city, with the site becoming a popular destination for the sick and dying in search of a cure. Many pilgrims would purchase the relatively cheap stone ampules, known as Menas ampules, to store holy water or oil that dripped from lamps within the monastery.

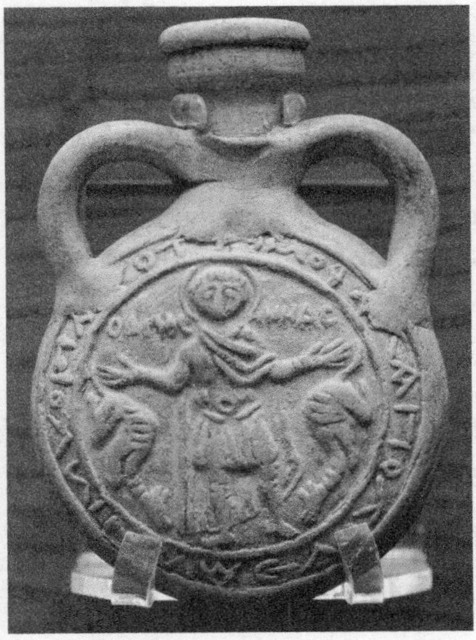

## Evolution of Medication Ampules

Ampules developed in the Roman Empire served more practical purposes. They were made larger and more durable, from thicker glass or strong clay, and stored and transported large quantities of perfumed oils and liquid ointments. These ancient perfume bottles, shown above, were known as **unguentaria**, and some modern perfume bottles still retain the elongated neck and round base that characterized these early ampules.

Over the centuries, ampule prototypes retained their characteristic long necks. However, their size diminished as these flasks were used to both hold and, sometimes, measure precise amounts of medications. For example, medication-filled ampules were common items in a field medic's bag during military conflicts. Due to their small size and ease of portability, these ampules were carried onto battlefields, where a reliable form of transport for medicines was critical to a soldier's survival.

During the Civil War, ampules containing morphia (morphine) were used to alleviate the pain of wounded soldiers during treatment and transport.

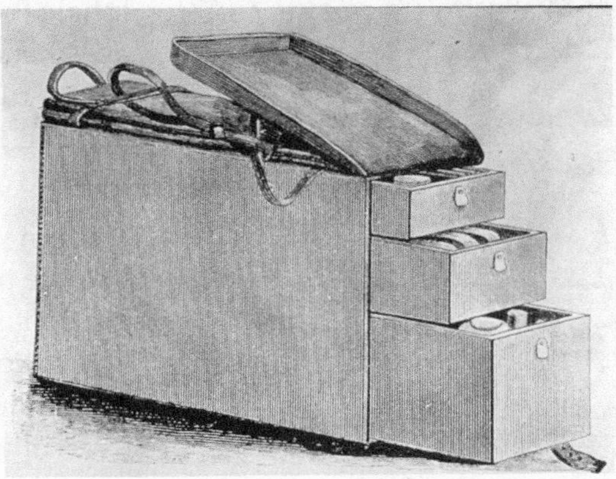

Allegedly, after the war was over, more than 400,000 soldiers became addicted to the pain-relieving effects of morphine—so much so that the term *soldier's disease*, referring to a morphine addiction, became part of the medical lexicon. (However, this claim of widespread addiction has been a subject of controversy.) In addition to morphine, ampules containing chloroform, an anesthetic, were used during Civil War field amputations. The chloroform ampules were crushed, releasing anesthetic vapors that would induce an altered state of consciousness in the wounded. After the Civil War, the use of medication-filled ampules on battlefields continued into the next century, as wartime medical personnel relied on its practical applications in difficult situations.

## Modern Glass Ampules

As medicine evolved and became standardized during the nineteenth century, physicians and pharmacists had a greater need to preserve and transport sensitive medications that were subject to mold and deterioration. In response to that need, French pharmacist Stanislas Limousin invented the modern glass ampule with a breakable head in 1886. Limousin filled an open container with medication and then fused a thin piece of glass to its opening, thereby sealing the container. This process formed an airtight closure that could easily be broken, allowing access to the container's contents. The sealed ampules became popular among traveling physicians, who used them to carry injectable solutions or inhalant sedatives and anesthetics such as ether and chloroform. Inhalation ampules were also popular with midwives in the first half of the twentieth century. The midwives would crush the gauze- or cotton-wrapped ampules, allowing the release of chloroform fumes into the air. Expectant mothers would then inhale the anesthetic vapors to dull the senses.

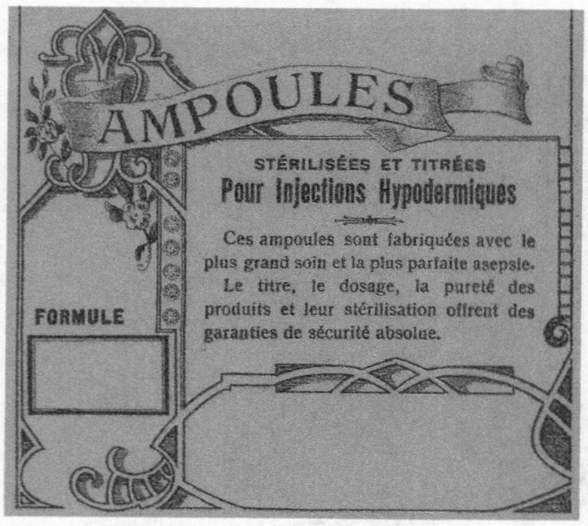


Modern ampule production is now a worldwide industry. While some smaller-scale labs still fill and seal ampules by hand, most pharmacies, labs, and hospitals rely on drug manufacturing companies that utilize large, automated production lines to efficiently and consistently package sterile medications in ampules. Large machines along an assembly line in a sterile manufacturing plant fill the short lengths of glass tubing, then rotate the tubing as the top is formed with gas torches (bearing a high-temperature oxygen flame) and the base of the neck is slightly grinded to create a fragile area for snapping. The ampule must be rotated evenly to ensure a symmetrical and consistently strong seal. Before the ampule is finally sealed, a stream of inert gas, such as nitrogen or carbon dioxide, is sometimes injected to displace all remaining air within the container and therefore prevent decomposition of the ampule's contents. The seal is then immediately created, usually by melting glass at the tip of the ampule's neck to close the opening (tip sealing) or by heating the neck and slowly pulling or stretching it as the ampule rotates (pull sealing).

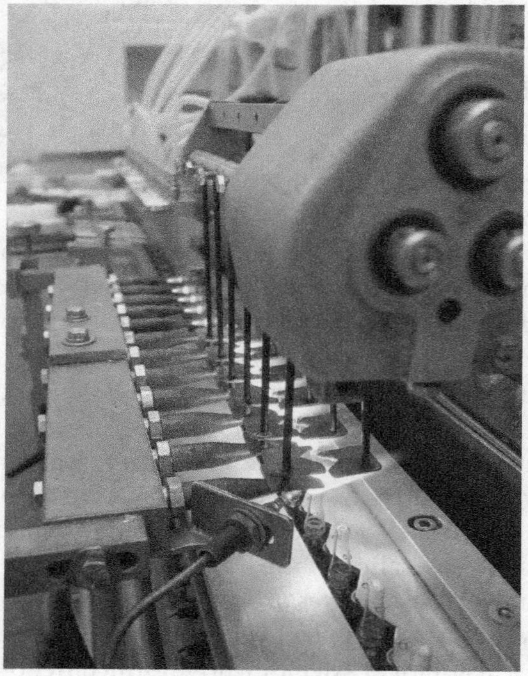

Today's ampules provide a simple and effective storage system for sterile parenteral medications and therefore are frequently used in the sterile compounding process. Consequently, IV technicians and pharmacists need to be familiar with the components and contents of ampules as well as the guidelines for their safe handling.

# Part 1: Concepts

Ampules are made from thin, medical-grade glass tubing and are manufactured as sterile containers for specific medications, many of which are incompatible with the rubber or PVC components found in most vials. During the manufacturing process, the medication (either in a liquid or powdered form) is placed into the glass tube, and then the top is melted to form a hermetic seal. The application of intense heat combined with the pull of gravity creates the ampule's unique elongated shape.

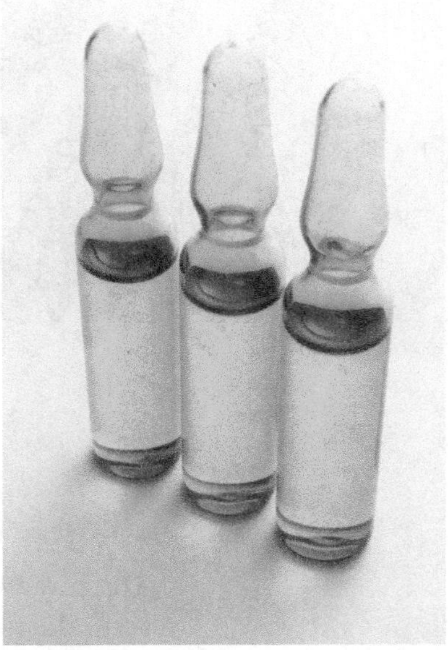

Medication ampules.

## Opening of Ampules

An ampule is designed so that the neck is either scored or made of thinner glass, called a **break ring**. To open an ampule, an IV technician applies pressure to either the scored area or the break ring of the tapered neck, which breaks off the head of the ampule. Once the ampule is opened, and prior to injecting the medication into the compounded sterile preparation (CSP), the solution must be filtered by passing it through a single-direction **filter needle**. This specialty needle removes any minute glass fragments that may have fallen into the ampule's fluid during the opening process.

It is essential to the safety of both patients and healthcare personnel to carefully follow aseptic technique protocol when opening and using ampules, and to properly filter all ampule medications during sterile compounding procedures.

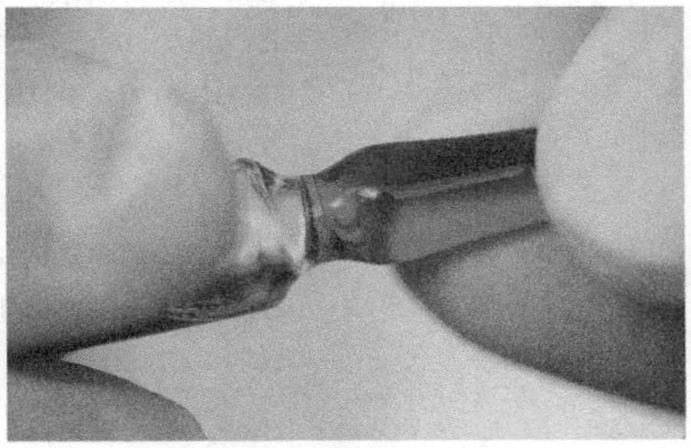

Break ring of an ampule.

## Contents of Ampules

Ampules most often contain sterile medications, such as promethazine or epinephrine, for parenteral administration. Occasionally, ampules contain a sterile powdered medication that requires the IV technician to reconstitute the powder with a sterile diluent prior to drawing it up into a syringe for parenteral administration. However, the vast majority of ampules for parenteral use contain a liquid, injectable medication that may be withdrawn from the ampule into a syringe. Therefore, all subsequent references to ampules in this chapter discussion refer to ampules containing liquid medications.

In general, ampule medications range in volume from as little as 1 mL to as much as 20 mL. The fragile nature of the glass ampule renders it incapable of safely storing larger fluid volumes. For the most part, the medication contained within a single ampule is sufficient to provide the necessary dose for a single intravenous piggyback (IVPB) or IV drip. Occasionally, due to the patient's size or condition, a larger dose is required, which then necessitates the use of two or more ampules to provide the dose needed for a single CSP.

**POINTER**

Occasionally, you may encounter an ampule whose neck is not scored. For this type of ampule, the drug manufacturer supplies a thin, metal file that you will use to gently score the ampule neck. Score the neck evenly around its entire circumference. Once you have scored the ampule neck, follow standard procedures for opening the ampule and withdrawing the medication.

## Administration of Ampule-Based Preparations

Ampule-based preparations may be administered by intramuscular (IM) injection or, more often, intravenously. For the latter administration route, a medication from an

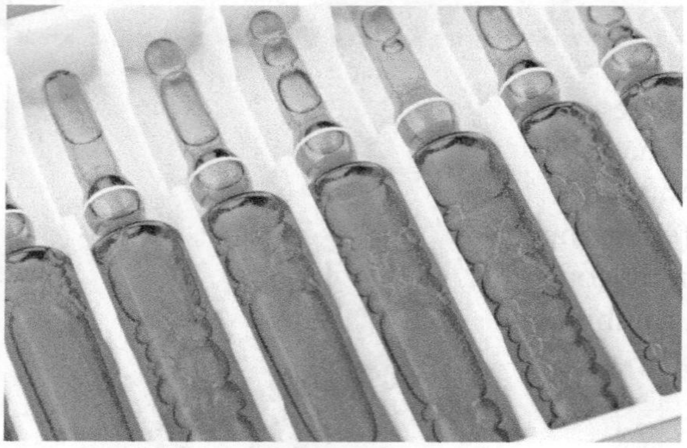

Container of fluid-filled ampules.

ampule is injected into an IV or IVPB base solution. The resulting CSP is then administered to the patient intravenously, according to a specific administration rate or dosing schedule ordered by the prescriber. The majority of ampule-based CSPs are IVPBs. Similar to IVPBs prepared from medications supplied in vials, those prepared from medications supplied in ampules are also administered by piggybacking them through IV tubing attached to a primary IV solution, or through a heparin lock. Therefore, the pharmacy must consider the physical and chemical properties of ampule medications, including compatibility and stability, when determining the appropriate IVPB base solution and volume. (For assistance on determining IVPB base solution type and volume, see Chapter 9.)

## Properties of Ampule Medications

The physical and chemical properties of ampule medications vary widely. Some ampule medications have an acidic pH value, a higher osmotic pressure, or a higher tonicity (referred to as hypertonic medications). However, as is the case with vial medications, once the ampule medication is injected into an IVPB base solution, the resulting CSP has physical and chemical properties that are generally isotonic, isoosmotic, and pH neutral. In some circumstances, a parenteral medication that is neutral despite being diluted in an IVPB base solution will be administered over a long period—at a very slow rate—to avoid any and all potential problems related to phlebitis or other administration risks. For instance, the medication gentamicin, which is generally isotonic and pH neutral, is administered by IVPB over a period of at least 60 minutes to avoid potential problems due to **ototoxicity** or **nephrotoxicity**, which may result from rapid administration of the medication.

## Risks of Parenteral Preparations

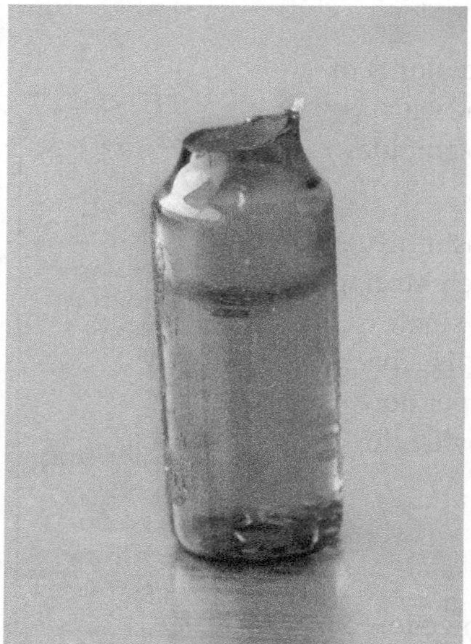

Glass shards inside an opened ampule.

Understanding the properties of parenteral products makes IV technicians aware of the potential risks associated with the preparation and administration of these solutions. Because parenteral medications circulate through the blood supply, the introduction of pathogens during sterile compounding can jeopardize the health and safety of patient recipients. Therefore, IV technicians must follow strict aseptic technique in the preparation of CSPs. (For more information on the preparation risks of CSPs, see Chapter 8.)

***Preparation Risks*** A preparation risk unique to ampule-based preparations is the presence of broken glass during the opening of an ampule. Broken glass can create a hazardous situation for both the patient and the IV technician. During the breaking process, minute shards of glass are commonly deposited in the contents of the ampule. Consequently, all ampule medications must be passed through a filter needle so that glass particles do not transfer into the CSP—a situation that would be harmful for patient recipients. Opening an ampule may also cause injury to the IV technician or create a dangerous work environment under the hood. Therefore, to reduce the risk of injury to sterile compounding personnel, special precautions must be followed when working with ampules. These precautions are discussed later in this chapter.

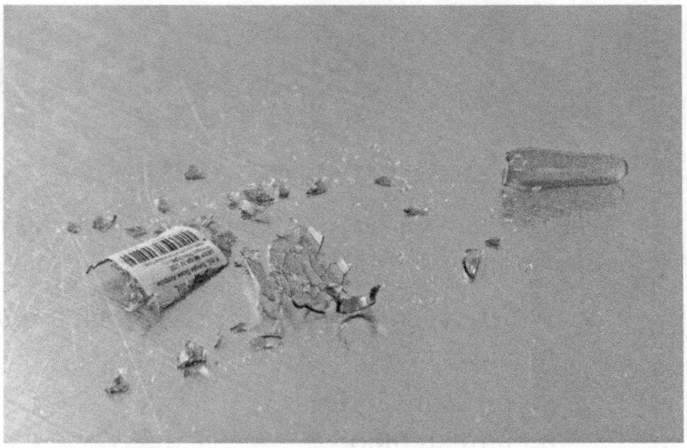

Improperly broken ampule on the hood surface.

***Administration Risks*** The administration of parenteral therapy involves potential complications that may lead to injury or, possibly, death for patient recipients. Therefore, *all* patients receiving parenteral fluids should be monitored for the following complications:

- nosocomial infection
- allergic reaction (including anaphylaxis)
- phlebitis
- tissuing
- embolism
- extravasation
- cellulitis
- Stevens-Johnson syndrome
- nephrotoxicity

CSPs prepared from ampules have similar preparation and administration risks as those prepared from vials. As is the case with all CSPs, the most common risks associated with ampule medications include phlebitis, allergic reaction, nosocomial infection, and medication-specific side effects, such as GI upset or drowsiness.

## USP Chapter <797> Guidelines for Ampule-Based Preparations

During preparatory and compounding procedures of ampules, the IV technician must adhere to the overarching principles set forth in USP Chapter <797>. These guidelines are reinforced in each facility's P&P manual. In accordance with these guidelines, sterile compounding personnel must pay strict attention to aseptic technique protocol both in the anteroom and clean room. Any breach in protocol may result in medication errors, sepsis, or, possibly, death for patient recipients. Therefore, as an IV technician, you bear primary responsibility for the preparation and integrity of the CSPs. With that in mind, only those personnel who have been specially trained, process validated, and certified in sterile product preparation and aseptic technique should be allowed to compound sterile preparations. Part 2 of this chapter guides you through the discovery and demonstration of proper aseptic technique when preparing liquid, injectable ampule medications for use in an IVPB.

# Concepts Self-Check

## Check Your Understanding

*Write your answers on a separate sheet of paper, as modeled in these examples:* 1d; 2c; 3b; *etc. Check your answers using the Answer Key in Appendix A.*

**1.** Which types of substances have been found in ancient ampules?
   a. medicinal oils
   b. human blood
   c. sterile medications
   d. all of the above
   e. only *a* and *b*

**2.** The unique shape of the ampule is created by employing which of the following elements?
   a. heat and gravity
   b. heat and light
   c. light and gravity
   d. gravity and positive pressure

**3.** Which of the following conditions is a risk unique to ampule preparations?
   a. ototoxicity
   b. exposure to broken glass
   c. nephrotoxicity
   d. exposure to pathogens

**4.** Which of the following statements is most true with regard to filtering an ampule-based preparation?
   a. A single-direction filter needle should be used.
   b. A bi-directional filter needle should be used.
   c. A single-direction HEPA filter should be used.
   d. A bi-directional HEPA filter should be used.

**5.** With regard to preparing ampules, which procedure is the most dangerous?
   a. transporting the ampule
   b. swabbing the ampule
   c. opening the ampule
   d. withdrawing medication from the ampule

## Apply Your Knowledge

*On a separate sheet of paper, write your answers to the questions posed in the paragraph below. Use complete sentences and take time to create a thorough and thoughtful response. Check your answers against the Answer Key in Appendix A.*

In Part 1 of this chapter, you learned that sterile compounding personnel must break open a glass ampule to access the medication it contains. With that in mind, how might the worker be affected by the incorrect opening or handling of an ampule? How might a patient be affected by the incorrect opening and handling of an ampule?

# Part 2: Training

*Before performing this lab, review the Sterile Compounding Area Procedures listed on pages 162–163 at the end of the Unit 2 opener, and preview the accompanying process validation checklist in Appendix D.*

## Understand the Resources and Supplies

USP Chapter <797> prescribes a number of special requirements for the preparation of ampule-based, small-volume parenteral products. This chapter and the corresponding lab provide supplies and procedures that are in alignment with the directives set forth in USP Chapter <797>.

### Essential Supplies

The vast majority of sterile compounding procedures require the same essential supply items to be available for use in both the anteroom and the clean room. For the anteroom, these supplies include a medication order and a CSP label; a standard calculator; a pen; a permanent, felt-tip marker; large and small plastic bags; aseptic garb; a sterile gown; presaturated, aseptic cleaning wipes; sterile, foamed 70% isopropyl alcohol (IPA); a waste container; and a transport vehicle. (Various other compounding supplies, such as those needed for aseptic hand washing and hood cleaning, are necessary supplies, but, for the purposes of this lab, are not included on the Essential Supplies list.) In the clean room, essential supply items include sterile, foamed 70% IPA; sterile, powder-free gloves; sterile 70% IPA swabs; a sharps container; a waste container; and a laminar airflow hood.

### Procedure-Specific Supplies

In addition to the previously listed essential supplies, each sterile compounding procedure requires supply items specific to the procedure being performed. The type, number, and amount of procedure-specific supply items are determined by the IV technician prior to performing the procedure, based on information provided on the CSP label and the medication additive label. After reading these labels, the IV technician performs one or more calculations that reveal the number and volume of additives needed to prepare the CSP. This information, in turn, dictates the number, size, and types of syringes needed for the procedure.

The process of compounding ampule-based preparations in this procedural lab involves the manipulation of regular needles and—in particular—an ampule, a filter needle (or filter straw or disc), and an IVPB base solution. Familiarity with the appearances of these items as well as any specific handling requirements is essential in sterile compounding procedures.

**POINTER**
Single-use containers are sometimes called single-dose vials (SDVs). SDVs may be either vials without preservatives, opened ampules, or syringes.

***Ampule*** The unique shape of the glass ampule makes the components of the ampule easy to identify. The base of the ampule, called the **ampule body**, is the largest portion of the ampule, and it is the area that contains the sterile fluid. The uppermost part of the ampule body, just before it starts to narrow, is sometimes referred to as the **ampule shoulder**. The narrowest portion of the ampule is the **ampule neck**, which must be broken in order to access the fluid within. The **ampule head** is the

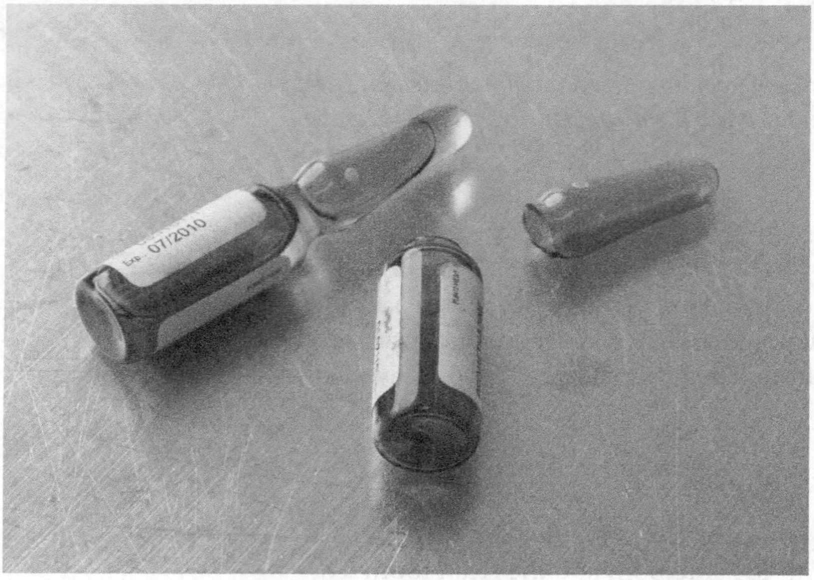

An unopened ampule next to a properly opened ampule.

small glass bulb located above the neck. Once the neck has been broken and the ampule head removed, the ampule is then considered to be an **open container** and should, therefore, be treated as a **single-use container**.

**Handling of an Ampule** An ampule preparation requires special handling considerations due to its packaging—a sealed glass container whose contents can only be accessed by breaking open the neck of the container. Therefore, it is imperative for sterile compounding personnel to open the ampule correctly, as glass shards from an improperly opened ampule may damage the HEPA filter, contaminate the hood's work surface or the contents of the ampule, and/or injure the worker.

There are a number of methods that IV technicians use to open an ampule safely. While employing these methods may seem to provide a certain degree of protection to the worker, these techniques may create more problems than they solve. For instance, some technicians prefer to place a piece of sterile gauze or a sterile 70% IPA swab over the neck of an ampule while it is being broken. However, using a piece of gauze prevents the worker from being able to see the ampule neck, which may result in improper hand placement during the breaking process and, ultimately, the potential for injury from broken glass. Using an IPA swab while breaking an ampule causes alcohol to seep onto the ampule's glass exterior, creating a slippery surface. As a result, the worker may not be able to maintain a firm grip on the ampule while opening it. In fact, anything placed over the neck of an ampule may potentially create touch or shadow contamination. Some IV technicians slip small plastic caps called **ampule breakers** over the heads of the ampules to safely open them. Ampule breakers provide a slight increase in worker safety, but they create additional expense, are not always readily available, and require additional time to use.

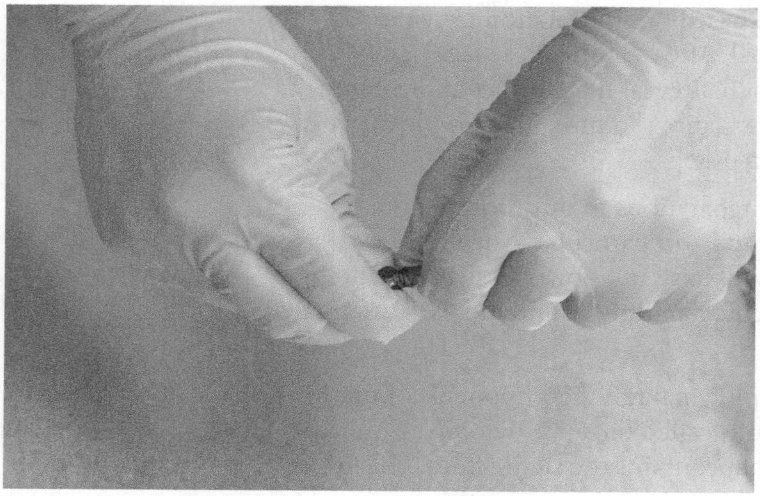
IV technician preparing to open an ampule.

Because of the risks just mentioned, many IV technicians prefer to simply open an ampule with their gloved hands. Provided the ampule is opened using proper aseptic technique—which is explained in detail in the procedural section of this chapter—this method is safe, efficient, and cost effective.

***Filter Needle and Filter Straw*** In addition to ampule-based preparations, some other compounding situations, such as total parenteral nutrition preparations, require that the medication or CSP be filtered prior to patient administration. There are a number of different filters—including filter needles, filter straws, and filter discs—that may be used during sterile compounding procedures. Each filter has a particular compounding situation for which it is most appropriately used. Refer to Chapters 3 and 13 of this textbook for information on filter types and the compounding situations in which they are used.

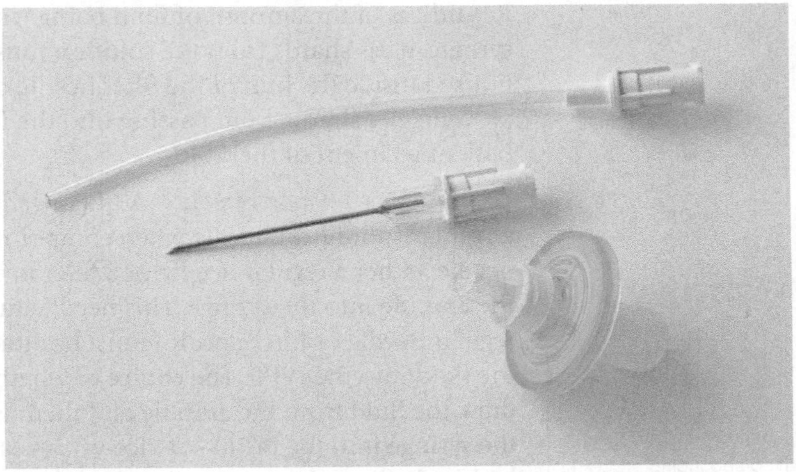

A filter straw, filter needle, and filter disc used in sterile compounding procedures.

When working with ampules, the type of filter most commonly used is a 5-micron filter needle. This type of needle looks exactly like a regular needle, except there is a small internal filter housed within the hub of the needle. A filter needle effectively removes particles, such as glass shards, that may have entered the ampule's contents when it was opened. Because of its unique design, a filter needle may only be used to either *withdraw* fluid from the ampule or *inject* the fluid from the syringe into a reservoir, such as an IV or IVPB. Therefore, this needle is commonly referred to as a single-direction filter needle.

**BE AWARE**

The single-direction filter needle may *not* be used to both withdraw and inject fluid.

When withdrawing a large amount of fluid (a volume greater than 5 mL) from an ampule, some IV technicians use a single-direction **filter straw**. This sterile, hollow, plastic tube attaches to a syringe and contains a 5-micron filter. As the IV technician withdraws fluid from the ampule through the filter straw into a syringe, glass shards are trapped in the filter. After the fluid has been withdrawn from the ampule and the filter straw has been removed from the syringe, a regular needle is attached to the syringe and the fluid may be injected into the IVPB.

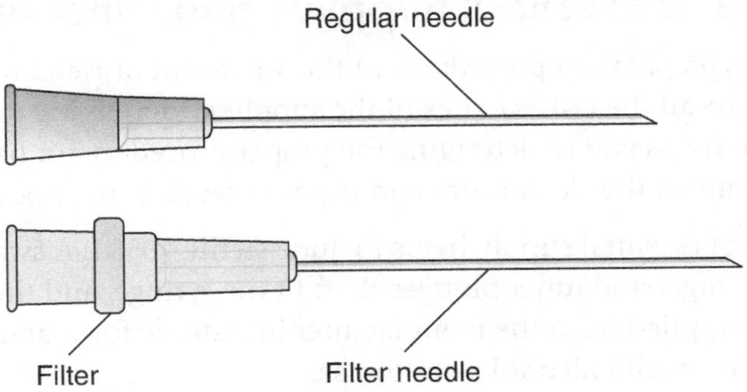


**FIGURE 10.1**

**Comparison of a Regular Needle and a Filter Needle**

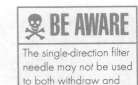

Regardless of the amount of fluid being withdrawn from the ampule into the syringe, glass shards from the solution must be trapped by the small internal filter housed inside the hub of the filter needle or filter straw. Using one of these devices prevents the shards from passing into the IVPB, which would be harmful to the patient recipient of the CSP.

**Handling of a Filter Needle** A filter needle is always used in conjunction with a regular (nonfilter) needle when compounding ampule-based preparations. One needle, either a regular needle or a filter needle, is used to withdraw the solution from the ampule into the syringe. This needle must then be removed, and a new needle (a regular needle or filter needle) must be attached to the syringe tip prior to injecting the fluid into the IVPB. The choice of whether to first use the regular needle to withdraw the fluid from the ampule and then use the filter needle to inject the fluid from the syringe into the IVPB—or vice-versa—is dependent upon the viscosity of the fluid within the ampule and the directives set forth within a facility's P&P manual. In general, sterile compounding personnel find it easier to use a regular needle to withdraw the medication from the ampule and a filter needle to expel the fluid from the syringe into the IVPB. Specifically, using a filter needle to withdraw a viscous solution from an ampule can be an arduous task: The thick fluid does not move well through the filter needle, making withdrawal difficult for the worker, and the fluid movement itself can create foam, skewing the true fluid measurement within the syringe.

**POINTER**

Some facilities prefer that the filter needle be used first, followed by a regular needle, during certain sterile compounding procedures. Refer to your facility's P&P manual for guidelines on the use of a filter needle.

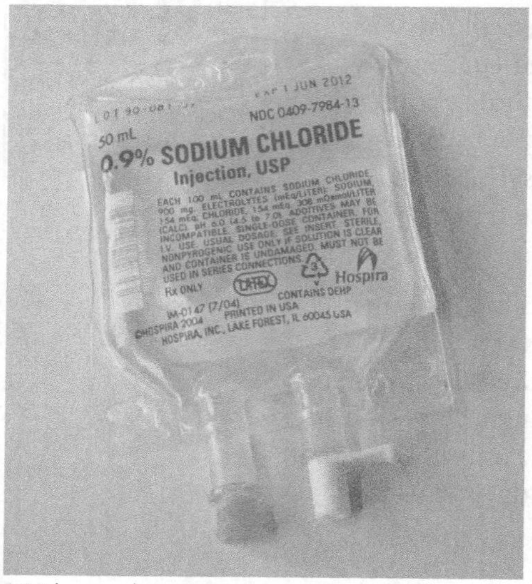


IVPB base solution.

The use of both a regular needle and a filter needle during the compounding of ampule-based preparations must be verified by an instructor or a pharmacist. To facilitate this verification check, it is best practice to place the used needle, once it has been capped and removed from the syringe tip, onto the hood's work surface—along with the ampule body, the filled and capped syringe, and the IVPB.

***IVPB Base Solution*** For ampule-based preparations, the IV technician uses an IVPB base solution bag with a tail injection port. Whether using a regular needle or a filter needle, the IV technician should insert the needle directly into the injection port without regard to the position of the needle bevel and without creating any bend to the needle.

## Critical Sites of Essential Supplies and Ampules

Before beginning preparatory procedures in the anteroom or clean room, the IV technician must recall the critical sites of the supplies. Identifying the critical site of each supply item helps you to determine the proper procedure for handling the item once you have entered the clean room and begin to work in the hood.

The critical sites of essential supply items include sterile 70% IPA swabs, the syringe tip, the piston plunger and inner plunger shaft of the syringe, and the needle. These critical sites are supplied from the manufacturer in a sterile form and should, therefore, not be swabbed with alcohol prior to use.

The critical sites of the procedure-specific supplies used for the Chapter 10 procedural lab include the injection port of the IVPB base solution, the ampule neck (the area swabbed prior to opening the ampule), and the opening into the body of the ampule after removing the head (see Figure 10.2). These critical sites must be swabbed with sterile 70% IPA prior to needle insertion to decrease the likelihood of contaminating the solution during injection or withdrawal procedures. In addition to these supplies, the Chapter 10 procedural lab also requires the use of a filter needle. Unlike the other procedure-specific supplies, the filter needle is provided from the manufacturer in a sterile form and therefore should never be swabbed with IPA.

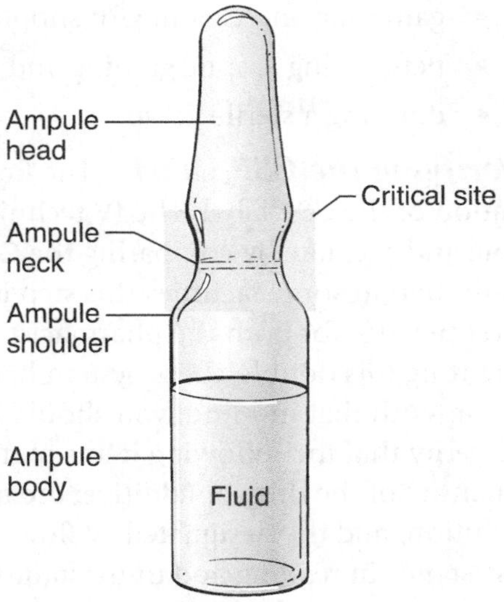


FIGURE 10.2

**Critical Site of a Glass Ampule**

After identifying the critical sites of all supply items, care must be taken not to taint the critical site of any supply item through touch contamination, shadowing, or incorrect placement of the item within the hood. (For additional assistance on the handling of critical sites of sterile compounding supplies, refer to Chapter 3 of this textbook.)

# Preview the Lab Procedure

*The following material provides a brief overview of the lab procedure that you will perform. First, read the* Preview the Lab Procedure *section. Then read each step of the* Procedural Lab *section carefully, visualizing every action. Next, reinforce your understanding of the process by watching the demonstration video. Once you are in the lab, your instructor will demonstrate the procedure, and then you will perform the procedure by following the steps in the* Procedural Lab *section. Practice the lab procedure multiple times. After sufficient practice, you will complete the lab procedure for process validation by your instructor.*

***Note:*** *This procedural lab requires the use of a basic, open-sided, horizontal laminar airflow hood. For pharmacies that do not have this type of hood, IV technicians should consult the* Instruction Guide *provided by the hood's manufacturer or their facility's P&P manual to determine which procedures may need to be adjusted to suit their hood.*

**POINTER**

Sterile compounding personnel must comply with certain restrictions when working in the anteroom and clean room areas. These restrictions include no gum chewing, horseplay, or food or drink in both the anteroom and clean room, and no hair spray, perfume, makeup, artificial or polished nails, or jewelry in the sterile compounding environment.

## Anteroom Preparatory Procedures

Because preparation for the sterile compounding process begins in the anteroom, that transition area provides a space for implementing the standard pharmacy protocols discussed in Chapters 3–6 of this textbook, including:

- verifying the CSP label against the medication order
- performing correct pharmacy calculations to determine type, size, and number of supply items needed

- gathering and cleaning of supplies
- performing aseptic garbing and hand washing
- donning a sterile gown

***Verifying the CSP Label*** The first step in the preparation of an IVPB is verification of the CSP label. The IV technician should check that the CSP label is legible and accurate by comparing the CSP label to the prescriber's medication order. Although in some facilities this step is performed by the pharmacist, it is considered best practice for both the pharmacist and IV technician to perform this task. Implementing this double-check system helps to reduce the likelihood of a medication error. With that in mind, you should compare the medication order to the CSP label to verify that the following items match exactly: the name, strength, and amount or quantity of the drug or additive; the name, concentration, and volume of the base solution; and the designated IV flow rate or administration time. (For additional assistance in reading and understanding medication orders, labels, and common abbreviations, refer to Chapter 4 and Appendix B of this textbook.)

***Performing Pharmacy Calculations*** Once you have verified the accuracy of the CSP label, you need to determine the type, size, and number of supply items needed for the procedure. Using information gleaned from the CSP label and the label on each medication or additive, calculate the desired volume of each additive or ingredient to be used in the procedure. The **desired volume** is the volume that you must withdraw from the ampule to deliver the dose ordered by the prescriber. (For additional assistance on performing calculations, refer to Chapter 5 of this textbook.)

***Gathering and Cleaning Supplies*** After performing the calculations, place the CSP label into a small plastic bag, place the medication order into a large plastic bag, and seal both bags. You should then gather the necessary supplies, including an appropriately sized syringe for the desired volume needed, and obtain a transport vehicle—such as a stainless-steel cart, basket, or a tray—to facilitate an easy transfer of supplies into and out of the clean room.

Wipe down or spray the exterior surface of every supply item, as well as the transport vehicle, with an appropriate cleaning agent. Place the cleaned supply items into the transport vehicle. (For additional assistance in gathering and cleaning supplies, refer to Chapter 8 of this textbook.)

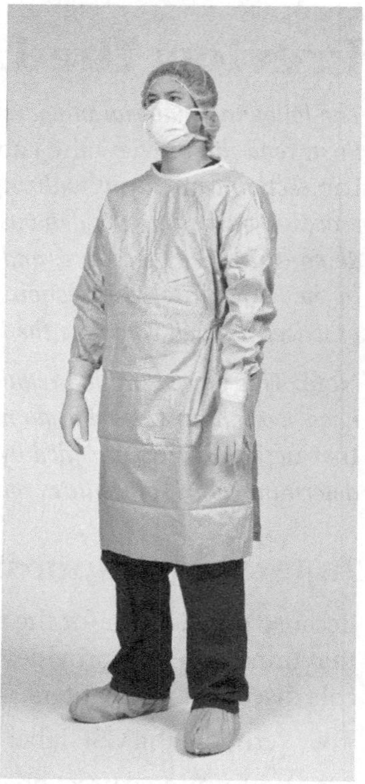

An IV technician wearing aseptic garb.

***Donning PPE*** Now that you have assembled your clean supplies, you must put on personal protective equipment (PPE). First, remove visible jewelry and ensure that you are properly attired for working in the clean room. Then put on aseptic shoe covers, a hair cover, a face mask, and, if appropriate, a beard cover. Lastly, don a sterile gown. (For additional assistance in aseptic garbing, refer to Chapter 6 of this textbook.)

Due to time constraints, you will not perform aseptic hand-washing procedures during this procedural lab. Keep in mind that, in sterile compounding practice, aseptic hand-washing procedures are mandatory and must be performed prior to donning a sterile gown.

## Clean Room Preparatory Procedures

When preparing ampule-based preparations for patient administration, sterile compounding personnel must diligently follow established pharmacy clean room protocols as well. These protocols, discussed in Chapters 6 and 7, include:

- cleansing hands with sterile, foamed 70% IPA
- donning sterile gloves
- cleaning the hood

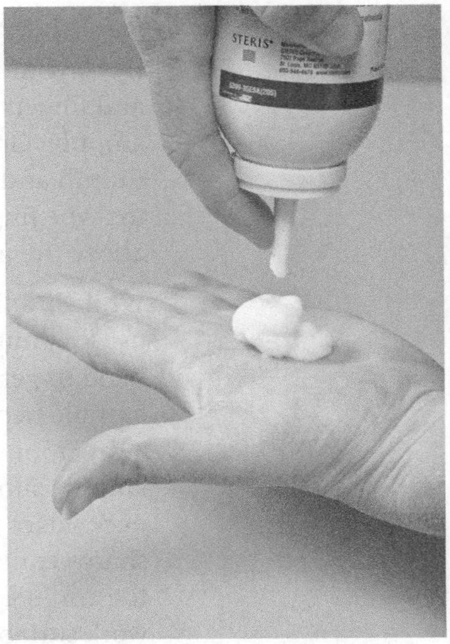

Cleansing hands with sterile, foamed 70% IPA in preparation for gloving.

Once the preparatory steps have been completed, ampule-based compounding procedures may begin.

Upon entering the clean room, place the transport basket or tray onto a clean shelf, table, or countertop. If the transport vehicle used is a cart, wheel it so that it is positioned away from the hood prefilter. Cleanse your hands and forearms with sterile, foamed 70% IPA and allow them to dry thoroughly. Don sterile gloves according to standard aseptic technique procedures. (For additional assistance on the procedure for donning sterile gloves, refer to Chapter 6 of this textbook.)

Due to time constraints, you will not perform hood-cleaning procedures during this procedural lab. Keep in mind that, in sterile compounding practice, hood-cleaning procedures are mandatory and must be performed prior to sterile compounding and at the intervals prescribed by USP Chapter <797>.

***Arranging and Preparing Supplies in the Hood*** Once the hood has been cleaned, you must transfer the clean supplies from the transport vehicle or clean countertop to certain areas of the hood. Place small supply items—such as the regular needle, filter needle, syringe, and alcohol swabs—in the outer six-inch zone of the hood. Place the ampule into the direct compounding area (DCA) of the hood. Tear open the IVPB base solution dust cover. Remove the IVPB base solution from the dust cover and place the IVPB into the DCA. Discard the dust cover into an appropriate waste container. Be sure to place the critical sites of the IVPB and ampule so that they receive uninterrupted airflow from the HEPA filter.

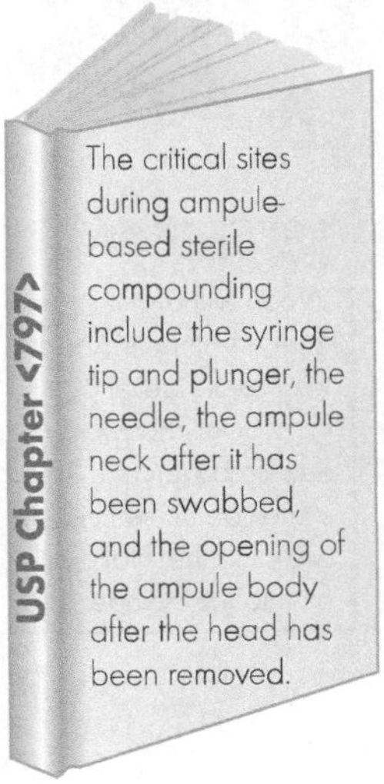

USP Chapter <797>
The critical sites during ampule-based sterile compounding include the syringe tip and plunger, the needle, the ampule neck after it has been swabbed, and the opening of the ampule body after the head has been removed.


## Ampule-Based Compounding Procedure

With the small supply items arranged in the outer six-inch zone and the ampule and IVPB bag placed in the DCA, you are ready to begin the ampule-based compounding procedure. Pick up the ampule and gently tap or swirl the container to clear the head and neck of fluid. Next, swab the neck of the ampule with a sterile 70% IPA swab, and then place the IPA swab onto the hood's work surface within the DCA. Prepare the syringe by aseptically attaching a regular needle. (*Note:* You will use a regular needle first and a filter needle second in this lab procedure, unless directed otherwise by your instructor. However, in practice, always refer to the established protocol of your facility's P&P manual.)

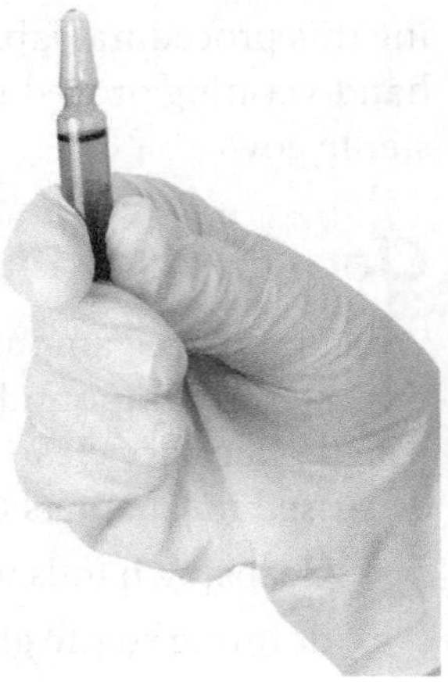

Now, hold the body of the ampule firmly but gently in your nondominant hand, so that your thumb and fingers are situated below the neck of the ampule. Grasp the head of the ampule between the thumb and forefinger of your dominant hand, so that the fingers of your dominant hand are situated above the ampule neck.

While holding your nondominant hand steady, use the thumb and forefinger of your dominant hand to gently but firmly snap the ampule neck. Always snap the ampule away from you, never toward you. The ampule should break cleanly at the neck. Place the ampule head into the sharps container. Temporarily place the ampule body onto the hood's work surface within the DCA so that the ampule's opening—now a critical site—receives uninterrupted airflow from the hood's HEPA filter.

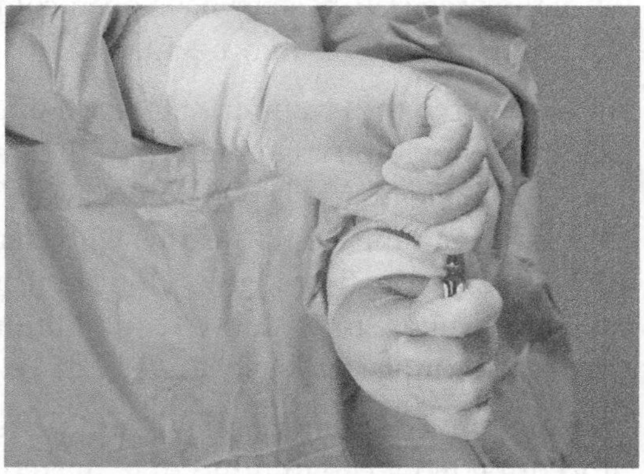

Correct hand placement for breaking a glass ampule.

**USP Chapter <797>**

When you are opening an ampule, place your hands toward the side of the hood, away from the HEPA filter. That way, glass shards from the broken ampule will not damage the HEPA filter.

**POINTER**

When withdrawing fluid from an ampule, keep the needle bevel pointing down. That way, the needle bevel remains immersed in the fluid, avoiding the intake of air into the syringe.

Grasp the barrel of the syringe in your dominant hand and then carefully remove the regular needle cap. Set the cap onto the sterile 70% IPA swab that you previously placed on the hood's work surface. Hold the ampule body with the thumb and forefinger of your nondominant hand, taking care not to touch or shadow the opening of the ampule at any time. With the needle bevel pointing down, insert the tip of the regular needle into the ampule so that it is completely immersed in the fluid inside the ampule.

While keeping the ampule in an *upright* position, and while maintaining the tip of the needle in the fluid within the ampule, pull back on the flat knob of the plunger with the thumb or forefinger of your dominant hand. (Note that you do not need to inject air into the ampule to equalize the pressure because the ampule is an open container.) Continue to pull back on the flat knob of the plunger until you have drawn at least 0.5 mL more than the desired volume. Remove your finger from the plunger knob, and grasp the syringe as you would a dart. Holding only the barrel of the syringe, carefully remove it from the ampule. Temporarily place the ampule body onto the hood's work surface within the DCA. Carefully recap the needle.

Hold the barrel of the syringe with the capped needle pointing upward. Tap the syringe barrel to force bubbles up toward the syringe tip (see Figure 10.3). Pull down slightly on the flat knob of the syringe to draw fluid from the needle into the syringe. Notice that this action creates a small air pocket at the tip of the syringe. Expel the air pocket from the syringe by using the thumb of your dominant hand to gently, and very slowly, push up on the flat knob just until the fluid in the syringe meets the "colored part" of the needle hub. Immediately release your thumb from the flat knob as soon as the fluid meets the needle hub to avoid the expulsion of fluid into the needle cap, a potentially dangerous situation.

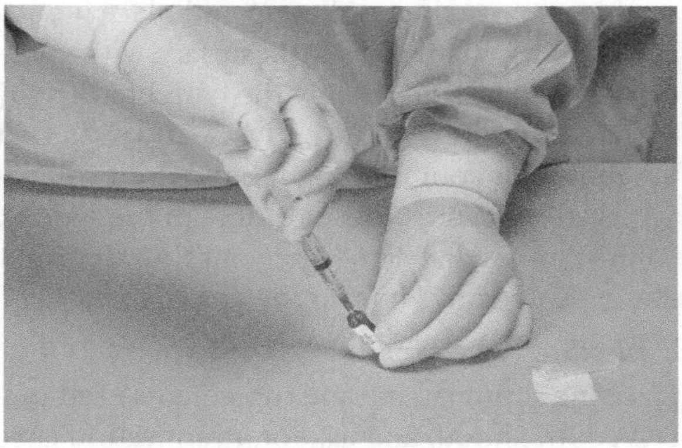

Correct technique for inserting a needle into a glass ampule.

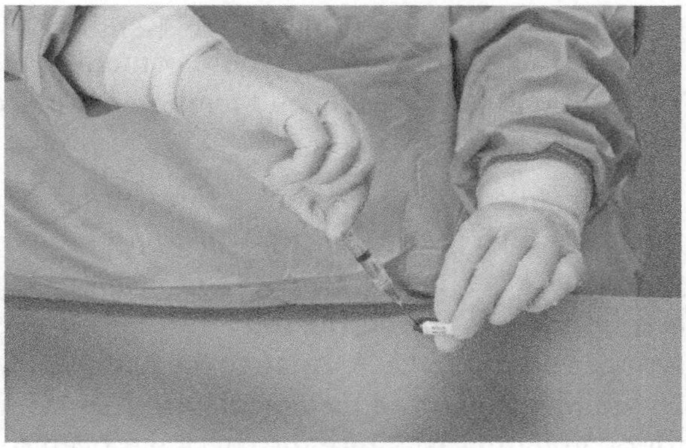

Withdrawal of fluid from a glass ampule.

**POINTER**

Keep the ampule in an upright, or nearly upright, position so that the fluid does not spill from the ampule onto the work surface. Unlike a vial, the ampule must not be inverted during withdrawal procedures.

**BE AWARE**

To avoid expelling fluid into the needle cap, always pull down on the plunger to remove fluid from the needle *after* tapping the syringe to dislodge air bubbles. Do not tap the syringe again after you have pulled down on the plunger.

Closely examine the filled and capped, bubble-free syringe. Determine which measurement point on the syringe barrel exactly matches the desired dose volume. If, at this point in the procedure, you already have the desired dose volume correctly drawn up in the syringe, temporarily place the syringe onto the hood's work surface within the DCA.

If you determine there is more fluid in the syringe than is necessary to deliver the desired dose volume, you must inject the excess fluid back into the ampule body. To

**FIGURE 10.3**

**Bubble Expulsion from a Syringe**

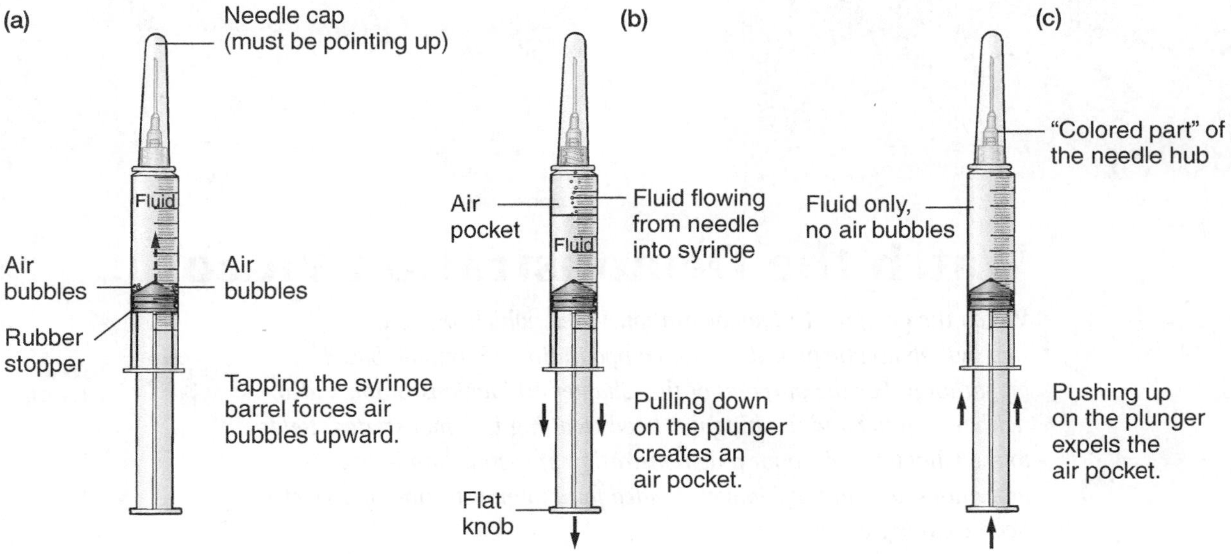

**POINTER**

Due to the potential for contamination, and the time involved in removing bubbles from a syringe, it is preferable to make only one withdrawal from the ampule. Draw up a small amount (in this case, 0.5 mL) of extra fluid when first withdrawing from the ampule. This extra fluid fills the space in the syringe previously occupied by air bubbles.

do this, remove the needle cap and place it onto the alcohol swab. Brace the ampule body against the hood's work surface with your nondominant hand. With your dominant hand, grasp only the barrel of the syringe and carefully insert the needle tip back into the ampule body. Gently push on the flat knob of the plunger with the thumb of your dominant hand until you have expelled the excess fluid and have achieved the desired dose volume in the syringe. Once you have the desired dose volume, immediately release your thumb from the flat knob. Holding the syringe like a dart, remove it from the ampule and carefully recap the needle. Temporarily place the capped syringe onto the hood's work surface within the DCA.

Place the supply items and ingredients used in the preparation of the CSP into the DCA of the hood, and ask for a verification check by your instructor or a pharmacist. Once the check has been completed, grasp the syringe with your nondominant hand, and use your dominant hand to pull down slightly on the flat knob of the plunger, thereby drawing any fluid contained in the regular needle into the syringe. Twist off the entire needle and temporarily place it onto the hood's work surface within the DCA.

**BE AWARE**

In practice, never place an uncapped needle or an unwrapped, capped needle onto the hood surface as this would cause contamination of the needle.

Hold the filled syringe in your dominant hand, with the syringe tip pointing toward the HEPA filter. Without setting down the syringe, use your fingers to open the filter needle package. Taking care not to touch or shadow the syringe tip or needle hub, aseptically twist the needle hub onto the syringe tip. Temporarily place the capped syringe within the DCA. Arrange the items and ingredients used for the CSP—including the used, capped regular needle—for a verification check by your instructor or a pharmacist. Once the check has been completed, use aseptic technique to inject the medication into the IVPB bag. Examine the bag for leakage and evidence of incompatibility. If neither issue is present, label the IVPB and affix an IVA seal over the injection port.

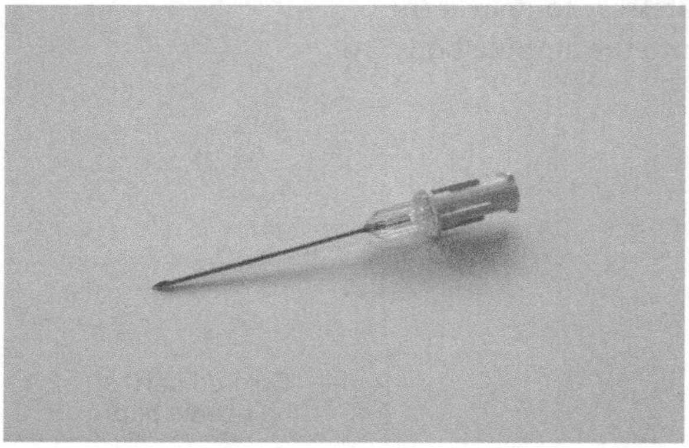

Uncapped filter needle.

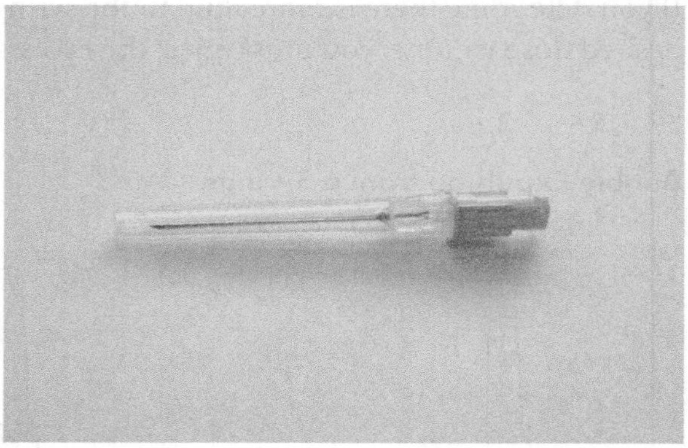

Capped filter needle.

# Watch the Demonstration Video

*Watch the Chapter 10 Demonstration Video, which shows the step-by-step aseptic procedures for compounding an ampule-based preparation. For the purposes of the Chapter 10 Demonstration Video, neither aseptic hand washing nor hood cleaning is demonstrated. Refer to the Chapter 6 video for a demonstration of aseptic hand-washing procedures, and to the Chapter 7 video for a demonstration of correct hood-cleaning procedures.*

Training Videos DVD

# Procedural Lab

*This lab walks you through the step-by-step actions that you must follow to properly compound ampule-based preparations using aseptic technique. Take your time. Work through each step methodically and with close attention to detail.*

***Note:*** *For the purposes of this procedural lab, you will not perform aseptic hand-washing or hood-cleaning procedures unless directed to do so by your instructor. Should your instructor ask you to perform these procedures, refer to Chapter 6 for instructions on aseptic hand washing and to Chapter 7 for directions on correct hood cleaning.*

***Note:*** *For step 1 below, please refer to Chapter 4 for a reminder of the step-by-step procedures required for medication order and CSP label verification. For steps 2 and 3, refer to Chapter 5 for pharmacy calculation procedures. For steps 4–8, refer to Chapter 3 for a reminder of the process for gathering and cleaning supplies. For steps 9–15, refer to Chapter 6 for step-by-step aseptic garbing, hand-washing, and gloving procedures. You should perform steps 1–12 and steps 45–47 in the anteroom. Perform steps 13–44 in the clean room.*

## Supplies

### *Essential Supplies*

To complete the Unit 2 procedural labs, you will need to ensure that various essential anteroom and clean room supplies such as those listed in Table 10.1 are available for your use.

**Table 10.1 Essential Anteroom and Clean Room Supplies for Sterile Compounding**

| |
|---|
| **Anteroom Supplies** |
| medication order and CSP label<br>calculator<br>pen<br>permanent, felt-tip marker<br>plastic bags (small and large)<br>aseptic garb, including shoe covers, hair cover, face mask, and beard cover (if appropriate)<br>sterile gown<br>presaturated, aseptic cleaning wipes<br>sterile, foamed 70% IPA<br>waste container<br>transport vehicle (optional) |
| **Clean Room Supplies** |
| sterile, foamed 70% IPA<br>sterile, powder-free gloves<br>sterile 70% IPA swabs, individually packaged × 2<br>sharps container<br>waste container<br>laminar airflow hood |

### *Procedure-Specific Supplies*

In addition to the supplies listed in Table 10.1, gather the following items specific to the Chapter 10 ampule-based procedural lab:

- promethazine 50 mg/2-mL ampule
- 3-mL Luer-lock syringe
- regular needle (nonfilter, nonvented needle, either 18 or 19 gauge)
- filter needle
- dextrose 5% in water ($D_5W$) 100-mL IVPB
- IVA seal (optional)

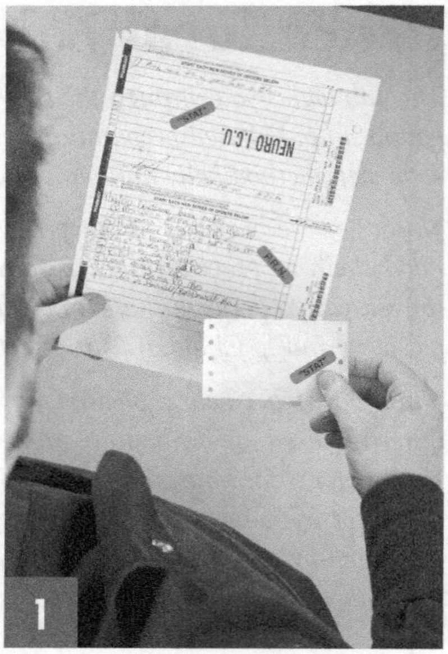


## Procedure

### *Verifying the Label*

1. Review the CSP label to verify that all of the information on the label matches the medication order. To help you with this task, compare the CSP label (see Figure 10.4) to the medication order and patient ID label (see Figure 10.6).

FIGURE 10.4

**CSP Label for Promethazine**

****Intravenous Piggyback****
Mercy Hospital
**Pt. Name:** Flores, Jaime **Room:** 831
**Pt. ID#:** 2088722 **Rx#:** 61131

**Promethazine 30 mg**
**Dextrose 5% in Water ($D_5W$) 100 mL**
**Rate: over 20 min**

Expires ______
Tech ______
RPh ______

Keep refrigerated –
warm to room temperature before use.

### *Calculating Desired Volume*

2. Read the label on the promethazine ampule (see Figure 10.5) to determine the concentration of the drug.
3. Perform calculations based on the promethazine dosage information that is provided on the CSP label, and the promethazine concentration from the ampule label. Assume that the ampule label indicates that promethazine has a concentration of 50 mg/2 mL. Use the following formula to calculate the dose:

$$\frac{50 \text{ mg}}{2 \text{ mL}} = \frac{30 \text{ mg}}{x \text{ mL}}$$

*Cross-multiply, then divide to solve for $x$ (the desired dosage volume) for each dose.

(For additional assistance, refer to Chapter 5 for step-by-step dosage calculation procedures.)

FIGURE 10.5

**Promethazine Label**

NDC 00000-000-00 25288
**Promethazine**
FOR INJECTION, USP
**50 mg/2 mL**
(25 mg/mL)
For IM or IV use

Sterile, nonpyrogenic
Preservative-free

Each mL contains 25 mg of promethazine.

**Must be diluted prior to IV use. Administer IV doses over ≥ 20 minutes.**

**Protect from light**

EMCP PHARMACEUTICALS
St. Paul, MN 55102
LOT: MANLAB11
Exp: 06/2017

**FIGURE 10.6**

**Daily Order**

**ID#:** 2088722
**Name:** Flores, Jaime
**DOB:** 3/2/55
**Room:** 831
**Dr.:** Valkema, Michelle

**MERCY HOSPITAL**
**PHYSICIAN'S MEDICATION ORDER**

**BEAR DOWN ON HARD SURFACE WITH BALLPOINT PEN**

GENERIC EQUIVALENT IS AUTHORIZED UNLESS CHECKED IN THIS COLUMN

ALLERGY OR SENSITIVITY TO NKDA

NONE KNOWN ☐ SIGNED:

DIAGNOSIS

COMPLETED OR DISCONTINUED

| DATE | TIME | ORDERS | PHYSICIAN'S SIG. | | NAME | DATE | TIME |
|---|---|---|---|---|---|---|---|
| 10/21/2014 | 3:31 PM | | | | | | |
| | | Height 5' 10" Weight 169 lbs | | | | | |
| | | DC p.o. promethazine | | | | | |
| | | Δ to promethazine 30 mg IVPB q 6 hours prn N/V | | | | | |
| | | | M. Valkema, MD | | | | |

PHARMACY COPY

### *Gathering and Cleaning Supplies*

4. Place the medication order into the large plastic bag and the CSP label into the small plastic bag. Gather all supply items listed in the supply section of the procedural lab.
5. Open the package of aseptic cleaning wipes. Remove one or, if necessary, more wipes, and thoroughly wipe down the entire transport vehicle.
6. Place the used wipes in the waste receptacle.
7. Remove a new aseptic cleaning wipe and wipe down the exterior surface of the IVPB bag's dust cover. Place the cleaned IVPB into the transport vehicle. Place the used wipe in the waste receptacle.
8. Repeat the cleaning procedure outlined in step 7 with each of the remaining supply items.

### *Garbing*

**POINTER**

During aseptic garbing, best practice is to reapply sterile, foamed 70% IPA to your hands after donning shoe covers and again after donning a hair cover.

9. Don shoe covers.
10. Put on a hair cover.
11. Don a face mask and beard cover (if appropriate).

    *Note:* For the purposes of this training lab, you will skip the mandatory aseptic hand-washing procedure.
12. Don a sterile gown.
13. Use a transport vehicle to bring all supply items, including an unopened package of sterile, powder-free gloves, into the clean room.
14. Place the transport vehicle onto a clean surface or countertop within the clean room. If a cart is used, position it so that it does not interrupt airflow into the hood prefilter.
15. Apply sterile, foamed 70% IPA to your hands. Allow them to air-dry and then don sterile gloves.

    *Note:* For the purposes of this training lab, you will skip the mandatory hood-cleaning procedure.

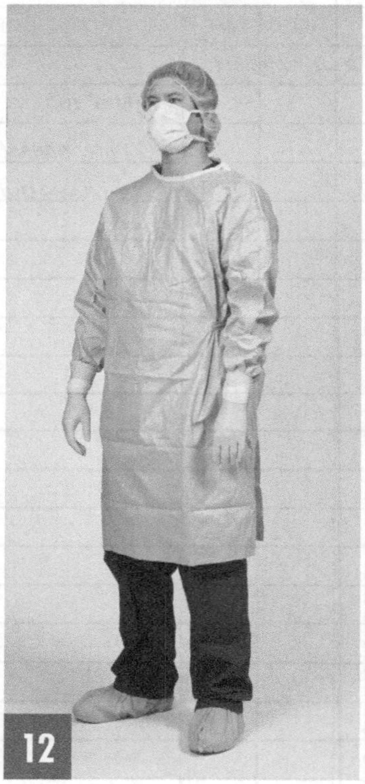


### *Compounding an Ampule-Based Preparation*

16. Tear open the dust cover and remove the IVPB. Place the IVPB into the DCA of the hood, and the dust cover into the waste receptacle. Place the ampule into the DCA as well. Then set the small supply items—such as the needles, syringe, and IPA swabs—into the outer six-inch zone of the hood.

17. Gently tap or swirl the ampule so that the head and neck are free of fluid and all of the medication is contained in the body of the ampule.

18. Tear open a sterile, 70% IPA swab while holding it within the DCA. Sterilize the neck of the ampule, and then place the used swab onto the hood's work surface within the DCA. Place the empty swab package in the discard pile.

19. Remove a 3-mL Luer-lock syringe from its outer wrap. If necessary, remove the cap from the tip of the syringe. Prepare the syringe by aseptically removing the needle from its packaging and attaching it to the syringe. Cap the syringe and then temporarily place it onto the hood's work surface within the DCA. Place the syringe's outer wrapper into the discard pile.

**POINTER**

During the opening of an ampule, maintain a firm hold of the ampule with the thumb and index finger of your nondominant hand to avoid dislodgement. Apply just enough pressure to avoid breaking the ampule's thin glass walls.

### *Opening the Glass Ampule*

20. Gently but firmly hold the body of the ampule with the thumb and index finger of your nondominant hand, curling the remaining three fingers around the body of the ampule to help stabilize it. Verify that the fingers of this hand are situated below the neck of the ampule.

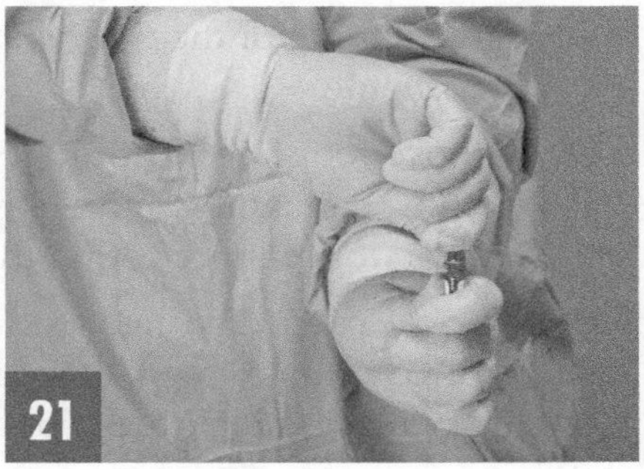


21. Place your dominant hand so that the thumb and forefinger have a firm grasp on the head of the ampule. Verify that the fingers of this hand are above the neck of the ampule.

22. Keeping your arms and fingers steady, use your dominant hand to apply pressure to the neck of the ampule with a quick snapping motion of the wrist. The ampule should break at the neck.

23. Put the head of the ampule into the sharps container. Temporarily place the body of the ampule onto the hood's work surface within the DCA so that the ampule's opening—now a critical site—receives uninterrupted airflow from the hood's HEPA filter.

**BE AWARE**

Before snapping the neck of the ampule, verify that the fingers of your hands are positioned away from the neck of the ampule, to avoid potential injury. During the opening process, snap the ampule away from you and toward the side of the hood, to avoid damaging the HEPA filter with glass shards.

### *Withdrawing the Correct Drug Volume from the Ampule*

24. Holding the barrel of the syringe with your dominant hand, remove the cap of the needle, and place the needle cap onto the swab with the opening pointing toward the hood's HEPA filter.

25. Rotate the barrel of the syringe so that the needle bevel is pointing down. Stabilizing the ampule with your nondominant hand, carefully insert the needle into the ampule.

**POINTER**

Be sure that the tip of the needle is maintained within the fluid inside of the ampule. When withdrawing from ampules, the needle bevel should be pointed down to keep the bevel in contact with the fluid inside of the ampule.

**POINTER**
The amount of extra fluid you withdraw from the ampule is determined by the syringe size: For 1-mL, 3-mL, and 5-mL syringes, draw up approximately 0.5 mL of extra fluid; for 10-mL syringes or larger, draw up approximately 1 mL of extra fluid.

**POINTER**
As you draw up fluid into the syringe and the ampule becomes empty, it may be necessary to tip the ampule slightly to bring fluid into the shoulder of the ampule where it can be reached more easily by the tip of the needle.

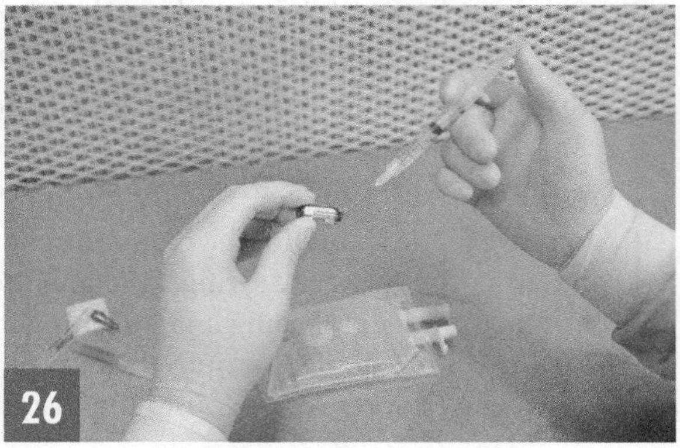

26

**26.** Use the fingers of your dominant hand to pull back on the flat knob of the plunger, gradually drawing fluid into the syringe. Continue to pull back on the plunger until the syringe contains approximately 0.5 mL more than the desired dose. (In this procedural lab, our desired 30-mg dose requires 1.2 mL—plus approximately 0.5 mL extra, for a total of approximately 1.7 mL.) Drawing up a small amount of extra fluid will assist you with bubble removal (see step 28) and helps ensure you have enough fluid for the dose without having to make another withdrawal from the ampule.

**27.** Remove your fingers from the plunger. Grasp the barrel of the syringe as you would a dart, and remove it from the ampule. Place the ampule body onto the hood's work surface within the DCA. Carefully recap the needle.

**28.** Turn the capped syringe so that the needle tip points upward. Tap the syringe to force air bubbles up toward the syringe tip. Continue to tap on the barrel of the syringe until all of the bubbles have been forced to the syringe tip.

**29.** Use your dominant hand to pull down slightly on the plunger to draw fluid from the needle into the syringe, thereby creating a small air pocket at the tip of the syringe. Slowly push up on the plunger to expel all air from the syringe. Release the plunger immediately once the fluid in the syringe comes into contact with the hub of the needle to avoid expelling fluid into the needle cap. *Note:* Refer to Figure 10.3 on page 305 for the proper procedure to remove bubbles from a syringe.

**30.** Look closely at the filled syringe to determine how much fluid it contains. If the syringe contains the exact volume needed for the desired dose, skip step 31 and proceed to step 32. If the syringe does not contain the exact volume needed for the desired dose, proceed to step 31.

**31.** To remove excess fluid from the syringe, carefully insert the needle back into the ampule and use the plunger to push any excess fluid into the ampule. Keeping your eye on the graduations on the syringe barrel, push the plunger down slowly and stop when you reach the correct volume. (In this procedural lab, the 30-mg dose requires 1.2 mL.) Release your thumb from the plunger, grasp the syringe at the barrel, and slowly remove it from the ampule.

**32.** Carefully recap the needle.

**33.** Hold the barrel of the syringe with your nondominant hand, so that the needle tip is pointing toward the ceiling. Use the thumb and forefinger of your dominant hand to pull down slightly (approximately 0.5 mL) on the plunger so that the fluid is drawn from the needle into the syringe, creating a small air pocket at the tip of the needle.

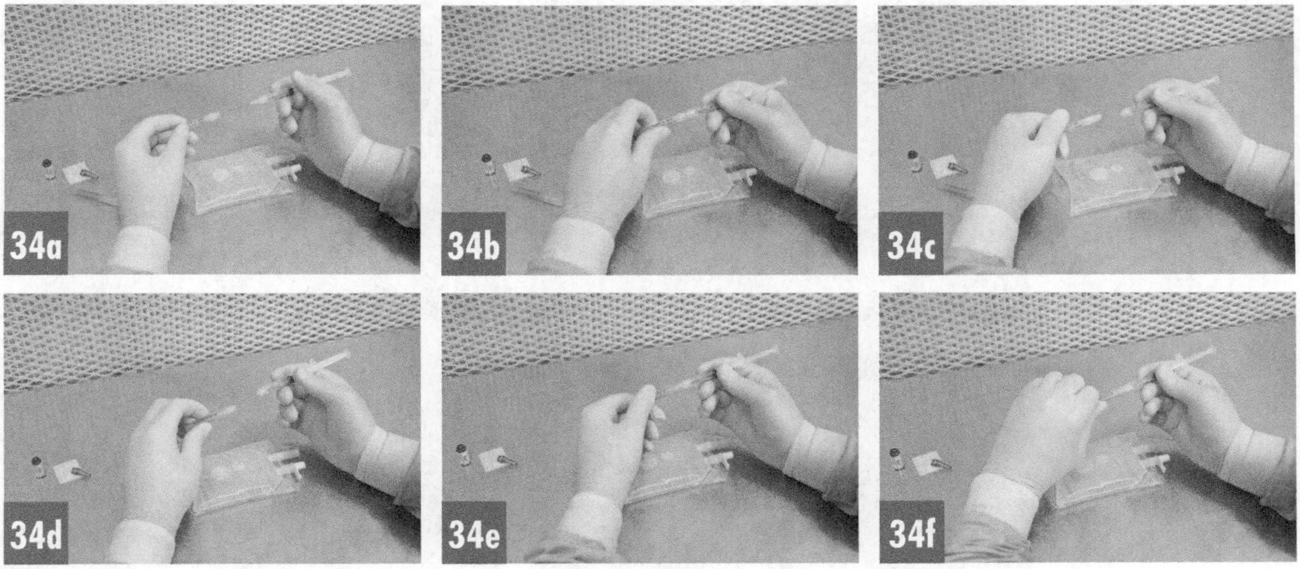


34. Twist off the entire, capped regular needle and place it temporarily onto the hood's work surface, next to the body of the ampule. Aseptically open the filter needle package, and attach the needle to the syringe. Place the syringe wrapper into the discard pile. Slowly push up on the plunger to remove air bubbles from the syringe. Verify that the syringe now contains the desired dose—in this case, 1.2 mL.

35. Arrange the filled syringe with attached, capped filter needle; the ampule; the used regular needle; and the IVPB on the hood's work surface for a verification check by the pharmacist or your instructor.

### *Injecting the Medication into the IVPB*

36. Once the verification check has been completed, rearrange items within the DCA so that the IVPB injection port and the filter needle-and-syringe unit receive uninterrupted airflow from the HEPA filter.

37. Open a new IPA swab and sterilize the injection port of the IVPB. Place the swab on the hood's work surface directly under the injection port.

38. Pick up the filter needle-and-syringe unit, and hold the barrel of the syringe in your dominant hand, as you would a dart. Remove the cap of the filter needle and place the needle cap onto the alcohol swab that you previously placed on the hood's work surface (see step 18).

39. Hold the injection port of the IVPB steady with your nondominant hand, taking care to avoid shadowing or touching the injection port. Then insert the needle straight into the injection port. Take care not to puncture the sidewall of the injection port.

**POINTER**

When inserting a needle into the injection port of an IVPB, it is not necessary to consider the direction in which the bevel faces. The needle should be inserted straight into the bag without angling or bending the needle.

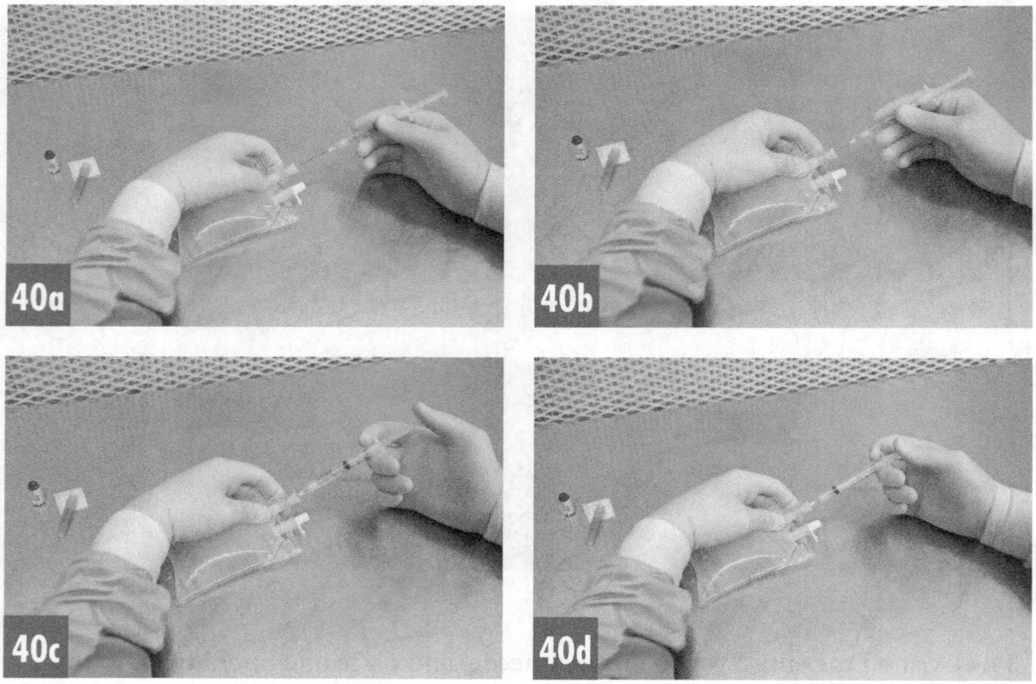

40a 40b 40c 40d

**40.** Inject the medication into the IVPB bag by pressing on the flat knob of the plunger with the thumb or forefinger of your dominant hand.

**41.** Holding only the barrel of the syringe, carefully remove the filter needle-and-syringe unit from the IVPB. Place the needle-and-syringe unit into the sharps container without recapping the needle.

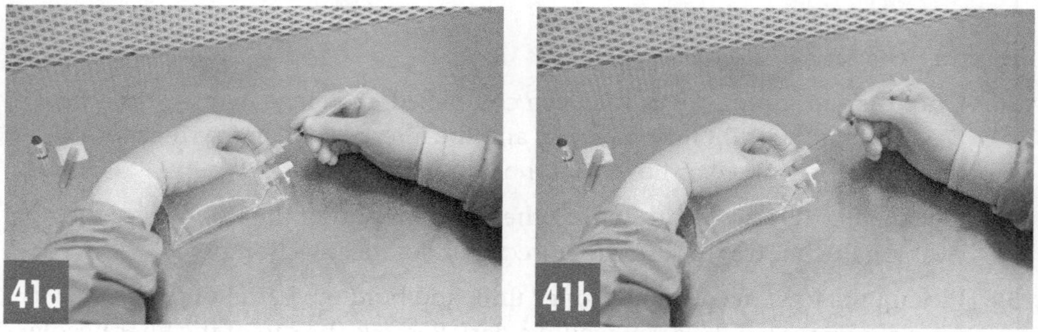

41a 41b

**42.** Squeeze the IVPB bag and examine it for leaks, precipitate, or evidence of incompatibility. If there are no signs of these issues, cover the injection port with an IVA seal.

**43.** Remove the correct CSP label from the plastic bag and affix the label to the IVPB bag.

### *Cleaning Up After the Procedure*

**44.** Place the waste from the discard pile into the regular waste container. Place the ampule, the regular needle, the filter needle, and the syringe into the sharps container. Place the labeled CSP and any remaining supply items into the transport vehicle, and return the vehicle to the anteroom.

**45.** In the anteroom, complete the compounding procedures by using a permanent, felt-tip pen to record your initials in the proper location on the CSP label.

**46.** Remove your PPE according to the standard protocol outlined in Chapter 6. Return any unused supply items to their proper locations.

**47.** Ask for a final verification check from the pharmacist or your instructor.

# Process Validation Checklist

*Your instructor will use the process validation checklist provided in Appendix D to evaluate your technique for this lab. In order to receive ACPE certification, and prior to making CSPs for patient use, you must correctly perform each component of the lab procedure. Review the Chapter 10 lab and thoroughly practice each of the steps prior to your evaluation.*

# Part 3: Assessment

## Chapter Summary

- An ampule is a flame-sealed, glass container with a tapered neck; it is used as a sterile reservoir for certain parenteral medications.
- Ampules are used to supply medications that are incompatible with certain materials used in the manufacturing of vials, such as plastic, polyvinyl chloride, or rubber. Ampule medications may be administered by several parenteral routes, including IV, IVPB, IV push, or IM.
- Ampules present a unique risk to both the patient recipient and the IV technician due to broken glass. Glass shards may enter the solution when the ampule head is removed, creating a potentially dangerous situation for the patient. In addition, the IV technician opening the ampule is at risk for injury from both breaking and handling the broken ampule within the hood.
- The primary components of the ampule are the head, neck, shoulder, and body. The ampule neck is tapered and scored so that it may be broken and the head removed, allowing access to the fluid in the body of the ampule.
- Once opened, an ampule is a single-use container (sometimes referred to as an SDV), which must be disposed of immediately after use.
- A number of methods may be used to open ampules, including using an alcohol swab, sterile gauze, gloved hands, or an ampule breaker. Each method has both advantages and disadvantages. The method used by an IV technician should be based on several factors, including safety, personal preference, and the guidelines set forth in the facility's P&P manual.
- A single-direction, 5-micron filter needle should be used to filter the solution prior to injecting it into the CSP.
- Two needles must always be used in the preparation of an ampule: one regular needle and one filter needle. Bacause glass shards become trapped within the needle's filter, a filter needle may not be used to *both* draw up the fluid from an ampule and inject the medication into an IVPB bag.
- Whether to first use a regular needle or a filter needle to withdraw fluid from the ampule is based on the viscosity and volume of the fluid being prepared, the preference of the IV technician, and the policies of the facility.
- Anteroom preparatory procedures include verifying the CSP label against the medication order, performing calculations, gathering and cleaning supplies, donning aseptic garb, aseptic hand washing, and donning a sterile gown.
- Clean room preparatory procedures include donning sterile gloves, cleaning the hood, and using aseptic technique to prepare the ampule-based CSP within the DCA of the hood.
- Critical sites that must be considered during ampule preparation procedures include the ampule neck, the open ampule (once the head has been removed), the syringe tip and plunger, the uncapped needle, and the IVPB injection port.
- The needle, syringe, and open ampule should never be contaminated by touch or shadow contamination, or by swabbing with sterile 70% IPA.
- The ampule neck and IVPB injection port must be swabbed with sterile 70% IPA and should never be contaminated by touch or shadowing after they have been sterilized.
- To avoid injury, always confirm that the fingers and hands are placed away from the ampule neck prior to removing the ampule head.
- When withdrawing fluid from the ampule, draw up at least 0.5 mL more than the desired volume (making sure the needle-and-syringe unit is pointed directly downward into the ampule liquid), cap the needle, tap the syringe to force bubbles to the tip of the syringe, and then pull down on the plunger immediately before expelling excess air. Any extra fluid in the syringe should be returned to the ampule.

- To change needles, hold the recapped, filled needle-and-syringe unit so that the tip is pointing upright; then pull down slightly on the flat knob of the plunger (to clear the needle of fluid), remove the capped needle, aseptically attach a new needle, and expel any excess air.
- Insert the needle-and-syringe unit straight into the IVPB injection port, taking care to avoid the side wall of the injection port.
- Place the final used needle-and-syringe unit and broken ampule components into the sharps container.
- Inspect the CSP for leakage and particulate matter. Label the CSP and apply an IVA seal.
- Upon return to the anteroom, record your name and the date on the CSP label. Aseptically remove your PPE.

# Key Terms

**ampule** a small container made of thin, medical-grade glass; usually used as a reservoir for certain sterile parenteral medications

**ampule body** the reservoir that holds sterile fluid within a glass ampule

**ampule breaker** a small plastic cap that fits over the head of an ampule and is used to snap the ampule neck, thus reducing the risk of glass cuts

**ampule head** the uppermost part of a glass ampule that must be removed by an IV technician to access the fluid within the ampule body

**ampule neck** the tapered area of the ampule that separates the body and head of the ampule; where the ampule must be broken to remove the ampule head

**ampule shoulder** the uppermost part of the ampule body, just prior to where the ampule narrows at the neck

**break ring** a ring of thin glass around the neck of an ampule, intended to make breaking the neck and opening the ampule easier

**critical site** an area of a supply item that must not be touched and to which airflow from the HEPA filter should never be interrupted; these areas include the needle, syringe tip and plunger, injection port, ampule neck, and the opening of the ampule body

**desired volume** the volume of a medication or solution component that must be drawn up in order to provide the prescribed dose

**filter needle** a specialty needle containing a filter (typically 5 microns) in the hub; this single-direction needle is used to *either* withdraw medication from an ampule *or* inject fluid from a syringe into a reservoir such as an IVPB bag

**filter straw** a thin plastic tube that looks like a straw and attaches to a syringe, just as a needle does; the tube contains a filter, so that any glass shards or other impurities will be trapped in the straw as liquid is drawn through it and into the syringe

**nephrotoxicity** an effect caused by a medicine that is toxic or otherwise damaging to the kidneys

**open container** a container that is not sealed airtight, such as a syringe or an open ampule

**ototoxicity** an effect caused by a medicine that is toxic or otherwise damaging to a component of the inner ear, potentially resulting in deafness

**single-use container** (also referred to as a single-dose vial, or SDV) a container that, once opened, cannot be resealed airtight, thus allowing bacteria and other contaminants easy access; types of SDVs include syringes, opened ampules, and vials that do not contain preservatives

**tear bottle** an ancient flask that was filled with the tears of a mourner and buried alongside the dead as a symbol of love and respect; also known as a *lachrymatory*

**unguentaria** ancient containers that were used to hold liquid ointments or perfumed oils

**viscosity** the quality or degree of being viscous or having a sticky consistency

## Check the Basics

*On a separate sheet of paper, write your answers as modeled in these examples: 1d; 2c; 3b; etc.*

**1.** Which of the following correctly lists the components of an ampule from top to bottom?
  a. head, face, neck, body
  b. head, neck, shoulder, body
  c. body, neck, shoulder, head
  d. head, body, shoulder, neck

**2.** Which of the following statements regarding ampule preparations is true?
  a. One regular needle and one filter needle must be used; the same needle may not be used to both withdraw and inject fluid.
  b. A single needle may be used to withdraw and inject fluid, provided that it is a single-direction filter needle.
  c. One regular needle and one vented needle must be used; the same needle may not be used to both withdraw and inject fluid.
  d. A single, regular needle may be used to withdraw and inject fluid.

**3.** Which of the following tasks must you perform prior to opening an ampule?
  a. Remove the fluid from the ampule body.
  b. Shake the ampule to be sure the medication is well mixed.
  c. Remove the fluid from the ampule head by tapping or swirling the ampule.
  d. Swab the ampule body.

**4.** Once the neck of the ampule has been broken, the ampule is considered to be which type of container?
  a. a closed, single-use container
  b. a closed, multiple-use container
  c. an open, single-use container
  d. an open, multiple-use container

**5.** What is the most common type of filter needle used in ampule preparation?
  a. HEPA filter
  b. 0.2-micron filter
  c. 0.5-micron filter
  d. 5-micron filter

**6.** With regard to breaking the ampule, which statement is true?
  a. The fingers of the dominant hand should grip the ampule neck; the fingers of the nondominant hand should grip the ampule body.
  b. The fingers of the dominant hand should be below the ampule neck; the fingers of the nondominant hand should be above the ampule neck.
  c. The fingers of the dominant hand should grip the ampule body; the fingers of the nondominant hand should grip the ampule neck.
  d. The fingers of the dominant hand should be above the ampule neck; the fingers of the nondominant hand should be below the ampule neck.

**7.** With regard to withdrawing fluid from an ampule, which statement is true?
  a. There is no need to inject air into the ampule since it is an open container.
  b. There is no need to inject air into the ampule since it is a collapsible container.
  c. Add an amount of air equal to the volume needed to be withdrawn.
  d. Add an amount of air 0.5 mL more than the volume needed to be withdrawn.

**8.** How should the needle bevel be positioned when withdrawing from an ampule?
  a. The needle bevel should be pointed up.
  b. The needle bevel should be pointed down.
  c. There is no bevel on a filter needle.
  d. none of the above

**9.** During ampule withdrawal, when should air bubbles be removed from the syringe?
  a. after the fluid-filled syringe has been removed from the ampule and the needle has been recapped
  b. while the fluid-filled syringe is still situated in the ampule
  c. after the fluid has been injected into the IVPB
  d. after the regular needle has been attached

10. When preparing for a verification check, which items should be arranged on the hood?
    a. the filled syringe with capped filter needle and the capped, used regular needle
    b. the ampule body
    c. the IVPB
    d. all of the above

## Make Connections

*On a separate sheet of paper, write your answers to the following three questions, using complete sentences and making sure your answers are thorough and thoughtful. Note that the third question requires Internet access.*

1. An ampule preparation requires the worker to break glass to withdraw the medication. What procedure would you follow if you cut yourself while opening an ampule? Would you follow the same procedure if you believed that you had cut yourself but there was no visible blood? Why or why not?

2. The procedure for removing bubbles from a filled syringe directs you to tap the syringe to force bubbles up toward the syringe tip. You are then instructed to pull down slightly on the flat knob of the plunger, immediately before expelling the air pocket from the syringe. Pulling down on the flat knob must be the *last step* before expelling the air pocket. What is the rationale behind this specific order? What might be the result if you were to tap on the syringe and then expel the air pocket without first pulling down on the flat knob?

3. Go to the website for the Occupational Health and Safety Administration (OSHA). Access the Regulations tab. Click on the link for *Bloodborne Pathogens—Standard 1910*. Scroll down to Standard 1910.1030(d)(2)(vii)(A) and read the information. The Chapter 10 Procedural Lab requires you to recap a needle prior to removing it or before preparing a filled syringe for a verification check. Based on what you read, is the recapping of a needle during sterile compounding a breach of standard 1910.1030(d)(2)(vii)(A)? Why or why not?

## Meet the Challenge

***Scenario*** This "snapping" activity will give you the opportunity to experiment with four different methods of opening an ampule.

***Challenge*** Your instructor has a handout outlining the supplies and steps for an activity centered around opening an ampule. This procedure takes your understanding of how to open an ampule to a deeper level. To meet this challenge, ask your instructor for the handout and give it a try, either as an individual, in small groups, or as a class.

### ADDITIONAL RESOURCES

*Go to the Paradigm Internet Resources Center at* www.paradigmcollege.net/sterilecomp *to access live links related to these Chapter 10 topics:*

+ Standards for worker safety
+ Articles on glass particle contamination and opened ampules
+ Step-by-step procedures for ampule use and handling

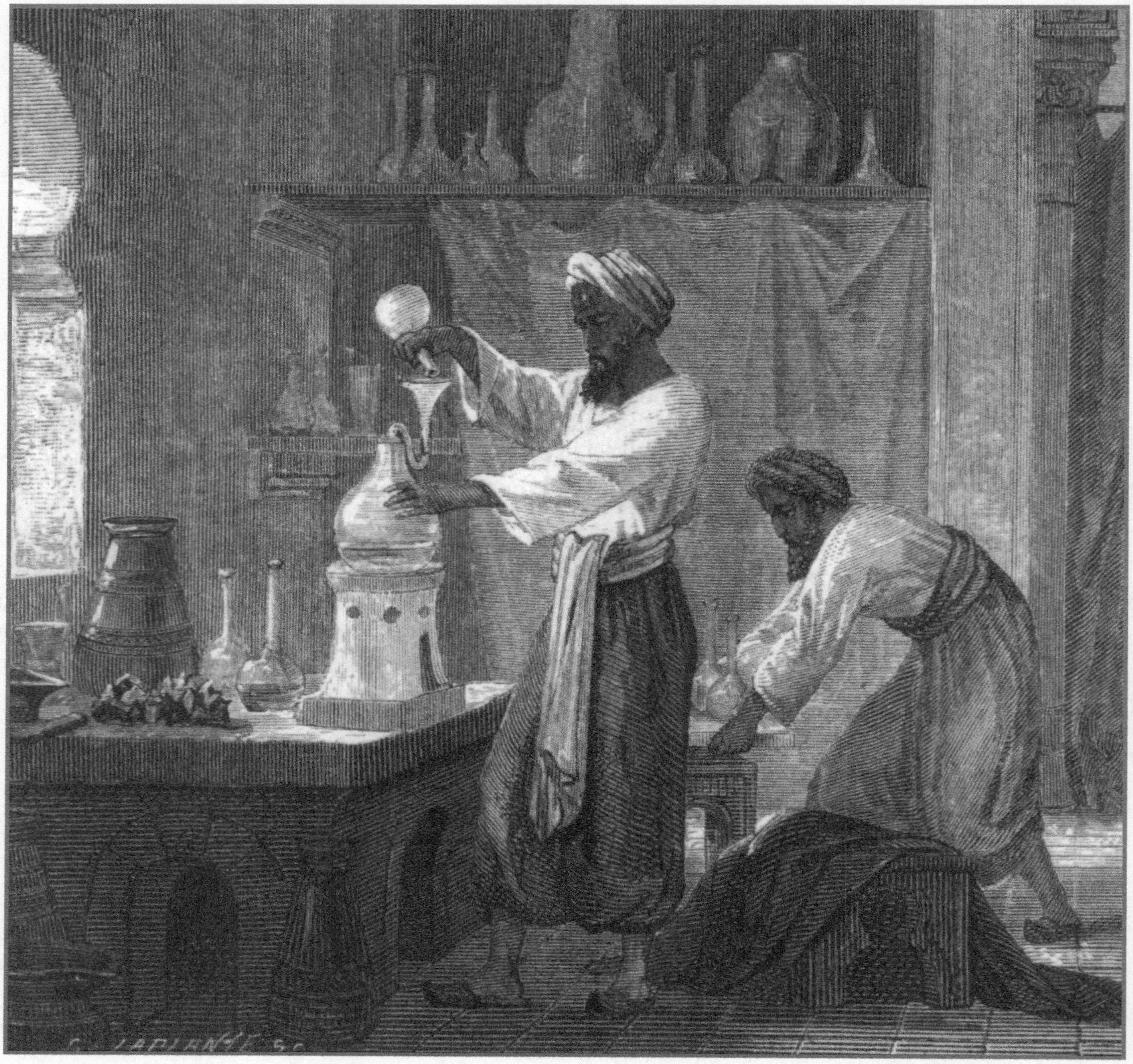

# Chapter 11

# Narcotic Preparations

## Learning Objectives

- Gain an awareness of the history of narcotic medications.
- Understand the legal regulations and procedures that must be followed when preparing various controlled substances for parenteral administration.
- Identify the USP Chapter <797> procedures that must be performed when preparing narcotic compounded sterile preparations (CSPs).
- Demonstrate correct technique in the preparation of narcotic CSPs.

The term narcotic is derived from the Greek word *narkoun*, which means "to make numb." Historically, it referred to any substance that could relieve pain, dull senses, or induce sleep. The history of narcotic medications is as old as the history of pharmacy, and even the history of medicine itself. Some natural and synthetic narcotic compounds are still used today, whereas others have a strictly historical or literary significance. For example, water lilies have been used for thousands of years by Asian, African, and European cultures for stomach illnesses and skin conditions, as well as for pain relief. While the term *water lily* has been used to refer to dozens of different aquatic plants, some scholars believe that the white lotus, or Egyptian lotus (the white-flowered *Nymphaea*), is the pleasure- and sleep-inducing plant ingested by the famous Lotus Eaters in Homer's *The Odyssey*. Ancient Egyptians believed that same plant gave them strength and, therefore, created ceremonial perfumes from its extracts.

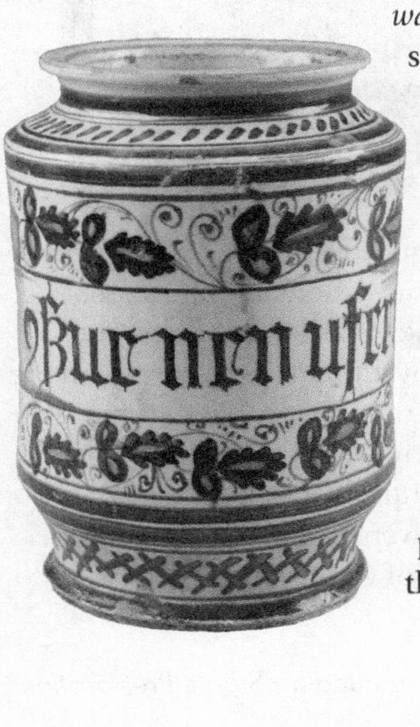

### Opium Poppy

Although the water lily and white lotus plants were recognized by early cultures for their pain-relieving qualities, the **opium poppy**—or *Papaver somniferum*—was discovered to have more potent analgesic properties and became a highly sought-after medicinal cure. The opium poppy plant is thought to be the originator of all narcotics and, to this day, is the primary source of most natural narcotic substances.

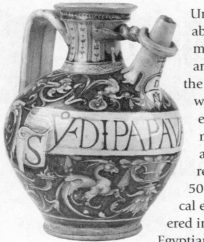

Unmatched in its ability to elevate mood, induce sleep, and relieve pain, the opium poppy was well-known among early Mesopotamian civilizations, according to papyrus records dating from 5000 BCE. Archaeological evidence has uncovered images of poppies in Egyptian hieroglyphics as well as in artifacts buried in the tombs of pharaohs. These early Middle Eastern cultures relied on harvesters to gather the spent poppy heads and scrape their capsules. This scoring process would release a milky-white sap called **latex**. Once collected, the sticky exudate, or raw opium, was added to food (such as poppy cakes) or drunk as a beverage (such as juice). The raw opium was found to be a particularly effective painkiller, and this natural medicinal remedy became a leading export to Europe and other regions of Asia.

## Opium Use Among Ancient Civilizations

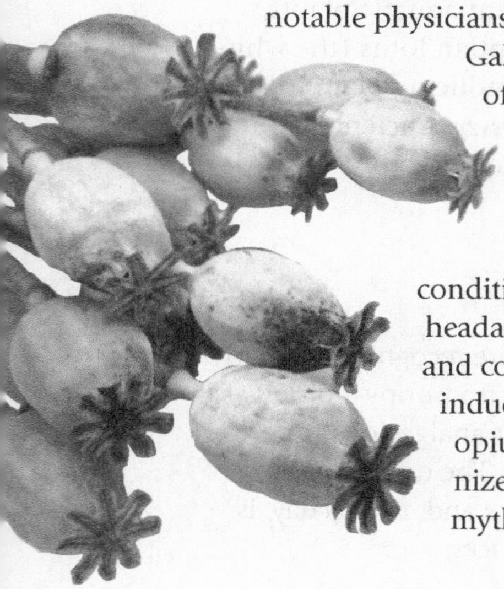

With the introduction of the opium poppy in Europe and Asia, the popularity of this medicinal plant grew—and so did its applications. Ancient Greek and Roman practitioners used crude drugs compounded from the opium poppy to quiet children and soothe pain. Indeed, two of their most notable physicians—Hippocrates and Galen—were advocates of opium use, prescribing the extract for not only pain relief and sleeplessness but also for a host of other conditions, such as asthma, headaches, epilepsy, fevers, and coughs. In fact, the sleep-inducing qualities of the opium poppy are recognized in their cultures' mythology: The Greek gods Hypnos (god of sleep) and Morpheus (god of dreams) are frequently depicted wearing or carrying the poppy flower, as is the Roman god of sleep, Somnos. These early civilizations also recognized the toxic properties of opium, with documented evidence pointing to its use as a poison—particularly among the elderly. An opium overdose led to respiratory depression and, eventually, cessation of respirations.

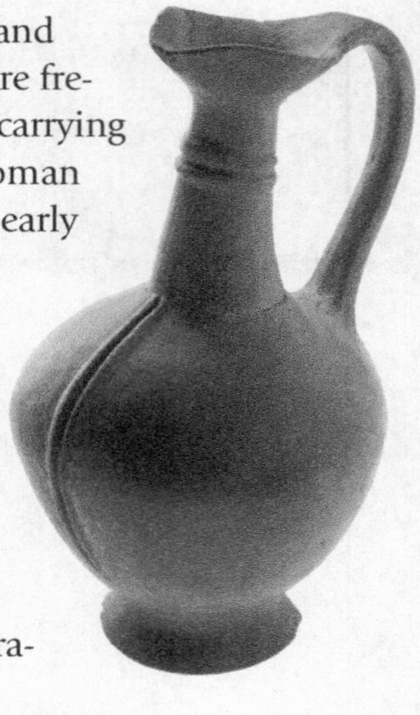

Opium was introduced to Western Asia in the eighth century through Middle Eastern and European trade. Britain became the main exporter of opium (which was grown in the fields of India); in return, the British merchants imported tea from China. With Asia's thriving opium import business, access to opium-based products became widespread. Asian practitioners prescribed opium regularly to alleviate the pain associated with medical conditions and surgical procedures. Outside of medical practices, individuals self-medicated by ingesting, drinking, and—later—smoking opium derivatives to alter their physical conditions or psychological states. Opium became one of the most widely used drugs in Asia, contributing to the drug's cultural association with this continent.

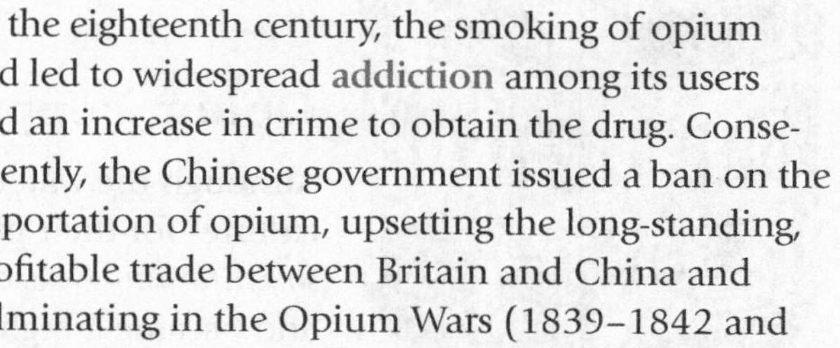

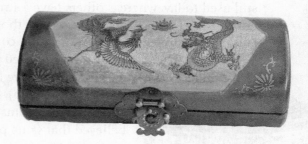

By the eighteenth century, the smoking of opium had led to widespread **addiction** among its users and an increase in crime to obtain the drug. Consequently, the Chinese government issued a ban on the importation of opium, upsetting the long-standing, profitable trade between Britain and China and culminating in the Opium Wars (1839–1842 and 1856–1860). By the advent of the twentieth century, roughly a quarter of China's population was

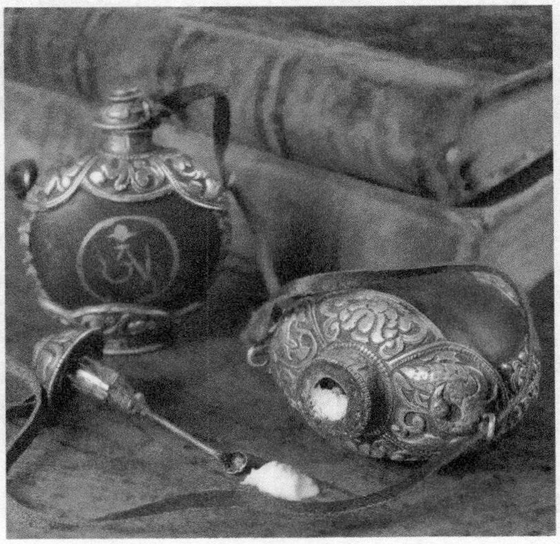

addicted to smoked opium. In fact, many Chinese immigrants to America during this period brought their addictive lifestyle to their adopted homeland and established **opium dens**—or establishments where addicts could smoke opium in a social setting.

## Laudanum, an Early Medicinal Opiate

As opium use spread around the world, experimentation with the poppy plant's extracts led to the discovery of several medicinal remedies. In the sixteenth century in Europe, **laudanum**—a preparation made from combining ground opium powder with alcohol—was used to soothe pain, calm nervousness, and elevate mood. An early formulation of laudanum was two ounces of opium, one ounce of saffron, and a drachm of cloves and cinnamon dissolved in a pint of wine. These added ingredients masked the bitter taste of the opium, making ingestion of the drug more palatable. By the nineteenth century, laudanum had spread to America and was used to alleviate pain from migraines, cure intestinal upset, and induce sleep. This opiate also became a commonly prescribed elixir for fussy, colicky, or teething children. Brands such as Godfrey's Cordial and Mrs. Winslow's Soothing Syrup were pitched to exasperated parents looking for some relief for their children—as well as for themselves.

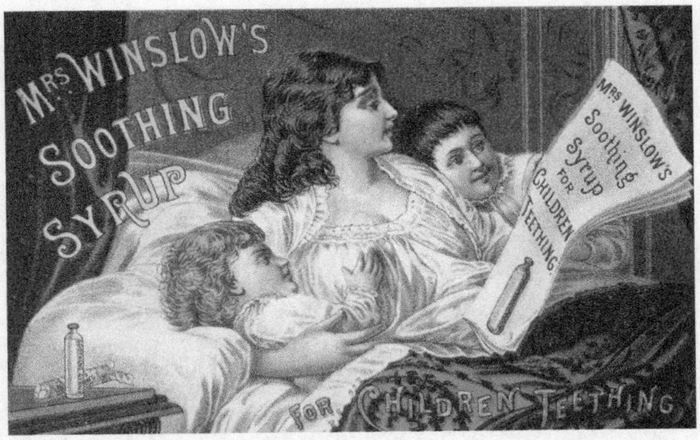


## Extraction of Morphine

In 1804, German pharmacist Friedrich Wilhelm Sertürner isolated the **alkaloid** morphine from the opium poppy. He named the substance morphium after Morpheus, the Greek god of dreams. **Morphine**, as the opiate derivative is called today, was used to treat patients suffering from acute pain and in need of quick relief. Available in oral forms, morphine was marketed under various names, including Papine (named after the opium poppy's plant species). Morphine became even more popular with the invention of the hypodermic needle in the middle of the nineteenth century, which allowed the drug to be administered in an injectable form. Ampules of morphine were commonly used by medics during the Civil War to alleviate soldiers' pain and suffering from injuries or field amputations. This practice supposedly led to widespread addiction among its military ranks. Today, morphine is a powerful narcotic (in fact, ten times more powerful than opium) that continues to be prescribed by healthcare professionals to alleviate moderate to severe pain.

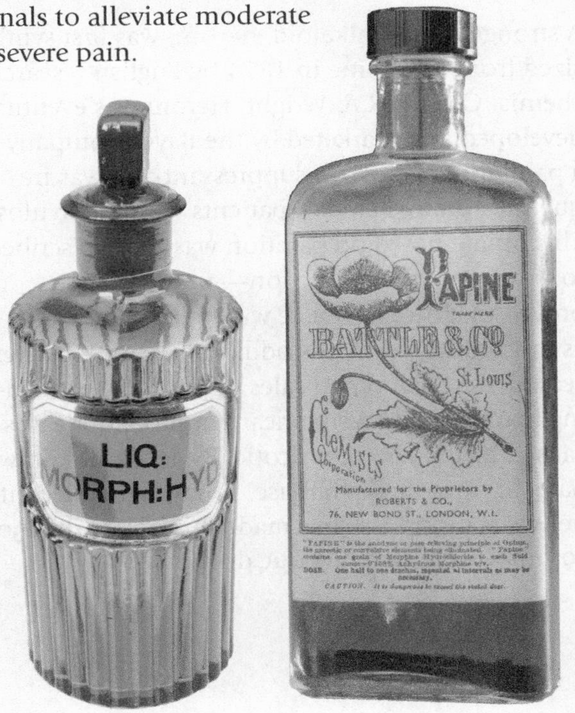

## Emergence of Codeine, Paregoric, and Heroin

A milder opiate alkaloid, **codeine**, was isolated from morphine in 1832 by French chemist Pierre-Jean Robiquet. This oral preparation had analgesic and antitussive properties and consequently was prescribed for pain relief and cough suppression. Codeine continues to be used in both prescription and over-the-counter medications and, according to the World Health Organization, is the most commonly used drug in the world.

Another mild opiate popular in the nineteenth century was **paregoric**, a camphorated tincture of opium that was used as an **anodyne**, or a medication for pain. This household remedy contained two grains of powdered opium mixed with anise oil, benzoic acid, camphor, and glycerin and was used to treat diarrhea, relieve pain from teething, and suppress coughing.

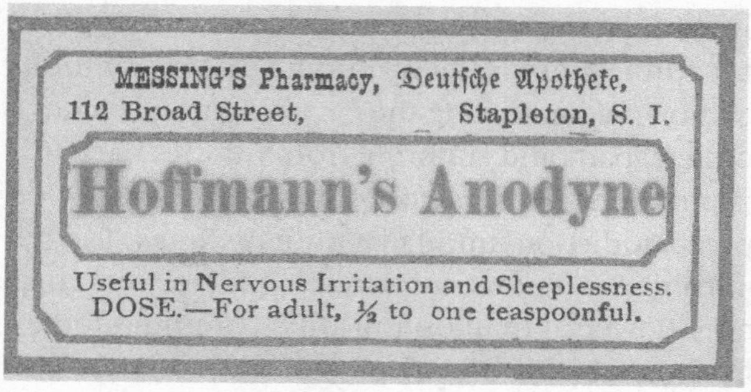


A stronger opiate alkaloid, **heroin**, was first synthesized from morphine in 1874 by English research chemist Charles R.A. Wright. Heroin was eventually developed and marketed by the Bayer Company as a painkiller and cough suppressant and was frequently administered to patients with tuberculosis. This opiate-based preparation was also prescribed to treat morphine addiction— until research proved that the substance was twice as powerful as morphine and highly addictive. In 1903, Bayer ceased production and sales of products containing heroin due to a significant number of deaths caused by the potent narcotic. By 1924, heroin was banned from medicinal use. Today, heroin's continued recreational use has made this opiate the most commonly abused narcotic drug.

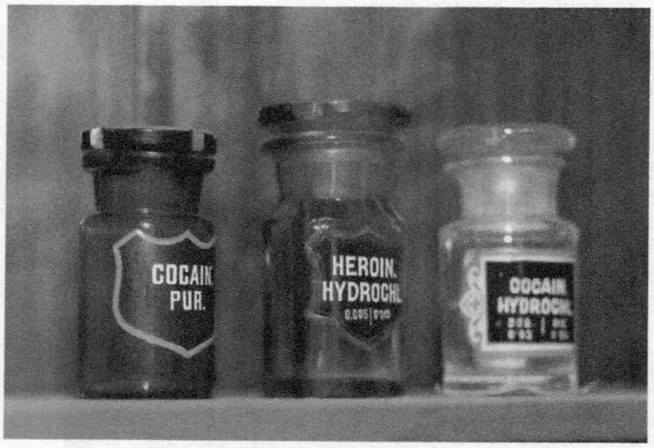


## Coca Plant and Cocaine

With the dawning of the twentieth century, a number of other plant substances began to be widely used for both medicinal and recreational purposes. The plant *Erythroxylum coca*, whose leaf contains the alkaloid **cocaine**, became a key ingredient in a number of over-the-counter products. A recognized local anesthetic, cocaine dates back to approximately 3000 BCE when indigenous South American tribes would bury bags of coca with the dead to sustain them in the afterlife. Coca produced a feeling of **euphoria**, and native South American Indians would often chew the leaves to alleviate the exhaustion felt at the high altitudes of the Andes Mountains.

The euphoric effects of coca came to the attention of the world with the publication of a book extolling the virtues of the plant. The author of the book, a nineteenth-century Italian doctor named Paolo Mantegazza, had himself experienced the effects of coca while living in Peru. Cocaine quickly became a component in several patented medicines, including cough syrups, various tonics, and throat lozenges. Cocaine also was an ingredient in coca wine and a "temperance drink" known as Coca-Cola. In

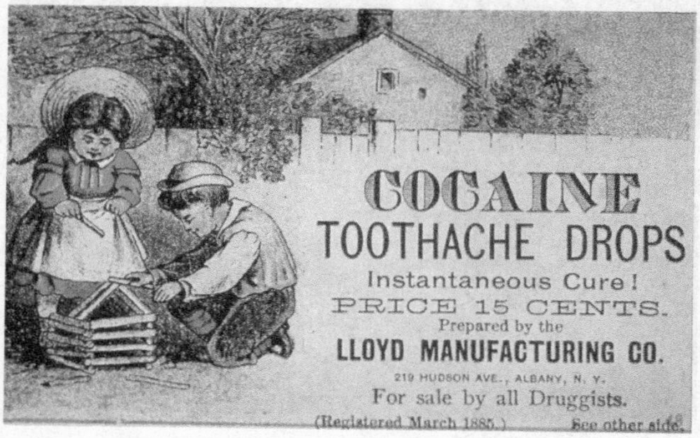

fact, for more than two decades, cocaine was part of the formula for this soft drink, until mounting concerns over the effects of cocaine forced the manufacturer to switch to using caffeine instead.

## Cannabis Plant and Marijuana

Another medicinal plant native to the Asian continent shares a similar history to the *Papaver somniferum* plant: the **Cannabis**, or the plant source of **marijuana**. The use of the cannabis plant can be traced back to 2737 BCE and the documents of Chinese emperor Shen Nung. In his papers, the emperor refers to marijuana tea, a concoction brewed from the cannabis plant and prescribed for individuals suffering from gout, arthritis, or malaria. Other ancient documents provide evidence that some early civilizations in the Far East ate the seeds of the cannabis plant. These seeds were also discovered in sacrificial vessels found in ancient tombs in China. The presence of the cannabis seeds supposedly welcomed the dead into the afterlife. In India, prior to 1000 BCE, the Aryan religion considered cannabis to be a gift from the gods because it was believed to lower fevers, improve judgment, and lead to a long and healthy life.

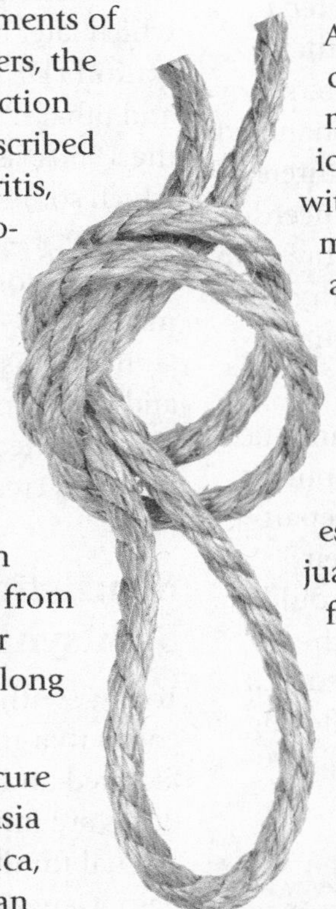

The idea of using the cannabis plant to cure various ailments quickly spread across Asia and to the neighboring continent of Africa, eventually finding its way to the European continent in 500 CE. There, the roots of the plant were used in poultices for skin inflammation and burns, and the oil was used to treat coughs, urinary incontinence, and muscle spasms.

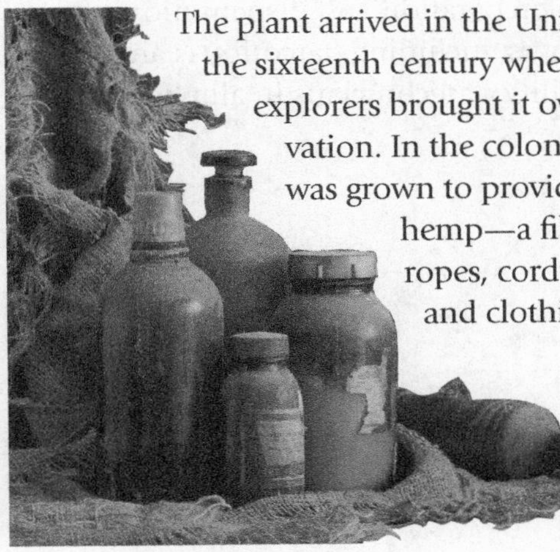

The plant arrived in the United States in the sixteenth century when European explorers brought it over for cultivation. In the colonies, cannabis was grown to provide a source of hemp—a fiber used in ropes, cording, burlap, and clothing. By the end of the nineteenth century, hemp became a significant cash crop, particularly among the southern states. Cannabis also became an ingredient in a number of medicinal preparations and was listed in the 1854 U.S. Dispensatory as a narcotic. The medication was frequently prescribed for women to ease childbirth pain and treat gynecological conditions. The medical uses of cannabis declined at the end of the nineteenth century as consumers turned to faster-acting injectable drugs and opiate-based derivatives to treat their illnesses.

At the beginning of the twentieth century, cannabis was viewed by the medical community as more of an intoxicant than a medication. This changing perception, coupled with the new federal narcotics regulations, moved the drug out of mainstream medicine and into an alternative form of medicine.

In the 1920s, alcohol prohibition encouraged individuals to pursue other means of achieving a euphoric state, and marijuana was the **recreational drug** of choice. Marijuana clubs, known as tea pads, were established, allowing users to smoke marijuana in a social setting. Like the opium dens from the previous century, club participants smoked to induce relaxation and create a sense of euphoria.

By 1937, the U.S. government passed the Marihuana [sic] Tax Act, which required that all individuals using marijuana for medicinal purposes had to register and pay a tax of $1 per ounce, and those individuals using marijuana for nonmedicinal purposes had to register and pay a tax of $100 per ounce. Needless to say, the legislation largely failed, and cannabis was removed from the U.S. Pharmacopeia and Formulary in 1941.

## Regulation of Opiate Narcotics

Although the dangers of opiate use were documented as early as the beginning of the nineteenth century, opiate addiction became an international health concern at the beginning of the twentieth century. The patented medicines containing opiate extracts were widely advertised by their manufacturers, touting their "cure-all" properties, and consumers fell victim to their addictive qualities.

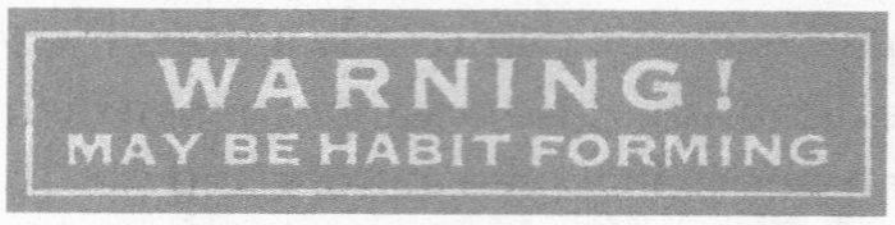


In 1906, President Theodore Roosevelt called for a conference among nations to examine the opium trade. Out of that conference—and several subsequent conferences—the U.S. Congress recognized the need for regulation of opiate narcotics. In 1914, Congress passed the Harrison Narcotic Act, a form of legislation that imposed controls for the preparation and distribution of opium, coca, and their derivatives. This act required that manufacturers, importers, pharmacists, and physicians who handled narcotics be licensed. However, the manufacturers of patented opiate preparations did not need a license as long as their remedies did not contain "more than two grains of opium, or more than one-fourth of a grain of morphine, or more than one-eighth of a grain of heroin in one avoirdupois ounce."

In addition, legislators passed a narcotics stamp tax, requiring manufacturers and distributors to purchase a narcotics stamp from the Treasury Department that was affixed to the packaging of their products. That way, the federal government could track the narcotics trade industry. However, the passage of this legislation inadvertently served as a catalyst for the creation of underground trafficking networks for illegal opiate narcotics.

In 1930, the U.S. government developed the **Federal Bureau of Narcotics** to oversee and enforce regulations related to the import, export, and taxation of narcotics. At the same time, there were growing concerns in the United States that narcotics could be addictive. Consequently, the generally accepted opinion on narcotics was that they should only be used in the proven treatment of disease. Many people feared the side effects of these drugs—specifically, mental illness and violent outbursts—and the repercussions of such side effects on society. Certain outspoken individuals went so far as to predict that drugs would lead to the downfall of society.

In 1968, the Federal Bureau of Narcotics merged with the **Bureau of Narcotics and Dangerous Drugs**, which later became the **Drug Enforcement Administration (DEA)**. Meanwhile, concerns about narcotics and other illicit drugs continued to grow throughout the 1960s, as protests against the Vietnam War—which some believe were fueled by the **drug counterculture**—and a significant number of deaths from drug overdose led to action by the federal government. In 1970, the United States enacted the **Controlled Substances Act (CSA)** to provide oversight and restriction regarding the prescription and use of all controlled substances, including narcotics. The DEA was created in 1973 to enforce the CSA.

## Synthetic and Semisynthetic Narcotics

Today, **synthetic narcotics** and **semisynthetic narcotics** that mimic the effects of opiates are manufactured and closely regulated by the DEA. These drugs are important products in the pharmaceutical arsenal for the management of moderate to severe pain. Generic names of these medications include hydrocodone, hydromorphone, meperidine, methadone, propoxyphene, and oxycodone, to name a few. Their misuse has become a growing problem in the twenty-first century; therefore, diligent record keeping of the preparation and dispensation of controlled substances, including narcotics, is an important responsibility of technicians in all pharmacy settings.

# Part 1: Concepts

Controlled substances, such as narcotic analgesics, are widely prescribed to patients in the hospital setting to control pain that is not relieved by analgesics such as acetaminophen or ibuprofen. Not all controlled substances are narcotics. Controlled substances may be found in stimulant, steroid, hallucinogen, antianxiety, and other drug classifications and are subject to the rules of the CSA.

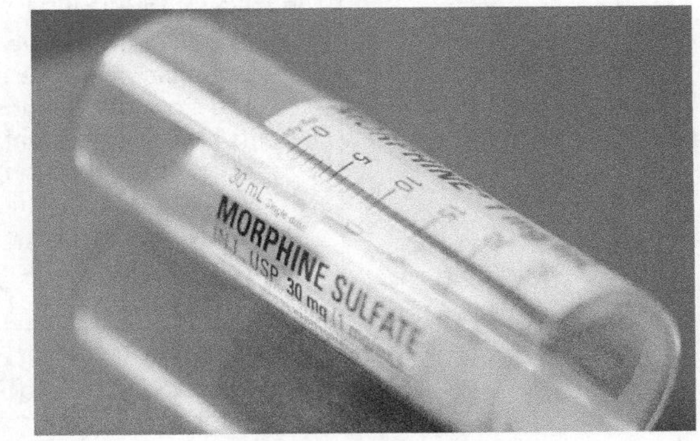

Morphine, a Schedule II controlled substance.

The CSA classifies controlled substances according to their potential for abuse and addiction. The most commonly prescribed oral narcotics fall into the Class III (C–III) category, whereas the most commonly prescribed injectable narcotics fall into the Class II (C–II) category. Most **narcotic CSPs** prepared by IV technicians are comprised of a C–II narcotic mixed with a base solution (such as normal saline [NS]). These narcotic preparations are then administered by a nurse via syringe pump, epidural cassette, or LVP.

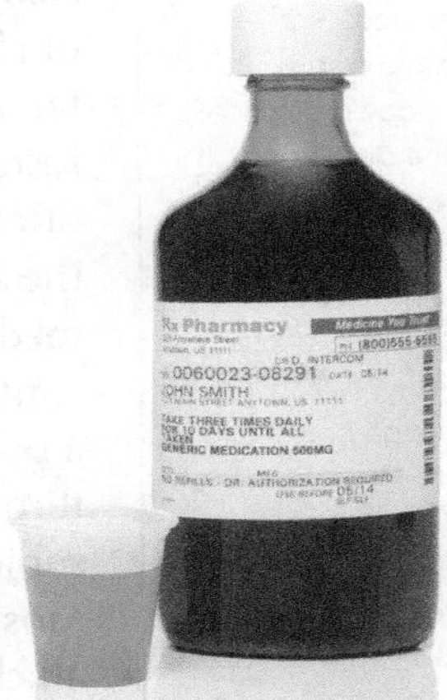

Prescription cough medicine with codeine, a Schedule V controlled substance.

## Drug Schedules

The CSA organizes controlled substances into five **drug schedules** or classes based on their **potential for abuse and addiction**. These drug schedules, including examples that fall into each class, are outlined in Table 11.1 below. When establishing these controlled substance classifications, the DEA considers a number of factors, as shown in Table 11.2.

In addition to these federal regulations enforced by the DEA, each individual State Board of Pharmacy provides guidelines and oversight regarding the prescribing and dispensing of **controlled substances**.

**Table 11.1 Drug Schedules Under the Controlled Substances Act of 1970***

| Schedule | Manufacturer's Label Stamp | Abuse Potential | Examples |
|---|---|---|---|
| I | C–I | Highest potential for abuse; no accepted medical use | Heroin, LSD, marijuana |
| II | C–II | High potential for abuse; may lead to severe physical or psychological dependence or addiction | Cocaine; codeine; dextroamphetamine; fentanyl; hydrocodone; hydrocodone combination products (hydrocodone combined with acetaminophen, aspirin, or ibuprofen); hydromorphone; levorphanol; meperidine; methylphenidate; morphine; oxycodone; racemorphan |
| III | C–III | Less potential for abuse or addiction than C–II | Codeine (when combined with acetaminophen, aspirin, or ibuprofen); ketamine |
| IV | C–IV | Less potential for abuse or addiction than C–III | Diazepam, lorazepam, phenobarbital, zolpidem |
| V | C–V | Lowest potential for abuse or addiction | Liquid (p.o.) codeine or opium preparations combined with nonnarcotic analgesic, antitussive, or antidiarrheal ingredients |

* Information for Table 11.1 can be found in the DEA Regulations, 21 C.F.R. Sections 1308.11 through 1308.15.

**Table 11.2 Determinants for a Drug's Schedule Classification**

| The DEA considers the following factors when classifying a controlled substance: |
|---|
| • Its actual or relative potential for abuse<br>• Scientific evidence of its pharmacological effects, if known<br>• The state of current scientific knowledge regarding the drug or other substance<br>• Its history or current pattern of abuse<br>• The scope, duration, and significance of abuse<br>• What, if any, risk there is to the public health<br>• Its level of psychic or physiological dependence liability<br>• Whether the substance is an immediate precursor of a substance already controlled under this title |
| Information for Table 11.2 can be found in the Controlled Substances Act, 21 USC Section 811, Authority and Criteria for Classification of Substances. |

**POINTER**

Refer to the Controlled Substances Act, the State Board of Pharmacy regulations (for the state in which you are working), and your facility's P&P manual to determine specific regulations related to controlled substance prescriptions and record keeping. Occasionally, a state law or facility procedure is somewhat different from a federal CSA law. In pharmacy, whenever two laws conflict, you must follow whichever law is more stringent.

Procedures regarding controlled substances also vary somewhat among the different types or classes of pharmacy, such as retail, hospital, nuclear, and mail-order pharmacies. For instance, community or retail pharmacies often stock C–III through C–V medications on the shelf along with **noncontrolled substance** medications. In this type of environment, C–II controlled substances must be tracked using a **perpetual inventory system**; however, C–III through C–V controlled substances are often subject to less stringent tracking requirements. Most institutional or hospital pharmacies store all classes of controlled substances under a **double-lock system**. Institutional pharmacies generally track all scheduled substances using a perpetual inventory system.

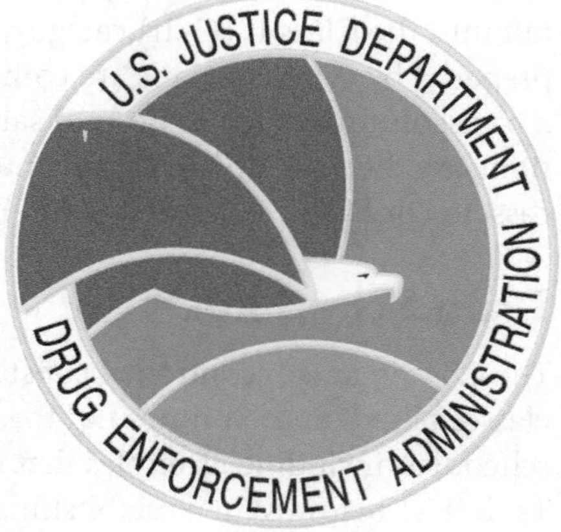


Seal of the Drug Enforcement Administration, the federal regulatory organization that enforces the Controlled Substances Act.

**POINTER**

Although not all controlled substances are narcotics, the term *narcotics* is widely used in pharmacy to describe policies, procedures, and materials related to all controlled substances. For instance the terms *narcotic room, narcotic technician, narcotic book,* and *narcotic diversion* all apply to the use of controlled substances, not just to those drugs within the narcotic drug class.

## Properties of Narcotic CSPs

The most commonly prepared controlled substance CSPs are narcotic-based CSPs. The physical and chemical properties of narcotic medications vary widely. Most narcotics have chemical properties that are generally isotonic, isoosmotic, and pH neutral. Occasionally, narcotics have an acidic pH value or are hypertonic or hyperosmotic. In those instances, the narcotic must be injected into an intravenous (IV) or IV piggyback (IVPB) base solution; the resulting CSP has physical and chemical properties that are generally isotonic, isoosmotic, and pH neutral.

## Potential Complications of Parenteral Therapy

The administration of parenteral medications involves certain potential complications that may lead to injury or, possibly, death for patient recipients. Therefore, all patients receiving parenteral therapy should be monitored for the following complications:

- nosocomial infection
- allergic reaction (including anaphylaxis)
- phlebitis

- tissuing
- embolism
- extravasation
- cellulitis
- Stevens-Johnson syndrome
- nephrotoxicity

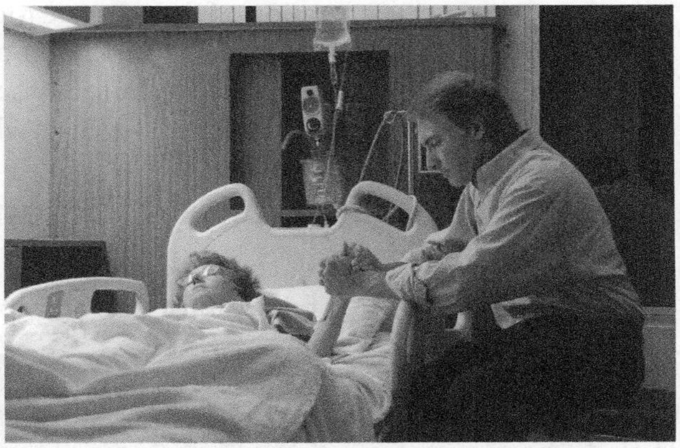

Patient receiving a narcotic preparation in a hospice setting.

In addition to the potential complications posed by all CSPs, narcotics have a chemical property that poses other unique risks. Often, patients with end-stage cancer or other terminal diseases sometimes build up a **narcotic tolerance** to the narcotic medications used to control their pain. Occasionally, a patient's tolerance builds to the point at which pain cannot be controlled by oral, topical, intramuscular (IM), or IV push narcotic analgesics. In these instances, the IV technician may be required to prepare an LVP preparation by injecting a C–II narcotic, such as **hydromorphone** or morphine (sometimes in a large quantity), into an IV base solution using standard aseptic technique. Typically, IV technicians compound this type of LVP. In the hospital, **hospice**, or **home healthcare** setting, nursing personnel typically administer the compounded preparation to the patient.

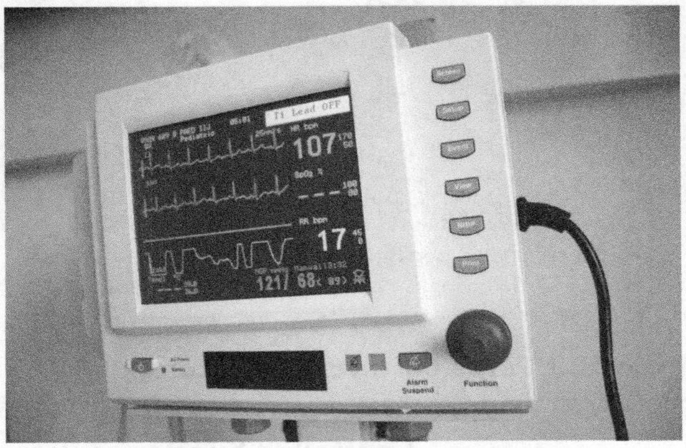


Cardiac monitor recording a patient's heart rate and respirations.

Patients receiving high-dose narcotics face a heightened risk from **central nervous system (CNS) depression.** The CNS directs the functions of all organs and tissues of the body. Narcotic analgesics cause the recipient's heart rate and respirations to slow down and, in the case of even a slight overdose, can lead to cardiac or respiratory arrest. Therefore, patients receiving narcotic medications must be closely monitored to prevent a potentially fatal reduction in their respiratory or cardiac functions.

In light of these potential complications, IV technicians must adhere to strict aseptic technique, controlled substance storage, and diligent record keeping when preparing narcotic CSPs. Likewise, healthcare personnel must vigilantly follow strict aseptic technique during the administration of narcotic CSPs to patients.

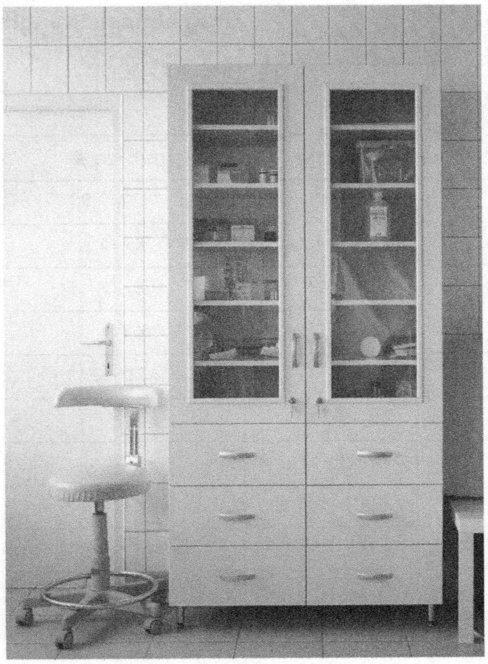

A locked narcotics cabinet.

## Controlled Substance Storage

Controlled substances carry various levels of risk with regard to their potential for drug abuse and **controlled substance diversion**, or narcotic diversion. Proper controlled substance storage is essential in mitigating these risks. In the institutional setting, all controlled substances within the pharmacy are kept in the **narcotic room** under a double-lock system. In larger institutions, a full-time pharmacy technician is often responsible for operation of the narcotic room (also referred to as the narcotic vault or cabinet, or the controlled substance room, vault, or cabinet). Smaller institutions may require the pharmacy technician to work with narcotics only on an as-needed basis or in special situations, such as when compounding narcotic CSPs.

## Controlled Substance Record Keeping

Proper controlled substance record keeping is also critical for reducing the possibility of drug abuse and controlled substance diversion. The technician responsible for handling controlled substances typically receives specialized on-the-job training. However, there is one aspect of controlled substance record keeping that all sterile compounding personnel should know: the use of a **perpetual inventory record**.

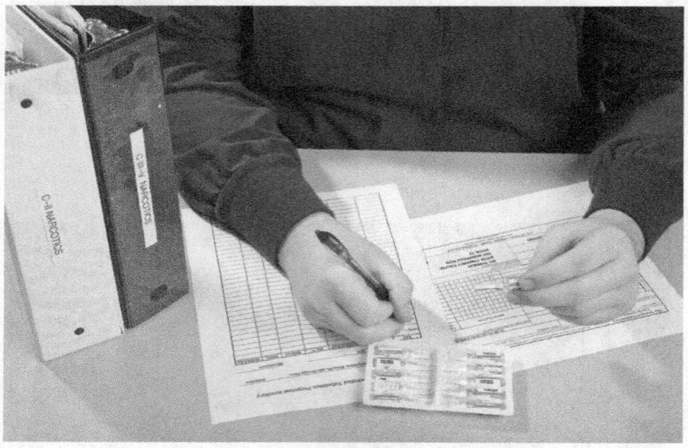

Perpetual inventory log books (one for C-II controlled substances and one for C-III through C-V controlled substances) used for controlled substances record keeping.

***Perpetual Inventory Log Book*** The **perpetual inventory log book** is an official, legal record with pages titled "Perpetual Inventory Record" or "Controlled Substance Record" (see Table 11.3).

The perpetual inventory record or log book is kept in the narcotic room or vault and is a record of all activity relating to the medications in the narcotic room. Every medication (capsule, tablet, syringe, dose cup, patch, suppository, vial, ampule, or milliliters), every

**Table 11.3 Perpetual Inventory Record**

**Controlled Substance Perpetual Inventory Record** (C-II)

Morphine 10 mg/mL Prefilled Syringe
**Drug Name, Strength, and Dosage Form**

000000-0000
**NDC**

EMCP Pharmaceuticals
**Manufacturer**

| | Date | Invoice # | Dept/Unit or Rx # | Qty +/- | Balance | Initials | Verified By |
|---|---|---|---|---|---|---|---|
| 1 | 7/15/2015 | BB888727-9980 | n/a | 200 | 200 | LMC | P.J., RPh |
| 2 | 7/16/2015 | n/a | 5E Floor Stock | 10 | 190 | LMC | P.J., RPh |
| 3 | 7/16/2015 | n/a | 663577 | 10 | 180 | LMC | P.J., RPh |
| 4 | 7/16/2015 | n/a | 4W Floor Stock | 10 | 170 | LMC | P.J., RPh |
| 5 | 7/17/2015 | BB8876392-8873 | N/A | 100 | 270 | V.V. | L.L., RPh |
| 6 | 7/17/2015 | N/A | 887309 | 5 | 265 | V.V. | L.L., RPh |
| 7 | 7/18/2015 | N/A | 256663 | 50 | 215 | V.V. | L.L., RPh |
| 8 | 7/18/2015 | n/a | 339287 | 30 | 185 | LMC | L.L., RPh |
| 9 | 7/20/2015 | BB267883-9989 | N/A | 100 | 285 | C.B. | TVG, RPh |
| 10 | | | | | | | |
| 11 | | | | | | | |
| 12 | | | | | | | |

medication strength (indicated by the number of milligrams per dose [10-mg tablet, 500-mg capsule, 25-mg patch, or 50-mg syringe]), and every controlled substance brought into the narcotic room (such as when new stock is received from the drug wholesaler) must be added to the perpetual inventory record. Every controlled substance that leaves the narcotic room—for example, to fill **floor stock**, prepare an epidural cassette, or compound a PCA syringe—must be signed out and subtracted from the perpetual inventory record. This process is referred to as a **narcotic sign-out**, or a controlled substance sign-out. In effect, the drug form and strength of every controlled substance is entered and maintained within the perpetual inventory log book.

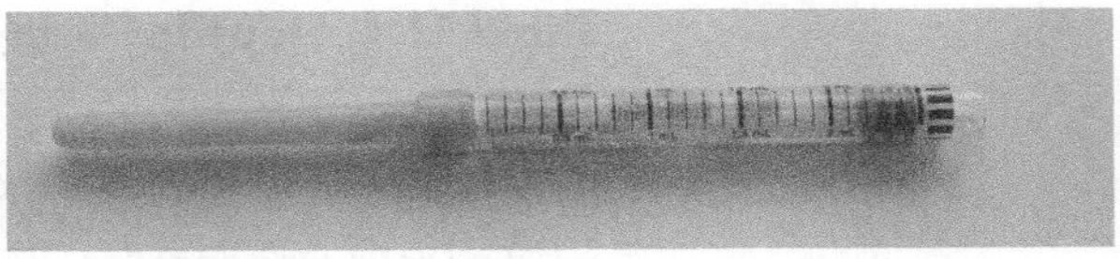

Morphine prefilled syringe.

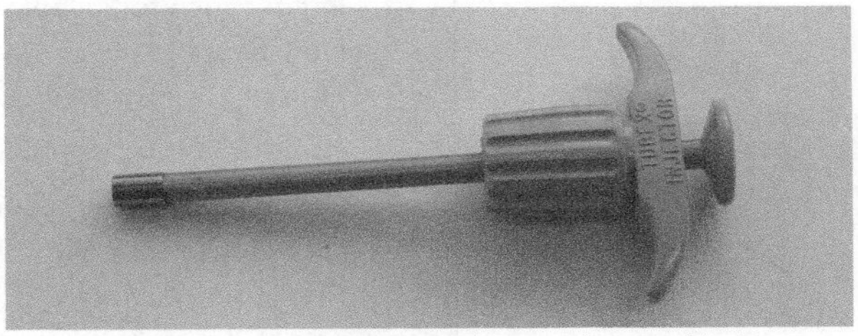

Tubex injector used to administer medications from prefilled syringes.

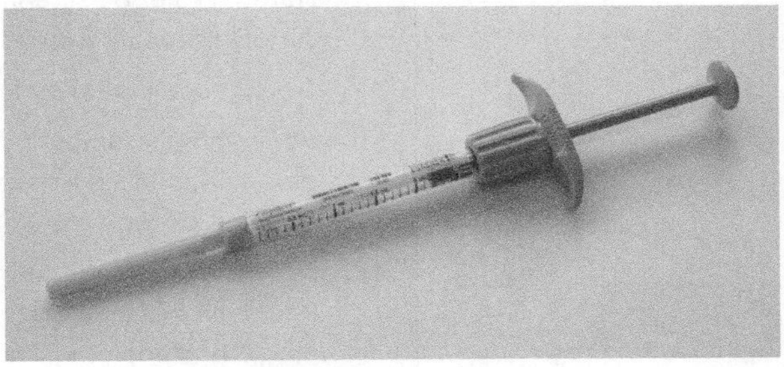

Morphine prefilled syringe attached to Tubex injector.

Should sterile compounding personnel ever have to remove a narcotic from the narcotic room in order to prepare a CSP, they must know the proper record-keeping procedure using the perpetual inventory record. That procedure begins with using the correct log book. There is one perpetual log book for C–II controlled substances and a different perpetual log book for C–III through C–V controlled substances. Refer to Table 11.4 for the proper procedures to follow when using the perpetual inventory record.

***Error Correction in the Perpetual Inventory Log Book*** In most facilities, pharmacy personnel will record an entry or addition to the log in black ink, and record withdrawals or negative balances (within the "Qty +/–" column only) in red ink. Personnel should never erase, scribble over, or use correcting tape or fluid to cover transcription errors. Instead, technicians should note an error by drawing a single line through the entire entry and placing their circled initials next to the text with the strike-through line. Following this error correction process is critical, for the perpetual inventory log book is an official document that may be reviewed by agencies such as the state board of pharmacy and the DEA.

***Security and Disposal of Controlled Substances*** To provide the utmost security, sterile compounding personnel should always ensure that the narcotics, the keys to the narcotic room, and all narcotic records are kept in their control while working in the narcotic room, working with perpetual inventory records, and compounding narcotic preparations. If a **discrepancy** is discovered while creating a record in the perpetual inventory log book, IV technicians must immediately report it to their instructor or pharmacist.

IV technicians must also properly dispose of unused controlled substance solutions after completing sterile compounding procedures. For this type of controlled substance waste, technicians should inject the unused solution into the sharps container or down the drain of the anteroom sink (due to environmental concerns, your facility may take additional, specific precautions when disposing of such narcotics). In order to prevent narcotic diversion, all narcotic waste procedures must be recorded in the perpetual inventory record and must be observed by a **narcotic waste witness**. Refer to the facility's P&P manual for specific narcotic waste disposal procedures.

**POINTER**

Some of the controlled substances administered in a hospital setting are supplied from their manufacturers in prefilled glass or plastic syringes. At an interval directed by the medication order, the nurse attaches the prefilled narcotic syringe to the Tubex injector and administers the medication to the patient by either the IM or IV push route.

**POINTER**

Although this chapter provides instruction for a perpetual inventory record-keeping system that uses a written or "hard copy" format, some facilities use a computerized system. Should your pharmacy use a different type of perpetual inventory system, consult your facility's P&P manual for procedures related to its use.

**Table 11.4 Steps for Using the Perpetual Inventory Record**

1. Open the perpetual log book to find the perpetual inventory record for the narcotic needed to prepare the CSP. Using a black pen, record the date in the column titled "Date."
2. Leave the space for "Invoice #" blank, as this column is used for filling floor stock narcotics.
3. In the space for "Dept/Unit or Rx #," write the name and room number of the patient on the CSP label.
4. Go to the "Quantity +/− " column. Using a red pen, record the amount or quantity of the narcotic you will need to remove from the narcotic room to prepare the CSP.
5. Using a calculator, subtract the quantity you recorded in step 4 from the existing balance in the balance space from the most recent (previous) entry in the perpetual inventory record. Then, using a black pen, record the new balance in the "Balance" column.
6. Locate the shelf or bin within the narcotic room in which the narcotic needed for the CSP is stored. *Note:* Be sure that you have the correct narcotic concentration. Most manufacturers supply narcotics in several different strengths.
7. Count each vial or syringe of this medication.
8. Verify that the amount you counted on the shelf or in the bin matches the balance that you determined in step 5. Remove the number of vials or syringes needed to prepare the CSP from the storage shelf or bin.
9. If the actual count (that which remains in the storage bin) matches the existing balance (that which is indicated by the number you wrote in the "Balance" column), you have properly completed the narcotic sign-out. You may now return to the anteroom to begin the narcotic CSP procedure.
10. If the balance on hand does *not* match the existing balance, you have discovered a discrepancy. Consult your instructor or pharmacist for the procedures to resolve a narcotic discrepancy.

***Note:*** Refer to the *Pharmacy Labs for Technicians: Building Skills in Pharmacy Practice* by Jason Sparks and Lisa McCartney for in-depth, step-by-step instruction in narcotic record keeping.

**POINTER**

Some facilities limit pharmacy controlled substances access to pharmacists, and do not allow pharmacy technicians to add or remove controlled substances from the perpetual inventory logs. Refer to your facility's P&P manual to determine the narcotic procedures for your pharmacy.

## Patient-Controlled Analgesia

In addition to understanding the storage, record-keeping, and disposal guidelines for controlled substances, IV technicians need to be familiar with several different controlled substance CSPs and their preparation, including LVPs used for chronic, severe pain control as well as **epidurals** and **patient-controlled analgesia (PCA)**. For training purposes, the procedural lab of this chapter focuses on the preparation of a PCA syringe.

A PCA provides narcotic pain control, or **narcotic analgesia**, for hospitalized patients. Most often used on a short-term basis to control postoperative pain, a PCA is administered via a preprogrammed syringe pump. The pump allows a patient to self-administer a dose of the medication intravenously by pressing a handheld controller. To avoid dosage errors, the PCA pump is preprogrammed to lock out the patient if a dose is requested before the scheduled time. Experience has shown that patient control of analgesia leads to less narcotic use and, therefore, less potential for issues related to drug tolerance or side effects.

## USP Chapter <797> Guidelines for Controlled Substance CSPs

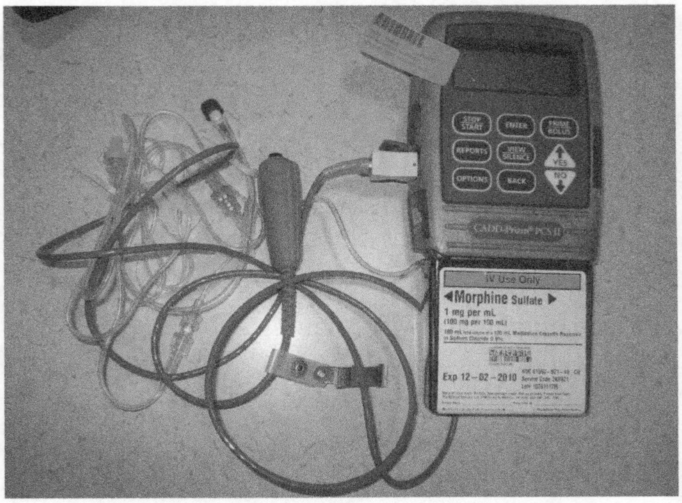

PCA infusion pump for postoperative IV administration of morphine.

In addition to the detailed record-keeping mandates for controlled substances, there are a number of other procedures that must be carefully followed while compounding controlled substance preparations. These procedures are presented in USP Chapter <797> and are reinforced in each facility's P&P manual. Sterile compounding personnel must pay strict attention to aseptic protocols both in the anteroom and clean room. Any breach in these protocols may result in medication errors, sepsis, or, possibly, death for patient recipients. Therefore, as an IV technician, you bear primary responsibility for the preparation and integrity of the CSPs. With that in mind, only those personnel who have been specially trained, process validated, and certified in aseptic technique and sterile product preparation should be allowed to compound CSPs. Part 2 of this chapter guides you through the discovery and demonstration of proper aseptic technique in a PCA syringe preparation.

# Concepts Self-Check

## Check Your Understanding

*Write your answers on a separate sheet of paper, as modeled in these examples:* 1d; 2c; 3b; *etc. Check your answers using the Answer Key in Appendix A.*

**1.** Which plant is the primary source of most natural narcotic substances?
   a. *Erythroxylum coca*
   b. *Nymphaea*
   c. *Papaver somniferum*
   d. *Cannabis*

**2.** Which of the following narcotics are derivatives of the opium poppy?
   a. paregoric, codeine, laudanum
   b. cocaine, cannabis, LSD
   c. opium, morphine, heroin
   d. all of the above
   e. both *a* and *c*

**3.** Which schedule of controlled substances has no accepted medical use?
   a. C–I
   b. C–II
   c. C–III
   d. C–IV
   e. C–V

**4.** The DEA was developed to oversee and enforce which federal act?
   a. the PCA
   b. the DEA
   c. the CSP
   d. the CSA

**5.** Controlled substance CSPs most often involve compounding medications using narcotics from which schedule?
   a. C–I
   b. C–II
   c. C–III
   d. C–IV
   e. C–V

## Apply Your Knowledge

*On a separate sheet of paper, write your answers to the questions posed in the paragraph below. Use complete sentences and take time to create a thorough and thoughtful response. Check your answers against the Answer Key in Appendix A.*

In Part 1 of this chapter, you learned that, in addition to aseptic technique, narcotic CSPs require strict adherence to legal regulations and record keeping. With that in mind, what is the rationale for handling controlled substances in a different manner than other prescription drugs? What is the rationale for handling C–II drugs differently than C–III through C–V drugs?

# Part 2: Training

*Before performing this lab, review the Sterile Compounding Area Procedures listed on pages 162–163 at the end of the Unit 2 opener, and preview the accompanying process validation checklist in Appendix D.*

## Understand the Resources and Supplies

USP Chapter <797> prescribes a number of special requirements for narcotic preparations. This chapter and the corresponding lab provide resources and supplies that are in alignment with the directives set forth in USP Chapter <797>.

### Essential Supplies

Most sterile compounding procedures require the same essential supply items to be available for use in both the anteroom and the clean room. For the anteroom, these supplies include a medication order and CSP label; a standard calculator; a pen; a permanent, felt-tip marker; large and small plastic bags; aseptic garb; a sterile gown; presaturated, aseptic cleaning wipes; sterile, foamed 70% isopropyl alcohol (IPA); a waste container; and a transport vehicle (optional). (Various other compounding supplies, such as those needed for aseptic hand washing and hood cleaning, are necessary supplies but, for the purposes of this lab, are not included on the Essential Supplies list.) In the clean room, essential supply items include sterile, foamed 70% IPA; sterile, powder-free gloves; sterile 70% IPA swabs; a sharps container; a waste container; and a laminar airflow hood.

### Procedure-Specific Supplies

In addition to the previously listed essential supplies, each sterile compounding procedure requires supply items specific to the procedure being performed. The type, number, and amount of procedure-specific supply items are determined by the IV technician prior to performing the procedure, based on information provided on the CSP label and the medication additive label. After reading these labels, the IV technician performs one or more calculations that reveal the number and volume of additives needed to prepare the CSP. This information, in turn, dictates the number, size, and types of syringes needed for the procedure.

***Controlled-Substance Perpetual Inventory Log Book*** A standard controlled-substance perpetual inventory log book (in this instance, the type used for the record keeping of C–II narcotics) is required for the compounding of narcotic CSPs. In this chapter's procedural lab, you'll specifically need to log your use of meperidine 50 mg/mL in 2-mL vials. Record the withdrawal of the number of vials needed to prepare the desired dose of the PCA.

***PCA Supply Items*** To prepare the PCA in the procedural lab, you need to be familiar with vials and their handling techniques (see Chapter 8). Regular needles and syringes of various sizes are also required to separately draw up the 0.9% sodium chloride (or normal saline [NS]) diluent and the narcotic. Lastly, you need to obtain a Luer-to-Luer connector, a supply item that will aid the transfer of contents from one syringe into another syringe; a syringe cap for the PCA syringe; and an IVA syringe seal.

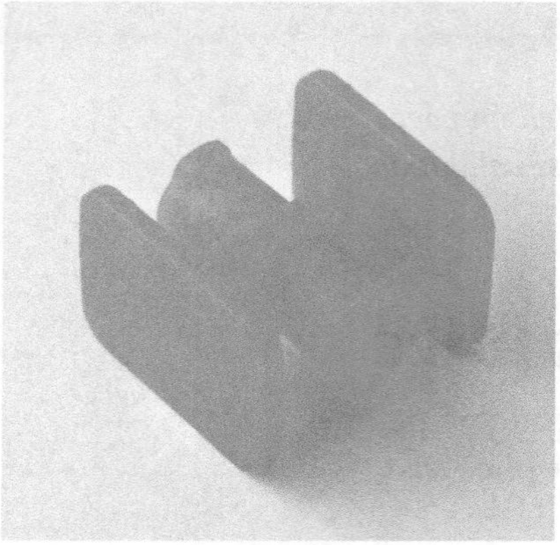

Luer-to-Luer connector that joins the tips of two syringes.

**Luer-to-Luer Connector** A **Luer-to-Luer connector** is a small plastic device used to join the tips of two syringes. This connector is comprised of a short (approximately ½″ long) tube with a Luer-lock at each end. You must remove the needle from one syringe and then fasten that syringe onto the Luer-lock at one end of the connector. Next, remove the needle from the second syringe and then fasten that syringe onto the Luer-lock at the other end of the connector. The fluid is then easily injected from one syringe into the other through the center tube connecting the two Luer-locked ends of the Luer-to-Luer connector.

Take care when using the Luer-to-Luer connector, as both ends are critical sites that must never be touched or shadowed. Some brands of Luer-to-Luer connectors have a small plastic cap on each end, which must be removed prior to use. However, most connectors do not have these protective caps. Therefore, it is imperative that you aseptically attach a syringe to each end without ever placing the uncapped Luer-to-Luer connectors or the uncapped needle-and-syringe unit onto the hood's work surface.

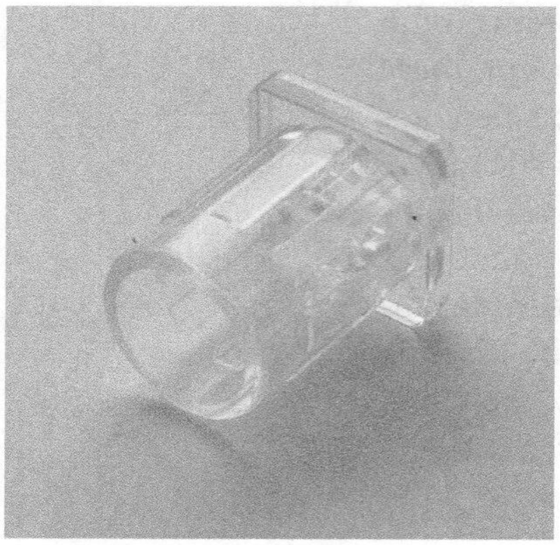

A syringe cap.

**Syringe Cap** Upon completion of the PCA compounding procedures, you need to attach a sterile, plastic cap, called a **syringe cap**, to the tip of the PCA syringe. Using gentle downward pressure, attach the syringe cap to the tip of the filled syringe by slipping the open end of the syringe cap over the tip of the syringe and screwing it onto the Luer-lock threads of the syringe hub.

**IVA Syringe Seal** An **IVA syringe seal** is an adhesive seal that is often affixed to a syringe cap to provide evidence of tampering should anyone attempt to remove the seal prior to patient administration. Although the application of this seal is optional, best practice indicates its placement during narcotic preparation.

***IVPB Base Solutions*** The IVPB base solution bag is the same type of bag used for other vial-based IVPBs: a bag with a tail injection port. When inserting a needle into the injection port of an IVPB, insert the needle directly into the injection port without regard to the position of the needle bevel and without creating any bend to the needle.

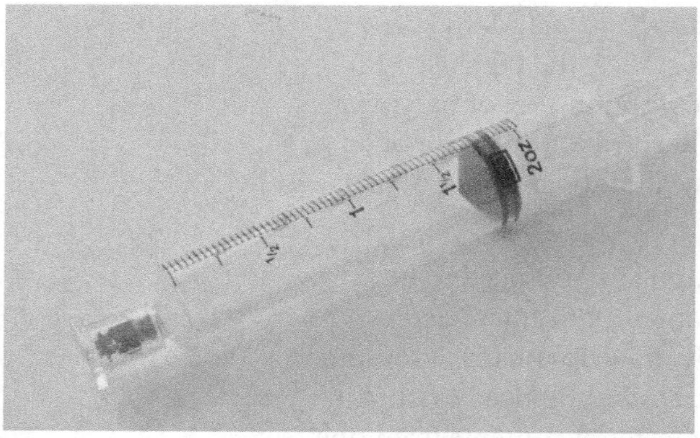

A syringe cap placed on a PCA syringe.

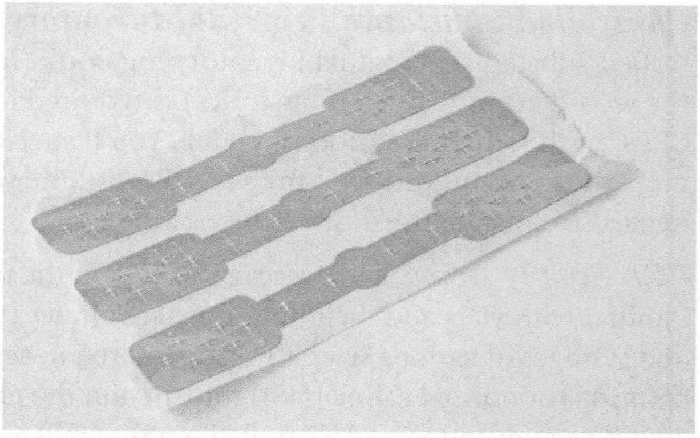

IVA syringe seals.

## Critical Sites of Essential Supplies and PCA Supplies

Before beginning preparatory procedures in the anteroom or clean room, the IV technician must recall the critical sites of the supplies. Identifying the critical site of each supply item helps you to determine the proper procedure for handling the supply item once you enter the clean room and begin working in the hood.

The critical sites of essential supply items include sterile 70% IPA swabs, the syringe tip, the piston plunger and inner plunger shaft of each syringe, and the needles. These critical sites are supplied by the manufacturer in sterile form and should, therefore, not be swabbed with alcohol prior to use.

The critical sites of the PCA supplies used for the Chapter 11 procedural lab include the injection port of the IVPB base solution and the vial top. These critical sites must be swabbed with sterile 70% IPA prior to needle insertion to decrease the likelihood of contaminating the solution during injection or withdrawal procedures.

In addition to these supplies, the Chapter 11 procedural lab also instructs you in the proper use of a Luer-to-Luer connector and a syringe cap. These are sterile supply items that should never be swabbed with IPA. All compounding procedures require that you take care to avoid tainting the critical site of any of the supply items through touch contamination, shadowing, or incorrect placement of the item within the hood.

# Preview the Lab Procedure

*The following material provides a brief overview of the lab procedure that you will perform. First, read the* Preview the Lab Procedure *section. Then read each step of the* Procedural Lab *section carefully, visualizing every action. Next, reinforce your understanding of the process by watching the demonstration video. Once you are in the lab, your instructor will demonstrate the procedure, and then you will perform the procedure by following the steps in the* Procedural Lab *section. Practice the lab procedure multiple times. After sufficient practice, you will complete the lab procedure for process validation by your instructor.*

*Note: This procedural lab requires the use of a basic, open-sided, horizontal laminar airflow hood. For pharmacies that do not have this type of hood, IV technicians should consult the* Instruction Guide *provided by the hood's manufacturer or their facility's P&P manual to determine which procedures may need to be adjusted to suit their hood.*

> **POINTER**
> Sterile compounding personnel must comply with certain restrictions when working in the anteroom and clean room areas. These restrictions include no gum chewing, horseplay, or food or drink in both the anteroom and clean room, and no hair spray, perfume, makeup, artificial or polished nails, or jewelry in the sterile compounding environment.

## Anteroom Preparatory Procedures

As you already know, the preparation for the sterile compounding process begins in the anteroom. This transition area provides a space for implementing the standard pharmacy protocols discussed in Chapters 3–6 of this textbook, including:

- verifying the CSP label against the medication order
- performing correct pharmacy calculations to determine type, size, and number of supply items needed
- gathering and cleaning of supplies
- performing aseptic garbing and hand washing
- donning a sterile gown

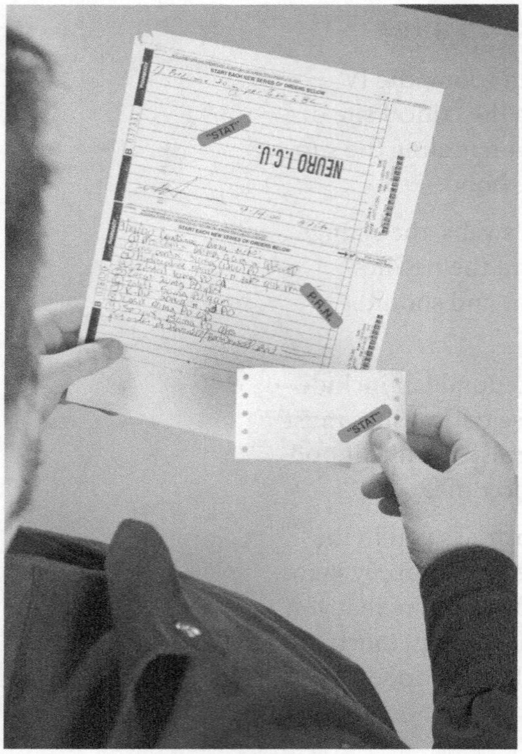

An IV technician verifying the medication order with the CSP label.

***Verifying the CSP Label*** Compare the medication order to the controlled substance CSP label to verify that all information on the CSP label matches the medication order exactly. Once you have verified the accuracy of the controlled substance CSP label, you need to determine the type, size, and number of supply items needed for the procedure.

***Performing Pharmacy Calculations*** Using information gleaned from the controlled substance CSP label and the narcotic vial label, calculate the desired volume. The **desired volume** is the volume you must withdraw from the narcotic vial to deliver the dose ordered by the prescriber. In addition to dosage calculations, the Chapter 11 procedural lab requires basic mathematical calculations to properly record the withdrawal of the narcotic in the perpetual inventory log book. Use the procedures identified in Table 11.4 to sign out the controlled substance required to prepare the CSP from the narcotic room. Read the CSP label to determine the amount of NS you need to draw up to prepare the CSP. (For additional assistance on performing calculations, refer to Chapter 5 of this textbook.)

***Gathering and Cleaning Supplies*** After performing the calculations and recording the withdrawal of the narcotic in the perpetual inventory log book, place the CSP label into the small plastic bag, place the medication order into the large plastic bag, and seal both bags. Then gather the necessary supplies, including an appropriately sized syringe for the desired volume needed. Obtain a transport vehicle—such as a stainless-steel cart, basket, or tray—to facilitate an easy transfer of supplies into and out of the clean room.

Wipe down or spray the exterior surface of every supply item, as well as the transport vehicle, with an appropriate cleaning agent. Place the cleaned supply items into the transport vehicle.

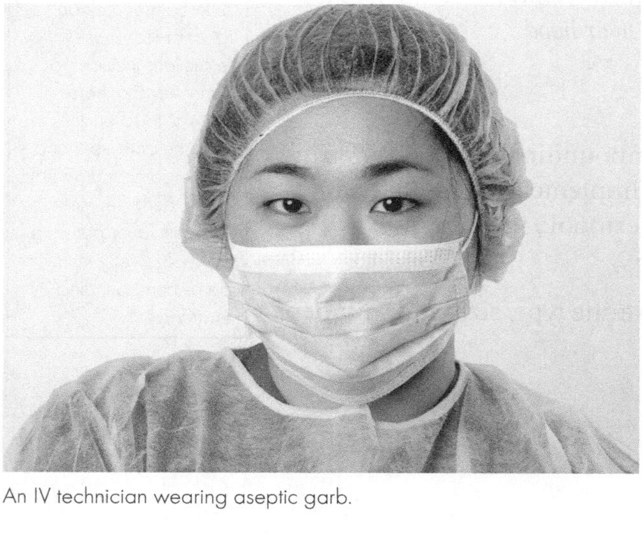

An IV technician wearing aseptic garb.

***Donning PPE*** Now that you have assembled your clean supplies, you must put on personal protective equipment (PPE). First, remove visible jewelry and ensure that you are properly attired for working in the clean room. Then put on aseptic shoe covers, a hair cover, a face mask, and, if necessary, a beard cover. Lastly, don a sterile gown.

Due to time constraints, you will not perform aseptic hand-washing procedures during this procedural lab. Keep in mind that, in sterile compounding practice, aseptic hand-washing procedures are mandatory and must be performed prior to donning a sterile gown.

## Clean Room Preparatory Procedures

When preparing controlled substance preparations for patient administration, sterile compounding personnel must diligently follow established pharmacy clean room protocols as well. These protocols, discussed in Chapters 6 and 7, include:

- cleansing hands with sterile, foamed 70% IPA
- donning sterile gloves
- cleaning the hood

Once the preparatory steps have been completed, narcotic PCA syringe compounding procedures may begin.

Upon entering the clean room, place the transport basket or tray onto a clean shelf, table, or countertop. If the transport vehicle used is a cart, wheel it so that it is positioned away from the hood prefilter. Cleanse your hands and forearms with sterile, foamed 70% IPA and allow them to dry thoroughly. Don sterile gloves according to standard aseptic technique procedures.

**POINTER**

Refer to Chapter 6 for procedures related to the use of sterile, foamed 70% IPA and the donning of sterile gloves.

Due to time constraints, you will not perform hood-cleaning procedures during this procedural lab. Keep in mind that, in sterile compounding practice, hood-cleaning procedures are mandatory and must be performed prior to beginning sterile compounding procedures and at intervals prescribed by USP Chapter <797>.

***Arranging and Preparing Supplies in the Hood*** Once the hood has been cleaned, you must transfer the clean supplies from the transport vehicle or clean countertop to certain areas of the hood. Place small supply items—such as the vials, needles, Luer-lock syringes, Luer-to-Luer connector, syringe cap, and alcohol swabs—within the outer six-inch zone of the hood. Remove the dust cover of the IVPB base solution, and dispose of the dust cover into an appropriate waste container. Then place the IVPB into the direct compounding area (DCA) of the hood, or at least six inches inside of the hood. Be sure to place the injection port of the IVPB bag so that it receives uninterrupted airflow from the high-efficiency particulate airflow (HEPA) filter. Swab the injection port of the IVPB, and then place the IPA swab onto the hood's work surface within the DCA.

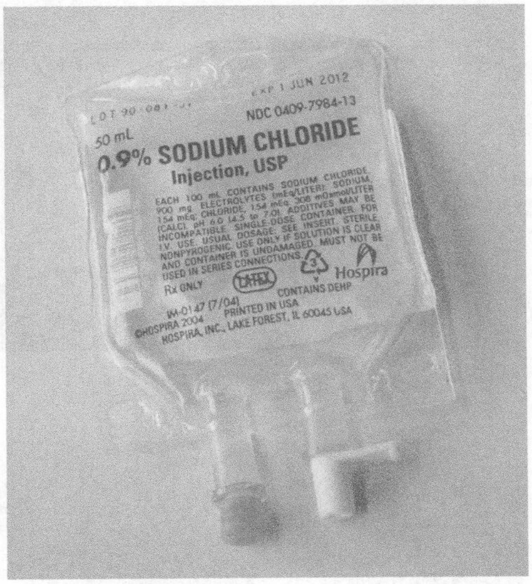

IVPB bag base solution.

## Narcotic PCA Syringe Compounding Procedure

With the small supply items arranged in the outer six-inch zone and the large supply items placed in the DCA, you are ready to begin the narcotic PCA syringe compounding procedure. Within the DCA, aseptically attach a regular needle to a 60-mL Luer-lock syringe. Without drawing air into the syringe, and without regard to the direction of the needle bevel, aseptically insert the needle into the IVPB injection port. Take care not to puncture the side wall of the injection port.

**POINTER**

The IVPB bag expands when fluid is injected and collapses when fluid is withdrawn, preventing pressure from building up within the IVPB. Therefore, you do not need to create positive pressure, as you would when withdrawing from a vial.

With the IVPB remaining on the hood's work surface, firmly grasp the barrel of the syringe with your nondominant hand, as you would the throttle of a motorcycle or the handlebar of a bicycle. *Note:* The unusual "motorcycle throttle" hand position

**POINTER**
Some IV technicians prefer to hang the IVPB bag from one of the stainless-steel hooks on the hood's hang bar while performing IVPB or IV withdrawal procedures. The method you choose is a matter of personal preference.

provides you with the best level of support while you forcefully pull down on the plunger flat knob with your dominant hand. When withdrawing fluid, take care not to pull down on the plunger so forcefully that it dislodges from the syringe. Brace the syringe barrel against the hood's work surface. Grasp the flat knob of the plunger with your dominant hand and forcefully pull back on the plunger until you have drawn up slightly more than the desired volume of NS (in this lab, approximately 41 mL). Use appropriate technique to remove bubbles and excess fluid from the syringe and then verify the correct volume within the syringe. (For additional assistance on bubble removal from a syringe, see Chapter 10 of this textbook.) Then place the filled and capped NS syringe onto the hood's work surface next to the empty IVPB.

**POINTER**
Be sure that all of the vials are arranged within the DCA so that the vials' rubber tops receive uninterrupted airflow from the HEPA filter throughout the compounding procedure.

Place all of the remaining supply items into the outer six-inch staging area of the hood. Bring each meperidine vial into the DCA. Remove the flip-top caps of the meperidine vials and then disinfect the vials' rubber tops with an IPA swab.

Assemble a new syringe and capped needle in such a way as to avoid touch contamination and shadowing of the syringe tip and the needle hub. After removing the needle cap and placing it on an alcohol swab, use aseptic technique to insert the needle into the first meperidine vial, and then use positive pressure and the milking technique to withdraw the entire contents of the vial into a 10-mL syringe. Remove the needle-and-syringe unit from the first vial and immediately insert it into the second vial. Draw the contents of the second vial into the syringe using the milking technique. ***Note:*** You are only required to inject air into the first vial. Once you have drawn the contents of the first vial into the syringe, the liquid within the syringe will provide enough positive pressure to perform the milking technique on the remaining vials. Repeat the milking procedure until you have withdrawn the correct volume of meperidine into the syringe. Cap the syringe and then place the filled and capped narcotic syringe next to the meperidine vials on the hood's work surface within the DCA, immediately adjacent to the NS syringe and empty IVPB. Await a verification check by your instructor or a pharmacist.

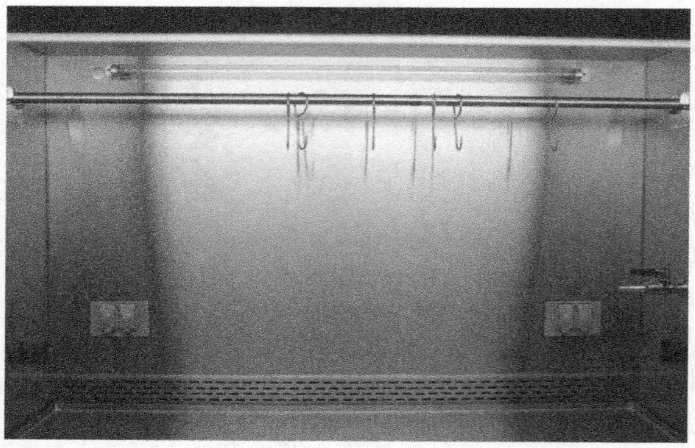
Laminar airflow hood with hang bar and hooks.

After the verification check, aseptically remove the needle from the narcotic syringe and carefully attach one end of a Luer-to-Luer connector to the tip of the filled narcotic syringe. Place the needle into the sharps container. Then remove the needle and aseptically attach the NS syringe to the other end of the Luer-to-Luer connector. Place the needle into the sharps container. Push down on the flat knob of the plunger of the syringe containing the narcotic while simultaneously pulling down on the flat knob of the plunger of the NS syringe. This action transfers the narcotic into the NS syringe. Once the narcotic has been completely transferred and any air bubbles have been removed, detach the filled PCA syringe (now containing both NS and the narcotic) from the Luer-to-Luer connector. Aseptically attach a syringe cap to the tip of the

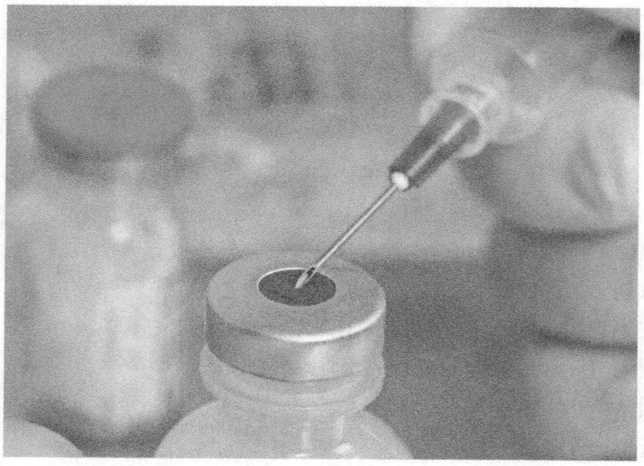
An IV technician piercing a vial's rubber top to withdraw medication; note the red flip-top cap covering the vial in the background.

PCA syringe. Place the empty syringe with attached Luer-to-Luer connector into the sharps container. Finally, label the compounded PCA syringe and place an IVA syringe tip seal over the syringe cap, extending it from one side of the syringe barrel and over the syringe tip before attaching to the other side of the syringe barrel.

Upon completion of the PCA syringe compounding procedure, dispose of used vials and supply items in the appropriate waste containers. If there is any remaining fluid in the meperidine vials, draw it up and summon a pharmacist to witness your narcotic waste disposal. ***Note:*** Consult your instructor or pharmacist to determine procedures related to recording controlled substance waste in the perpetual inventory log book. The pharmacist or narcotic technician typically records controlled substance waste in the perpetual log. Place the labeled PCA syringe and any unused supply items into the transport vehicle, and return these items to the anteroom. Record the date and your initials on the CSP label. Remove PPE in the order and manner described in Chapter 6 of this textbook.

# Watch the Demonstration Video

*Watch the Chapter 11 Demonstration Video, which shows the step-by-step aseptic procedures for compounding a narcotic PCA syringe preparation. For the purposes of the Chapter 11 Demonstration Video, neither aseptic hand washing nor hood cleaning is demonstrated. Refer to the Chapter 6 video for a demonstration of aseptic hand-washing procedures, and to the Chapter 7 video for a demonstration of correct hood-cleaning procedures.*

Training Videos DVD

# Procedural Lab

*This lab walks you through the step-by-step actions that you must follow to properly compound a narcotic PCA syringe preparation. As with most sterile compounding procedures, there are several ways that a PCA syringe may be aseptically prepared. The Chapter 11 procedural lab presents one possible scenario for PCA syringe preparation and offers you the opportunity to practice using a Luer-to-Luer connector. Take your time. Work through each step methodically and with close attention to detail.*

***Note:*** *For the purposes of this procedural lab, you will not perform aseptic hand-washing or hood-cleaning procedures unless directed to do so by your instructor. Should your instructor ask you to perform these procedures, refer to Chapter 6 for instructions on aseptic hand washing and to Chapter 7 for directions on correct hood cleaning.*

***Note:*** *For step 1 below, please refer to Chapter 4 for a reminder of the step-by-step procedures required for medication order and CSP label verification. For steps 2, 3, and 5; refer to Chapter 5 for pharmacy calculation procedures. For step 4, refer to Table 11.4 for proper narcotic sign-out procedures. For steps 6–10, refer to Chapter 3 for a reminder of the process for gathering and cleaning supplies. For steps 11–17, refer to Chapter 6 for step-by-step aseptic garbing, hand-washing, and gloving procedures. Perform steps 1, 5–14, and 62–63 in the anteroom; perform steps 2–4 in the narcotic room; and perform steps 15–61 in the clean room.*

## Supplies

### *Essential Supplies*

To complete the Unit 2 procedural labs, you will need to ensure that various essential anteroom and clean room supplies such as those listed in Table 11.5 are available for your use.

**Table 11.5 Essential Anteroom and Clean Room Supplies for Sterile Compounding**

| Anteroom Supplies |
|---|
| medication order and CSP label |
| calculator |
| pen |
| permanent, felt-tip marker |
| plastic bags (small and large) |
| aseptic garb, including shoe covers, hair cover, face mask, and beard cover (if appropriate) |
| sterile gown |
| presaturated, aseptic cleaning wipes |
| sterile, foamed 70% IPA |
| waste container |
| transport vehicle (optional) |
| **Clean Room Supplies** |
| sterile, foamed 70% IPA |
| sterile, powder-free gloves |
| sterile 70% IPA swabs, individually packaged × 2 |
| sharps container |
| waste container |
| laminar airflow hood |

### *Procedure-Specific Supplies*

In addition to the supplies listed in Table 11.5, gather the following items specific to the Chapter 11 narcotic PCA syringe procedural lab:

- perpetual inventory log book containing a record for meperidine 50 mg/mL, 2-mL vials
- regular needles × 2
- meperidine 50 mg/mL, 2-mL vials × 5
- 10-mL Luer-lock syringe
- 60-mL Luer-lock syringe
- Luer-to-Luer connector
- 0.9% sodium chloride or normal saline (NS) IVPB, 50-mL bag
- sterile, 70% IPA swabs, individually packaged × 2
- syringe cap
- IVA syringe seal (optional)

## Procedure

### *Verifying the Label*

1. Review the CSP label to verify that all of the information on the label matches the medication order. To help you with this task, compare the CSP label (see Figure 11.1) to the medication order and patient ID label (see Figure 11.2). Then bring the CSP label into the narcotic room.

**FIGURE 11.1**

**CSP Label for Meperidine 500 mg**

****PCA Syringe****
Memorial Hospital

**Pt. Name:** Tou Her **Room:** 540
**Pt. ID#:** 73623662 **Rx#:** 25441

**Meperidine 500 mg**
**Sodium Chloride 0.9% (NS) 50 mL**
**For patient controlled anesthesia via programmed syringe pump**

Expires ______
Tech ______
RPh ______

Not for direct IV push administration – FOR PCA USE ONLY.

### *Calculating the Desired Narcotic Volume*

2. Look at the CSP label to determine the desired dose of the narcotic meperidine. Find the narcotic in its storage area within the narcotic room. Read the meperidine drug vial label to determine the concentration needed.
3. Perform the calculations based on the narcotic dose provided on the CSP label and the meperidine concentration from the vial label. Assume the narcotic drug vial label indicates that meperidine has a concentration of 50 mg per 1 mL. Use the following formula to calculate the dose:

$$\frac{50 \text{ mg}}{1 \text{ mL}} = \frac{500 \text{ mg}}{x \text{ mL}}$$

*Cross-multiply, then divide to solve for $x$ (the desired dosage volume) for each dose.

(For additional assistance, refer to Chapter 5 for step-by-step dosage calculation procedures.)

FIGURE 11.2

**Daily Order**

| | |
|---|---|
| **ID#:** 73623662<br>**Name:** Tou Her<br>**DOB:** 11/30/59<br>**Room:** 540<br>**Dr.:** Samuel Richter | **MEMORIAL HOSPITAL**<br>**PHYSICIAN'S MEDICATION ORDER**<br>BEAR DOWN ON HARD SURFACE WITH BALLPOINT PEN |

GENERIC EQUIVALENT IS AUTHORIZED UNLESS CHECKED IN THIS COLUMN

| ALLERGY OR SENSITIVITY TO *Shellfish, Bactrim, Morphine*<br>NONE KNOWN ☐ SIGNED: | DIAGNOSIS | COMPLETED OR DISCONTINUED |
|---|---|---|

| DATE | TIME | ORDERS | PHYSICIAN'S SIG. | NAME | DATE | TIME |
|---|---|---|---|---|---|---|
| | | | | | | |
| | | *Height 5' 11"    Weight 179 lbs* | | | | |
| | | *Diet: NPO until 10 PM and then clear liquids as tolerated.* | | | | |
| | | *Activity: OOB w/assistance for first 24 hrs post-op then ad lib* | | | | |
| | | *Vitals: q4h, call for temp >101 degrees or any other complications* | | | | |
| | | *Meds:* | | | | |
| | | *IV fluids: NS @ 125 mL/hr until taking po well and then DC* | | | | |
| | | *PCA orders: meperidine 500 mg/50 mL NS* | | | | |
| | | *Patient-controlled dose: 10–30 mg* | | | | |
| | | *Lockout: 15 minutes* | | | | |
| | | *4-hour limit: 250 mg* | | | | |
| | | | | | | |
| | | *DC PCA when taking po well; then start Vicodin 5 mg, one or two tabs,* | | | | |
| | | *q6h prn for pain* | | | | |

PHARMACY COPY

### *Signing Out the Narcotic*

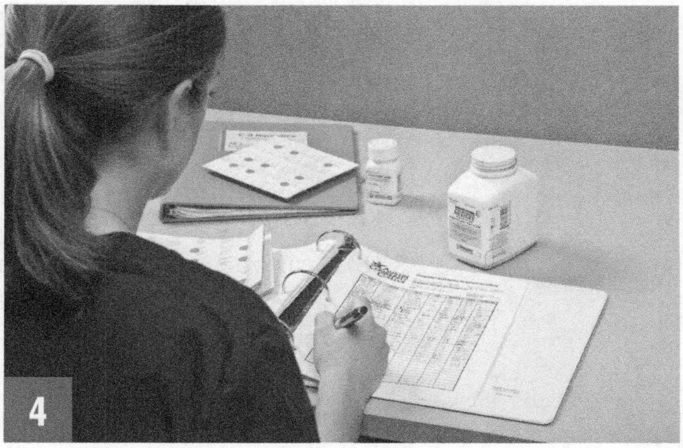

4. Follow the steps outlined in Table 11.4 to sign out the volume of meperidine that you calculated in step 3. ***Note:*** Due to time constraints, your instructor may direct you to skip this step for the purpose of this training lab. Consult with your instructor to determine the appropriate course of action.

### *Calculating the Desired NS Volume*

5. After returning to the anteroom, perform a calculation to determine the volume of NS you need to draw up to make the CSP. To do so, subtract the volume that you determined in step 3 from the total volume of the PCA syringe—in this case, 50 mL. Given that you determined the CSP requires 10 mL of narcotic, determine the desired volume of NS with this simple calculation:

   50 mL – 10 mL = 40 mL (amount of NS necessary to make the CSP)

### *Gathering and Cleaning Supplies*

6. Place the medication order into the large plastic bag and the CSP label into the small plastic bag. Gather all of the remaining items on the Chapter 11 supply list.
7. Open the package of aseptic cleaning wipes. Remove one or, if necessary, more wipes, and thoroughly wipe down the entire transport vehicle.
8. Place the used wipes in the waste receptacle.
9. Remove a new aseptic cleaning wipe and wipe down the exterior surface of the IVPB bag's dust cover. Place the cleaned IVPB bag into the transport vehicle. Place the used wipe in the waste receptacle.
10. Repeat the cleaning procedure outlined in step 9 for each of the remaining supply items.

### *Garbing*

11. Don shoe covers.
12. Put on a hair cover.
13. Don a face mask and beard cover (if appropriate).

    *Note:* For the purposes of this training lab, you will skip the mandatory aseptic hand-washing procedure.

14. Don a sterile gown.
15. Use a transport vehicle to bring all supply items, including an unopened package of sterile, powder-free gloves, into the clean room.
16. Place the transport vehicle onto a clean surface or countertop within the clean room. If a cart is used, position it so that it does not interrupt airflow into the hood prefilter.

**POINTER**

During aseptic garbing, best practice is to reapply sterile, foamed 70% IPA to your hands after donning shoe covers and again after donning a hair cover.

17. Apply sterile, foamed 70% IPA to your hands. Allow them to air-dry and then don sterile gloves.

    *Note:* For the purposes of this training lab, you will skip the mandatory hood-cleaning procedure.

### *Withdrawing from the IVPB Bag*

18. Tear open the dust cover and remove the IVPB bag. Place the IVPB into the DCA of the hood, and the dust cover into the waste receptacle. Place the remaining supply items—such as needles, syringes, IPA swabs, and vials—into the outer six-inch staging area of the hood.
19. Position the injection port of the IVPB bag so that it receives uninterrupted airflow from the HEPA filter. Tear open an IPA swab within the DCA. Swab the injection port of the IVPB, and then place the IPA swab on the hood's work surface within the DCA.
20. Remove a 60-mL syringe from its outer wrap, and place the wrapping in the discard pile in the outer six-inch zone of the hood. Prepare the syringe by aseptically removing a regular needle from its packaging and attaching it to the syringe tip. Place the needle's outer wrapping in the discard pile.
21. Grasp the barrel of the syringe as you would a dart. Remove the needle cap and place it onto the alcohol swab on the hood's work surface. Stabilize the injection port of the IVPB with the thumb and forefinger of your nondominant hand, and then carefully insert the needle directly into the center of the injection port.

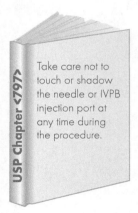

USP Chapter <797>

Take care not to touch or shadow the needle or IVPB injection port at any time during the procedure.

22. Allow the IVPB bag to rest on the hood's work surface. Firmly grasp the barrel of the syringe with your nondominant hand, as you would the throttle of a motorcycle. Brace the syringe barrel against the hood's work surface. Grasp the flat knob of the plunger with your dominant hand and forcefully pull the plunger toward you. Without lifting the IVPB-and-syringe unit from the hood's work surface, continue to brace the syringe barrel while simultaneously and steadily maintaining the plunger in this retracted position (similar to the retraction of an arrow within a bow just prior to the release of the arrow). Notice that the fluid from the IVPB rapidly transfers into the syringe.
23. Continue to hold the plunger in this retracted position until approximately 35 mL of fluid has been transferred from the IVPB bag into the syringe. Once you have reached that fluid measurement, decrease the intensity of your retraction of the plunger. Continue to gently retract the plunger's flat knob until approximately 41 mL of NS is contained in the syringe.
24. Hold the IVPB in your nondominant hand and the barrel of the syringe in your dominant hand. While keeping the needle completely inserted in the IVPB, use a clockwise motion (a counterclockwise motion if you are left-handed) to invert the IVPB so that the needle-and-syringe unit is below the IVPB.
25. Move your nondominant hand to hold the syringe barrel. Use your dominant hand to forcefully tap the syringe barrel to force bubbles up toward the tip of the syringe. Once all of the bubbles have been transferred to the tip of the syringe, slightly pull down on the plunger's flat knob so that a small pocket

(approximately 2 mL) of air is created at the syringe tip. Without re-tapping the syringe barrel, push up on the flat knob to expel the air pocket and excess fluid into the attached IVPB bag.

**26.** Verify that you have the desired volume of NS in the bubble-free syringe. Hold the IVPB bag with your nondominant hand and the syringe barrel with your dominant hand. Using a counterclockwise motion (a clockwise motion, if you are left-handed), return the IVPB with attached needle-and-syringe unit to the hood's work surface.

**27.** Hold the IVPB with your nondominant hand; grasp the barrel of the syringe with your dominant hand, as you would a dart. Carefully remove the needle-and-syringe unit from the IVPB. Recap the needle using aseptic technique. Temporarily place the filled-and-capped syringe, along with the empty IVPB bag, on the hood's work surface within the DCA.

### *Withdrawing the Narcotic Using the Milking Technique*

**28.** Place the meperidine vials within the DCA. Remove the flip-top cap from each vial. Place the plastic caps in the discard pile. Arrange the vials within the DCA so that each vial's rubber top receives uninterrupted airflow from the HEPA filter. Open an IPA swab and swab the top of each vial. Place the IPA swab on the hood's work surface within the DCA.

**POINTER**

Some facilities allow the IV technician to swab several vial tops consecutively with the same IPA swab, provided that the alcohol has not evaporated from the swab and that the swab has not been placed on the hood's work surface, removed from the DCA, or otherwise contaminated. Other facilities require that a new swab be used for each vial top. Consult your facility's P&P manual to determine the proper swabbing procedures for your pharmacy.

**29.** Remove the 10-mL syringe from its outer wrap, and place the outer wrapping in the discard pile. Prepare the syringe by aseptically removing a regular needle from its outer wrapping and attaching the capped needle to the syringe tip. Place the needle's outer wrapping in the discard pile.

**30.** Pull down on the flat knob of the syringe to draw a volume of air into the syringe equal to or slightly less than the volume you wish to withdraw from the vial (in this lab, 2 mL).

**31.** With your dominant hand, grasp the syringe barrel and hold it as you would a dart. Use your nondominant hand to remove the needle cap by pulling it carefully but firmly off the needle. Place the needle cap on top of the alcohol swab on the hood's work surface, with the open end of the cap pointing toward the HEPA filter.

**32.** Use the fingers of your dominant hand to rotate the barrel of the syringe so that the bevel of the needle points up toward the ceiling.

**33.** Using your nondominant hand, brace the first meperidine vial against the hood's work surface. Lay the tip of the needle, bevel up, onto the center of the vial's rubber top.

**POINTER**

Take care to hold the vial and syringe so that the critical areas—the area from the tip of the syringe to the neck of the vial, including the entire needle and the vial's rubber top—receive unobstructed airflow from the HEPA filter at all times.

**34.** Insert the needle into the vial using proper aseptic technique to avoid coring the vial's rubber top.

**35.** Hold the meperidine vial with your nondominant hand. Hold the syringe, with needle firmly inserted into the vial, with your dominant hand. Invert the vial, using a clockwise motion (a counterclockwise motion if you are left-handed), so that the needle-and-syringe unit is below the vial.

**36.** Use the thumb of your dominant hand to gradually push up on the flat knob of the plunger to inject a small amount of air (approximately 1 mL) into the

**POINTER**

When withdrawing fluid from a vial, keep the tip of the needle near the interior neck of the vial so that a steady stream of fluid is drawn into the the syringe. Such attentive positioning of the needle helps to avoid drawing excess air into the syringe.

meperidine vial, creating a slight positive pressure within the vial. Release your thumb from the plunger and allow fluid to flow into the syringe. Repeat this milking process until you have withdrawn the entire contents of the vial into the syringe.

37. Without removing the bubbles, and while keeping the needle firmly inserted in the vial, use a counterclockwise rotation (a clockwise rotation if you are left-handed) to return the vial and syringe to the original starting position, with the upright vial braced against the hood's work surface and the dominant hand holding the syringe barrel. Continue to brace the vial with your nondominant hand. Grasp the barrel of the syringe and slowly remove the needle-and-syringe unit from the medication vial. Remember to avoid touching the plunger or flat knob of the syringe at any time while removing it from the vial.
38. Repeat steps 33–37 to withdraw the meperidine from vials two through four into the 10-mL syringe.
39. Repeat steps 33–36 to withdraw the meperidine from vial five into the 10-mL syringe.
40. While ensuring that the needle remains entirely within the last meperidine vial, brace the vial between the thumb and forefinger of your nondominant hand, allowing the syringe barrel to rest against your palm. Be sure that this palm faces the HEPA filter, ensuring proper airflow to the critical site. Then tap the barrel of the syringe with the fingers of your dominant hand to force air bubbles within the fluid up toward the tip of the syringe. Take care not to bring your dominant hand between the critical site and the HEPA filter at any time.
41. Push up on the flat knob of the plunger with the thumb of your dominant hand to expel the air bubbles gathered near the tip of the syringe and any extra fluid.
42. Verify that the syringe now contains the desired amount of meperidine (in this lab, 10 mL).
43. While keeping the needle firmly inserted in the vial, use a counterclockwise rotation (a clockwise rotation if you are left-handed) to return the vial and syringe to the original starting position, with the upright vial braced against the hood's work surface and the dominant hand holding the syringe barrel. Continue to brace the vial with your nondominant hand. Grasp the syringe barrel and slowly remove the needle-and-syringe unit from the medication vial. Remember to avoid touching the plunger or flat knob of the syringe at any time while removing it from the vial.
44. Carefully recap the needle and place the capped needle-and-syringe unit, now filled with meperidine, onto the work surface within the DCA.
45. Arrange the filled syringe (with attached, capped needle) and the meperidine vials on the hood's work surface within the DCA. Position them adjacent to the NS syringe and empty IVPB bag. Ask for a verification check by your instructor or a pharmacist.

### *Transferring the Narcotic into the NS Syringe Using a Luer-to-Luer Connector*

46. Once the verification check has been completed, arrange both filled syringe-and-needle units within the DCA so that they receive uninterrupted airflow from the HEPA filter.
47. Grasp the meperidine syringe in your dominant hand as you would a dart. Twist off the capped needle and place it into the sharps container. Carefully manipulate the syringe within your dominant hand so that the syringe tip remains pointed toward the HEPA filter and your thumb and forefinger are free to use.
48. While keeping the syringe tip pointed toward the HEPA filter, use your nondominant hand and the thumb and forefinger of your dominant hand to carefully peel open the outer package of the Luer-to-Luer connector. Remove the connector from the package, taking care not to touch or shadow either end of the Luer-lock connector at any time during the procedure.
49. Twist the meperidine syringe onto one end of the Luer-to-Luer connector. Manipulate the syringe with your dominant hand so that the open end of the Luer-lock connector, which is now attached to the meperidine syringe, remains pointed toward the HEPA filter, but in such a way that you have free use of the thumb and forefinger of your dominant hand.
50. Grasp the barrel of the NS syringe with your nondominant hand. While pointing the open end of the Luer-lock connector toward the HEPA filter, use the thumb and forefinger of your dominant hand to twist off and remove the capped needle from the NS syringe. Dispose of the capped needle in the sharps container. Then, using a twisting motion, attach the NS syringe to the open end of the Luer-to-Luer connector.

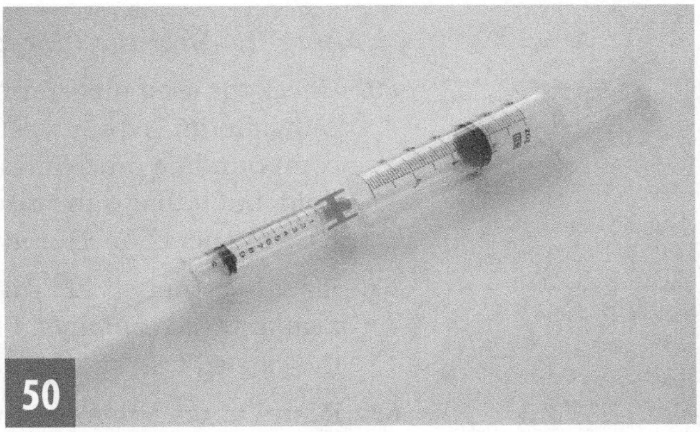

50

51. Invert the syringes, which are connected to each end of the Luer-lock connector, using a clockwise motion, so that the meperidine syringe is on top of the NS syringe.
52. Inject the meperidine into the NS syringe by gently pushing down on the flat knob of the meperidine syringe with your nondominant hand; simultaneously pull down on the plunger of the NS syringe with your dominant hand.
53. Keep the barrel of the meperidine syringe inverted so that it is on top of the NS syringe. Once all of the meperidine has been transferred into the NS syringe, tap the barrel of the NS syringe to force air bubbles up toward the syringe tip. Once all of the bubbles have been forced to the syringe tip, pull down on the flat knob of the NS syringe, creating a small pocket (approximately 2 mL) of air at the tip of the syringe. Carefully expel the air and any excess fluid from the NS syringe by gently pushing up on the flat knob until only 50 mL of bubble-free fluid remains in the syringe.

54. Verify that you have the desired final PCA volume (50 mL):

    40 mL of NS + 10 mL of meperidine = 50 mL PCA (final volume)

55. Temporarily place the PCA syringe, with attached Luer-to-Luer connector and meperidine syringe, onto the hood's work surface within the DCA.
56. Aseptically open a package of sterile syringe caps within the DCA.
57. Pick up the PCA syringe with attached Luer-to-Luer connector and meperidine syringe. With your dominant hand, hold the barrel of the PCA syringe as you would a dart. Unscrew the PCA syringe from the Luer-to-Luer connector and immediately insert the tip of the PCA syringe into one of the syringe caps. Screw the tip of the syringe into the syringe cap to attach it. Place the empty meperidine syringe with attached Luer-to-Luer connector into the sharps container.
58. Remove an IVA syringe seal from its release paper. Attach one end of the IVA seal to the barrel of the syringe near the point at which the syringe begins to taper toward the syringe tip. Drape the IVA seal across the syringe cap and attach the other end of the seal to the opposite side of the syringe barrel.
59. Remove the CSP label from the plastic bag and affix the CSP label to the barrel of the PCA syringe so that it does not cover any of the graduation markings.

### *Cleaning Up After the Procedure*

60. Check the used meperidine syringe to determine if there is a visible, significant amount (typically > 0.5 mL) of narcotic remaining in the syringe. In most compounding procedures, there will *not* be a significant amount of remaining fluid, but if that is the case, place the empty meperidine syringe with attached Luer-to-Luer connector into the sharps container.
61. Place the empty IVPB, empty meperidine vials, and used IPA swabs into the regular waste container. Place the used needle into the sharps container. Place the labeled CSP and any remaining supply items into the transport vehicle.
62. Return to the anteroom to begin the compounding completion procedures. Record your initials and the date in the proper location on the CSP label. Return any supply items to their proper storage locations. Remove your PPE according to the standard protocol outlined in Chapter 6.
63. Ask for a final verification check from your instructor or the pharmacist.

**POINTER**

The definition of a "significant amount" and the procedures related to its disposal and subsequent record keeping vary among facilities. If there is a significant amount (typically > 0.5 mL) of fluid remaining in the narcotic syringe, summon your instructor to witness the narcotic waste disposal. While your instructor is watching, inject the remaining fluid into the sharps container by pushing firmly on the flat knob of the plunger.

# Process Validation by Instructor

*Your instructor will use the process validation checklist provided in Appendix D to evaluate your technique for this lab. In order to receive ACPE certification, and prior to making CSPs for patient use, you must correctly perform each component of the lab procedure. Review the Chapter 11 lab and thoroughly practice each of the steps prior to your evaluation.*

# Part 3: Assessment

## Chapter Summary

- The opium poppy plant is thought to be the originator of all narcotics and is the primary source of all controlled substances. Extracts of the opium poppy include opium, paregoric, laudanum, morphine, codeine, and heroin.
- Cocaine is derived from the plant *Erythroxylum coca,* whereas marijuana is derived from the *Cannabis* plant.
- In 1968, the Federal Bureau of Narcotics merged with the Bureau of Narcotics and Dangerous Drugs, which would later become the DEA.
- In 1970, the United States created the CSA to provide oversight and restriction on the prescription and use of all controlled substances, including narcotics. The DEA is responsible for enforcing this act.
- Sterile compounding personnel make CSPs to provide narcotic pain control, or narcotic analgesia. The types of controlled substance CSPs prepared by IV technicians are LVPs, epidurals, and PCAs.
- The CSA classifies controlled substances into five schedules or classes based on their potential for abuse or addiction. C–I controlled substances have no approved medical use; C–II controlled substances have a high potential for abuse or addiction; C–III controlled substances have less potential for abuse or addiction than C–II; C–IV controlled substances have less potential for abuse or addiction than C–III; C–V controlled substances have the lowest potential for abuse or addiction.
- Class A pharmacies often stock C–III through C–V medications on the shelf, along with noncontrolled substance medications. In this type of environment, C–II controlled substances must be tracked using a perpetual inventory system; however, C–III through C–V medications are often subject to less stringent tracking requirements.
- Most Class C pharmacies store all classes of controlled substances under a double-lock system. Class C pharmacies generally track all scheduled substances using a perpetual inventory system.
- Most controlled substances are narcotics, a class of drugs that may cause CNS depression. Patients receiving narcotics must be closely monitored for this condition.
- The perpetual inventory log book is an official, legal record with pages titled "Perpetual Inventory Record" or "Controlled Substance Record." The perpetual log book is a record of all activity relating to the medications in the narcotic room.
- For security purposes, be sure that controlled substances, narcotic storage keys, and narcotic records are kept under strict control. Immediately report drug discrepancies or evidence of suspected drug diversion to the pharmacist in charge.
- When signing out controlled substances, complete every section on the perpetual inventory log sheet, use black pen, double-check your math, and verify that the actual amount on hand matches the amount on the perpetual inventory log sheet.
- Anteroom preparatory procedures include verifying the CSP label with the medication order, performing calculations, gathering and cleaning supplies, donning aseptic garb and a sterile gown, and aseptic hand washing.
- Clean room preparatory procedures include donning sterile gloves, cleaning the hood, and using aseptic technique to prepare the narcotic-based CSP within the DCA of the hood.
- In addition to essential supply items, controlled substance CSPs sometimes require the use of syringe caps, Luer-to-Luer connectors, and IVA syringe seals.

# Key Terms

**addiction** physical and psychological dependence on a chemical substance such as a narcotic

**alkaloids** a group of naturally occurring, nitrogen-based compounds

**anodyne** a medication used to treat pain

**Bureau of Narcotics and Dangerous Drugs** a U.S. government agency created to oversee issues related to dangerous drugs; merged with the Federal Bureau of Narcotics to become the DEA

***Cannabis*** the plant source of the controlled substance marijuana

**central nervous system (CNS) depression** a physiological degradation of the CNS that results in decreased autonomic functions, such as breathing and heart rate

**cocaine** a controlled substance known to produce feelings of euphoria and increased stamina

**codeine** an opium derivative; a C–II narcotic that may be a C–III narcotic when combined with an analgesic (such as acetaminophen with codeine) or a C–V narcotic when combined with a cough suppressant

**controlled substance** any drug classified by the CSA as having a potential for abuse and addiction ranging from Schedule V (C–V) to Schedule I (C–I)

**controlled substance diversion** evidence found during perpetual inventory record-keeping procedures that indicates a controlled substance is missing or has been improperly logged out of the perpetual inventory record; this situation requires immediate notification of a pharmacist or supervisor; can also refer to the use or sale of a drug for nonmedical purposes or to individuals other than for whom the drug was prescribed; also known as *narcotic diversion*

**Controlled Substances Act (CSA)** the 1973 federal act that created five schedules or classes of controlled substances based on a drug's potential for abuse or addiction; the act restricts access, sale, and prescription of controlled substances, as well as defines penalties for the illegal possession and/or use of controlled substances

**desired volume** the amount of a drug or ingredient that must be drawn up to provide the prescribed dosage

**discrepancy** any difference or disagreement between the actual narcotic count and the balance listed in the controlled substances perpetual inventory record; an error in math and/or transcription in a perpetual narcotic record; may be evidence of drug diversion and requires immediate notification of a pharmacist or supervisor

**double-lock system** a system often employed in hospital pharmacies in which all controlled substances are stored behind two separate locks (i.e., a locked narcotic room within a locked pharmacy)

**drug counterculture** a segment of society (most notably college students and peace activists) known to indulge in various drugs in the early 1960s to late 1970s, when narcotics and other illicit drugs were readily accessible

**Drug Enforcement Administration (DEA)** the federal agency responsible for overseeing all regulations related to controlled substances

**drug schedule** the classification of a controlled substance medication based on the drug's potential for abuse or addiction; one of the five controlled substance classifications; also known as *drug class*

**epidural** a type of narcotic CSP administered intrathecally; often used during labor and delivery

***Erythroxylum coca*** the plant source of cocaine

**euphoria** an overwhelming feeling of happiness and well-being that may be induced by some controlled substances

**Federal Bureau of Narcotics** the first U.S. government agency charged with enforcement of controlled substance regulations

**floor stock** medications replenished by the pharmacy and stored on the nursing unit, often in locked, automated-dispensing machines that provide tracking of drug distribution

**heroin** a derivative of the opium poppy; a Schedule I narcotic with a high potential for abuse

**home healthcare** at-home hospice care or other types of healthcare for patients with terminal illnesses or other conditions requiring long-term treatment

**hospice** care for patients with end-stage disease, either at home or in a healthcare facility; hospice staff often provide pain-control treatment during the last stage of a terminal illness

**hydromorphone** a synthetic narcotic derived from the opium poppy plant

**IVA syringe seal** an adhesive seal that is affixed to a syringe cap to provide evidence of tampering prior to patient administration

**latex** the milky white sap of the opium poppy capsule that, once dried, creates raw opium

**laudanum** a narcotic derived from the opium poppy plant

**Luer-to-Luer connector** a sterile supply item consisting of a small, plastic device with a Luer-lock syringe adaptor at each end; used to transfer sterile fluid from one syringe to another

**marijuana** a controlled substance known to produce feelings of relaxation and euphoria when smoked or ingested

**morphine** a synthetic narcotic derived from the opium poppy plant

**narcotic** a class of mostly opium-based drugs used to treat pain or induce sleep; a drug listed on the DEA schedule of controlled substances

**narcotic analgesia** narcotic pain control

**narcotic CSPs** compounded sterile preparations—such as LVPs, IVPBs, PCAs, and epidural cassettes—that contain one or more controlled substance ingredients

**narcotic room** a locked area within the pharmacy where controlled substances are stored; also known as the *narcotic vault* or *narcotic cabinet*

**narcotic sign-out** the process of recording the withdrawal of one or more controlled substance doses from the perpetual inventory log sheet or perpetual inventory record

**narcotic tolerance** the resistance that builds up in the patient's body after continual use of narcotics over an extended period, often leading to a need for a higher amount of the drug to provide the same effect

**narcotic waste witness** a healthcare worker (such as a pharmacist, certified pharmacy technician, or nurse) authorized to witness the destruction of controlled substances

**noncontrolled substance** any medication not classified by the CSA as having a potential for abuse or addiction

**opium den** a place where illegal narcotics such as opium are sold and self-administered

**opium poppy** the plant source of most narcotics; the pods of this plant are scraped to collect raw opium, a natural substance used to provide pain relief; also known as *Papaver somniferum*

***Papaver somniferum*** the opium poppy plant; used to provide pain relief in ancient societies

**paregoric** an opium-based liquid pain medicine; camphorated tincture of opium

**patient-controlled analgesia (PCA)** a type of narcotic CSP that allows the patient to self-administer a closely controlled amount of IV pain medication based on a preset dose ordered by a prescriber

**perpetual inventory log book** a book, computer, or file in which controlled substance records are regularly updated and constantly maintained

**perpetual inventory record** a document or record of controlled substances; also known as a *perpetual inventory*

**perpetual inventory system** a method of continually recording additions and withdrawals of controlled substances from a pharmacy's stock

**potential for abuse and addiction** the likelihood that a drug or class of drugs may lead to abuse or drug addiction; the potential for a drug to be used for a purpose, person, or in a manner other than that which it is prescribed; the overuse or illegal sale of a drug, often a narcotic; controlled substances are classified on a schedule from I–V, with Schedule I controlled substances having no accepted medical use, and Schedule V controlled substances having the least potential for abuse or addiction

**recreational drug** a drug, such as a controlled substance, that is used for personal enjoyment; a drug used for a person or purpose other than for whom or what it was prescribed

**semisynthetic narcotic** a drug, such as hydromorphone, that is refined or derived from the opium poppy; a partially man-made narcotic

**synthetic narcotic** a narcotic made entirely in a laboratory setting; a drug that mimics a natural substance such as opium, but that is not made from the substance; a man-made narcotic

**syringe cap** a sterile, plastic or rubber cap placed on the syringe tip instead of a needle; protects personnel during transport

## Check the Basics

*On a separate sheet of paper, write your answers as modeled in these examples: 1d; 2c; 3b; etc.*

**1.** What is the name of the supply item sometimes used to transfer fluid from one syringe to another without the use of a needle?

a. PCA syringe
b. repeater pump
c. syringe cap
d. Luer-to-Luer connector

**2.** Which of the following critical sites must be swabbed with sterile 70% IPA prior to use?

a. vial's rubber top, IVPB injection port
b. needle, syringe cap
c. Luer-to-Luer connector, syringe cap
d. all of the above

**3.** Which of the following critical sites should never be touched, shadowed, or swabbed with alcohol?

a. vial's rubber top, IVPB injection port
b. needle, syringe tip
c. Luer-to-Luer connector, syringe cap
d. both *a* and *b*
e. both *b* and *c*

**4.** Which supply item is used to cover the tip of a PCA syringe after sterile compounding?

a. Luer-to-Luer connector
b. syringe cap
c. IVA syringe seal
d. regular needle

**5.** With regard to withdrawal from an IVPB bag, which of the following statements is true?

a. The needle should be inserted with the bevel pointing up.
b. The needle should be inserted with the bevel pointing down.
c. An amount of air equal to the volume to be withdrawn should be injected into the IVPB bag.
d. No air should be injected into the IVPB bag.

**6.** With regard to removing bubbles from a syringe, what is the *last* thing you must do, immediately before expelling the air pocket?

a. Tap the syringe.
b. Pull down on the plunger.
c. Adjust the volume in the syringe.
d. Remove the needle-and-syringe unit from the vial.

**7.** With regard to the perpetual inventory record, which of the following statements is true?

a. Transcription errors should be indicated with a single strike-through line and your circled initials.
b. Black ink should be used for entries and additions to the record; red ink should be used for withdrawals and to indicate a negative balance.
c. If the actual narcotics count does not match the existing balance, you have discovered a discrepancy that must be resolved.
d. all of the above

**8.** Which of the following calculations would you use to determine the volume of NS that must be drawn up to prepare the PCA?

a. narcotic volume – the total volume of PCA = volume of NS
b. number of narcotic vials – the total volume of PCA = volume of NS
c. total volume of PCA – the narcotic volume = volume of NS
d. narcotic volume × PCA volume / total volume = volume of NS

**9.** What is the schedule of the narcotic used to prepare the CSP in the procedural lab?

a. C–II
b. C–III
c. C–IV
d. C–V

**10.** The PCA pump is preprogrammed to _________ the patient, thus preventing a potential drug overdose if the pump's dosing button is pushed too early.

a. inject
b. lock out
c. freeze
d. stop

# Make Connections

*On a separate sheet of paper, write your answers to the following three questions, using complete sentences and making sure your answers are thorough and thoughtful. Note that the third question requires Internet access.*

1. Upon the completion of the PCA compounding procedure, you discover that 0.8 mL of meperidine remains in the narcotic syringe. What is the best course of action to take in light of this discovery? Would you follow a different course of action if you had discovered that there was 0.4 mL of meperidine remaining in the narcotic syringe? Why or why not?

2. While signing out a narcotic for CSP preparation, you discover that the narcotic count does not match the existing balance. You immediately bring the discrepancy to the attention of a more experienced senior technician, who directs you to "erase the existing balance from the perpetual inventory record, and then write in the correct amount so that the numbers match." What is the best course of action? Would you follow a different course of action if a pharmacist had given you the same direction? Why or why not?

3. Go to the DEA Office of Diversion Control website at http://www.deadiversion.usdoj.gov/. Select the *Inside Diversion Control* tab, then click *About Us*. Read the information on this webpage. According to this website, what is meant by *drug diversion*? With that understanding, read the following scenario and address the follow-up questions: During the course of your pharmacy duties, a member of the nursing staff tells you that she suspects a coworker has been removing small quantities of narcotics from the unit's automated drug dispensing machine in order to sell them. How should you respond? Would you respond differently if the person told you the coworker was personally taking the narcotic to control her pain due to a chronic disease? Would you respond differently if the person who told you the information asked you to "keep it confidential"?

# Meet the Challenge

***Scenario*** This "undercover" activity will give you the opportunity to discover several errors in narcotic transcription on a perpetual inventory record.

***Challenge*** Your instructor has a handout outlining the supplies and steps for an activity centered around finding the transcription errors on a perpetual inventory record. This procedure takes your understanding of the perpetual inventory log book to a deeper level. To meet this challenge, ask your instructor for the handout and give it a try, either as an individual, in small groups, or as a class.

## ADDITIONAL RESOURCES

*Go to the Paradigm Internet Resources Center at* www.paradigmcollege.net/sterilecomp *to access live links related to these Chapter 11 topics:*

- Information on drug diversion and drug diversion prevention and reporting
- Information on the CSA
- Detection of drug abuse, addiction, and diversion

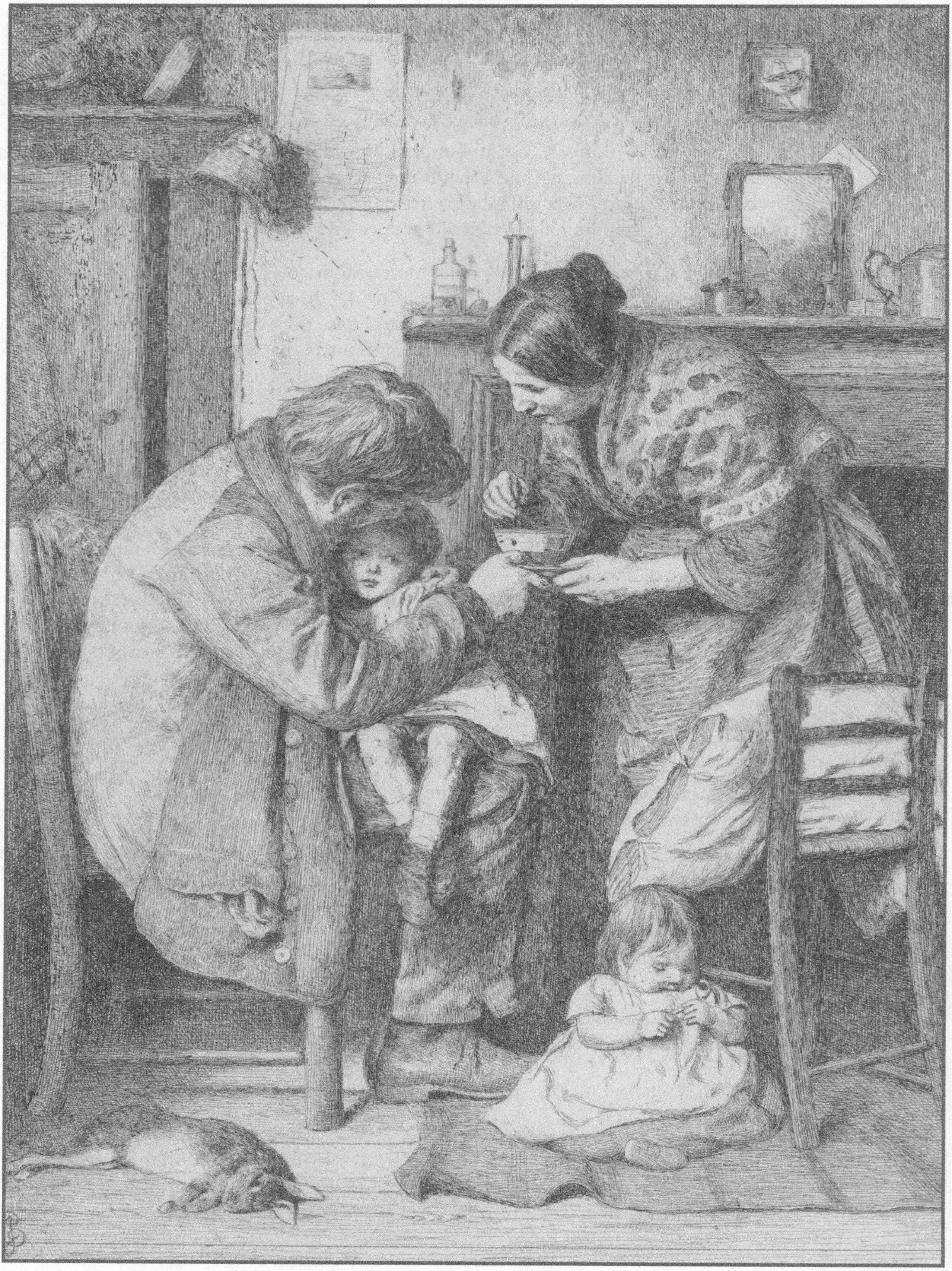

# Chapter 12

# Pediatric Preparations

## Learning Objectives

- Recognize the origins of pediatric medicine and pharmacy.
- Identify the special situations and actions that must be considered when preparing medicine for pediatric use.
- Identify the USP Chapter <797> procedures that must be performed when compounding pediatric preparations.
- Demonstrate correct technique in preparing a pediatric special dilution.

Pediatrics, or the care and treatment of children, derives from the Greek words *pais,* meaning "child," and *iatros,* meaning "healer or physician." The specialty of pediatrics is relatively new to the medical community. Although there are a number of historical records that discuss various childhood illnesses and diseases, it wasn't until the eighteenth and early nineteenth centuries that the medical treatment of children became more specialized and eventually branched off from adult medicine into its own field.

## Early History of Pediatrics

Throughout history, the healthcare of children has rested primarily with family members. For more serious illnesses that affected children or young relatives, family caregivers sought help from shamans, herbalists, and respected maternal figures whose healing practices were well-known in the community. With little understanding of **pediatric anatomy and physiology**, these untrained practitioners could sometimes do little for this vulnerable patient population, which led to widespread mortality among children. Chronically ill children were often abandoned in church sanctuaries and left to the care of religious advisors.

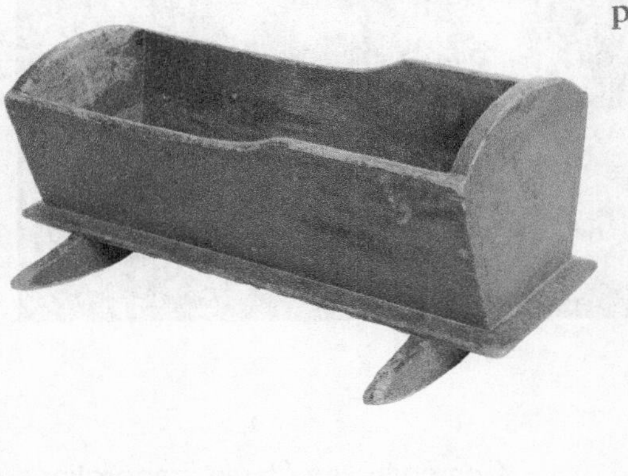

As knowledge of human anatomy increased, recognition of many childhood conditions became evident in ancient records. Included in these records is the Ebers Papyrus (1500 BCE), which discusses treatment for diseases

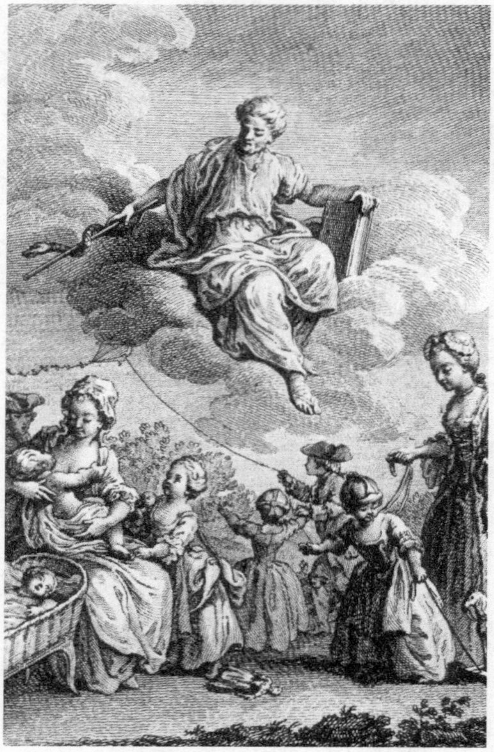

of the eye as well as a cure for intestinal worms; writings from the Greek physician Hippocrates, which present treatments for diarrhea, asthma, and mumps, as well as the care of children's teeth; and documents from the Greek practitioner Galen, which detail treatments for pneumonia and rickets. However, it wasn't until the first century that the first book dedicated solely to the treatment of children, *The Diseases of Children*, was recorded. Written by Persian pharmacist and physician Abu Bakr Muhammad ibn Zakariya al-Razi (also known as Razis or Rhazes), this publication addressed such childhood diseases as smallpox and measles, laying the foundation for the specialization of pediatric medicine. Because of his groundbreaking work, Rhazes has been referred to as the "Father of Pediatrics."

In the second century, Greek physician Soranus wrote a manuscript detailing several childhood diseases. The manuscript also contained separate sections on the daily care of children, including topics such as the feeding, bathing, and swaddling of infants. However, Soranus's recommendations—like those of his medical predecessors—remained largely unknown to the general population. Dissemination of information was primarily by word of mouth, and it would be many centuries before the invention of movable type. Consequently, most parents were left to rely on their own nurturing instincts as well as the medical advice of established community leaders when caring for their children's health.

With the invention of the printing press in 1440 in Europe, scholars began publishing their medical research and observations and gained access to information from their counterparts across the continent. Several books categorizing pediatric diseases, symptoms, and their treatments were printed during this time. Bagallarder's *Little Book on Disease in Children*, an Italian book published in 1472, was the first printed book on pediatrics. The first English-language book that exclusively covered children's health was *The Boke of Chyldren* by English physician Thomas Phaire. His book discussed childhood conditions such as head lice and parasitic worms, as well as "small pockes and measles, watching out of measure (wakefulness), bredying of teeth, colyke and rumbling of the guttes . . . ."

## Treatments and Immunizations for Childhood Diseases

In the seventeenth century, English physician Thomas Sydenham advocated commonsense treatments, such as fresh air and plenty of cool fluids, for children afflicted with scarlet fever, measles, and other common diseases. Sydenham's methods dramatically improved the outcomes of his youngest patients, as well as the medical community's understanding of these diseases. In fact, Sydenham had moderate success in treating one of the deadliest diseases of his lifetime: smallpox.

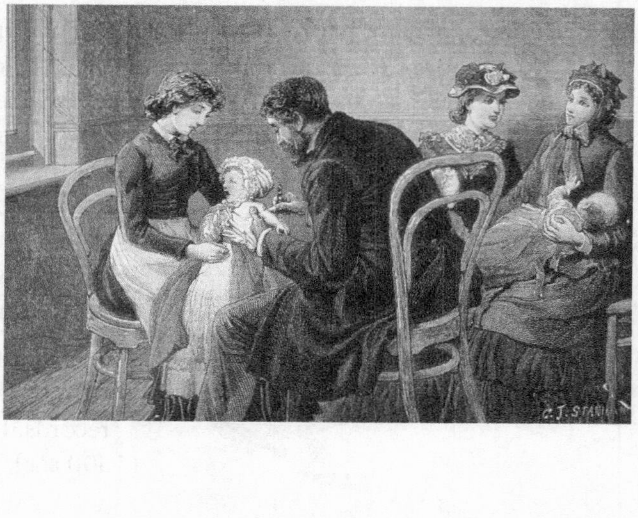

**Smallpox**, a disease that dates back to 10,000 BCE in Africa, was epidemic in Europe during the seventeenth century. Its name was derived from the small pockmarks (or pox) that scarred the faces of its victims. This devastating disease was passed through direct contact with an infected individual and soon became the scourge of humankind, resulting in the deaths of thousands. Many children fell victim to the "speckled monster" well into the eighteenth century, with more than three-quarters of infants in cities such as London and Berlin succumbing to the disease. In response to this epidemic crisis, medical practitioners tried a variety of treatments, including the common practice of blood-letting. However, the medical community would soon discover that the only cure for smallpox was prevention.

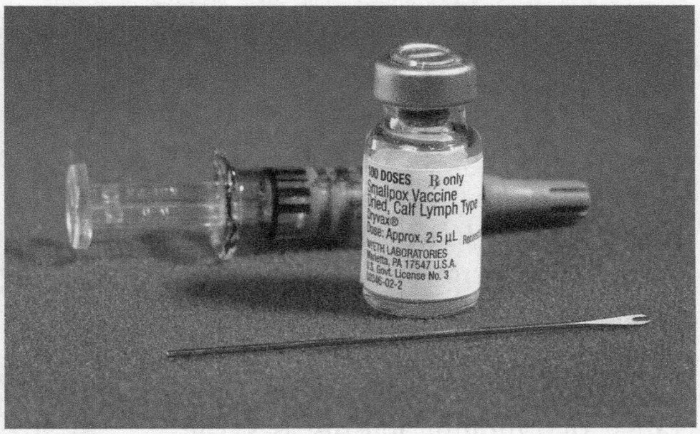


In 1796, Dr. Edward Jenner, an English physician and scientist, theorized that perhaps the treatment for smallpox rested with *cowpox*, a poxvirus that primarily affected cows but was occasionally transferred to human caregivers. Jenner's theory was based on his observation that dairymaids who suffered from cowpox did not contract smallpox. Jenner concluded that exposure to cowpox might allow a child to develop an immunity to smallpox. He tested his theory by collecting cowpox matter from a dairymaid's skin lesion and rubbing the exudate into a scratch on the arm of an eight-year-old boy—the son of his gardener. Over the following months, the young boy was repeatedly exposed to smallpox but never developed the disease. Jenner recorded his findings in a 1798 publication, in which he discussed the inoculation procedure and introduced the word "vaccination," a term derived from the Latin word *vacca*, meaning "cow." His research and further experiments eventually led to a **smallpox vaccine**, which was heralded as one of the wonder drugs of the nineteenth century. Today, smallpox has been virtually eradicated.

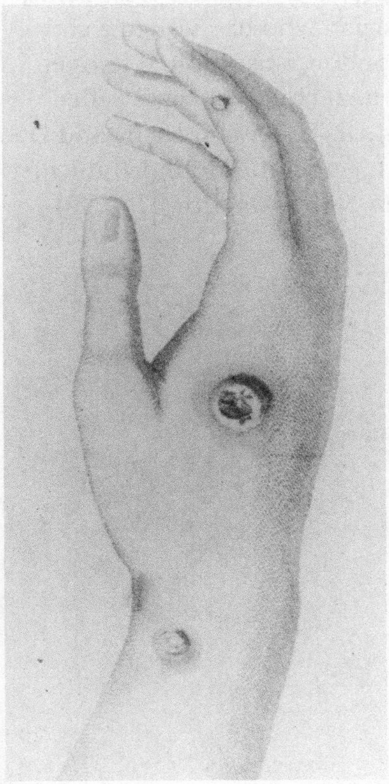

Jenner's work with the smallpox vaccine paved the way for other childhood immunizations to be developed from live, **attenuated viruses**. In particular, the emergence of vaccines for diphtheria and poliomyelitis spared the lives of many children during the twentieth century. Diphtheria, a disease that affected more than 10,000 children at one time, is now all but eradicated due to routine vaccination of children. Poliomyelitis, or polio, another common childhood disease that often resulted in paralysis or death, reached epidemic proportions in the United States in the 1950s, when incidence skyrocketed to 58,000 in 1952. A polio vaccine developed by Jonas Salk proved to be successful in preventing polio, and in 1955, a mass campaign to vaccinate children was launched. By 1957, the number of polio cases had fallen to 5,600. By 1961, the number was only 161, and in 1994 the Americas were declared polio-free.

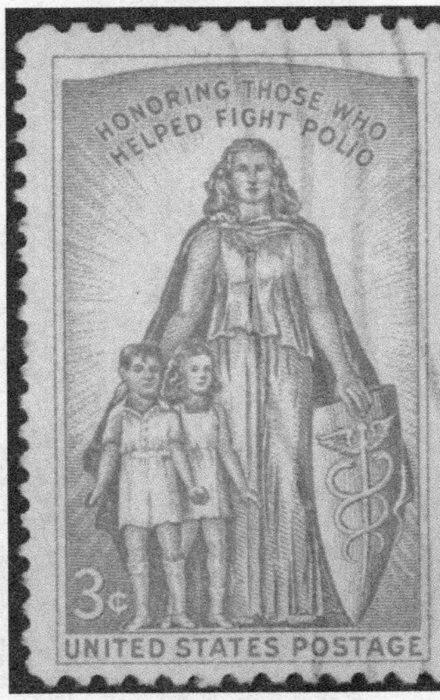

## Early Children's Hospitals

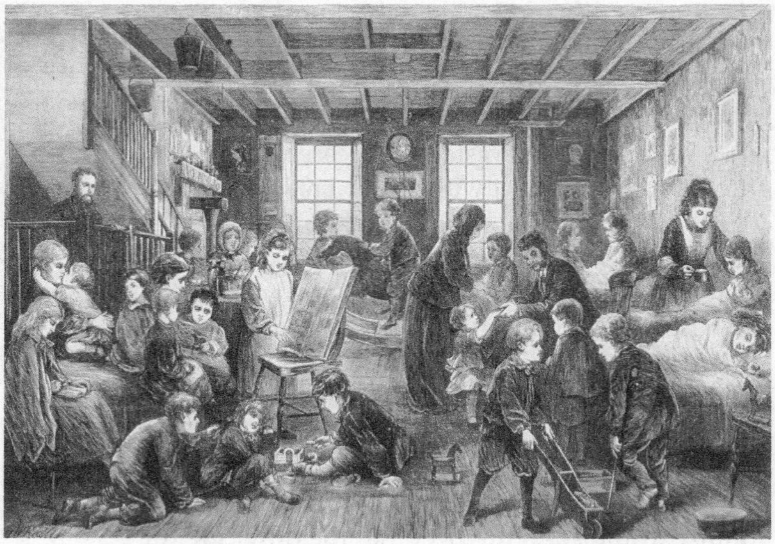

The spread of infectious diseases among children could certainly be attributed to societal changes in Europe and the United States in the nineteenth century. The rise of industrialization led to increasingly crowded living conditions and widespread poverty. Children themselves worked in close quarters in factories, making them susceptible to a variety of communicable diseases. The crowded conditions, poor nutrition, and lack of adequate healthcare proved to be a deadly combination for children. In response to the high mortality rate of children, children's hospitals were established to treat the unique healthcare needs of poverty's most vulnerable victims.

The first children's hospital was The Hospital for Sick Children in London, England, which was established in 1852. The hospital opened with only 10 beds, but it soon grew to be one of the world's leading children's hospitals, in part because of attention from English writer Charles Dickens. Dickens wrote an article called "Drooping Buds" for the magazine *Household Words* and published it the same year that The Hospital for Sick Children opened. In the article, he drew attention to the high infant mortality rate in London and praised the hospital for being dedicated to healing children. He later gave financial support to the hospital, allowing it to avoid bankruptcy.

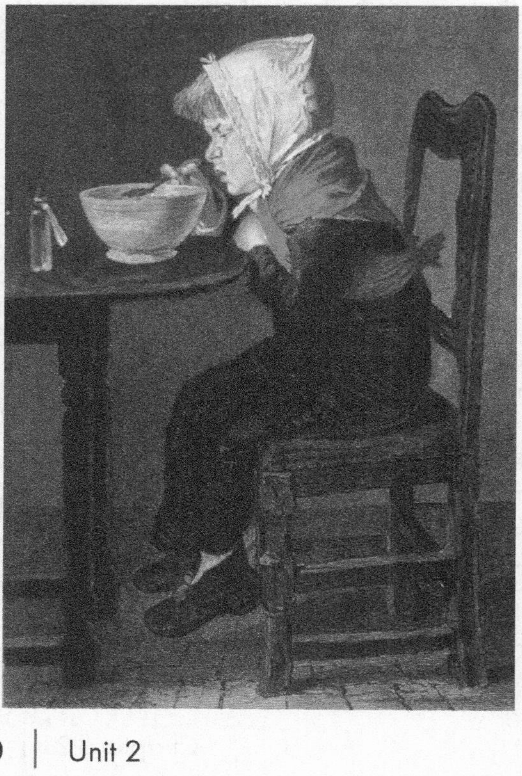

With the influx of immigrants and the spread of industrialization across the Atlantic, the United States took its cue from England and established the first pediatric hospital in 1855 in Philadelphia. At the time, Philadelphia's youngest citizens were dying in record numbers from several infectious diseases, including smallpox, tuberculosis, typhoid, and scarlet fever. Dr. Francis West Lewis, a Philadelphia physician who had visited a children's hospital in London, was inspired to open his own hospital to treat children. Lewis called upon his colleagues, Dr. T. Hewson Bache and Dr. R.A.F. Penrose, and together they founded the first children's hospital in North America: The Children's Hospital of Philadelphia. The hospital had 12 beds and a dispensary and catered to the illnesses and injuries of children. Children's Hospital of Philadelphia, or CHOP, is still in operation today and is ranked as one of the top children's hospitals in the nation.

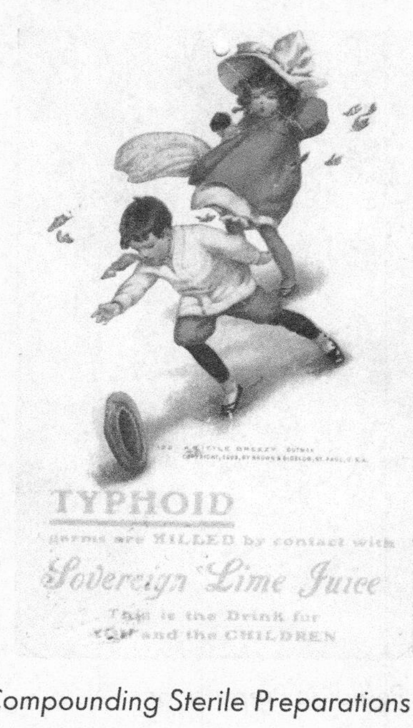

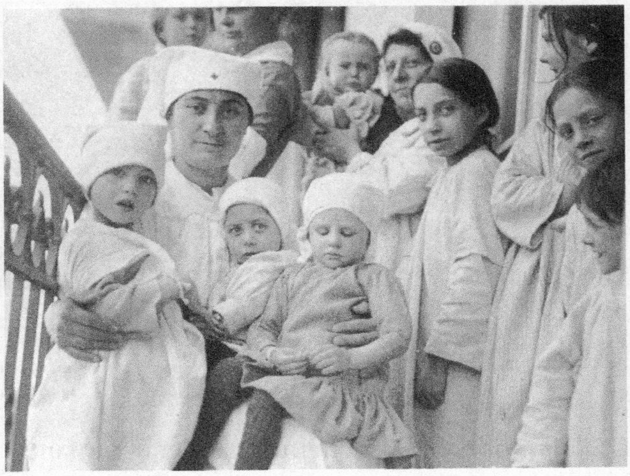

Soon after the establishment of this hospital, other major urban areas, such as New York, Chicago, and Boston, followed suit. Several of these children's hospitals were affiliated with religious organizations and employed a live-in hospital matron to oversee patient care and a staff of nuns to provide nursing services. Children were often isolated from their families for weeks at a time during their hospitalization. Upon discharge, the children would typically be moved to a convalescent home where they could benefit from nutritious food and outdoor, fresh-air excursions.

Although early children's hospitals mainly provided supportive care, by the close of the nineteenth century, these facilities offered medical and surgical services. A number of nineteenth-century physicians made notable contributions to the advancement of pediatric medicine in the United States, including Dr. John Forsyth Meigs (1818–1882), who practiced medicine in Philadelphia; Dr. Luther Holt (1855–1924), who practiced in New York City; and Dr. William M. Marriott (1885–1936), who practiced in St. Louis, Missouri. One of the most notable early contributors to pediatric medicine was Dr. Abraham Jacobi (1830–1919), who trained in Germany and in 1853 moved his pediatric practice to New York City, where he taught pediatric medicine to students at New York Medical College. Jacobi's contributions in the emerging field of pediatrics earned him the title "Father of American Pediatric Medicine." Each of these early practitioners authored numerous medical journals, pioneered research, and developed teaching modalities based on the belief that children have a unique **physiology** and require medical treatment and medicine specifically developed for children. With the establishment of the American Pediatric Society in 1888, society finally acknowledged the unique healthcare needs of children, and the field of pediatric medicine became a recognized medical specialty.

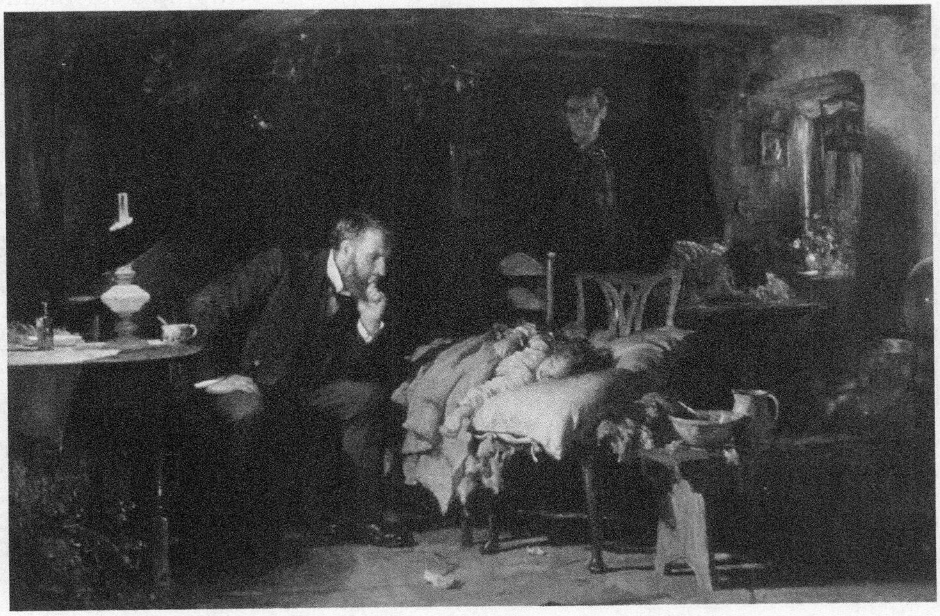

## Pediatric Medicine Today

During the twentieth century, the field of pediatric medicine rapidly expanded, establishing its own identity in the medical arena. Educational institutions began to offer coursework and practice for physicians in pediatrics. The individuals who completed these studies became **pediatricians**, or doctors who specialize in the development, treatment, and diseases of children. Today's pediatricians must have a minimum of 11 years of higher education: four years of college, followed by four years of medical school, a one-year pediatrics internship, and a two-year pediatrics residency. Pediatricians who become board-certified in pediatrics may use the designation FAAP (or F.A.A.P.), meaning Fellow of the American Academy of Pediatrics.

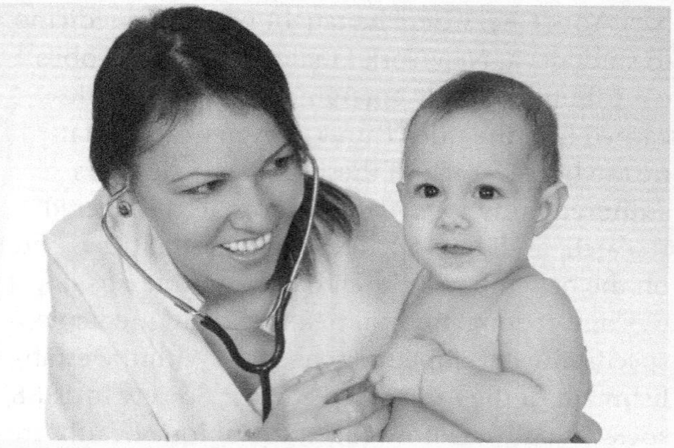

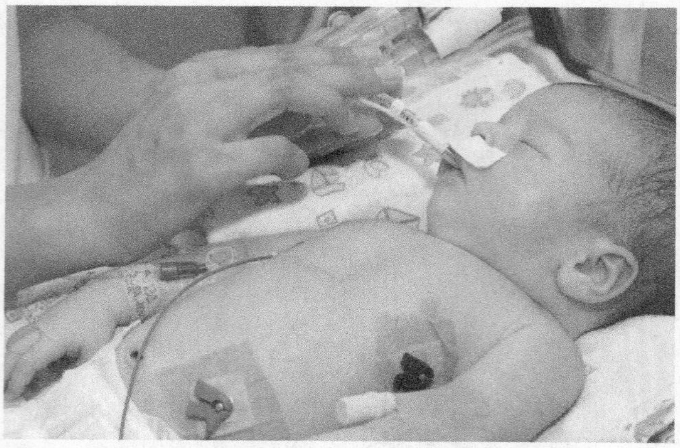

The practice of pediatrics has also grown to include many subspecialties, such as pediatric emergency medicine, pediatric cardiology, developmental-behavioral pediatrics, and pediatric endocrinology. Two other pediatric subspecialties focus on the oldest and youngest members of this patient population: adolescent medicine and neonatal-perinatal medicine. Adolescent medicine emphasizes the care of patients from ages 11–18, including studies on eating disorders, reproductive medicine, substance abuse, sexually transmitted diseases, and mental health. Neonatal-perinatal medicine focuses on newborns. The word *neonatal* is derived from the Latin words *neo* (meaning "new") and *natal* (meaning "birth" or "born"). **Neonatologists** specialize in the treatment of **neonates** (or infants under one month of age) who need critical care due to **premature** birth, **congenital defects**, infections, or birth trauma. These newborn specialists must fulfill the same education and training requirements as pediatricians, plus complete an additional three-year fellowship in **neonatology**. This area of specialization has become increasingly important as advances in technology and pharmaceuticals over the past 50 years have increased the survival rate of premature infants born as early as 22 weeks' **gestation**. Two notable developments in neonatal care include the invention of the **mechanical ventilator** in the 1950s and the discovery of the class of drugs known as **pulmonary surfactants**. Both of these developments have helped compensate for the immature lungs of neonates, increasing their chances of survival. Infants receiving treatment by a neonatologist are usually critically ill and hospitalized in a **neonatal intensive care unit (NICU)**.

In addition to the NICU, many hospitals have pediatric units as well as **pediatric intensive care units (PICUs)** that specialize in the treatment of infants and children. More recently, entire hospitals singly dedicated to the treatment of infants and children have become commonplace, especially in large cities. These specialized care sites recognize the unique requirements of children and offer state-of-the-art equipment sized for smaller patients and personnel who are educated and trained in treating children's physical, mental, and emotional needs. In the hospital setting, **clinical pharmacists** work closely with pediatricians and neonatologists to recommend appropriate drug therapy, monitor **clinical outcomes**, and perform **drug utilization review**. Pharmacists must be familiar with **pediatric physiology** as well as drug disposition, dosage modification procedures, and **pharmacotherapeutic treatment** of the pediatric patient.

## Pharmacy and Pediatrics

With the diversification of medicine and rapid advancements in drug therapy in the twentieth

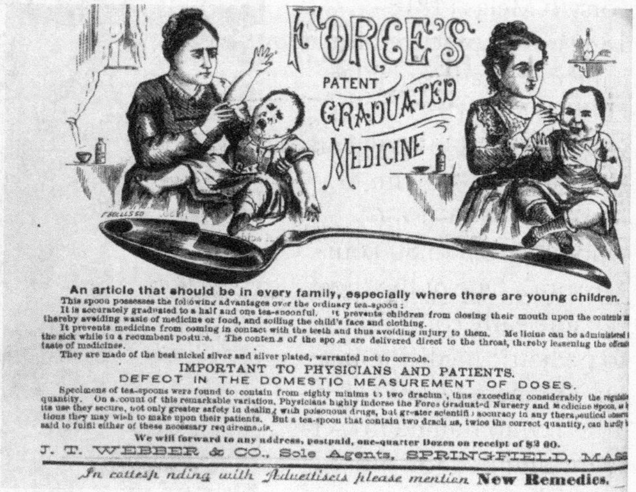

century, the medical and pharmaceutical fields worked toward increased specialization in the treatment of specific patient populations and disease states. For pediatric patients, changes in drug therapy came slowly. Up until the early 1970s, the primary consideration for pediatric drug therapy had to do with adjusting adult medication doses so that they were appropriate for a child's considerably smaller body size. Many different rules were developed to calculate the proper medication dose for a child. These rules were often inaccurate and inconsistent and have since been replaced with more accurate methods of dosing. (For additional information on the history of pediatric dosing methods, refer to Chapter 5 of this textbook.)

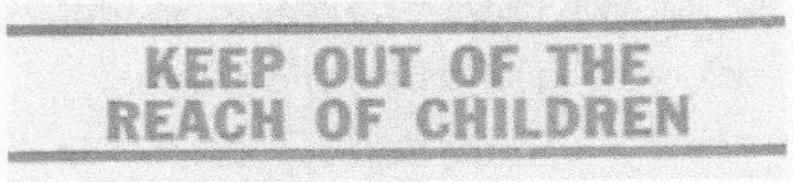
KEEP OUT OF THE
REACH OF CHILDREN

Although adult medications continue to be adjusted for use in pediatric patients, many drug companies have channeled significant resources toward the research and development of medications formulated specifically for pediatric patients. These pediatric medications offer several benefits: For patients, these formulations offer an easier delivery method and an improved taste; for pharmacy personnel, they allow accurate dose titration, thus reducing the incidence of medication errors and drug toxicity.

Pharmacy practices have also undergone significant changes in the preparation and dispensation of pediatric medicine. In 1979, pharmacists recognized the need for medication practices that were specifically geared toward the treatment of pediatric patients. They discussed their concerns at an **American Society of Health-System Pharmacists (ASHP)** Midyear Clinical Meeting, which led to the inclusion of pharmacy directors of pediatric hospitals to the organization. In 1986, this group formed the **Pediatric Pharmacy Administrative Group (PPAG)** to promote pediatric pharmacy research as well as advocacy of pediatric pharmacy issues, such as decreasing pediatric medication errors.

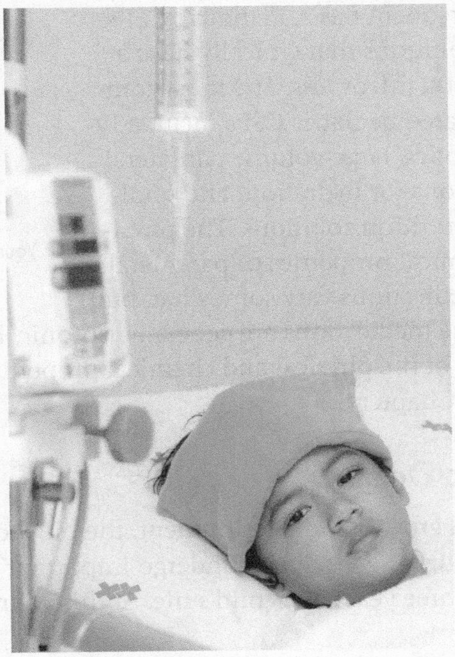

## Pediatric Specialization

Pharmacy education and accreditation have also responded to the outgrowth of pediatric medicine by offering increased clinical education for pharmacists in the areas of pediatric and neonatal drug therapy. In July 2000, the **Accreditation Council for Pharmacy Education (ACPE)** officially adopted standards that required pharmacy students to earn a **Doctor of Pharmacy degree (PharmD)**, rather than a Bachelor of Science (BS) degree. This change was driven in part by the desire for greater specialization in areas such as pediatric and neonatal drug therapy. Some pharmacy students further specialize with advanced certification in **pediatric pharmacy**.

Along with the increased education and training of pharmacists in pediatric medicine, pharmacy technicians also have the opportunity for advanced training in this specialty. Some hospital pharmacies, as well as a number of pharmacy technician training programs, now offer advanced pharmacy technician training and certification, with an emphasis in pediatric and neonatal pharmacy procedures, or a specialization in the preparation of pediatric compounded sterile preparations (CSPs) using strict aseptic technique.

Like other sterile products, pediatric CSPs must be prepared in strict accordance with correct compounding and aseptic technique protocols. In addition, pediatric preparations require several special considerations during the compounding process, including dosage volume adjustments and specialized ingredients and supply items. This chapter provides the background information, aseptic technique details, and specific sequence of sterile compounding procedures to be used in the preparation of a pediatric special dilution for intravenous (IV) administration.

# Part 1: Concepts

Pediatric medicine—or a branch of medicine concerned with the treatment of infants and children up to approximately age 18—is its own primary care specialty due to the special needs of its patient population. Aside from the obvious anatomical differences of body size and weight, children also have distinct physiologies that set them apart from adults. Specifically, the internal organs, tissues, and cells of infants and children are in a constant state of change. These maturing body systems result in markedly different responses to medications due to variances in kidney and liver functions, as well as differences in cardiovascular and respiratory systems.

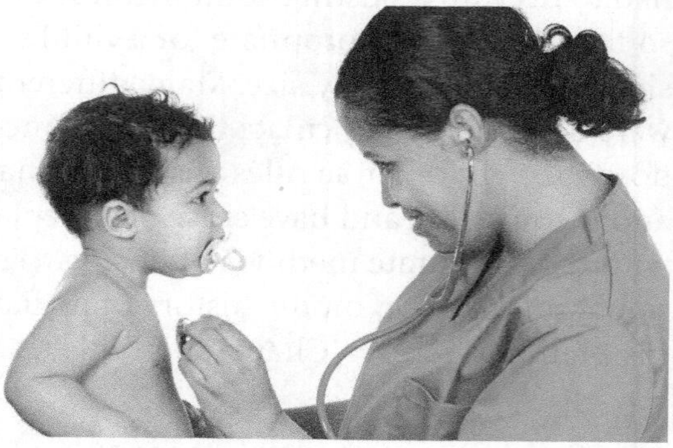

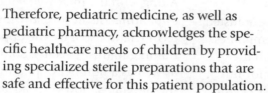

Physician caring for a pediatric patient.

Therefore, pediatric medicine, as well as pediatric pharmacy, acknowledges the specific healthcare needs of children by providing specialized sterile preparations that are safe and effective for this patient population.

## Pediatric CSPs

Because the vast majority of medications for pediatric and neonatal patients are administered intravenously, sterile compounding personnel prepare pediatric CSPs on a frequent basis. **Pediatric CSPs** are sterile solutions that typically have a volume of 500 mL or less. The most commonly prepared pediatric CSPs include IV push antibiotics, large-volume parenteral (LVP) solutions for hydration, and total parenteral nutrition solutions. The physical and chemical properties of parenteral pediatric medications vary somewhat, but most of these medications are generally isotonic, isoosmotic, and pH neutral. (For an overview of the physical and chemical properties of parenteral medications in general, see Chapter 8.)

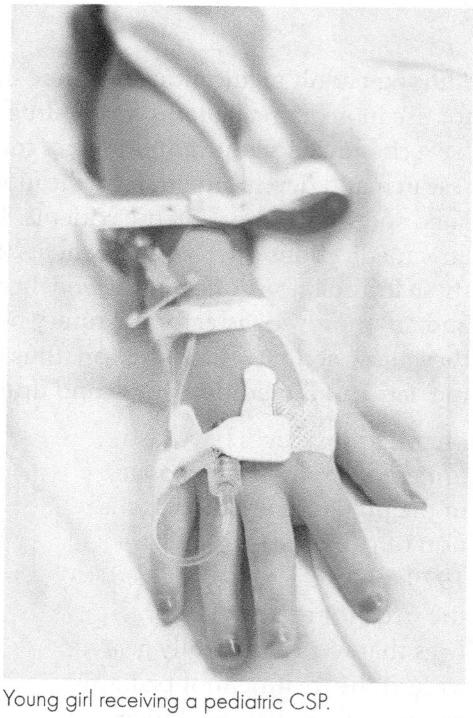

Young girl receiving a pediatric CSP.

## Pediatric Dosing

During child growth and development, the biochemical and physiological processes that control **drug disposition** undergo important changes. This is especially true for the first three years of a child's life. At this young age, drugs may be absorbed or eliminated more slowly or more rapidly than in adults. With that in mind, many factors must be considered when determining **pediatric dosing** for a patient, including:

- pediatric anatomy and physiology
- body weight or body surface area (BSA)
- age
- diagnosis
- drug disposition
- organ function

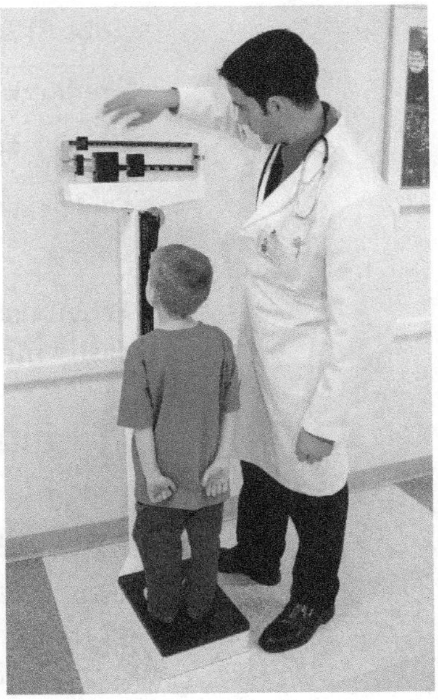

Young boy being weighed by a medical assistant.

## Pediatric Formulations

Pediatric dosing has long been based on **adult-strength formulations** of medications. Prescribers would simply modify the dosage of an adult medication to appropriately treat the smaller pediatric patient. This method of dosing continues to be used today, with prescribers using body weight or BSA to help them determine appropriate dosages for parenteral medications.

At times, however, the high concentrations of adult-strength medications make reduction to child-sized doses difficult (see Table 12.1). In these situations, the pediatric doses are such small volumes that they are hard to draw up accurately in a syringe. As a result, many manufacturers have reformulated certain adult-strength medications into diluted concentrations, or **pediatric-strength formulations**, making pediatric dose preparation easier and more accurate (see Table 12.2). Quite often, these pediatric-strength formulations must be even further diluted with a solution such as sterile water or normal saline (NS) prior to pediatric patient administration.

**POINTER**

A prescriber often consults a pharmacist to determine the appropriate pediatric dosage of an adult medication.

Regardless of whether the pediatric medication is based on an adult-strength formulation or a pediatric-strength formulation, all drugs for pediatric use are required to undergo studies prior to approval by the Food and Drug Administration. This federal law—included in a 2007 amendment to the Federal Food, Drug, and Cosmetic Act—was established, in part, to improve the safety and efficacy of pediatric medications.

**Table 12.1 Providing a Pediatric Dose from an Adult-Strength Medication**

| |
|---|
| **Adult Gentamicin Dosage** |
| An average gentamicin dose based on a patient's body weight is 2 mg/kg. Adult-strength gentamicin is supplied from the manufacturer in a concentration of 40 mg/mL. Based on this information, the dose needed for an 80-kg patient is 160 mg (2 × 80 = 160). To prepare the 160-mg dose, the IV technician must draw up 4 mL of gentamicin (160/40 = 4 mL). |
| **Pediatric Gentamicin Dosage** |
| An average gentamicin dose based on a patient's body weight is 2 mg/kg. Again, the adult-strength gentamicin is supplied from the manufacturer in a concentration of 40 mg/mL. Based on this information, the dose needed for a 1-kg neonate is 2 mg (2 × 1 = 2). To prepare the 2-mg dose, the IV technician must draw up 0.05 mL of gentamicin (2/40 = 0.05 mL). |

As the examples in Table 12.1 illustrate, using adult-strength gentamicin to draw up a pediatric dose may require a volume of gentamicin that is too small for the IV technician to accurately measure (in this case, 0.05 mL).

The same dose as the previous example is prepared in Table 12.2; however, in this situation, the IV technician uses *pediatric-strength* gentamicin to prepare the dose.

**Table 12.2 Providing a Pediatric Dose from a Pediatric-Strength Medication**

| Pediatric Gentamicin Dosage |
| --- |
| An average gentamicin dose is 2 mg/kg. Pediatric gentamicin is supplied from the manufacturer in a concentration of 10 mg/mL. Based on this information, the dose needed for a 1-kg neonate is 2 mg (2 × 1 = 2). To prepare the 2-mg dose, the IV technician must draw up 0.2 mL of gentamicin (2/10 = 0.2 mL). |

When using the pediatric-strength gentamicin to draw up this dose, the volume is easily measured with accuracy (in this case, 0.2 mL).

## Administration of Pediatric CSPs

Pediatric CSPs are primarily given as continuous IV infusions or as intermittent doses using the **IV push route of administration**.

***Continuous IV Infusion*** Many pediatric patients receive a continuous IV infusion during their hospitalization. Pediatric continuous IV infusions are generally comprised of an IV base solution to which an additive, such as potassium chloride, is injected during sterile compounding procedures.

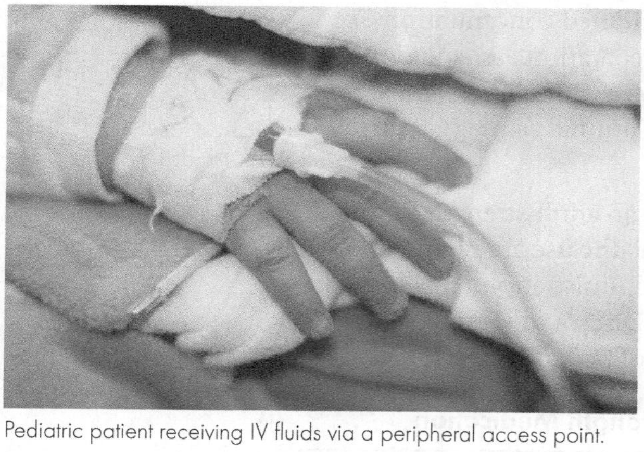

Pediatric patient receiving IV fluids via a peripheral access point.

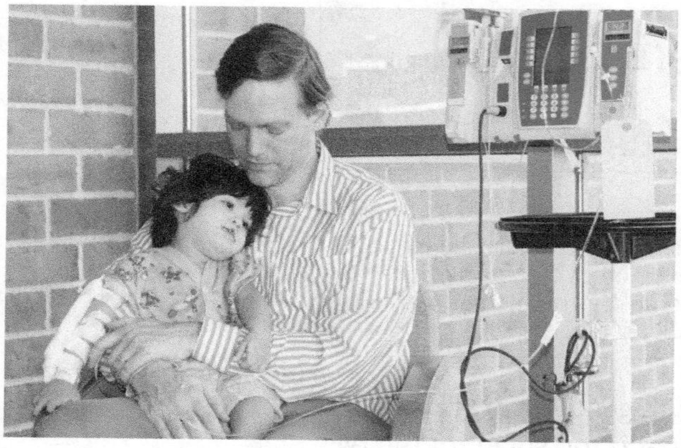

Young girl receiving IV push medications through a syringe pump.

ADMINISTRATION OF A CONTINUOUS IV INFUSION To administer a continuous IV infusion to patients age 2 or older, a peripheral **access point** is established. However, some pediatric patients, especially neonates, have fragile peripheral veins that may be difficult to access and maintain for IV administration purposes. For these patients, it may be more practical for the nursing staff to establish a central line or gain IV access through a **femoral line** or **umbilical line**.

Once an access point has been established, nursing personnel use an IV pump programmed to deliver the medication at a flow rate designated by the prescriber. The use of an IV pump helps to regulate the dosage, thus reducing the likelihood of inadvertent fluid overload. The continuous infusion CSP is typically given until the patient is discharged or until the prescriber writes an order to discontinue the IV.

***Intermittent CSP Administration*** Parenteral medications requiring intermittent dosing are commonly administered by the IV push route. Sterile compounding personnel frequently prepare pediatric IV push medications, especially in facilities that serve pediatric and neonatal patients. Medications used for pediatric IV push administration are supplied in several forms, including compounded syringes and empty evacuated containers.

**Compounded Syringes** **Compounded syringes** are syringes of medication that are compounded in the pharmacy and then sent to a nursing unit for patient administration. These syringes are typically sent without an attached needle; instead, a syringe cap is placed on the tip of the filled syringe during sterile compounding procedures. Using a syringe cap rather than a capped needle is a precautionary measure taken to avoid a needle stick from the accidental dislodgment of the needle cap during transport of the syringe. Once the syringe cap is attached, an **IVA syringe seal** is then placed over the cap to ensure that the contents of the syringe remain sterile and that they have not been subject to tampering prior to patient administration. At the time of medication administration, a nurse removes the syringe cap with attached IVA seal, attaches a sterile needle to the syringe, and administers the dose to the patient.

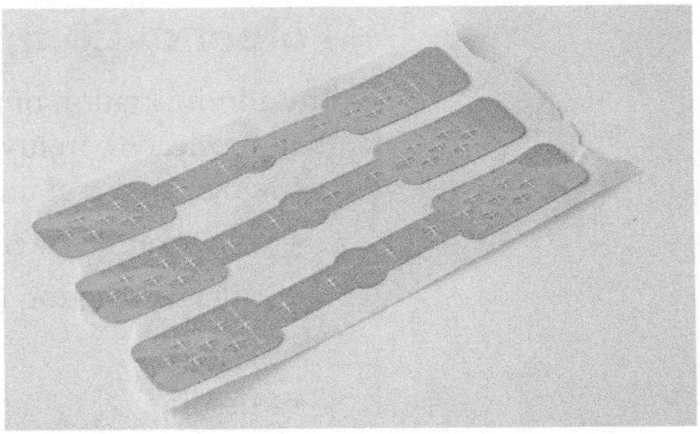
IVA syringe seals.

**Empty Evacuated Containers** Often, a pediatric IV push medication is compounded into patient-specific vials or empty plastic bags known as **empty evacuated containers (EECs)**. These special-dilution (SD) vials are commonly used in pediatric sterile compounding situations and are especially useful for neonatal patients whose size dictates further dilution of a pediatric-strength drug with preservative-free (PF) sterile water or NS. EECs typically contain a CSP, which is comprised of a sterile, injectable, PF medication and a diluent. Each vial generally contains enough medication for 24 hours of dosing for a single patient, depending on the stability of the CSP.

**POINTER**

Some EEC vials are limited to one-time use. Other EEC vials may be used for multiple-dose withdrawals over a period of 24 hours, provided that the medication is refrigerated. Consult your facility's P&P manual for guidance.

EECs have several advantages for nursing and pharmacy personnel:

- Unlike a compounded syringe, EECs can still be used if the patient dosage changes.
- EECs are either vials or bags, not syringes, which helps avoid accidental needle sticks during handling. The use of vials also lessens the risk of contamination of the medication that may occur during removal of the syringe cap and attachment of the needle.
- Because most patient recipients receive the same concentration of medication, preparing batches of EECs—rather than individual syringe doses—is easier and more convenient for pharmacy personnel.

One disadvantage of EECs is that they are more costly than the syringe dosage form. Another disadvantage is the potential for EEC or syringe contamination when the dose is drawn up just prior to administration.

**Administration of Pediatric Push Medications** Pediatric IV push medications should be administered either by a syringe pump or by the use of a buretrol or similar mechanism. A **buretrol** is a special type of tubing that contains a large, tube-shaped cylinder. The IV push medication is injected into the cylinder, where it mixes with a specific volume of fluid from the patient's primary IV solution. The diluted medication is then administered through the tubing via a pump programmed to slowly inject the medication over a preset period.

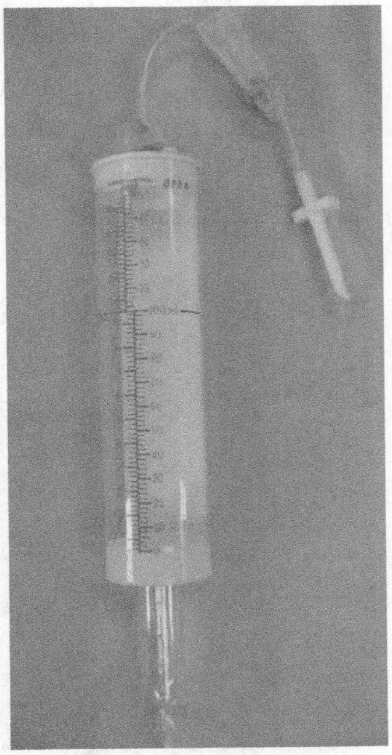
A buretrol used for intermittent administration of IV push medications to pediatric patients.

A buretrol or some similar type of chamber device is also used to administer the occasional pediatric medication with an acidic pH value or one that is hypertonic or hyperosmotic. Using one of these administration devices will result in a CSP that is generally isotonic, isoosmotic, and pH neutral.

## Potential Complications of Pediatric CSPs

The administration of parenteral medications involves certain potential complications that may lead to injury or, possibly, death for patient recipients. Therefore, all patients receiving parenteral therapy should be monitored for the following complications:

- nosocomial infection
- allergic reaction (including anaphylaxis)
- phlebitis
- tissuing
- embolism
- extravasation
- cellulitis
- Stevens-Johnson syndrome
- nephrotoxicity

**POINTER**
The administration of PF medications to neonates is a directive followed by all pharmacy facilities. However, the use of these medications for older infants and children varies among facilities. Most facilities include pediatric patients up to age five in this directive, but some facilities require *all* pediatric patients to receive PF medications. Consult your facility's P&P manual for guidance.

Other complications are specific to certain types of CSPs, and to varying degrees. For pediatric CSPs, there is an increased likelihood for overdose. Therefore, IV technicians need to be aware of both the preparation and administration risks associated with pediatric CSPs.

***Preparation Risks*** During the compounding of pediatric preparations, **pediatric CSP ingredients** must be considered. Due to the fragile and still-developing organ systems of children, especially neonates, preservatives such as benzyl alcohol (found in many multiple-dose vials [MDVs]) should not be used in compounding procedures. The bodies of neonates are unable to process this preservative. In fact, benzyl alcohol may cause damage to multiple organ systems, potentially triggering a life-threatening condition called **benzyl alcohol gasping syndrome**. For this reason, only **preservative-free (PF) ingredients** should be used in pediatric CSPs.

In addition to using PF ingredients, the compounding of pediatric CSPs requires additional oversight to ensure the accuracy of pharmacy calculations. Because of the small size and delicate nature of pediatric patients, even minor errors in dosage calculation of a pediatric CSP could be fatal. Therefore, extra caution should be taken to confirm the accuracy of all calculations. It is best practice to have three verification checks performed on the calculations for pediatric CSPs: In some facilities, two pharmacists and one IV technician perform the verification checks; in other facilities, one pharmacist and two IV technicians perform the checks. Consult your facility's P&P manual to determine the checking procedures for pediatric CSPs.

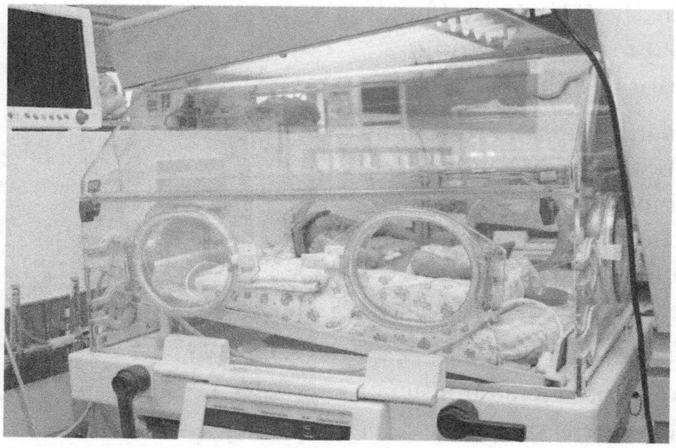

A neonatal patient in an incubator.

***Administration Risks*** Healthcare personnel must be vigilant during the administration of pediatric CSPs. Because children, especially neonates, are so small, the total volume of parenteral fluid being administered to this patient population must be significantly smaller than the fluid volumes given to adult patients. If too much fluid were to be administered to a neonate too quickly (generally referred to as **accidental rapid administration**), **hypervolemia**, cardiac arrest, or death may result. The cause of such an error is most commonly a nursing or IV pump error. Many hospitals avoid **accidental fluid overload** by enacting policies that prohibit the use of 1000-mL IV bags with pediatric patients. In addition, facilities limit the size of an IV bag to 250 or 500 mL for neonates. These precautionary measures eliminate the possibility of this dangerous administration error.

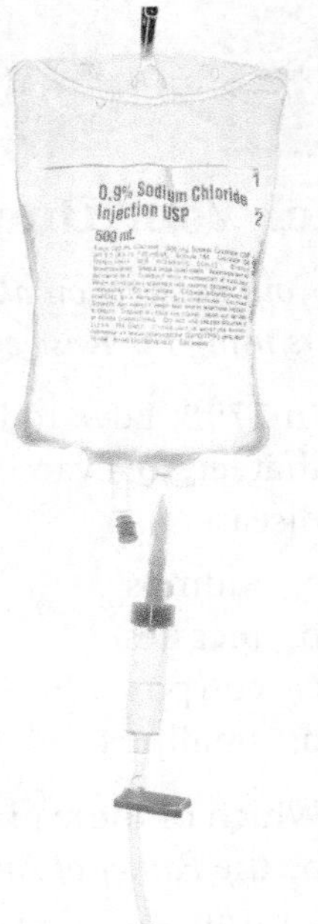

A 500-mL bag of IV fluid.

Children older than age five may receive some medications by the IV piggyback (IVPB) route of administration. The volume of the IVPB base solution used for children is usually 25 mL or 50 mL, compared with an IVPB volume of 100 mL or even 250 mL commonly given to adults. Children age five and younger usually receive intermittent medications by the IV push route of administration. These medications are often administered via syringe pump.

## USP Chapter <797> Guidelines for Pediatric CSPs

In light of these potential risks, IV technicians must adhere to strict dosage verification and aseptic protocols when preparing pediatric CSPs. Any breach in these protocols may result in medication errors, sepsis, or, possibly, death for patient recipients. Therefore, as an IV technician, you bear primary responsibility for the preparation and integrity of the CSPs. With that in mind, only those personnel who have been specially trained, process validated, and certified in aseptic technique and sterile product preparation should be allowed to compound sterile products. Part 2 of this chapter guides you through the discovery and demonstration of proper aseptic technique in the preparation of a pediatric special dilution.

**POINTER**

Some hospitals restrict the maximum pediatric IV bag size to 500 mL; other facilities restrict the maximum pediatric IV bag size to 250 mL. These guidelines may also vary according to whether the patient recipient is a neonate. Refer to your facility's P&P manual to determine the guidelines for maximum IV bag size.

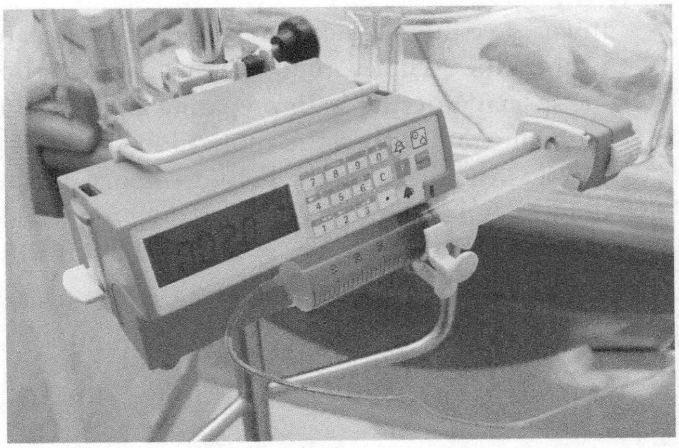

Neonatal patient receiving medications via a syringe pump.

# Concepts Self-Check

## Check Your Understanding

*Write your answers on a separate sheet of paper, as modeled in these examples:* 1d; 2c; 3b; *etc. Check your answers using the Answer Key in Appendix A.*

**1.** In 1798, Edward Jenner published research that led to a vaccine for which contagious disease?

a. mumps
b. measles
c. cowpox
d. smallpox

2. Which of these physicians is considered to be the *Father of American Pediatric Medicine*?

a. William M. Marriott
b. Luther Holt
c. Abraham Jacobi
d. John Forsyth Meigs

**3.** Which of the following must be considered when determining a pediatric dose?

a. the patient's weight or BSA
b. pediatric physiology and organ function
c. diagnosis
d. all of the above
e. both *a* and *b*

**4.** Accidental rapid administration of a 1-liter bag of IV fluids may lead to a condition called:

a. hypovolemia
b. hypervolemia
c. fluid overdose syndrome
d. fluid gasping syndrome

**5.** When using a vial of sterile, NS solution in the preparation of a neonatal CSP, which of the following abbreviations should be found on the diluent vial label?

a. MDV
b. $D_5W$
c. PF
d. NF

## Apply Your Knowledge

*On a separate sheet of paper, write your answers to the questions posed in the paragraph below. Use complete sentences and take time to create a thorough and thoughtful response. Check your answers against the Answer Key in Appendix A.*

In Part 1 of this chapter, you learned that pediatric CSPs require additional verification checks to confirm the accuracy of dosage calculations. The Chapter 12 procedural lab will introduce you to the special procedures for preparing and verifying pediatric CSPs. With that in mind, what is the rationale for handling the verification checks of pediatric CSPs in a different manner than other CSPs? Given the additional requirements and considerations for handling pediatric CSPs, do you think IV technicians preparing sterile products should be required to undergo additional training and certification before preparing pediatric CSPs? Why or why not?

# Part 2: Training

*Before performing this lab, review the Sterile Compounding Area Procedures listed on pages 162–163 at the end of the Unit 2 opener, and preview the accompanying process validation checklist in Appendix D.*

## Understand the Resources and Supplies

USP Chapter <797> prescribes a number of special requirements for the preparation of a pediatric special dilution. This chapter and the corresponding lab provide resources and supplies that are in alignment with the directives set forth in USP Chapter <797>.

### Essential Supplies

Most sterile compounding procedures require the same essential supply items to be available for use in both the anteroom and the clean room. For the anteroom, these supplies include a medication order and CSP label; a standard calculator; a pen; a permanent, felt-tip marker; large and small plastic bags; aseptic garb; a sterile gown; presaturated aseptic cleaning wipes; sterile, foamed 70% isopropyl alcohol (IPA); a waste container; and a transport vehicle. Various other compounding supplies, such as those needed for aseptic hand washing and hood cleaning, are necessary supplies, but, for the purposes of this lab, are not included on the Essential Supplies list. In the clean room, essential supply items include sterile, foamed 70% IPA; sterile, powder-free gloves; sterile 70% IPA swabs; a sharps container; a waste container; and a laminar airflow hood.

### Procedure-Specific Supplies

In addition to the previously listed essential supplies, each sterile compounding procedure requires supply items specific to the procedure being performed. The type, number, and amount of procedure-specific supply items are determined by the IV technician prior to performing the procedure, based on information provided on the CSP label and the medication additive label. After reading these labels, the IV technician performs one or more calculations that reveal the number and volume of additives needed to prepare the CSP. This information, in turn, dictates the number, size, and types of syringes needed to correctly withdraw the necessary ingredient volumes of the drug and diluent.

***Pediatric Special Dilution Supplies*** The process of compounding certain pediatric CSPs involves the manipulation of regular needles and, in particular, medication, diluent, and EEC vials. Familiarity with the appearance of these items as well as any specific handling requirements is essential to sterile compounding procedures. (For specific information on the use of regular needles and vial techniques, see Chapter 8.)

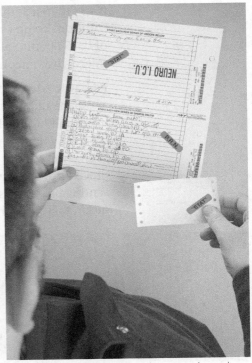

An IV technician verifying a medication order and a CSP label.

**FIGURE 12.1**

**A medication label indicating that the medication is for pediatric use and is preservative-free.**

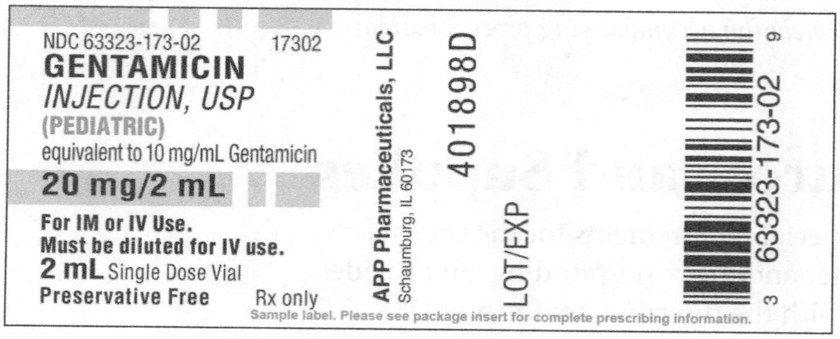

NDC 63323-173-02 17302
GENTAMICIN
INJECTION, USP
(PEDIATRIC)
equivalent to 10 mg/mL Gentamicin
20 mg/2 mL
For IM or IV Use.
Must be diluted for IV use.
2 mL Single Dose Vial
Preservative Free
Rx only
APP Pharmaceuticals, LLC
Schaumburg, IL 60173
401898D
LOT/EXP
3 63323-173-02 9
Sample label. Please see package insert for complete prescribing information.


**PF Gentamicin Vial** The drug used in this chapter's procedural lab must be pediatric-strength, PF gentamicin. To verify this information, the IV technician should check the vial's medication label for the word *Pediatric* (or *Pedi*), indicating that it is the pediatric-strength dose of gentamicin, and for the words *preservative-free* or the abbreviation *PF*, indicating that it is a preservative-free medication (see Figure 12.1).

**PF Diluent Vial** The type of diluent most often used when preparing pediatric CSPs is normal saline (NS). When compounding sterile products for neonatal use, the diluent must be preservative-free (PF) as well. Most pharmacies require the use of PF diluents for both neonatal and pediatric patients to avoid potential complications caused by the presence of a preservative such as benzyl alcohol. The type of PF NS diluent used for a pediatric CSP is generally supplied from the manufacturer in a single-use vial with a volume of either 10 mL or 30 mL.

**EECs** EECs are vacuum-sealed, sterile glass containers or empty polyvinyl chloride bags available in many sizes, including 2 mL, 5 mL, 10 mL, 20 mL, 30 mL, 50 mL, 100 mL, 150 mL, 250 mL, 500 mL, and 1000 mL. EECs are used to prepare **custom-made CSPs**, or CSPs that are compounded by IV technicians from scratch, using various components or ingredients that are not commercially available in the dosage, volume, or strength ordered by the prescribers. Occasionally, the base solution must be created from scratch as well. For example, if a medication order calls for *vancomycin 1 gram in 0.45 NS 250 mL IVPB*, but the pharmacy only stocks the base solution 0.45 NS in a 1000-mL bag, the IV technician is then required to make the IVPB base solution. To do so, she or he must transfer 250 mL of fluid from the 1000-mL bag of 0.45 NS into a 250-mL EEC, using secondary IV tubing. The IV technician then injects the vancomycin into the custom-made 0.45 NS 250-mL IVPB base solution.

**Pediatric special dilutions** provide accurate parenteral medication dosing for neonates and particularly small or young pediatric patients. To compound a custom-made CSP using an EEC, the IV technician draws up the appropriate volume of PF diluent and separately draws up the appropriate volume of medication. Once the ingredients have been checked, she or he injects the contents of both syringes into an EEC vial using procedures to properly vent the air pressure from the vial (see Chapter 8 for proper vial venting procedures). Upon completion of the sterile compounding process, the IV technician then seals the EEC vial's rubber top with a tamper-evident IVA seal. Finally, the prepared and labeled EEC vial is sent to the pediatric unit or NICU for patient administration.

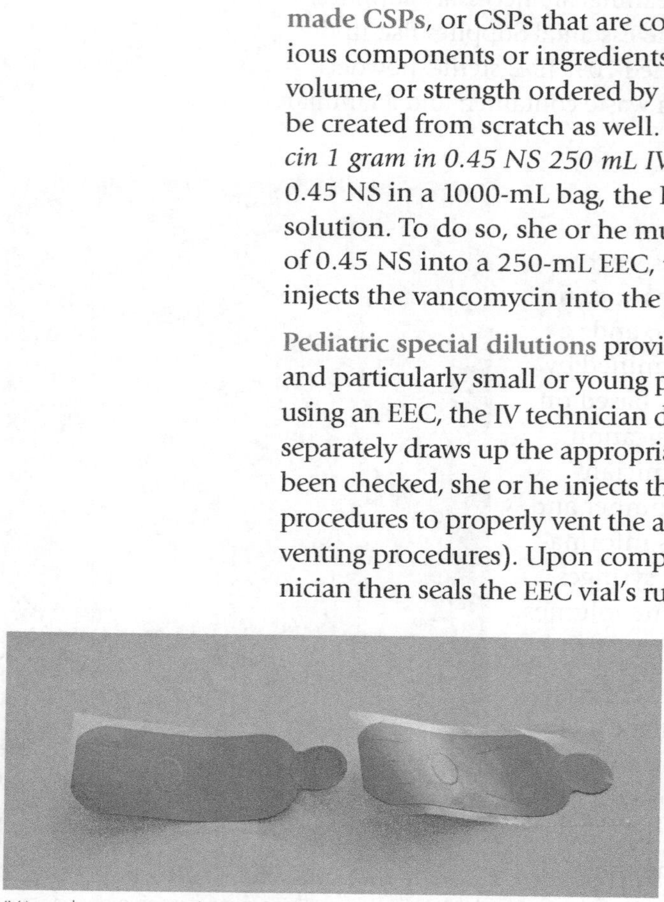

IVA seals prior to application to the vials' rubber tops.

Once the EEC arrives on the nursing unit—and just prior to the scheduled dose administration time—the nurse withdraws from the EEC vial the volume needed for one dose and places the filled syringe into a syringe pump. The pump then administers the medication to the patient over a specified period, usually 60 minutes.

In general, CSPs with PF ingredients are stable for a maximum of 24 hours. However, because the nurse withdraws from the vial in conditions that do not meet ISO Class 5 requirements (i.e., on the nursing unit and not in a laminar airflow hood), the EEC is considered a high-risk, immediate-use CSP once opened. Therefore, after withdrawal from the EEC, the dose must immediately be administered, and any remaining medication must be discarded.

## Critical Sites of Essential Supplies and Pediatric CSP Supplies

Before beginning preparatory procedures in the anteroom or clean room, the IV technician must recall the critical sites of the supplies (see Figure 12.2). Identifying the critical site of each supply item helps you determine the proper procedure for handling the supply item once you have entered the clean room and begin working in the hood.

The critical sites of essential supply items include the sterile 70% IPA swabs. The critical sites of the pediatric CSP preparation supplies include the regular needles, the syringe tip, the piston plunger, and the inner plunger shaft of the syringe. These critical sites are supplied by the manufacturer in a sterile form and should, therefore, not be swabbed with alcohol prior to use.

The critical sites of the other pediatric CSP supplies used for the Chapter 12 procedural lab include the rubber tops of the diluent vial and the PF gentamicin vial, as well as the rubber top of the EEC. These critical sites must be swabbed with sterile 70% IPA prior to needle insertion to decrease the likelihood of contaminating the solution during injection or withdrawal procedures.

After identifying the critical sites of all supply items, care must be taken not to taint the critical site of any supply item through touch contamination, shadowing, or incorrect placement of the item within the hood. (For additional assistance on the handling of critical sites of sterile compounding supplies, refer to Chapter 3 of this textbook.)

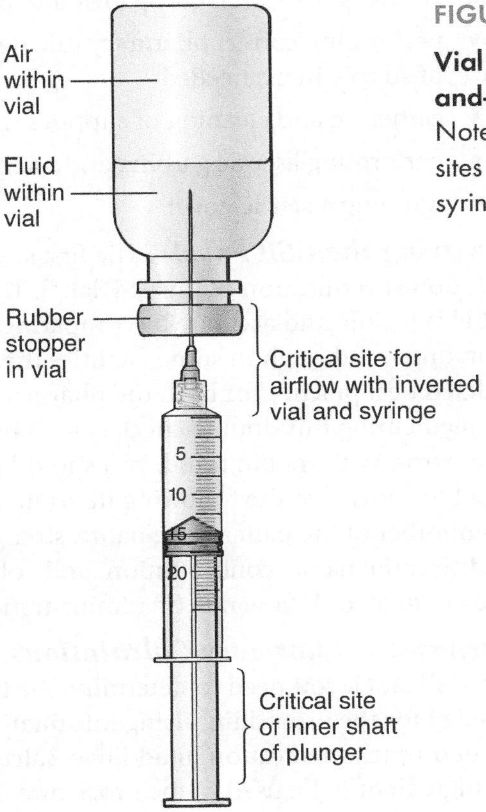


FIGURE 12.2

**Vial and Needle-and-Syringe Unit**
Note the critical sites of the vial and syringe.

# Preview the Lab Procedure

*There are many different compounding scenarios requiring CSPs for pediatric use. Some of those scenarios include the preparation of large-volume parenterals, small-volume parenterals, vials, ampules, IV push syringes, and narcotics. Refer to Chapters 8–11 for step-by-step procedures related to these types of compounding scenarios. The Chapter 12* Procedural Lab *instructs you in the proper procedure for preparing a pediatric special dilution in an EEC vial.*

*The following material provides a brief overview of the lab procedure that you will perform. First, read the* Preview the Lab Procedure *section. Then read each step of the* Procedural Lab *section carefully, visualizing every action. Next, reinforce your understanding of the process by watching the demonstration video. Once you are in the lab, your instructor will demonstrate the procedure, and then you will perform the procedure by following the steps in the* Procedural Lab *section. Practice the lab procedure multiple times. After sufficient practice, you will complete the lab procedure for process validation by your instructor.*

**POINTER**
Sterile compounding personnel must comply with certain restrictions when working in the anteroom and clean room areas. These restrictions include no gum chewing, horseplay, or food or drink in both the anteroom and clean room, and no hair spray, perfume, makeup, artificial or polished nails, or jewelry in the sterile compounding environment.

***Note:*** *This procedural lab requires the use of a basic, open-sided, horizontal laminar airflow hood. For pharmacies that do not have this type of hood, IV technicians should consult the* Instruction Guide *provided by the hood's manufacturer or their facility's P&P manual to determine which procedures may need to be adjusted to suit their hood.*

## Anteroom Preparatory Procedures

As you already know, the preparation for the sterile compounding process begins in the anteroom. This transition area provides a space for implementing the standard pharmacy protocols discussed in Chapters 3–6, including:

- verifying the CSP label against the medication order
- performing correct pharmacy calculations to determine type, size, and number of supply items needed
- gathering and cleaning of supplies
- performing aseptic garbing and hand washing
- donning a sterile gown

**POINTER**
Some facilities require verification of the CSP label by *three* pharmacy staff members. Consult your facility's P&P manual for guidance.

***Verifying the CSP Label*** The first step in the preparation of a pediatric special dilution is verification of the CSP label. The IV technician should check that the CSP label is legible and accurate by comparing the CSP label to the prescriber's medication order. Although in some facilities the pharmacist performs this step, it is considered best practice for both the pharmacist and IV technician to perform this task. Implementing this double-check system helps to reduce the likelihood of a medication error. With that in mind, you should compare the medication order to the CSP label to verify that the following items match exactly: the name, room number, and ID number of the patient; the name, strength, and amount or quantity of the drug or additive; the name, concentration, and volume of the base solution or diluent; and the designated IV flow rate or administration time.

***Performing Pharmacy Calculations*** Once you have verified the accuracy of the CSP label, you need to determine the type, size, and number of supply items needed for the procedure. Using information gleaned from the CSP label and the label on each medication or additive, calculate the desired volume for each additive or ingredient to be used in the procedure. The desired volume is the volume that you must withdraw from the PF gentamicin vial to deliver the dose ordered by the prescriber. In addition, you will need to perform a calculation to determine the volume of PF NS that you must draw up in order to prepare the CSP.

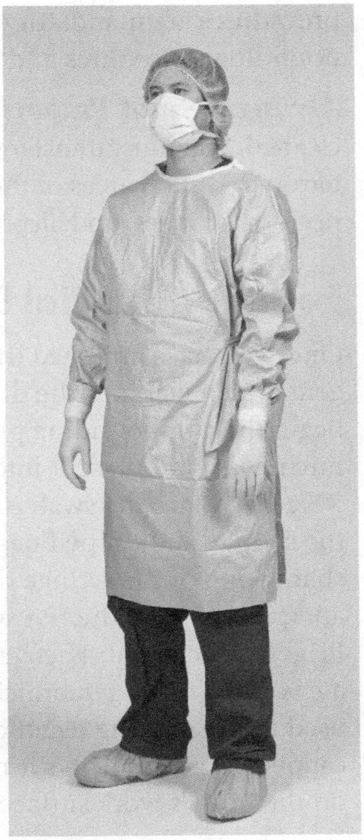

A fully gowned and gloved pharmacy technician.

***Gathering and Cleaning of Supplies*** After performing the calculations, place the CSP label into the small plastic bag, place the medication order into the large plastic bag, and seal both bags. Then gather the necessary supplies, including an appropriately sized syringe for the desired drug volume needed and a separate syringe for the diluent needed. Wipe down or spray the exterior surface of every supply item, as well as the transport vehicle, with an appropriate cleaning agent. Finally, place the clean supply items into the transport vehicle.

***Donning PPE*** Now that you have assembled your clean supplies, you must put on personal protective equipment (PPE). First, remove visible jewelry and ensure that you are properly attired for working in the clean room. Then put on aseptic shoe covers, a hair cover, a face mask, and, if appropriate, a beard cover. Lastly, don a sterile gown.

Due to time constraints, you will not perform aseptic hand-washing procedures during this procedural lab. Keep in mind that, in sterile compounding practice, aseptic hand-washing procedures are mandatory and must be performed prior to donning a sterile gown.

## Clean Room Preparatory Procedures

When preparing pediatric CSPs, sterile compounding personnel must diligently follow established pharmacy clean room protocols. These protocols, discussed in Chapters 6 and 7, include:

- cleansing hands with sterile, foamed 70% IPA
- donning sterile gloves
- cleaning the hood

Once the preparatory steps have been completed, pediatric special dilution compounding procedures may begin.

Upon entering the clean room, place the transport basket or tray onto a clean shelf, table, or countertop. If the transport vehicle used is a cart, wheel it so that it is positioned away from the hood prefilter. Cleanse your hands and forearms with sterile, foamed 70% IPA and allow them to dry thoroughly. Don sterile gloves according to standard aseptic technique procedures.

Due to time constraints, you will not perform hood-cleaning procedures during this procedural lab. Keep in mind that, in sterile compounding practice, hood-cleaning procedures are mandatory and must be performed prior to beginning sterile compounding procedures and at intervals prescribed by USP Chapter <797>.

***Arranging and Preparing Supplies in the Hood*** Once the hood has been cleaned, you must transfer the clean supplies from the transport vehicle or clean countertop to certain areas of the hood. Place small supply items—such as the vials, EEC, needles, syringes, and alcohol swabs—within the outer six-inch zone of the hood.

## Pediatric Special Dilution Compounding Procedure

Once you have arranged the supply items in the outer six-inch zone, bring the PF gentamicin vial into the direct compounding area (DCA). You are now ready to begin the compounding procedure. Remove the flip-top cap from the PF gentamicin vial, and place it into the discard pile. Swab the vial's rubber top with sterile 70% IPA. Place the swab on the hood's work surface within the DCA. Assemble the syringe and capped needle in such a way as to avoid touch contamination and shadowing of the syringe tip and the needle hub. After removing the needle cap and placing it on the IPA swab, use aseptic technique to insert the needle into the PF gentamicin vial. Then employ the milking technique to withdraw the appropriate volume of PF gentamicin into the syringe. (Refer to Chapter 8 for the procedures used in the milking technique and in bubble removal from a syringe.) The filled and capped PF gentamicin syringe should then be placed next to the PF gentamicin vial on the hood's work surface within the DCA.

Next, bring the PF NS (diluent) vial into the DCA, remove the flip-top cap, and swab the vial's rubber top with sterile 70% IPA. Assemble the empty syringe and capped needle aseptically, making sure to avoid touch contamination and shadowing of the syringe tip and the needle hub. After removing the needle cap and placing it on the alcohol swab, use aseptic technique to insert the needle into the diluent vial, and then employ the milking technique to withdraw the appropriate volume of diluent into the syringe.

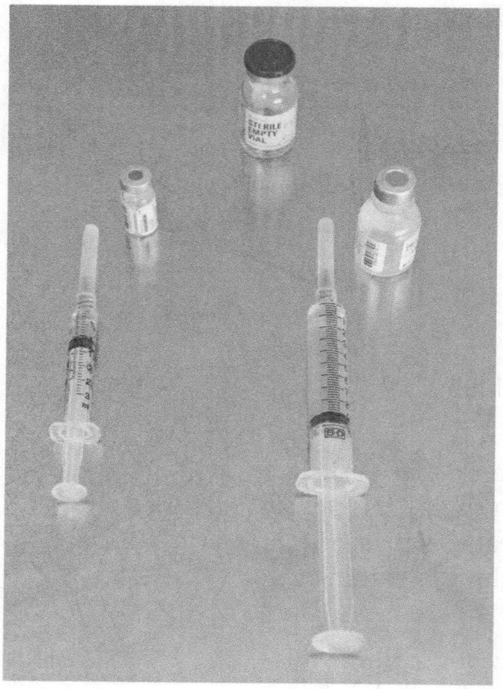

Filled diluent and medication syringes and vials positioned for a verification check.

In preparation for the verification check, position the filled and capped diluent syringe next to the diluent vial on the hood's work surface, immediately adjacent to the filled PF gentamicin syringe and PF gentamicin vial. Bring the EEC vial into the DCA and position it with the filled syringes, PF gentamicin vial, and NS vial on the hood's work surface. Place the small plastic bag containing the CSP label and the large plastic bag containing the medication order within the outer six-inch edge of the hood. Ask for a verification check.

After the verification check, reposition the EEC vial within the DCA so that the vial receives uninterrupted airflow from the HEPA filter and is away from supply items that might create air turbulence. Remove the flip-top cap, and then open a new sterile 70% IPA swab and clean the EEC vial's rubber top. Remove the cap from the PF gentamicin syringe and aseptically insert the needle into the EEC vial top. While keeping the EEC in contact with the hood's work surface, press down on the flat knob of the plunger to inject the PF gentamicin into the EEC vial. Remove your thumb from the flat knob of the plunger to allow air pressure from the EEC to be vented into the now-empty PF gentamicin syringe. Hold the syringe as you would a dart and carefully remove the needle-and-syringe unit from the EEC. Place the needle-and-syringe unit into the sharps container.

Open a new sterile 70% IPA swab and reswab the EEC vial's rubber top. Aseptically inject the diluent into the EEC vial. Vent air pressure from the EEC into the empty diluent syringe using the procedure described previously. Hold the syringe as you would a dart, and then carefully remove the needle-and-syringe unit and place it into the sharps container. Check the filled EEC for solution clarity. Finally, label the compounded pediatric special dilution EEC, and cover the EEC vial's rubber top with an IVA seal.

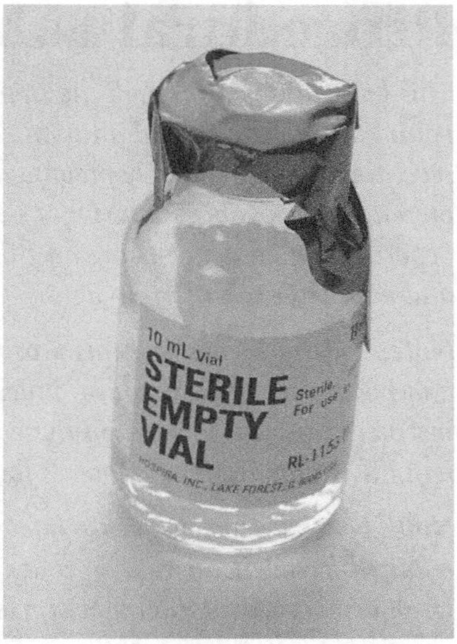

A filled EEC vial with an IVA seal over the vial top.

Upon completion of the pediatric special dilution compounding procedure, dispose of used vials and supply items in the appropriate waste container. Return the labeled pediatric special dilution EEC and any unused supply items to the transport vehicle and return them to the anteroom. Record the date and your initials on the CSP label. Remove PPE in the order and manner described in Chapter 6 of this textbook.

**POINTER**

Although the use of IVA seals with IV bags and syringes is considered optional, most facilities require that IVA seals be placed over the tops of EECs. This action helps to ensure the sterility and security of the EECs' contents during transportation and storage.

# Watch the Demonstration Video

*Watch the Chapter 12 Demonstration Video, which shows the step-by-step aseptic procedures for compounding a pediatric special dilution. For the purposes of the Chapter 12 Demonstration Video, neither aseptic hand washing nor hood cleaning is demonstrated. Refer to the Chapter 6 video for a demonstration of aseptic hand-washing procedures, and to the Chapter 7 video for a demonstration of correct hood-cleaning procedures.*

**Training Videos DVD**

# Procedural Lab

*This lab walks you through the step-by-step actions that you must follow to properly compound a pediatric special dilution. As with most sterile compounding procedures, there are several ways to aseptically prepare a pediatric special dilution. The Chapter 12 lab procedure presents one possible scenario for pediatric special dilution preparation and offers you the opportunity to practice using an EEC. Take your time. Work through each step methodically and with close attention to detail.*

***Note:*** *For the purposes of this procedural lab, you will not perform aseptic hand-washing and hood-cleaning procedures unless directed to do so by your instructor. Should your instructor ask you to perform these procedures, refer to Chapter 6 for instructions on aseptic hand washing and to Chapter 7 for directions on correct hood cleaning.*

***Note:*** *For step 1 below, please refer to Chapter 4 for a reminder of the step-by step procedures required for medication order and CSP label verification. For steps 2–6, refer to Chapter 5 for pharmacy calculation procedures. For steps 7–10, refer to Chapter 3 for a reminder of the process for gathering and cleaning supplies. For steps 11–18, refer to Chapter 6 for step-by-step aseptic garbing, hand-washing, and gloving procedures. Steps 1–14 and steps 43–44 should be performed in the anteroom. Steps 15–42 should be performed in the clean room.*

## Supplies

### *Essential Supplies*

To complete the Unit 2 procedural labs, you will need to ensure that various essential anteroom and clean room supplies such as those listed in Table 12.3 are available for your use.

**Table 12.3 Essential Anteroom and Clean Room Supplies for Sterile Compounding**

| |
|---|
| **Anteroom Supplies** |
| medication order and CSP label<br>calculator<br>pen<br>permanent, felt-tip marker<br>plastic bags (small and large)<br>aseptic garb, including shoe covers, hair cover, face mask, and beard cover (if appropriate)<br>sterile gown<br>presaturated, aseptic cleaning wipes<br>sterile, foamed 70% IPA<br>waste container<br>transport vehicle (optional) |
| **Clean Room Supplies** |
| sterile, foamed 70% IPA<br>sterile, powder-free gloves<br>sterile 70% IPA swabs, individually packaged × 3<br>sharps container<br>waste container<br>laminar airflow hood |

### *Procedure-Specific Supplies*

In addition to the supplies listed in Table 12.3, gather the following items specific to the Chapter 12 pediatric special dilution procedural lab:

- regular needle × 2
- 3-mL Luer-lock syringe × 2
- Pediatric gentamicin, 10-mg/mL vial (PF)
- 0.9% sodium chloride (NS), 10-mL vial (PF)
- EEC, 10-mL vial
- IVA seal

## Procedure

### *Verifying the Label*

1. Review the CSP label (see Figure 12.3) to verify that all information on the label matches the medication order (see Figure 12.5 on page 380).

FIGURE 12.3

**CSP Label for Gentamicin**

****Pediatric Special Dilution in EEC Vial****

Mercy Hospital

**Pt. Name:** Skyler Geiseler **Room:** PICU-12

**Pt. ID#:** 6627882 **Rx#:** 8836277

**SD Solution Concentration: Gentamicin (PF) 5 mg/mL 4-mL vial**

**Dosage: Gentamicin (PF) 7.5 mg/1.5 mL every 24 hours**

For IV push administration via syringe pump.
Administer over 60 minutes.

Expires ______
RPh ______
Tech ______

Preservative-free – for single-use only.

### *Calculating the Amount (mg) of PF Gentamicin*

2. Read the CSP label to determine the desired concentration and the desired total volume of the CSP.
3. Assuming that the CSP label calls for a desired concentration of 5 mg/mL and a desired total volume of 4 mL, perform a calculation to determine the number of milligrams needed to prepare the CSP:

$$\frac{5 \text{ mg}}{1 \text{ mL}} = \frac{x \text{ mg}}{4 \text{ mL}}$$

*Cross-multiply, then divide to solve for $x$ (the desired number of milligrams) for this pediatric special dilution. (For additional assistance, refer to Chapter 5 for step-by-step dosage calculation procedures.)

### *Calculating the Volume (mL) of PF Gentamicin*

4. Read the medication label for pediatric PF gentamicin to determine the drug concentration (see Figure 12.4).

FIGURE 12.4

**Medication Label for Pediatric PF Gentamicin**

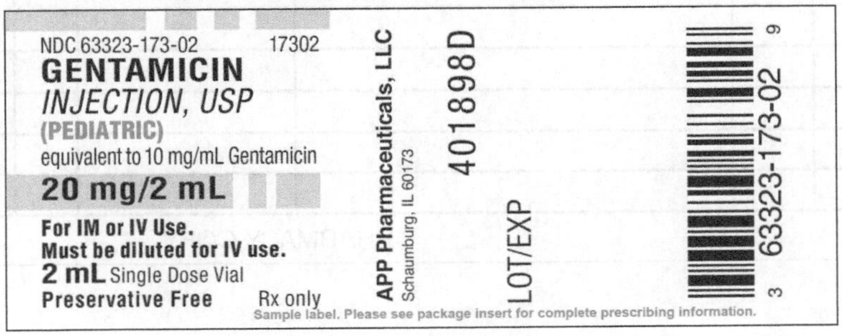
NDC 63323-173-02
17302
GENTAMICIN
INJECTION, USP
(PEDIATRIC)
equivalent to 10 mg/mL Gentamicin
20 mg/2 mL
For IM or IV Use.
Must be diluted for IV use.
2 mL Single Dose Vial
Preservative Free
Rx only
APP Pharmaceuticals, LLC
Schaumburg, IL 60173
401898D
LOT/EXP
3 63323-173-02 6
Sample label. Please see package insert for complete prescribing information.

FIGURE 12.5

**Daily Order**

**ID#:** 6627882
**Name:** Skyler Geiseler
**DOB:** 08/15/14
**Room:** PICU-12
**Dr.:** Marc Darrow

**MERCY HOSPITAL**
**PHYSICIAN'S MEDICATION ORDER**

**BEAR DOWN ON HARD SURFACE WITH BALLPOINT PEN**

GENERIC EQUIVALENT IS AUTHORIZED UNLESS CHECKED IN THIS COLUMN

ALLERGY OR SENSITIVITY TO *NKA*

NONE KNOWN ☐ SIGNED:

DIAGNOSIS

| DATE | TIME | ORDERS | PHYSICIAN'S SIG. | COMPLETED OR DISCONTINUED NAME | DATE | TIME |
|---|---|---|---|---|---|---|
| | | *Age: 45 days Wt: 1.8 kg* | | | | |
| | | *Resp. care to evaluate vent settings in a.m.* | | | | |
| | | *Vitamin K, bilirubin, lytes, CBC with morning labs* | | | | |
| | | *PICU house officer to evaluate central line placement ASAP* | | | | |
| | | *Change gentamicin dose to 7.5 mg IV q 24 hours* | | | | |
| | | *(note to pharmacy and nursing staff – okay to use standard gent. SD concentration of 5mg/mL)* | | | | |
| | | *Pharmacy to monitor pharmacokinetics per routine* | | | | |
| | | | *Marc Darrow, M.D.* | | | |
| | | | *9/30/14* | | | |

PHARMACY COPY

5. Assuming that the medication label indicates the concentration of the PF gentamicin is 10 mg/mL, perform a calculation to determine the amount in milliliters of PF gentamicin needed to prepare the CSP. (Use the answer from step 3 in your calculation here.)

$$\frac{10\text{ mg}}{1\text{ mL}} = \frac{20\text{ mg}}{x\text{ mL}}$$

*Cross-multiply, then divide to solve for $x$ (the desired dosage volume) for the CSP. (For additional assistance, refer to Chapter 5 for step-by-step dosage calculation procedures.)

> **POINTER**
> It is considered best practice to perform all pediatric CSP calculations twice to double-check your accuracy.

### *Calculating the Desired PF NS Volume*

6. Read the diluent label to verify that the diluent is preservative-free (see Figure 12.6). Then read the information on the CSP label to determine the total volume of the CSP. Perform a calculation to determine the volume of PF NS that you must draw up to make the CSP. Subtract the volume that you determined in step 5 (above) from the desired total volume of the pediatric special dilution—in this case, 4 mL. Given that you determined the CSP requires 2 mL of PF gentamicin, determine the desired volume of PF NS with this simple calculation:

4 mL – 2 mL = 2 mL (amount of PF NS necessary to make the CSP)

> **POINTER**
> When determining the necessary volume of a *diluent* (such as normal saline) for a pediatric stock solution, you will not consider the percent strength or concentration of the diluent. In this situation, you only need to determine the diluent volume; therefore, label information such as the *0.9% sodium chloride* is extraneous and not to be included in your calculation.

FIGURE 12.6

**Medication Label for PF NS**

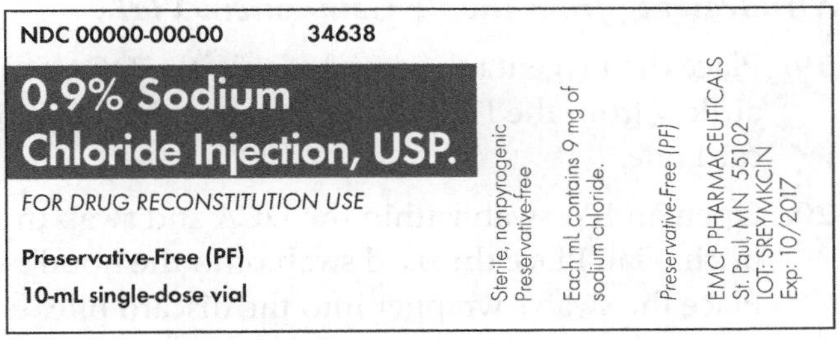

NDC 00000-000-00
34638
0.9% Sodium Chloride Injection, USP.
FOR DRUG RECONSTITUTION USE
Preservative-Free (PF)
10-mL single-dose vial
Sterile, nonpyrogenic
Preservative-free
Each mL contains 9 mg of sodium chloride.
Preservative-Free (PF)
EMCP PHARMACEUTICALS
St. Paul, MN 55102
LOT: SREYMKCIN
Exp: 10/2017


### *Gathering and Cleaning Supplies*

7. Place the medication order into the large plastic bag and the CSP label into the small plastic bag. Gather all supply items listed in the supply section of the procedural lab.
8. Open the package of aseptic cleaning wipes. Remove one or, if necessary, more wipes, and thoroughly wipe down the entire transport vehicle.
9. Place the used wipes in the waste receptacle.
10. Remove a new aseptic cleaning wipe and wipe down the exterior surface of each supply item. Place the cleaned supply items into the transport vehicle. Place the used wipes in the waste receptacle.

> **POINTER**
> During aseptic garbing, best practice is to reapply sterile, foamed 70% IPA to your hands after donning shoe covers and again after donning a hair cover.

### *Garbing*

11. Don shoe covers.
12. Put on a hair cover.

13. Don a face mask and beard cover (if appropriate).

    *Note:* For the purposes of this training lab, you will skip the mandatory aseptic hand-washing procedure.

14. Don a sterile gown.
15. Use a transport vehicle to bring all supply items, including an unopened package of sterile, powder-free gloves, into the clean room.
16. Place the transport vehicle onto a clean surface or countertop within the clean room. If you are using a cart, position it so that it does not interrupt airflow into the hood prefilter.

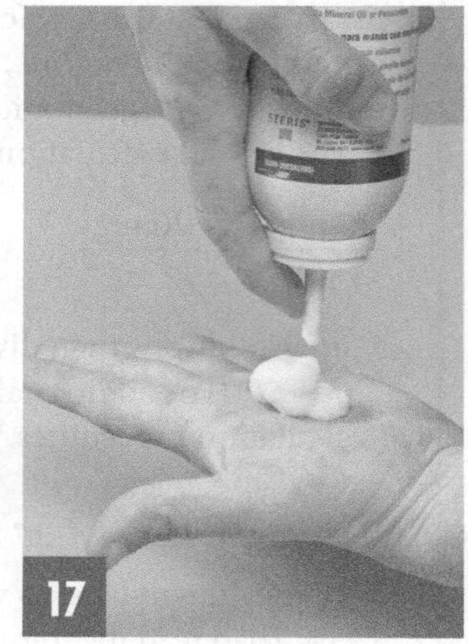

17

17. Apply sterile, foamed 70% IPA to your hands. Allow them to air-dry and then don sterile gloves.

    *Note:* For the purposes of this training lab, you will skip the mandatory hood-cleaning procedure.

18. Place all of the supply items needed for the procedure into the outer six-inch staging area of the hood.

***Withdrawing from the PF Gentamicin Vial***

19. Place the PF gentamicin vial within the DCA so that it receives uninterrupted airflow from the HEPA filter. Remove the flip-top cap and place it into the discard pile.
20. Open an IPA swab within the DCA and swab the rubber top of the PF gentamicin vial. Place the used swab onto the hood's work surface within the DCA. Place the swab's wrapper into the discard pile.
21. Prepare the first syringe by aseptically attaching a regular needle. Pull down on the flat knob to draw a volume of air into the syringe equal to or slightly less than the volume you wish to withdraw from the vial—in this case, 2 mL. Grasp the barrel of the syringe with your dominant hand, as you would a dart. Remove the needle cap and place it onto the sterile 70% IPA swab.
22. Using the thumb and forefinger of your nondominant hand, stabilize the PF gentamicin vial against the hood's work surface. Place the needle tip, bevel up, onto the PF gentamicin vial top. Use proper needle insertion technique to insert the needle into the PF gentamicin vial.

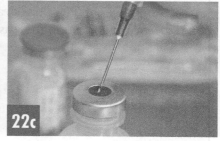

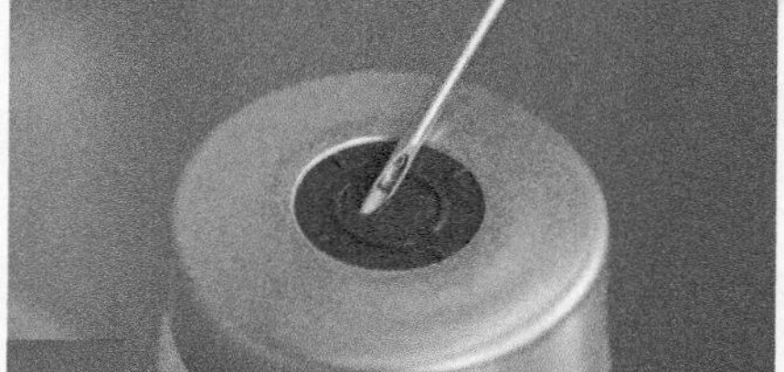

22a

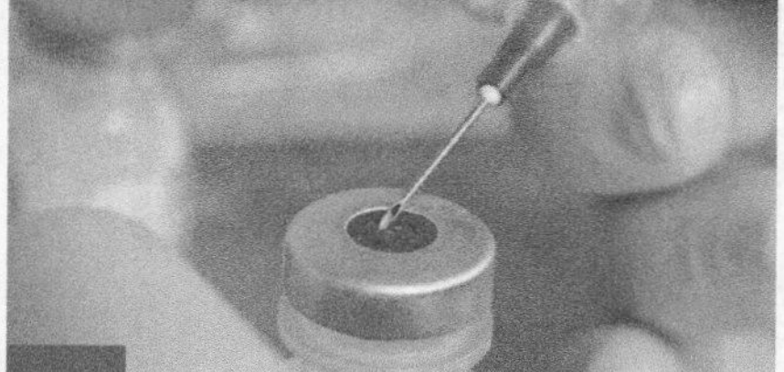

22b

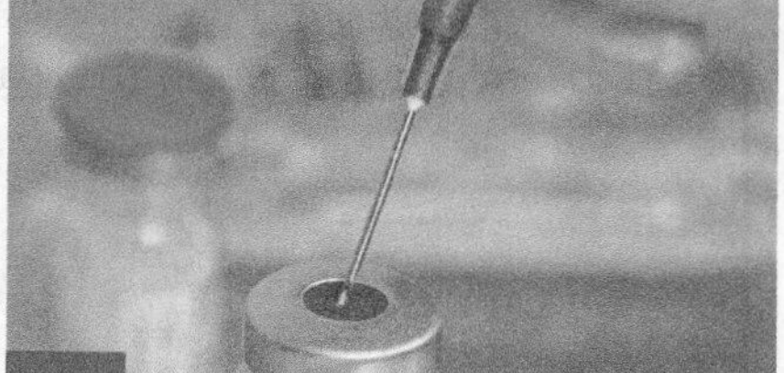

22c

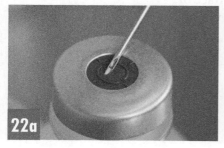

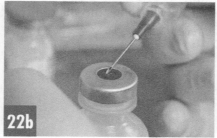

23. With your nondominant hand holding the vial and your dominant hand maintaining the needle in the vial, invert the vial using a clockwise motion (a counterclockwise motion if you are left-handed), so that the needle-and-syringe unit is now below the vial.

24. Use the thumb of your dominant hand to gradually push up on the flat knob of the plunger to inject a small amount of air (approximately 1 mL) into the PF gentamicin vial, creating a slight positive pressure within the vial. Release your thumb from the plunger and allow fluid to flow into the syringe. Repeat this milking process until you have withdrawn the desired volume of PF gentamicin into the syringe (in this case, 2 mL).

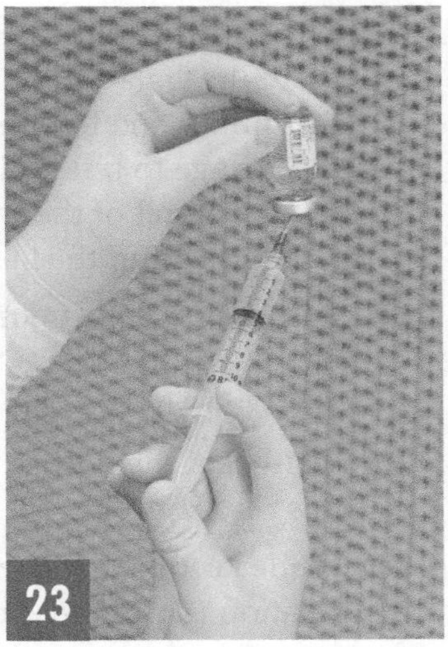
23

**POINTER**

Take care to hold the vial and syringe so that the airflow from the HEPA filter to the critical site—the area from the tip of the syringe to the neck of the vial, including the entire needle and the vial's rubber top—remains unobstructed at all times.

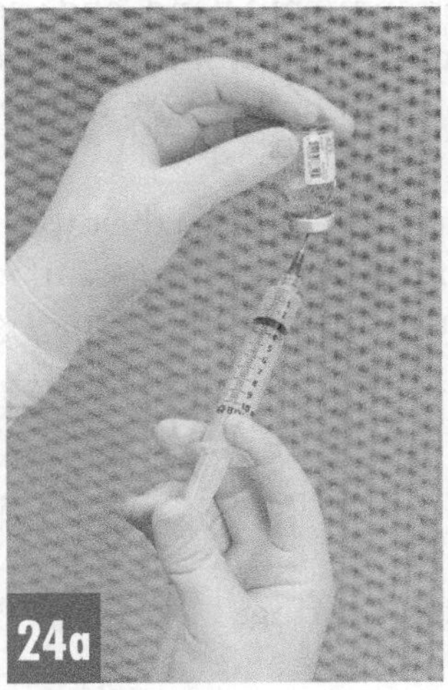
24a

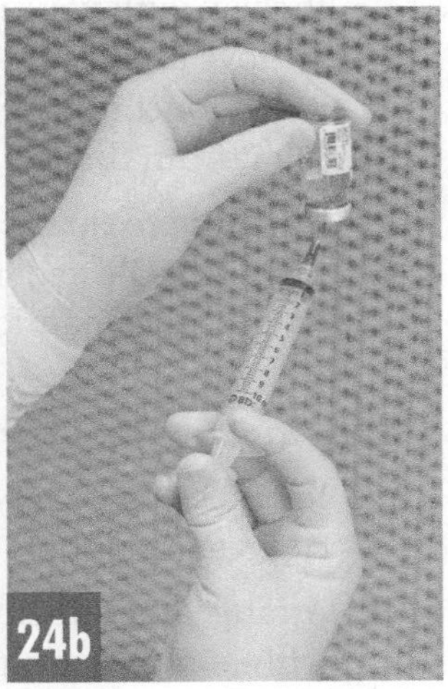
24b

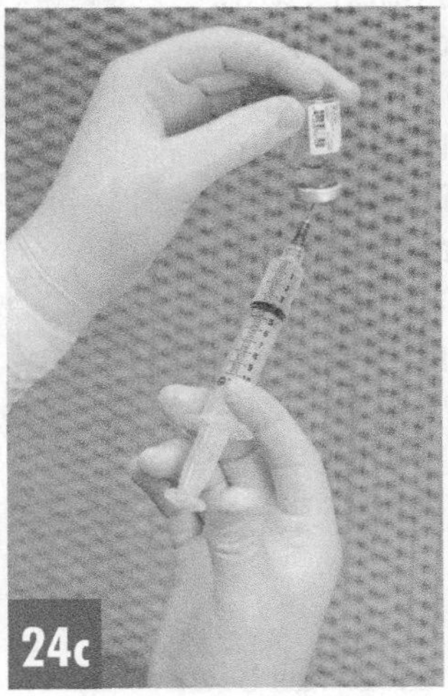
24c

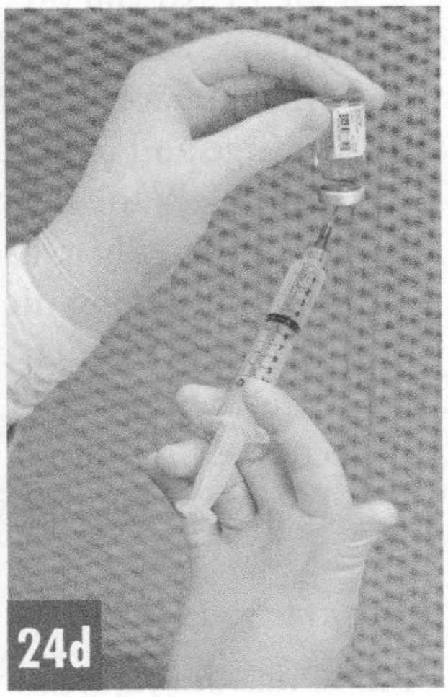
24d

> **POINTER**
> To properly perform the bubble-removal procedure, rotate your nondominant hand so that your palm faces the HEPA filter. As you hold the vial or brace the syringe against your palm, your hand should not block airflow to the critical site. You must take care to do this in such a way that your dominant hand does not come in between the critical site and the HEPA filter at any time.

**25.** While ensuring the needle remains entirely within the PF gentamicin vial, brace the vial—with needle and attached syringe inserted completely—between the thumb and forefinger of your nondominant hand, allowing the barrel of the syringe to rest against the palm of that hand. Using your dominant hand, tap the barrel of the syringe with the fingers of your dominant hand to force air bubbles within the fluid up toward the tip of the syringe.

**26.** Push up on the flat knob of the plunger with the thumb of your dominant hand to expel the air bubbles gathered near the tip of the syringe, along with any extra fluid.

**27.** Verify that the syringe now contains the desired amount of PF gentamicin (in this case, 2 mL).

**28.** While keeping the needle firmly inserted in the vial, use a counterclockwise rotation (a clockwise rotation if you are left-handed) to return the vial and syringe to the starting position, with the upright vial braced against the work surface and the dominant hand holding the syringe barrel. Continue to brace the vial with your nondominant hand, and use your dominant hand to slowly remove the needle-and-syringe unit from the medication vial. Remember to avoid touching the plunger or flat knob of the syringe at any time while removing it from the vial.

**29.** Carefully recap the needle and place the capped needle-and-syringe unit, now filled with PF gentamicin, onto the work surface within the DCA. Place the empty PF gentamicin vial next to the filled PF gentamicin syringe.

### *Withdrawing from the PF Diluent Vial*

**30.** Repeat steps 19–29 to draw up the correct amount of PF NS.

**31.** Arrange the diluent-filled syringe with attached, capped needle and the PF NS vial on the hood's work surface within the DCA. Position them adjacent to the PF gentamicin syringe and empty PF gentamicin vial. Place the EEC vial next to these items. Finally, place the small plastic bag containing the CSP label within the outer six-inch edge of the hood, directly in front of the items to be checked. Ask for a verification check by your instructor or a pharmacist.

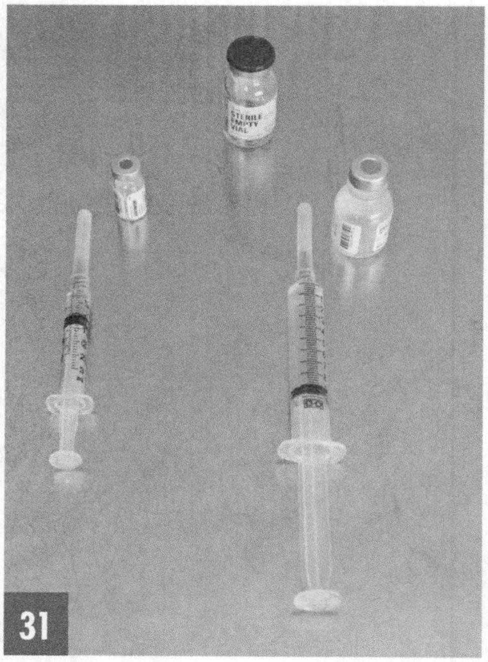

31

### *Preparing the CSP*

**32.** Once the verification check has been completed, arrange the filled syringe-and-needle units within the DCA so that they receive uninterrupted airflow from the HEPA filter.

33. Remove the flip-top cap from the EEC vial and set the vial into the DCA of the hood so that it receives uninterrupted airflow from the HEPA filter. Place the cap into the discard pile.

34. Open an IPA swab and use it to swab the rubber top of the EEC vial. Place the used swab onto the hood's work surface within the DCA.

35. Grasp the barrel of the PF gentamicin syringe with your dominant hand, as you would a dart. Remove the needle cap, and then place it onto the sterile 70% IPA swab.

36. Stabilize the EEC vial against the hood's work surface with your nondominant hand. Use proper needle insertion technique to insert the needle into the EEC vial.

37. Gently push down on the flat knob of the plunger with the thumb of your dominant hand until you have injected approximately 1 mL of PF gentamicin into the EEC vial. Release your thumb from the flat knob and allow built-up air pressure to transfer from the EEC vial into the syringe. Repeat this milking technique until all of the PF gentamicin has been injected into the EEC vial and an equivalent amount of positive air pressure has transferred into the syringe.

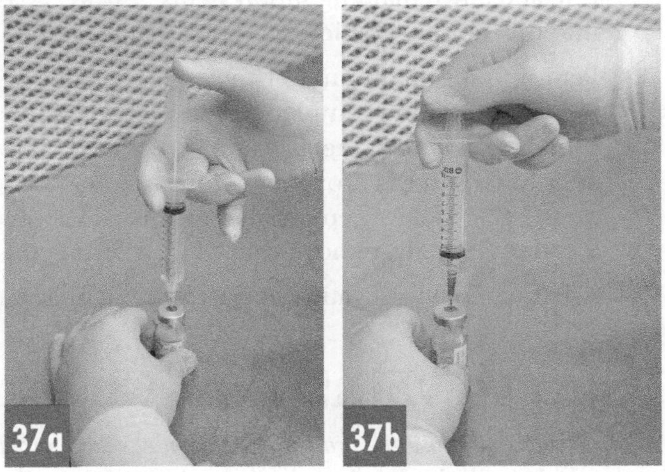
37a 37b

38. Grasping only the barrel of the syringe, use proper technique to remove the needle-and-syringe unit from the EEC vial. Place the needle-and-syringe unit into the sharps container.

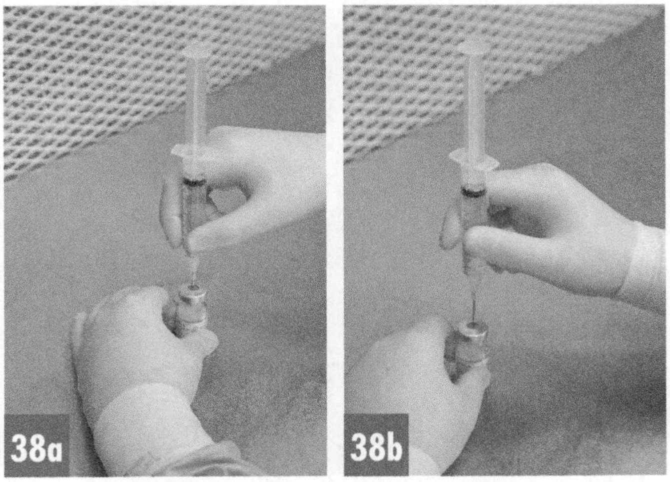
38a 38b

**POINTER**

When using the milking technique to inject a fluid into an EEC vial, the vial should remain upright on the hood's work surface with the needle-and-syringe unit positioned above the vial. Additionally, it is important to keep the tip of the needle near the interior neck of the vial to avoid drawing fluid back into the syringe, which may happen if the needle is situated near the bottom interior of the vial.

**POINTER**

Often the CSP label is too large to easily fit on the side of the EEC vial without obscuring or covering some of the information on the label. If this is the case, the label should be folded in half so that only the two ends of the CSP label are adhered to the vial. This is called "flagging" the label. Labeling the EEC vial in this manner allows the label to be affixed to the vial without obscuring any portion of the CSP label.

**39.** Repeat steps 34–38 using the diluent syringe.

**40.** Place an IVA seal over the filled EEC vial's rubber top.

**41.** Remove the CSP label from the plastic bag. Then affix the label to the EEC vial so that it does not come in contact with the EEC vial's rubber top or obscure any portion of the label.

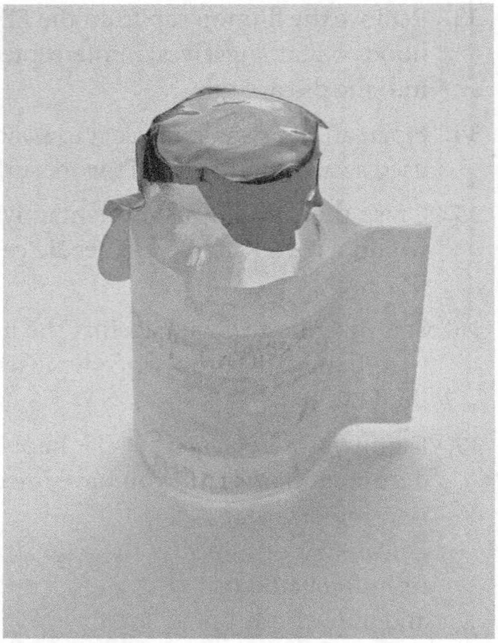

Filled and labeled EEC vial with an IVA seal over the vial top.

### *Cleaning Up After the Procedure*

**42.** Place the waste items into the proper waste container. Place the labeled CSP and any remaining supply items into the transport vehicle.

**43.** Return to the anteroom to begin the compounding completion procedures. Record the date and your initials in the proper location on the CSP label. Then return any unused supply items to their proper storage locations. Finally, remove your PPE according to standard procedures.

**44.** Ask for a final verification check from the pharmacist or your instructor.

# Process Validation Checklist

*Your instructor will use the process validation checklist provided in Appendix D to evaluate your technique for this lab. In order to receive ACPE certification, and prior to making CSPs for patient use, you must correctly perform each component of the lab procedure. Review the Chapter 12 lab and thoroughly practice each of the steps prior to your evaluation.*

# Part 3: Assessment

## Chapter Summary

- Pediatrics is a medical specialty focusing on the care and treatment of children.
- Pediatric medicine is different from adult medicine in several important ways, taking in to account the patient's physiology, body size, and weight, as well as kidney, liver, cardiovascular, and respiratory functions.
- Abu Bakr Muhammad ibn Zakariya al-Razi is called the "Father of Pediatrics" for treating childhood diseases such as smallpox and measles, and for having written the book *The Diseases of Children*.
- Dr. Thomas Sydenham wrote about treatments for children who were afflicted with scarlet fever, measles, epilepsy, and scurvy. Sydenham's work dramatically improved medical understanding of these diseases.
- In 1798, Dr. Edward Jenner's published pediatric research led to further experiments that eventually led to a smallpox vaccine, which was heralded as one of the wonder drugs of the nineteenth century.
- Nineteenth-century physicians who made notable contributions to the advancement of pediatric medicine include Dr. John Forsyth Meigs, Dr. Luther Holt, and Dr. William M. Marriott. New York physician Dr. Abraham Jacobi is considered the "Father of American Pediatric Medicine."
- The Pediatric Pharmacy Administrative Group (PPAG) promotes pediatric pharmacy research, advocacy, and medication-error reduction.
- Neonatology is a subspecialty of pediatrics dealing with premature babies and seriously ill infants younger than one month of age. Neonatologists specialize in the treatment of infants who need critical care due to premature birth, congenital defects, infections, or birth trauma. Most patients are hospitalized in the NICU.
- Specially trained clinical pharmacists work closely with prescribers to recommend appropriate drug therapy, monitor clinical outcomes, and perform drug utilization review. Pharmacists must be familiar with pediatric physiology, as well as drug disposition, dosage modification procedures, and pharmacotherapeutic treatment of neonatal and pediatric patients.
- Pediatric special dilutions are custom-made CSPs designed to provide accurate parenteral medication dosing for neonates and particularly small or young pediatric patients.
- Pharmacy personnel must ensure that parenteral medications are of an appropriate volume and strength for a pediatric patient. Medications with preservatives should not be used for neonatal or pediatric patients.
- Additional safeguards should be implemented for pediatric and neonatal CSPs to ensure that pharmacy calculations and all aspects of sterile compounding receive additional verification checks, as even minor errors may lead to harmful results for neonatal and pediatric patients.
- In addition to essential supplies, pediatric CSPs often require the use of EECs. Only PF ingredients should be used for these CSPs.
- Anteroom preparatory procedures include verifying the CSP label against the medication order, performing calculations, gathering and cleaning supplies, donning aseptic garb, performing aseptic hand washing, and donning a sterile gown.
- Clean room preparatory procedures include donning sterile gloves, cleaning the hood, and using aseptic technique to prepare the pediatric CSP within the DCA of the hood.

# Key Terms

**access point** the area of the body through which the vein is accessed by insertion of a needle or catheter

**accidental fluid overload** unintentional administration of excess IV fluid, which may result in electrolyte imbalance or hypervolemia

**accidental rapid administration** the administration of a drug too quickly, which could possibly result in patient death

**Accreditation Council for Pharmacy Education (ACPE)** a national agency for the accreditation of professional degree programs in pharmacy and providers of continuing pharmacy education

**adult-strength formulation** the most common strength of a drug as supplied by the drug's manufacturer; the strength of a drug that must be diluted (i.e., reduced in concentration or strength) prior to pediatric use

**American Society of Health-System Pharmacists (ASHP)** a pharmacy professional organization that provides advocacy, continuing education, and drug information for pharmacy professionals and that accredits pharmacy residency and pharmacy technician programs

**attenuated virus** a virus that is scientifically manipulated to reduce its pathogenic nature so it may be used to vaccinate against a disease without causing the disease; a "live" virus

**benzyl alcohol gasping syndrome** a condition caused by the injection of a preparation containing benzyl alcohol into neonatal patients; may result in severe respiratory distress or death

**buretrol** a type of tubing with a large chamber used to dilute and administer parenteral medications for pediatric IV therapy; also known as a *chamber device*

**clinical outcomes** the clinical monitoring of patient response to drug therapy (e.g., drug levels within the blood)

**clinical pharmacist** a pharmacist with specialized training in drug dosing, therapy, and pharmacokinetics

**compound syringe** a CSP that is prepared in a syringe final container so that it can be administered via a syringe pump or IV push route of administration

**congenital defect** a physical abnormality that is present at birth; birth defect

**custom-made CSP** a type of CSP in which all of the components are prepared from scratch; also called a *pediatric special dilution*

**Doctor of Pharmacy Degree (PharmD)** the level of education required to practice as a clinical pharmacist in the United States; the level of education required for all new pharmacy school graduates

**drug disposition** the body's process of absorbing, distributing, metabolizing, and excreting a drug

**drug utilization review** the pharmacist's monitoring of drug dosage and treatment to provide the most effective drug therapy and avoid medication errors, duplicate therapy, and side effects

**empty evacuated container (EEC)** a vacuum-sealed, sterile glass container or empty plastic bag used to prepare a custom-made CSP such as a pediatric special dilution

**femoral line** a large vein in the groin and leg that is sometimes used as an IV access point

**gestation** the length of time within the mother's womb, from conception to birth

**hypervolemia** a potentially fatal condition resulting from fluid overload

**IVA syringe seal** a tamper-evident foil seal affixed over a syringe cap

**IV push route of administration** intermittent parenteral medication injection from a syringe into an IV line or chamber

**mechanical ventilator** a machine that provides ventilation of the lungs for patients who are unable to breathe effectively on their own; greatly improves the survival chances of premature infants

**neonatal intensive care unit (NICU)** an intensive care unit that treats critically ill neonatal patients

**neonate** an infant under one month of age

**neonatologist** a specially trained physician who treats critically ill infants who need care due to premature birth, congenital defects, infections, or birth trauma

**neonatology** a subspecialty of pediatrics involving the medical treatment of premature babies, as well as seriously ill infants under one month of age

**pediatric anatomy and physiology** the structure and function of the various organs and organ systems of a pediatric patient

**pediatric CSP** a compounded sterile preparation formulated specifically for pediatric administration; a CSP comprised of medications or ingredients possessing a strength or formulation designed for use in neonates or children

**pediatric CSP ingredient** a sterile, preservative-free, pediatric-strength parenteral medication, additive, or solution component

**pediatric dosing** medication dosing specific to pediatric patients; medication dosing based on a child's size and physiology

**pediatrician** a physician who specializes in the treatment of children

**pediatric intensive care unit (PICU)** an intensive care unit specializing in the treatment of pediatric patients

**pediatric pharmacy** a pharmacy specialty related to the clinical drug therapy and treatment of neonatal and pediatric patients

**Pediatric Pharmacy Administrative Group (PPAG)** a pharmacy professional organization that promotes pediatric pharmacy research, advocacy, and research as well as standards for the reduction of pediatric medication errors

**pediatric physiology** the study and treatment of the unique bodily functions and responses of pediatric patients

**pediatrics** a branch of medicine concerned with the treatment of infants and children up to approximately age 18

**pediatric special dilution** a custom-made, preservative-free CSP that provides accurate medication dosage for neonatal or pediatric patients needing medication volume, strength, or concentrations not commercially available

**pediatric-strength formulation** medication supplied from the manufacturer in a strength or concentration designed for the treatment of children

**pharmacotherapeutic treatment** administration of medication that targets specific organisms or organ systems and that is tailored to the patient's physiology and disease state

**physiology** the study of the biological functions of the body and organ systems

**premature** human birth prior to 37 weeks of gestation in the mother's womb

**preservative-free (PF) ingredient** a CSP ingredient free of preservatives such as benzyl alcohol, an organic compound that can damage the still-developing organs of neonates and children

**pulmonary surfactants** a class of drugs that assists with the lung functions of premature infants, greatly improving their chances of survival

**smallpox** an infectious disease caused by a poxvirus and characterized by the formation of skin lesions that leave permanent pockmarks on the skin of its victims

**smallpox vaccine** a live virus vaccine used to prevent infection with the smallpox virus

**umbilical line** a catheter or IV line inserted into the umbilical artery of a neonate

## Check the Basics

*On a separate sheet of paper, write your answers as modeled in these examples: 1d; 2c; 3b; etc.*

**1.** What types of sterile compounding procedures may necessitate the use of an EEC?
a. transferring a specific amount of fluid from an LVP into a smaller container
b. preparation of custom-made IV or IVPB base solutions
c. pediatric special dilutions
d. both *a* and *c*
e. all of the above

**2.** When preparing a pediatric special dilution, where must you look to determine the desired concentration of the CSP?
a. the drug vial label
b. the CSP label
c. the PF NS label
d. all of the above

**3.** When preparing a pediatric special dilution, where must you look to determine the desired total volume of the CSP?
a. the drug vial label
b. the CSP label
c. the PF NS label
d. all of the above

**4.** When preparing a pediatric special dilution, where must you look to determine the concentration of the stock drug PF gentamicin?
a. the drug vial label
b. the CSP label
c. the PF NS label
d. all of the above

**5.** When preparing a pediatric special dilution, how should you determine the volume of diluent needed to prepare the CSP?
a. by subtracting the concentration of the stock drug from the desired concentration
b. by subtracting the volume of the stock drug from the desired total volume
c. by subtracting the volume of the stock drug from the desired concentration
d. none of the above

**6.** What does the abbreviation PF mean?
a. precipitate-free
b. pyrogen-free
c. preservative-free
d. parenteral fluid

**7.** In the procedural lab, what diluent is used in compounding the pediatric special dilution?
a. sterile water
b. PF sterile water
c. NS
d. PF NS

**8.** With regard to injecting fluid into an EEC, which of the following statements is true?
a. The vial should remain upright on the hood surface, and air should be vented from the vial into the empty syringe.
b. The vial should be inverted above the needle-and-syringe unit, and air should be vented from the vial into the empty syringe.
c. The vial should be shaken before the syringe is inserted.
d. The vial should be inverted above the needle-and-syringe unit, and air should be vented using a vented needle.

**9.** According to best practice principles, how many pharmacy personnel should verify the CSP label and medication order for pediatric CSPs?
a. 1
b. 2
c. 3
d. none of the above

**10.** What is the appropriate order of cleanup and completion procedures?
a. dispose of waste, remove gloves, return to the anteroom, record initials on label
b. dispose of waste, return to the anteroom, record initials on label, remove PPE
c. return to the anteroom, record initials on label, remove PPE, dispose of waste
d. record initials on label, remove gloves, dispose of waste, return to the anteroom

# Make Connections

*On a separate sheet of paper, write your answers to the following three questions, using complete sentences and making sure your answers are thorough and thoughtful. Note that the third question requires Internet access.*

1. Upon receiving a medication order and a corresponding CSP label, you notice that the pharmacist has written her dosage calculations on the medication order. Since the calculations are already written out and have been confirmed by a pharmacist, is it necessary for you to perform the calculations again? Why or why not?

2. When verifying the pharmacist's dosage calculations, you come up with a different answer than that which the pharmacist wrote on the medication order. What is the best course of action? Would you follow a different course of action if you knew that a second pharmacist had already verified the first pharmacist's calculations? Why or why not?

3. Go to the website of the Pediatric Pharmacist Administrative Group at www.ppag.org and then hover over the *Education & Programs* tab; from there, scroll down to the *Artemis Safety Initiative* tab and click on the tab. Read about the Artemis Safety Initiative. What is the Artemis Safety Initiative? Do you believe that this type of innovation significantly improves patient safety? Why or why not?

# Meet the Challenge

***Scenario*** This "diluting" activity will give you the opportunity to discover more information about pediatric special dilutions.

***Challenge*** Your instructor has a handout outlining a series of calculations, the type of which may be required to prepare a CSP for the smallest neonates (some of whom weigh less than 500 grams). Babies this size may require a special CSP known as a *micro-dilution*. This procedure takes your understanding of how to perform necessary calculations to prepare a CSP for the smallest neonates to the next level of comprehension. To meet this challenge, ask your instructor for the handout and give it a try, either individually, in small groups, or as a class. *Note:* This activity is most effective when performed in the classroom environment.

## ADDITIONAL RESOURCES

*Go to the Paradigm Internet Resources Center at* www.paradigmcollege.net/sterilecomp *to access live links related to these Chapter 12 topics:*

- Pediatric pharmacy research, advocacy, and medication error reduction
- Pediatric dosing and medical treatment

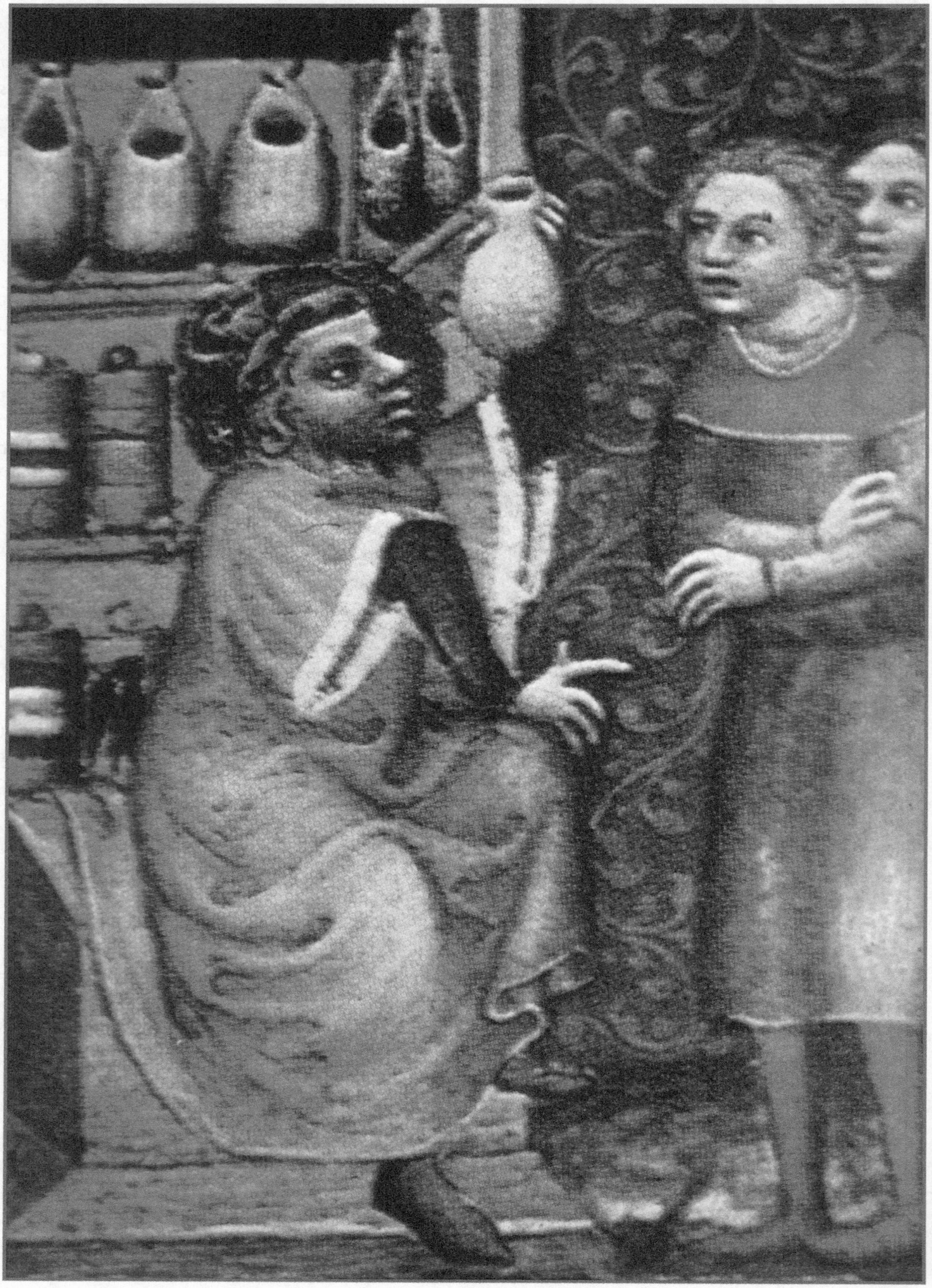

# Chapter 13

# Total Parenteral Nutrition

## Learning Objectives

- Recognize the origins of total parenteral nutrition.
- Identify the special situations and actions that must be considered when preparing total parenteral nutrition.
- Identify the risks associated with parenteral preparations.
- Identify the USP Chapter <797> procedures that must be performed when compounding total parenteral nutrition.
- Demonstrate correct technique in the preparation of a total parenteral nutrition solution.

Although enteral nutrition therapy is commonly used to treat seriously ill patients today, this practice is not a recent development. In fact, the beginnings of enteral nutrition can be traced back to ancient Egypt and the priest-physicians who practiced a combination of spiritual healing and herbal medicine to cure the illnesses of their fellow citizens.

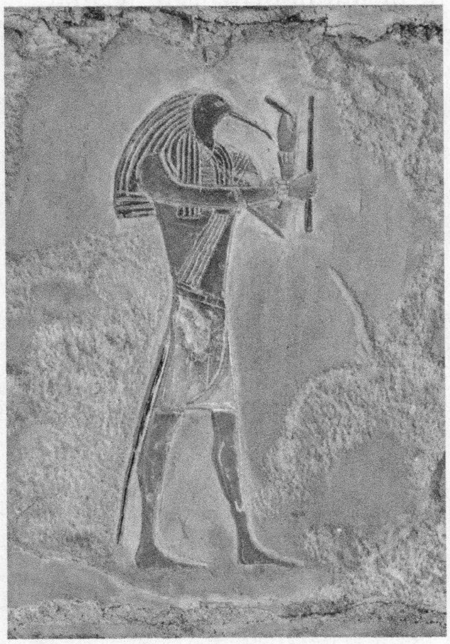

### Ancient Egyptian Medicine

As part of their therapeutic practice, early Egyptian physicians prayed to Thoth to provide healing powers for those who were ill. Thoth, the god of wisdom and inventor of medicine, was often depicted on ancient papyruses, hieroglyphics, and other excavated artifacts as having the head of an ibis, a sacred bird in Egypt. According to Egyptian legend, the ibis was the guardian of the country, protecting its people from evil forces such as plagues and serpents. In fact, thousands of mummified ibises have been discovered in the tombs of pharaohs.

Another legend of this primordial culture tells the story of ancient observers who witnessed an ibis taking up water in its curved beak and then inserting its beak into its rectum to cleanse it. This folklore reflected the cultures' rudimentary knowledge of human anatomy and physiology. Early Egyptians believed that a network of channels existed in the human body and converged into a

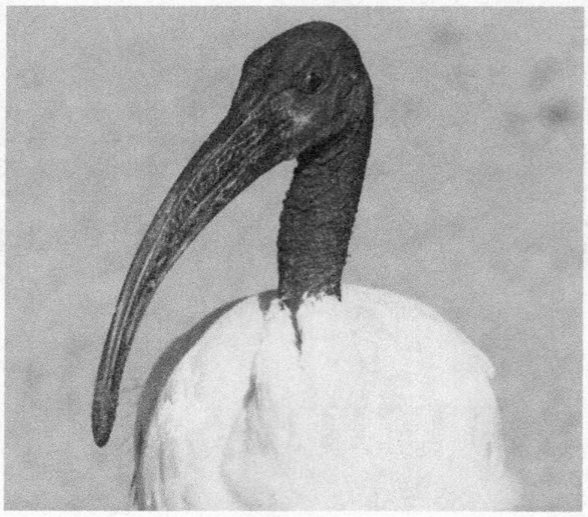

central location: the rectum. Consequently, these practitioners introduced their herbal remedies into the rectum, which—according to their theories—would then channel the fluids to different parts of the body. By feeding nutrient-rich solutions into the rectum, physicians thought that fluid balance within the body could be restored, thus promoting good health. So, like the sacred ibis, the cleansing of the bowel could cleanse the body of toxins that brought about disease.

The solutions that were injected into ill patients were typically a mixture of milk, broth, whey, and wine and were commonly prescribed to treat gastrointestinal disorders such as dysentery. Administered by practitioners through a hollow reed, animal bone, or horn, these solutions were introduced into the rectum via gravity or by the use of a primitive bulb syringe made from an animal bladder. More than 700 recipes for **rectal feedings**, or nutrient enemas, were documented in the Ebers Papyrus (1550 BCE) in the "book of the stomach."

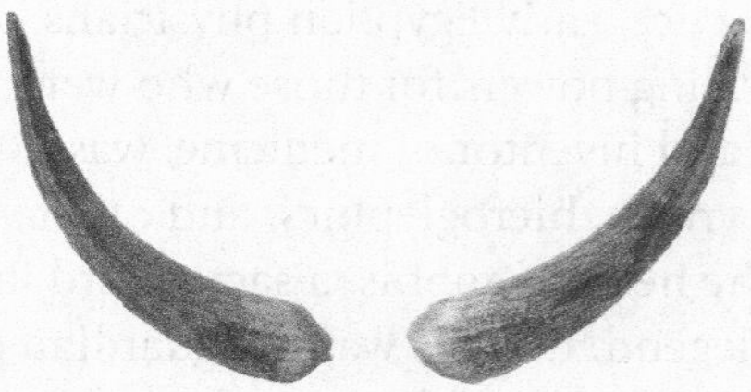

## Rectal Feedings and Wellness

Another proponent of the use of nutrient enemas was Greek physician Hippocrates. His collection of ancient medical texts, called the *Hippocratic Corpus*, details his theory that health could be restored or damaged by the consumption or lack of certain foods. Hippocrates understood the impact of nutrition on wellness, and he administered rectal feedings to his patients to treat their diseases, supplement their fluid losses, and improve their overall well-being. His rectal feeding tube consisted of a piece of pipe that was attached to an animal bladder.

Like Hippocrates, well-known second-century physician Galen also treated a number of disorders with rectal feedings consisting of water or a salt solution with, perhaps, honey or oil added. Galen would inject the solution into his patients using a crude syringe-like device called a **clyster**, similar to the ones shown below. The solution would then cleanse the bowel before nutrient-rich substances were instilled. Galen expanded upon the work of his predecessor, Hippocrates, by studying the body's response to various nutrients and, years later, wrote extensively about his theory that proper nutrition was necessary to maintain balance in the body.

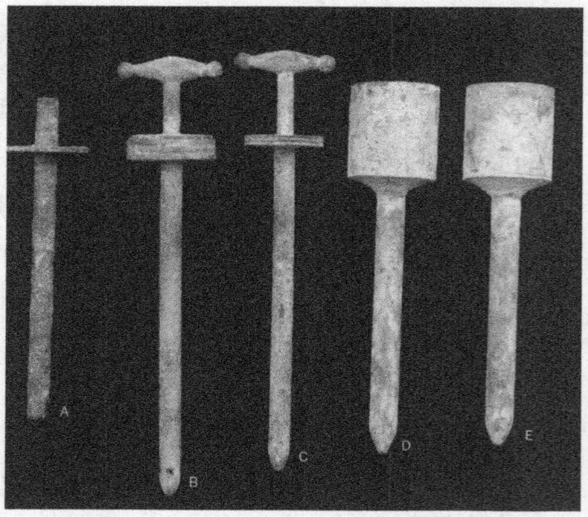


For many centuries after Galen's research, rectal enemas were used to restore health and meet the nutritional needs of ailing patients, with many physicians extolling the healthful benefits of regular rectal irrigation to remove the body's toxins. These enemas were administered through a clyster attached to a tube and some type of pump apparatus. Ironically, colon hydrotherapy became somewhat of a status symbol among the affluent during the seventeenth century.

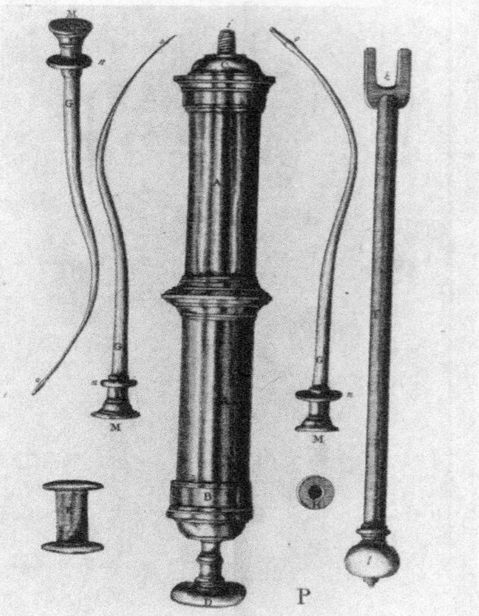

To maintain wellness and personal hygiene, socialites kept a collection of well-appointed clysters and hired a personal attendant to administer these rectal enemas—sometimes four or five times a day.

However, for those who were critically ill, administering nutrient-rich fluids through the rectum proved to be minimally effective. Although the lining of the colon is designed to absorb water during the digestive process, it is not meant to absorb nutrients, whose stores are severely depleted during illness, disease, surgery, or trauma. Researchers and physicians would spend the next several centuries exploring alternative methods of supplying nutrition to these patients.

## Beginnings of Parenteral Nutrition

Twelfth-century Muslim physician and surgeon Ibn Zuhr (commonly known as Avenzoar) was the first practitioner to attempt **parenteral nutrition**. To treat patients whose conditions precluded the ingestion of foods, Avenzoar recommended three methods of providing food: soaking the patient in a bath of tepid liquid (containing crushed herbs, grains, and flowers); administering liquid nutrients by way of an enema; or, on more desperate occasions, injecting liquid feedings directly into the stomach through a large needle. Although these first recorded efforts of parenteral nutrition were unsuccessful, Avenzoar's experiments, as well as those of other practitioners, paved the way for finding ways to feed malnourished patients who were too ill to eat.

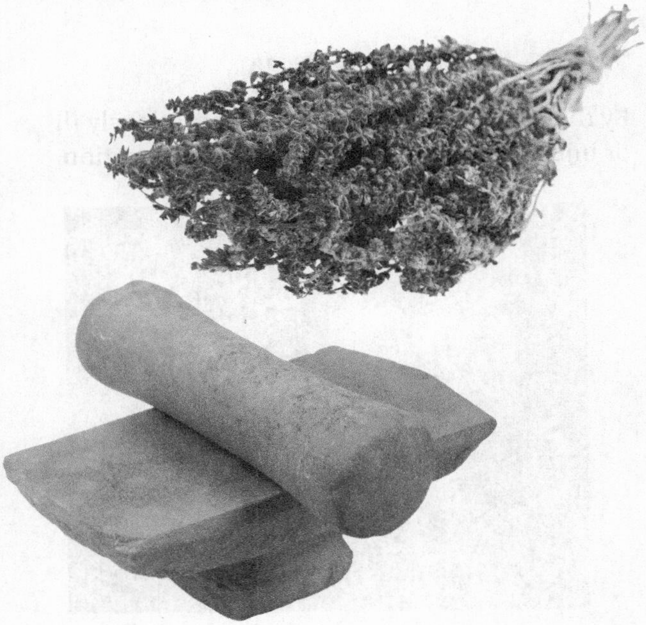

## Gastric Feeding Tubes

By the sixteenth and seventeenth centuries, **gastric feedings** became a common treatment modality for infirm patients unable to chew, swallow, or digest foods. Both orogastric and nasogastric tube apparatuses were constructed from animal bladders and animal bone covered with eel skin. The slippery, hollow bone was threaded either through the mouth or nose and down the esophagus. Then the fluid contained within the animal bladder would be pumped through the hollow bone and into the patient's stomach. Aside from animal bones, gastric tubes were also fashioned from flexible leather and malleable metals. The types of feeding solutions varied, but a typical solution might be comprised of jelly, milk, eggs, sugar, broths, and wine. Scottish surgeon and anatomist John Hunter is credited with successfully providing the first nasogastric feeding in 1790 to a stroke victim left paralyzed and unable to consume food.

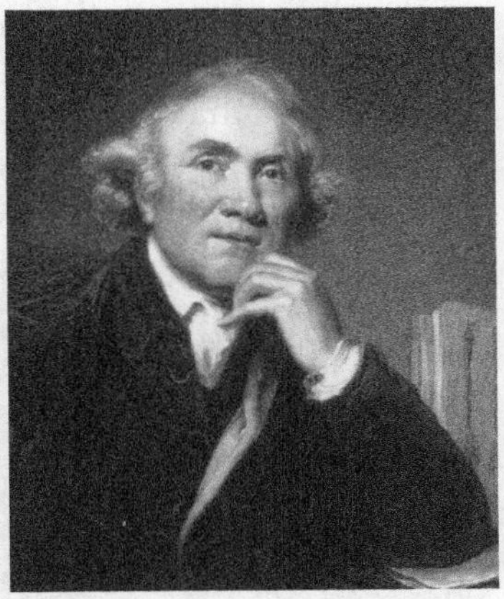

**Feeding funnels** were also employed in gastric feeding. These funnels were often used for patients after surgery or those who suffered a traumatic injury to the head or neck, impeding the intake of food. Other funnels, such as the one pictured here, were used to feed patients who were unable to chew or swallow due to cultural rituals, such as tattooing of the face. Regardless of the circumstances, the funnel was attached to a flexible tube that was inserted in the patient's mouth. The feeding solution was then poured into the funnel and through the tube into the patient's stomach.

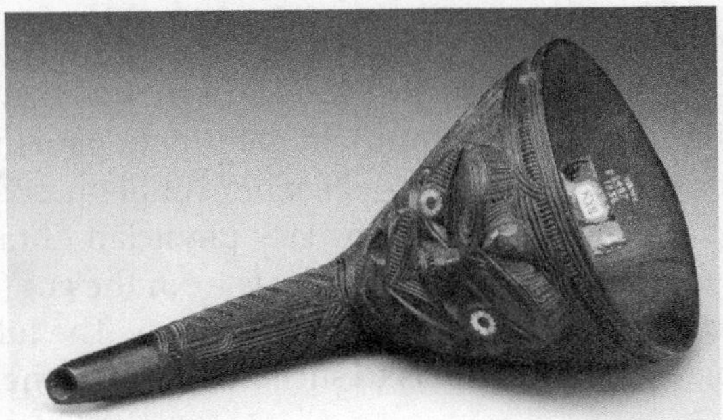

In the nineteenth century, nasogastric tubes—or tubes that were inserted in the nostril and down the esophagus—were used to administer gastric feedings. Several physicians prescribed gastric feedings for children who were diagnosed with diphtheria or croup. The feedings consisted of a variety of ingredients, including eggs, warm milk, beef-tea, even brandy and stimulants. Surprisingly, one physician suggested nasogastric feeding for "spoilt children, who, when ill, refuse food."

This concept of **force feeding** was also implemented in patients who suffered from mental disorders and, therefore, refused food, or those patients who had difficulty opening their mouths (due to tetanus) or swallowing (due to esophageal stricture). For these patients, an instrument, such as the feeding tube pictured below, was inserted into the mouth so that the crossbars held the mouth open. The feeding solution was then poured down the tube and into the stomach.

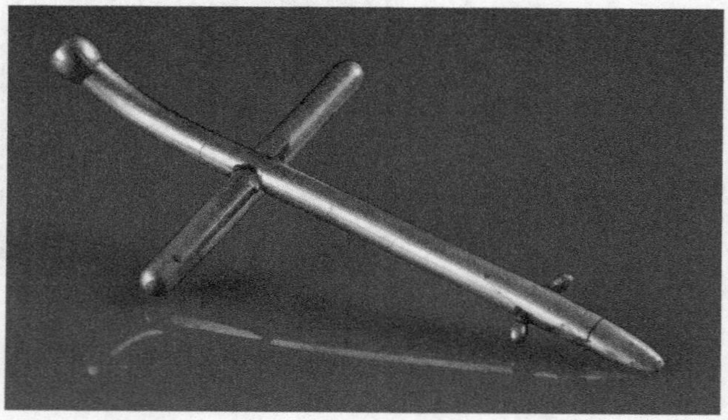

Rectal feeding solutions also continued to be popular in the nineteenth century. In fact, after his attempted assassination in 1881, U.S. president James Garfield was kept alive for 79 days on a rectal solution of beef broth, egg yolks, milk, whiskey, and opium. Unfortunately, rectal feedings cannot sustain life, and Garfield wasted away from his injury.

## Twentieth-Century Enteral Feedings

By the start of the twentieth century, innovations in supplies, such as the introduction of the **Levin tube** in 1921, made nutrient delivery to patients easier. The Levin tube—a flexible, rubber nasogastric tube—was invented by U.S. physician Abraham Levin to remove gastric contents from the gut (gastric decompression) after a laparotomy. The tube's single lumen connects to suction, allowing the drainage of gastric contents into a receptacle. The Levin tube continues to be used today for gastrointestinal feeding and aspiration, only now the tube is made from lightweight polyurethane material.

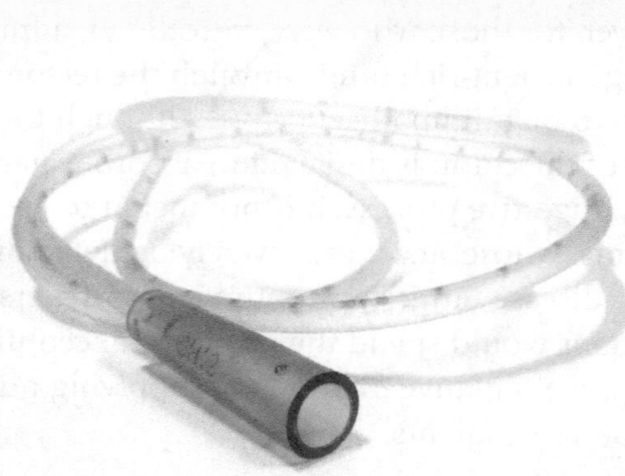

In 1937, Robert Elman and D. O. Weiner, two U.S. physicians, experimented with intravenous (IV) feeding of protein hydrolysates (an amino acid mixture) to five patients who could not digest protein, a substance responsible for the growth and repair of cells and tissues. Two of their patients had intestinal obstruction, and three patients had stomach cancer. Although the patient results were favorable, additional research was necessary for two reasons: The large volumes of solution needed to deliver the necessary caloric intake made the procedure difficult, and the use of a peripheral access site created local complications from the infusion. Still, their report in *The Journal of the American Medical Association* opened up the possibility of using an IV route to deliver nutritional therapy.

## The Emergence of TPN

By the 1940s, standard treatment of seriously ill or injured patients included the administration

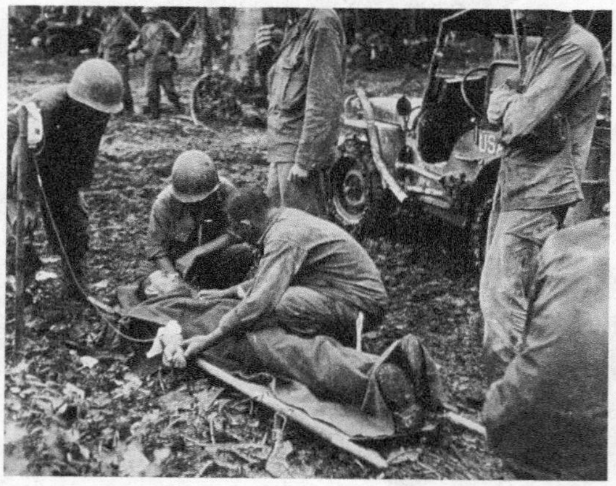

of IV medication. One of these medications was an amino acid mixture created by Merck and Co., Inc., a pharmaceutical company, to supplement the body's protein synthesis process. With the outbreak of World War II, this product was in high demand by physicians who sought ways to provide the rapid healing properties of protein to injured soldiers. The success of this amino acid supplement in maintaining the weight and nitrogen balance of these patients over an extended recovery period confirmed Elman's and Weiner's research that parenteral nutrition *could* sustain life.

During this same period, a breakthrough in the delivery of nutritional feedings occurred. Dr. Jonathan Rhoads, a prominent surgeon at the Hospital of the University of Pennsylvania, conducted studies to identify appropriate feeding solutions and delivery methods for malnourished patients after undergoing gastroenterostomies. After researching the positive effects of IV nutrient feedings on the development of puppies, Rhoads and his colleagues, Dr. Stanley Dudrick and Dr. Harry Vars, determined that five liters of dextrose 10% in water mixed with protein hydrolysates could deliver a sufficient number of calories to treat patients who were unable to eat. However, Rhoads was faced with two major complications: The infusion of a large volume of feeding solution resulted in fluid overload and pulmonary edema for the patient recipient, and the infusion of a smaller, more concentrated formula led to thrombosis of the patient's peripheral veins used in the fluid administration. Rhoads and his colleagues found that they could use a more concentrated formula if they delivered the IV feedings through a catheter placed in the **superior vena cava**.

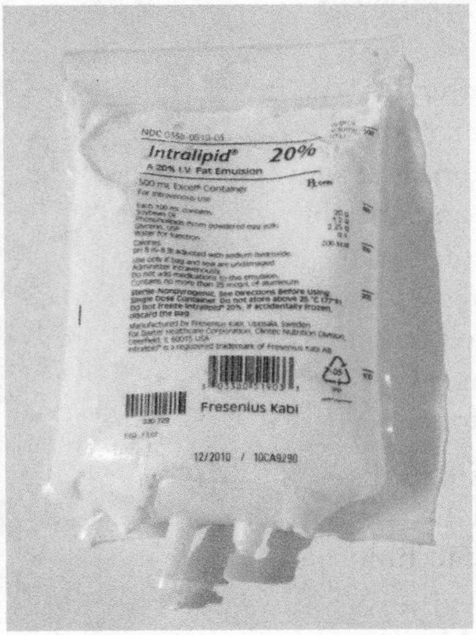


In 1966, Rhoads published his research on the subclavian administration of total parenteral nutrition, which he called **hyperalimentation** (or "hyperal"). In this method, a **central venous catheter (CVC)** is surgically inserted into the **subclavian vein**. The nutrient-rich solution is then safely administered through the CVC to the patient, virtually eliminating the problem of venous extravasation. Rhoads' discovery laid the foundation for **total parenteral nutrition (TPN)**, an IV therapy that provides nutritional support for patients who require a long-term alternative to enteral feeding.

## Innovative Formulas and Routes

By the 1960s, advances in nutritional formulas made IV feedings commonplace in the healthcare setting. In addition to replacing proteins and carbohydrates, lipids became part of the total parenteral nutrition formula in 1962 with the discovery of the first IV fat emulsion by Swedish professor Arvid Wretlind. Wretlind combined egg phospholipids, glycerin, and soybean oil, a mixture now marketed as Liposyn III or Intralipid. By the end of the decade, hospital pharmacies started to compound IV solutions of sterile water, dextrose, amino acids, and Liposyn, as well as an assortment of electrolytes, vitamins, and minerals, thus establishing modern-day TPN therapy.

Changes also occurred in the administration of tube feedings. Now, in addition to the use of a nasogastric tube and CVC catheter, a gastrostomy (G) tube and jejunum (J) tube allowed access to the stomach through a surgical

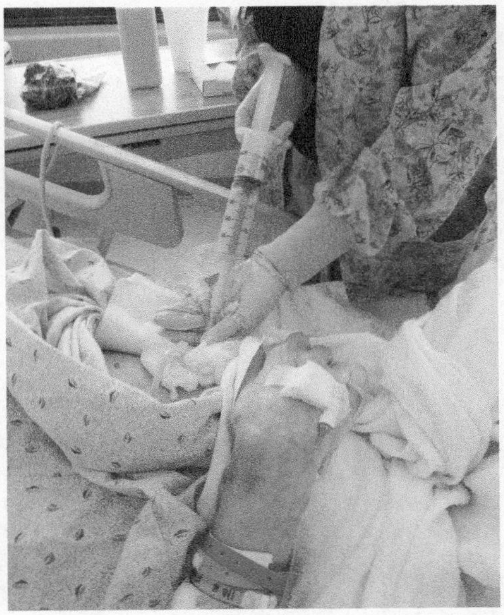

opening made in the skin of the abdomen. The liquid nutritional feedings could then be injected or infused into the tube and deposited into the stomach.

## Options for Delivery of Nutritional Solutions

In the late 1960s, home parenteral nutrition also became an option for patients who were discharged but in need of continued nutritional support. These patients took home the hospital supplies and powdered formulas that they needed to mix and subsequently administer their own enteral tube-feeding solutions—a lengthy procedure for these amateur "pharmacists."

Today, many patients self-administer enteral tube feedings but no longer need to mix the solutions themselves. Some manufacturers of IV nutrient solutions now provide premixed TPN bags and portable administration pumps that allow patients the freedom of mobility during the TPN feeding procedure. Patients and their caregivers are provided training in performing this procedure and are monitored closely by a team of healthcare professionals.

Still, many patients who receive TPN solutions—whether at home or in a healthcare facility—rely on sterile products compounded by IV technicians in pharmacy clean rooms.

## Responsibilities of IV Technicians in TPN Preparation

For sterile compounding personnel, proper procedures and strict aseptic technique must be followed when preparing TPN solutions. In addition to adhering to established protocols, TPN preparation requires sterile compounding personnel to have additional education and training in calculations, compounding procedures, and special equipment and ingredients. This chapter provides the background information, aseptic techniques, and specific sequence of sterile compounding procedures necessary for proper TPN preparation.

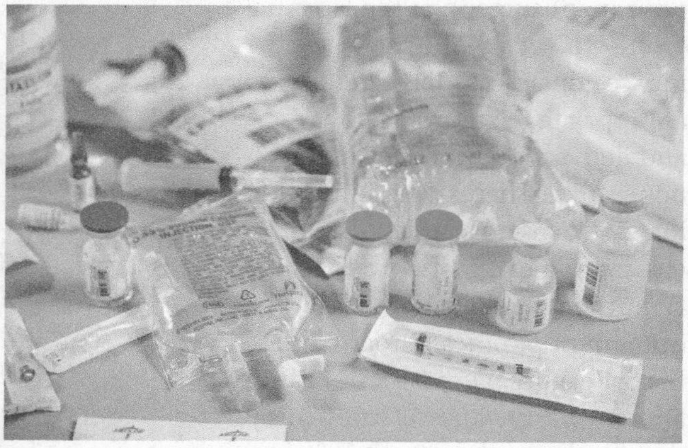

# Part 1: Concepts

Nutritional therapy is administered to patients who have a condition that prevents proper absorption of nutrients from food and/or medical conditions that render them unable to swallow or move food along the **gastrointestinal (GI) tract**. For patients unable to swallow (but who otherwise have healthy, working GI tracts), enteral nutrition may be administered via an artificial opening (see Figure 13.1). A liquid enteral product is poured into a feeding tube that, in turn, delivers nutrients directly into the GI tract. The feeding tube may be a **nasogastric (NG) tube**, a **gastric (G) tube**, or a **jejunum (J) tube**. An NG tube is a soft rubber or plastic tube inserted manually through a nostril and threaded down the esophagus and into the stomach. An NG tube is uncomfortable for a patient; therefore, this type of feeding tube is only for short-term use. If enteral feeding is necessary for more than a few days, a G tube or a J tube is surgically placed through the skin of the abdomen directly into the patient's stomach. If disease or injury of a component of the GI tract prohibits enteral feeding—i.e., the patient is unable to intake nutrition orally or by way of an enteral feeding tube—then parenteral nutrition may be prescribed.

FIGURE 13.1

**Enteral Feeding Tube Sites**

Insertion sites for NG, G, and J tubes.

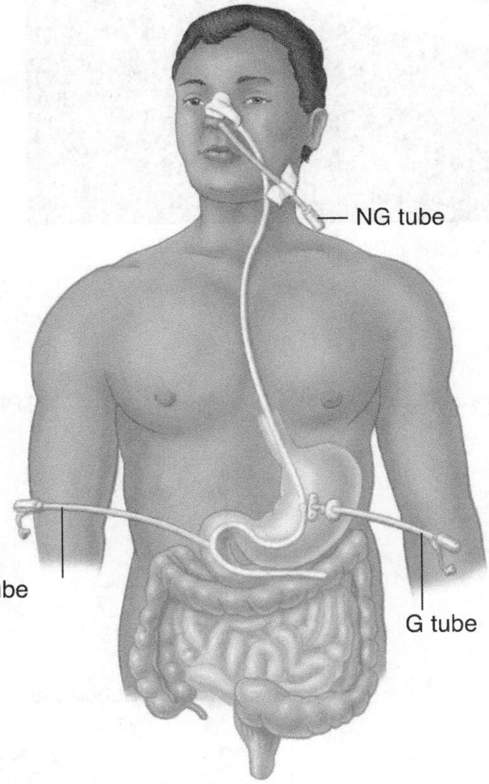


## Types of Parenteral Nutrition

Patients who require long-term (usually longer than one week) nutritional support, and who are unable to receive enteral feedings, may be prescribed parenteral nutrition. In the most general sense, there are two types of parenteral nutrition: temporary (also referred to as peripheral or partial parenteral nutrition) and complete (also referred to as total parenteral nutrition).

***Peripheral Parenteral Nutrition*** Also known as **partial parenteral nutrition** or PPN, this type of parenteral solution provides a portion of the daily calories, electrolytes, and hydration to a patient in need of nutritional supplementation. These solutions are administered to a patient on a temporary basis and are delivered through a peripheral vein until a central venous catheter (CVC) can be surgically inserted into a large vein in the patient's chest, neck, or abdomen. The long-term administration of PPN is rarely done due to the risk of extravasation. **Extravasation** is the discharge or escape of blood or some other fluid (such as an IV medication) from a vessel into the surrounding tissues. In parenteral nutrition therapy, infiltration of these highly acidic, hypertonic, and hyperosmolar solutions may cause tissue irritation or necrosis.

***Total Parenteral Nutrition*** The most commonly compounded parenteral nutrition solutions in the pharmacy, TPN solutions are generally comprised of highly concentrated dextrose and water solutions, which may be mixed with amino

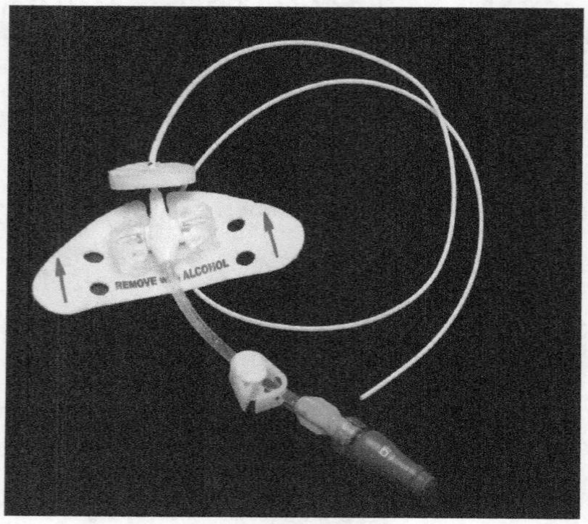


A PICC used in TPN administration.

acids (AA), fat emulsions, electrolytes, vitamins, and minerals. TPNs are administered into a large vein in the neck (internal or external jugular vein), the chest (subclavian vein), the groin (femoral vein), or the abdomen (umbilical vein)—the latter of which is used primarily for neonates. IV access into these large veins is accomplished by placing a CVC into the vein during a minor surgical procedure (see Figure 13.2). There are a number of different methods to insert a CVC, including **tunneled catheter** and **nontunneled catheter insertion** and **peripherally inserted central catheters (PICCs)**. In addition, there are many different types or brands of CVCs, all of which provide a port or injection site through which the TPN solution is administered into the patient's bloodstream. Some common CVCs include Hickman, BROVIAC, triple lumen, Quinton, PORT-A-CATH, and GROSHONG catheters.

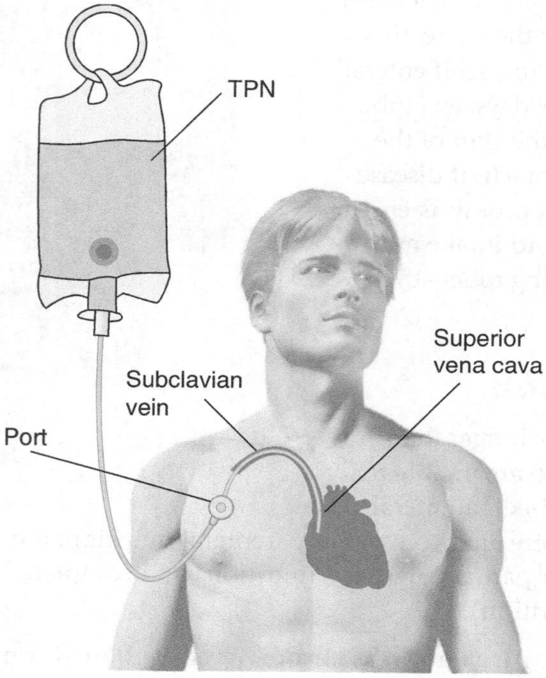


FIGURE 13.2

**CVC Placement for TPN Administration**

During a minor surgical procedure, a CVC is placed into a patient's subclavian vein and threaded into the superior vena cava. The TPN tubing is then attached to the port of the catheter, allowing the administration of the TPN solution directly into the subclavian vein.

## Indications for Prescribing TPN

TPN solutions are often administered in critical care settings; however, they may also be administered to home healthcare patients or other ambulatory patients requiring long-term nutritional support. Some medical conditions that may lead to the prescription of TPN include:

- diseases of the stomach, bowel, or GI tract, such as **Crohn's disease**, **short-bowel syndrome**, **ischemic bowel disease**, or **ulcerative colitis**
- any GI trauma or disease that results in **gastrectomy** or **colectomy**
- **congenital disorders** of the GI tract
- diseases such as cancer, stroke, or **acquired immune deficiency syndrome (AIDS)**

- severe cachexia, a type of malnutrition created by conditions such as marasmus or anorexia
- any type of trauma, treatment, or disease that impairs the patient's ability to intake nutrition by the oral or enteral route of administration (e.g., a GI tract condition or intensive, long-term radiation treatment to the throat region, which often inhibits the patient's ability to swallow)

## Formulation of TPN Solutions

TPN solutions provide a 24-hour supply of all nutrients needed for survival, and they must be prepared using sterile components and strict aseptic technique. In general, there are two common types of TPN formulas: the *2-in-1* solution and the *3-in-1* solution. A 2-in-1 TPN solution provides a 24-hour supply of all nutrients except fatty acids. In the case of most patients receiving 2-in-1 TPN solutions, fatty acids are administered separately and are not a component of the compounded TPN bag. The most common TPN formula is the 3-in-1 TPN solution. This formula provides all of the nutrients needed for a 24-hour period, including fatty acids in the form of Liposyn. The 3-in-1 TPN solution may be referred to as a *total nutrient admixture (TNA)*.

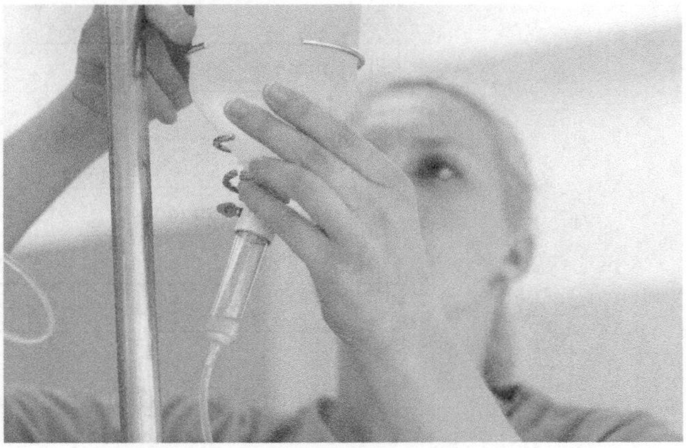

A nurse administering a 2-in-1 TPN solution.

Regardless of the formula, most TPNs are comprised of the same basic ingredients:

- sterile water, which provides hydration
- dextrose, which supplies the primary source of carbohydrates for calories and energy
- Aminosyn (amino acids or AA), which provides the molecular building blocks for protein synthesis
- Liposyn, which supplies essential fatty acids
- electrolytes, vitamins, and minerals, which provide the body with the nutrients needed for a myriad of chemical processes, including those that contribute to nerve, cell, and muscle functions

The last group of ingredients—electrolytes, vitamins, and minerals—are considered additives. In addition to several base components, most TPN solutions have a minimum of 5 additives, with some solutions comprised of as many as 50 additives.

## Guidelines for Ordering TPN

When ordering sterile TPN components, prescribers consider several factors, including the patient's age, diagnosis, kidney function, liver function, and electrolyte levels. Table 13.1, on page 402, provides a list of the typical TPN base components and additives, as well as the average requirements for an adult patient with normal kidney function. These requirements are for a 24-hour period and are based on the patient's body weight in kilograms, unless otherwise indicated on the table.

**Table 13.1 Adult TPN Base Components and Additives for a 24-Hour Period**

| TPN Base Component | Average 24-Hour Requirement |
|---|---|
| Sterile water | 35 mL/kg* |
| Dextrose (sugar) | 1.5 grams/kg |
| Aminosyn; amino acid (protein) | 2 grams/kg |
| Liposyn; lipid (fat) | ≤ 20 grams/day |
| **TPN Additives** | **Average 24-Hour Requirement** |
| Sodium | 1.5 mEq/kg |
| Potassium | 1.5 mEq/kg |
| Phosphate | 1.5 mEq/kg |
| Magnesium | 12 mEq/kg |
| Calcium | 12 mEq/kg |
| Trace mineral elements | 5 mL/day |
| Multivitamins | 10 mL/day |

* Per kg of an adult patient's body weight

Medications other than the typical TPN components are usually not added to a TPN solution due to the potential for incompatibility. However, the three exceptions to this guideline are 1) insulin, which is occasionally added to help maintain the patient's blood glucose level; 2) an $H_2$ antagonist such as ranitidine, which may be added to help prevent the formation of gastric ulcers; and 3) heparin, which may be added in a small quantity to help prevent clotting at the catheter site. Insulin, ranitidine, and heparin have been determined to be compatible with most TPN solutions. Trace minerals such as zinc, copper, manganese, or chromium may also be ordered individually or within a combined trace element solution, as necessary, per physician discretion.

***TPN Medication Order*** Due to the extensive amount of time, labor, and cost associated with TPN preparation, most facilities develop guidelines for prescribing nutritional therapy. Like other types of medication, the prescriber orders the components of the TPN solution by filling in a TPN order form (see Figure 13.3). The form is then sent to the pharmacy for compounding. Most facilities provide preprinted, standardized TPN order forms to ensure consistent and clear communication among healthcare personnel. The compounded preparation's CSP label, which may also be referred to as a TPN label, should match the information on the order form exactly (see Figure 13.4).

***TPN Flow Rate and Volume*** Generally, a 24-hour supply of adult TPN solution ranges in volume from 1000–4000 mL. A 24-hour supply of TPN solution for a neonate ranges from 100–500 mL. Larger pediatric patients may receive daily TPN volumes between 250–1500 mL. The volume of solution compounded by the pharmacy to provide a 24-hour supply to the patient is determined by the TPN flow rate ordered by the physician. For example, if a prescriber orders a rate of 100 mL/hr, the pharmacy provides a 2500-mL bag. The bag lasts 24 hours (the maximum hang time), and a new bag is hung at the same time each day.

## FIGURE 13.3

### Order Form

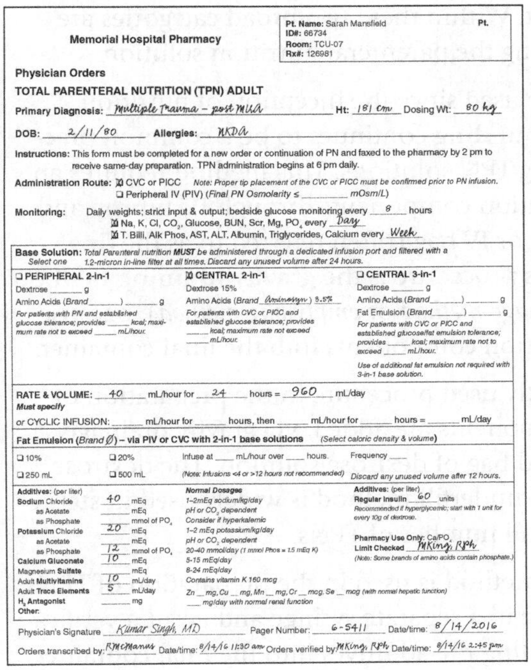

Memorial Hospital Pharmacy

Pt. Name: Sarah Mansfield Pt.
ID#: 66734
Room: TCU-07
Rx#: 126981

Physician Orders

TOTAL PARENTERAL NUTRITION (TPN) ADULT

Primary Diagnosis: Multiple Trauma – post MVA Ht: 181 cm Dosing Wt: 80 kg

DOB: 2/11/80 Allergies: NKDA

Instructions: This form must be completed for a new order or continuation of PN and faxed to the pharmacy by 2 pm to receive same-day preparation. TPN administration begins at 6 pm daily.

Administration Route: ☒ CVC or PICC *Note: Proper tip placement of the CVC or PICC must be confirmed prior to PN infusion.*
❑ Peripheral IV (PIV) (*Final PN Osmolarity ≤ ______ mOsm/L*)

Monitoring: Daily weights; strict input & output; bedside glucose monitoring every 8 hours
☒ Na, K, Cl, $CO_2$, Glucose, BUN, Scr, Mg, $PO_4$ every Day
☒ T. Bili, Alk Phos, AST, ALT, Albumin, Triglycerides, Calcium every Week

Base Solution: *Total Parenteral nutrition **MUST** be administered through a dedicated infusion port and filtered with a 1.2-micron in-line filter at all times. Discard any unused volume after 24 hours.*
*Select one*

| ❑ PERIPHERAL 2-in-1 | ☒ CENTRAL 2-in-1 | ❑ CENTRAL 3-in-1 |
|---|---|---|
| Dextrose ______ g | Dextrose 15% | Dextrose ______ g |
| Amino Acids (Brand______) ______ g | Amino Acids (Brand Aminosyn) 3.5% | Amino Acids (Brand______) ______ g |
| *For patients with PIV and established glucose tolerance; provides ______ kcal; maximum rate not to exceed ______ mL/hour.* | *For patients with CVC or PICC and established glucose tolerance; provides ______ kcal; maximum rate not exceed ______ mL/hour.* | Fat Emulsion (Brand______) ______ g |
| | | *For patients with CVC or PICC and established glucose/fat emulsion tolerance; provides ______ kcal; maximum rate not to exceed ______ mL/hour.* |
| | | *Use of additional fat emulsion not required with 3-in-1 base solution.* |

RATE & VOLUME: 40 mL/hour for 24 hours = 960 mL/day
***Must specify***

*or* CYCLIC INFUSION: ______ mL/hour for ______ hours, then ______ mL/hour for ______ hours = ______ mL/day

Fat Emulsion (*Brand Ø*) – via PIV or CVC with 2-in-1 base solutions (*Select caloric density & volume*)

| | | | |
|---|---|---|---|
| ❑ 10% | ❑ 20% | Infuse at ____ mL/hour over ____ hours. | Frequency ____ |
| ❑ 250 mL | ❑ 500 mL | (*Note: Infusions <4 or >12 hours not recommended*) | *Discard any unused volume after 12 hours.* |

| Additives: (per liter) | | Normal Dosages |
|---|---|---|
| Sodium Chloride | 40 mEq | *1–2mEq sodium/kg/day* |
| as Acetate | ______ mEq | *pH or $CO_2$ dependent* |
| as Phosphate | ______ mmol of $PO_4$ | *Consider if hyperkalemic* |
| Potassium Chloride | 20 mEq | *1–2 mEq potassium/kg/day* |
| as Acetate | ______ mEq | *pH or $CO_2$ dependent* |
| as Phosphate | 12 mmol of $PO_4$ | *20-40 mmol/day (1 mmol Phos = 1.5 mEq K)* |
| Calcium Gluconate | 10 mEq | *5-15 mEq/day* |
| Magnesium Sulfate | ______ mEq | *8-24 mEq/day* |
| Adult Multivitamins | 10 mL/day | *Contains vitamin K 160 mcg* |
| Adult Trace Elements | 5 mL/day | *Zn __ mg, Cu __ mg, Mn __ mg, Cr __ mcg, Se __ mcg (with normal hepatic function)* |
| $H_2$ Antagonist | ______ mg | *____ mg/day with normal renal function* |
| Other: | | |

Additives: (per liter)
Regular Insulin 60 units
*Recommended if hyperglycemic; start with 1 unit for every 10g of dextrose.*

Pharmacy Use Only: Ca/$PO_4$
Limit Checked MKing, RPh
*(Note: Some brands of amino acids contain phosphate.)*

Physician's Signature Kumar Singh, MD Pager Number: 6-5411 Date/time: 8/14/2016

Orders transcribed by: RMcManus Date/time: 8/14/16 11:30 am Orders verified by: MKing, RPh Date/time: 8/14/16 2:45 pm

## FIGURE 13.4

### CSP Label for TPN

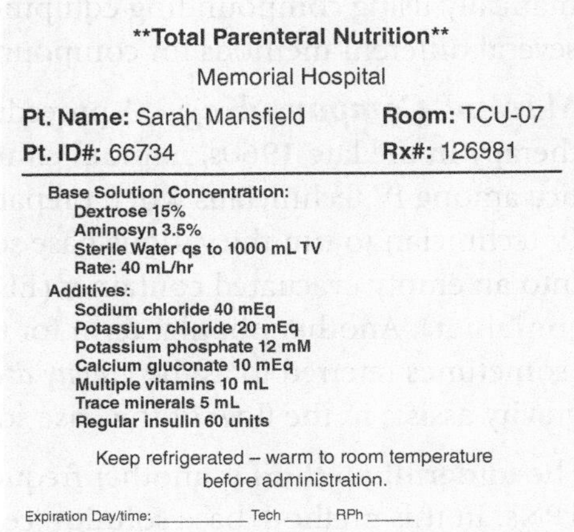

****Total Parenteral Nutrition****
Memorial Hospital

**Pt. Name:** Sarah Mansfield **Room:** TCU-07
**Pt. ID#:** 66734 **Rx#:** 126981

**Base Solution Concentration:**
**Dextrose 15%**
**Aminosyn 3.5%**
**Sterile Water qs to 1000 mL TV**
**Rate: 40 mL/hr**
**Additives:**
**Sodium chloride 40 mEq**
**Potassium chloride 20 mEq**
**Potassium phosphate 12 mM**
**Calcium gluconate 10 mEq**
**Multiple vitamins 10 mL**
**Trace minerals 5 mL**
**Regular insulin 60 units**

Keep refrigerated – warm to room temperature before administration.

Expiration Day/time:______ Tech______ RPh______

In general, the trace minerals and multivitamin (MVI) additives are the only two additives that are not affected by the TPN flow rate. These additives are already ordered by the prescriber in milliliters (typically 5 mL of trace minerals and 10 mL of MVI). Therefore, no matter what size TPN is prepared by the pharmacy, the volume of trace minerals and MVI additives ordered by the prescriber should be the amount drawn up to prepare the TPN solution. The rationale for handling these two additives differently from the other TPN additives—which are adjusted based on the TPN flow rate/TPN bag volume—is that they are the only TPN additives that are ordered *per day*. Because the TPN solution is designed for administration over a 24-hour period, the daily dose of trace minerals and MVI is administered over the 24 hours that the TPN bag is being infused, regardless of the TPN's total volume. The electrolyte additives are ordered *per liter* and, therefore, need to be adjusted to provide the desired dosage based on the TPN flow rate/TPN bag volume.

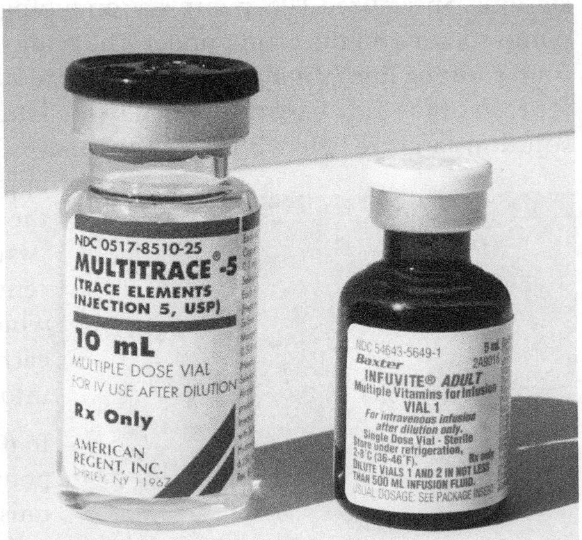


Unlike the electrolyte additives, the trace minerals and MVI additives are ordered per day and are not affected by the TPN flow rate.

**POINTER**

A TPN bag typically contains an additional 100–250 mL to cover any lag time that may occur in the transport of a new bag from the pharmacy to the hospital unit. This additional fluid ensures that the bag does not run dry in the interim.

## Compounding of TPN Solutions

In general, the preparation of TPN solutions is completed either manually or automatically using compounding equipment. Within these two broad categories are several different methods for compounding the parenteral nutrition solution.

***Manual Compounding*** A procedure used since the inception of nutrition therapy in the late 1960s, **manual compounding** continues to be a common practice among IV technicians when preparing TPN solutions. This method requires an IV technician to run the various base solution components through **IV tubing** and into an empty evacuated container (EEC) or IV bag (often referred to as the **final container**). Another popular term for this procedure is the **gravity draining method** (sometimes referred to as the *gravity drainage method* or *empty bag method*), because gravity assists in the flow of the base solution components into the final container.

The **underfill method** is another frequently used procedure in the preparation of TPNs. In this method, base solution components are added, via gravity drainage, to a commercially available, partially filled bag of dextrose solution. The dextrose bag then serves as the final container. The underfill method is widely used in sterile compounding facilities that prepare a small number of TPNs.

No matter which manual compounding method is used in the preparation of TPNs, IV technicians must draw up each additive in a separate syringe and await a verification check from a pharmacist before injecting the additives into the final container of base solutions.

***Automated Compounding*** The preparation of nutritional therapy can also be accomplished through the use of partially automated or fully **automated TPN compounding**. In **partially automated TPN compounding**, the TPN base solution is prepared using an **automated compounding device (ACD)**. The ACD—often called an *automated TPN compounder*, *automix*, or, simply, a *compounder*—rapidly fills the empty final container. The compounder is comprised of up to eight different **pump stations**. Specialized TPN pump station tubing is threaded through each of the pump stations on the compounder. The pump station tubing provides a separate source-tubing line (sometimes called a "lead") and color-coded **IV tubing spike** for each of the TPN base components (the latter of which are often called **source solutions** and are held within **source containers**). Each of the individual leads is approximately 12" long and merges (at the end opposite from the individual IV tubing spike) with the slightly larger, centralized TPN pump station tube, which automatically delivers fluid from each of the source containers directly into the final container.

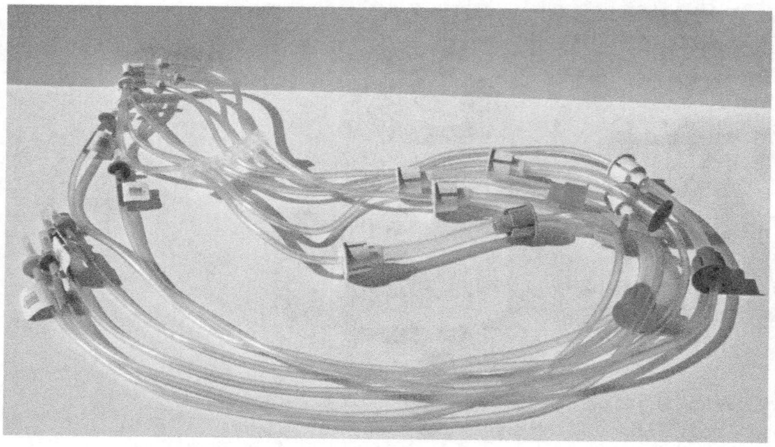
Six color-coded leads and tubing spikes used in an ACD.

In the partially automated TPN compounding method, the IV technician must still draw up each TPN additive in an individual syringe and, once checked by a pharmacist, manually inject the additives directly into the final TPN container. The partially automated TPN compounding method is frequently used in hospital and home infusion pharmacies, where a moderate number of TPN solutions are prepared each day.

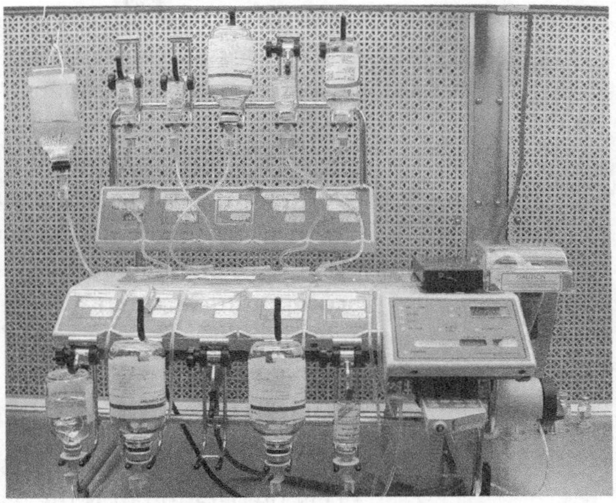
The micronutrient compounding device automatically injects electrolytes and most other additives into the final container.

Fully automated TPN compounding is a common procedure in facilities that prepare large numbers of TPN solutions each day. In this method, the TPN base solution is formulated using a TPN compounding device, such as an automix compounder, and the TPN electrolytes and most other additives are prepared by a special automated device called a micromix compounder (also known as a *micronutrient compounder*). The micromix compounder is separate from the automix compounder, but both devices are attached to the final container through special compounder tubing. The micromix compounder has between 6 and 12 individual pump stations and color-coded tubing-and-spike units. IV technicians must individually insert the tubing into each electrolyte or additive vial. The pump stations inject the prescribed amount of each additive into the final container.

The automix and micromix compounders are controlled by individual base control units, which may be manually or automatically programmed through the attached computer system. The automix and micromix systems have integrated computer software, which allows the IV technician or pharmacist to enter the TPN order into the computer. The computer then automatically programs the base control unit to deliver the appropriate volume of base solution components and, if necessary, electrolyte additives to the final container. The method used to measure the amount of each solution or additive pumped from the source container or vial into the final container may be either volumetric or gravimetric, depending on which brand of compounding device is used.

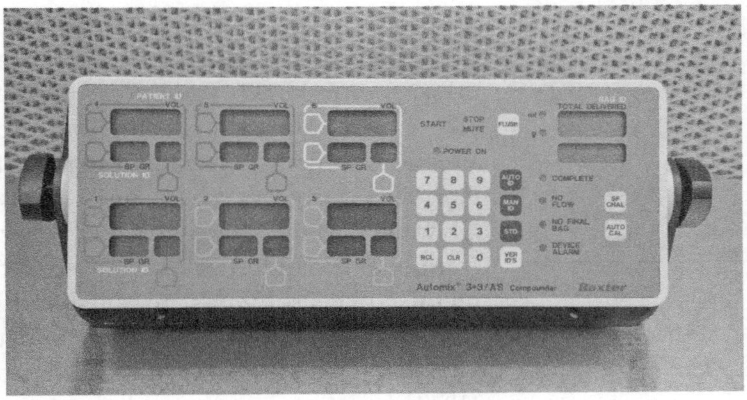
Base control unit used to program the automix TPN compounder.

***Benefits and Drawbacks of Manual and Automated Compounding Methods*** When determining which compounding method is most appropriate to use, sterile compounding facilities must consider the benefits and drawbacks of each procedure. Manual TPN preparation is generally the most cost-effective method of TPN compounding; however, this procedure is also very time-consuming and labor-intensive for sterile compounding personnel. Preparing the base solution, drawing up the separate additives, and using the gravity-draining method to empty the base solution components into the final container requires an extended period of time. In addition, the tasks required in manual preparation carry a greater risk for human error and possible contamination of the compounded sterile preparation (CSP).

The process of partially automated TPN preparation is considerably faster and more accurate than manual TPN preparation; however, it is significantly more expensive. Fully automated TPN preparation is by far the fastest and most accurate method of TPN preparation, though for many facilities the expense associated with this type of ACD is prohibitive. The specialized computer system, software, base compounder unit, automix and micromix compounders, as well as the specialized tubing and final containers required for ACDs, may cost approximately $25,000 per year to operate. In addition to the extensive cost associated with automated TPN compounders, the potential for power failure or equipment malfunction must be considered.

**USP Chapter <797>**

Facilities that use automated TPN compounding should have a contingency plan in place in the event of a power outage or equipment failure. Check your facility's P&P manual for guidelines, if appropriate.

## Cleaning and Calibration of the ACD

USP Chapter <797> requires that an ACD be cleaned and calibrated daily prior to TPN preparation. It is the responsibility of the performing technician to refer to the manufacturer's instructions or the facility's P&P manual for specific directions on the cleaning and calibration of the device and to record these tasks on an **ACD Cleaning and Verification Log Sheet** (see Figure 13.5). This log sheet is located in the anteroom and must be kept on file within the pharmacy for the lifetime of the equipment. Most automated TPN compounders are calibrated so that they are accurate within +/– 3 percent.

**POINTER**

A limited selection of premixed TPN solutions are available from a small group of manufacturers. These solutions are manufactured in such a way that nothing may be injected into the bag.

## Premixed TPN Solutions

While most TPN solutions are prepared by sterile compounding personnel, some facilities utilize premixed TPN solutions. Premixed TPN solutions are primarily used in home healthcare situations in which the patient requires long-term TPN therapy and has consistently stable lab values (so that no variation in TPN base components or additives is required). These premixed TPN solutions are called **multiple-channel TPN solutions**. Critically ill patients on TPN therapy often require a daily adjustment of TPN base components or additives in response to the patient's changing lab values or nutritional needs. Because neither the base components nor the ingredients in premixed bags may be adjusted, they are generally not used in the acute care setting.

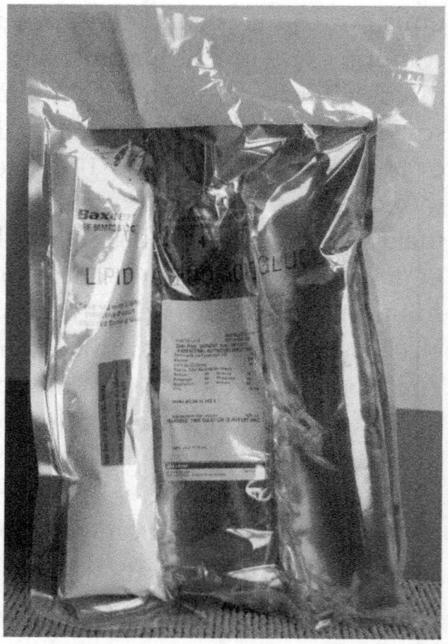

Premixed TPN solution used in the home healthcare setting.

## Preparation Risks of Parenteral Fluids

Understanding the properties of the multiple components of parenteral nutrition makes IV technicians aware of the potential risks associated with the preparation of TPN solutions. Because parenteral medications circulate through the blood supply, the introduction of pathogens during sterile compounding can jeopardize the health and safety of patient recipients. Therefore, IV technicians must follow strict aseptic

**FIGURE 13.5**

**ACD Cleaning and Verification Log Sheet**

# Automated Compounding Device (ACD) Cleaning and Verification Log Sheet

***Refer to the ACD manufacturer's recommendations and your facility's P&P manual to determine specific ACD cleaning and verification procedures. The ACD must be cleaned; new compounder tubing must be installed; and the gravimetric (or volumetric, if applicable) accuracy must be verified at least daily, as specified by USP Chapter <797>.***

| Date/Time | ACD Cleaned by (Initials) | Compounder Tubing Changed By (Initials) | ACD Calibration Performed by (Initials) | SIGNATURE |
|---|---|---|---|---|
| | | | | |
| | | | | |
| | | | | |
| | | | | |
| | | | | |
| | | | | |
| | | | | |
| | | | | |
| | | | | |
| | | | | |
| | | | | |
| | | | | |
| | | | | |
| | | | | |
| | | | | |
| | | | | |

technique in the preparation of TPNs. (For more information on the preparation risks of CSPs in general, see Chapter 8.)

***TPN Preparation Risks*** Aside from the risks common to all parenteral solutions, TPN preparation has a unique set of complications that explain its classification as a medium-risk compounding activity by USP Chapter <797>. These complications include a heightened risk of contamination and incompatibility issues.

CONTAMINATION To prepare a TPN solution, IV technicians must manipulate a number of supply items during the compounding process. Every time a needle pierces a vial's rubber top or the injection port of an IV bag, there is a risk of contamination of the CSP. Because TPN solutions are comprised of multiple solution components mixed with multiple additive components, the risk of contamination is greater with TPNs than it is with other CSPs.

INCOMPATIBILITY In addition to the risks associated with the procedure itself, the chemical makeup of TPN solutions makes them especially susceptible to **incompatibility** complications, including:

- **therapeutic incompatibility**, which occurs when two or more combined drugs result in a change in the effectiveness of one or both of the drugs upon administration
- **chemical incompatibility**, which occurs when two or more combined substances initiate a chemical change, possibly resulting in the decomposition of certain TPN components or an alteration of the pH of the TPN solution
- **physical incompatibility**, which occurs when two or more combined substances (either additives or the base solution components themselves) have a chemical interaction, resulting in a physical change to the end product

In general, therapeutic and chemical incompatibilities are not visible to healthcare personnel and may only be identified by **end-product testing**—an elective process that is both time-consuming and cost-prohibitive. Physical incompatibility within a TPN solution, however, is easily recognizable; evidence includes changes in color, separation or layering of the various components of the TPN solution, or **precipitation**.

In TPN preparation, the most commonly encountered physical incompatibility occurs between the additives phosphate and calcium. When injected concurrently into a TPN base solution, these additives cause the formation of a snowflake-like precipitate within the fluid. To avoid this incompatibility issue, sterile compounding personnel should add the phosphate first to the solution, followed by all of the remaining additives, except the calcium. The calcium additive should be injected last. Inserting additives in this order ensures that the phosphate is flushed into the base solution by the remaining additives prior to the addition of the calcium. Once this flushing process has occurred, the calcium may be safely added to the bag without forming a precipitate.

**POINTER**

Prescribers must order amounts of phosphate and calcium below the threshold at which incompatibility results. If excessive amounts of either phosphate or calcium are added to a TPN solution, a precipitate forms, regardless of the order of mixing or the amount of dilution within the bag.

***Note:*** Facilities may vary as to whether sterile compounding personnel are required to add the phosphate first and calcium last or vice versa. In either case, always separate these two additives from the other additives. In addition, most facilities require that additives containing color, such as MVI (which is orange), be added last (after the calcium additive) in order to more easily identify particulate matter problems within the TPN solution. Sterile compounding personnel should consult their facility's P&P manual to determine the specific mixing order protocol.

## Standard Mixing Protocols for TPN Preparation

All facilities should implement standard protocols for TPN preparation based on current, well-substantiated pharmacy reference materials. Protocols should specify appropriate ingredients and doses to ensure that all TPN components are both therapeutically and chemically compatible. These protocols should also provide guidelines on the mixing order of the TPN components—an important consideration for the safety of the final CSP. In general, the ingredient mixing order for TPNs is as follows: the base solution—dextrose, amino acids, sterile water, and then fatty acids—followed by the additives (in the order described on page 408).

## The Final Container

As mentioned earlier, the final container for a TPN solution is either an EEC or an empty bag. The glass EEC used in TPN preparation may have a special type of aluminum cap that must be removed prior to use. It is important to remove the cap very carefully and in a specific manner. Incorrect cap removal from an EEC may create a jagged edge on the aluminum cap, resulting in a possible injury to the person preparing the CSP. Because of this safety concern, an empty bag constructed of plastic or polyvinyl chloride (PVC) is more commonly used among sterile compounding personnel. This specialized bag has a hard plastic tail, which serves as the conduit for the pumped base solution. Although more costly than an EEC, a TPN bag is easier to handle during the sterile compounding process. (The various compounding methods and related supplies will be discussed later in this chapter.)

At the completion of TPN compounding procedures, the final container must be inspected for evidence of particulate matter or incompatibility. If any signs of these issues are present, the IV technician must consult the pharmacist to determine the source of the incompatibility and, if necessary, contact the prescriber to modify the TPN order so that one or more of the additives may be decreased or discontinued. A new TPN solution with the modified additives must then be prepared. If that is the case, the IV technician must reinspect the solution for signs of incompatibility.

If the final container is problem-free, sterile compounding personnel affix a CSP label to the final container and then either send the TPN to the nursing unit or place the container in the refrigerator or freezer for storage.

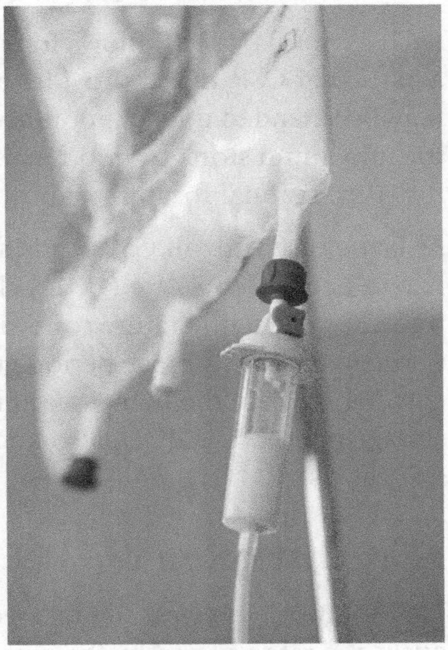

TPN solution containing fatty acids (Liposyn); notice the Liposyn has a white color, which makes it difficult to see particulate matter.

**BE AWARE**

Do not use TPN solutions that show evidence of incompatibility. Instead, contact the pharmacist for further directives.

## Storage of the Final Container

In general, prepared TPN solutions should be refrigerated (36° to 46° F [2°to 8° C]) and then removed from the refrigerator approximately 30 minutes before administration. During this time, the solution warms to room temperature. See Table 13.2 for information regarding TPN storage parameters.

**Table 13.2 USP Chapter <797> Medium-Risk CSPs—Maximum Storage Periods**

In the absence of passing a sterility test, the storage period of medium-risk CSPs cannot exceed the following time periods:

- Not more than 30 hours at controlled room temperature (68° to 77° F [20° to 25° C])
- Not more than 9 days at controlled cold (refrigerated) temperature (36° to 46° F [2° to 8° C])
- Not more than 45 days in a solid frozen state (-4° to 14° F [-25° to -10° C])

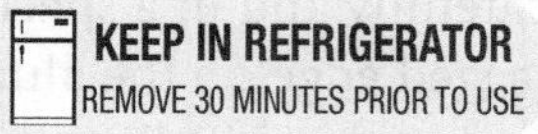
KEEP IN REFRIGERATOR
REMOVE 30 MINUTES PRIOR TO USE

Many facilities set maximum storage periods slightly less than the maximum storage periods provided by USP Chapter <797>. For instance, it is very common for compounding facilities to set the maximum storage period for medium-risk CSPs as follows:

- Not more than 24 hours at controlled room temperature
- Not more than 7 days at controlled cold (refrigerated) temperature
- Not more than 30 days in a solid frozen state

Such a "grace period" allows for easier tracking of the storage expiration dates for a particular CSP. It also provides a small window in which the facility storage time may be extended due to an unforeseen circumstance (while still remaining within the maximum storage period mandated by USP Chapter <797>). Refer to your facility's P&P manual for information regarding medium-risk CSP storage periods.

As is the case with all CSPs, TPN solutions prepared using strict aseptic technique have a **beyond-use date (BUD)** clearly marked on the CSP label. The BUD is determined by the temperature conditions under which the TPN is stored in comparison to the maximum storage period guidelines provided by your facility. Under no circumstances may the BUD exceed the USP Chapter <797> guidelines for maximum storage period. The BUD, also known as the expiration date, must be included on all CSP labels.

## Administration of TPN Solutions

TPN solutions are typically infused through a CVC and are administered continuously at a rate ordered by the prescriber. Because the catheter is placed directly into a major blood vessel and may remain in place for a week or longer, nursing personnel must exercise proper care of the catheter. On at least a daily basis, staff must cleanse the catheter site, appropriately flush the catheter, and check the catheter site for swelling, heat, discharge, redness, and other signs of infection.

Patients on TPN therapy must also be closely monitored to ensure that they receive adequate nutrition, maintain balanced electrolyte levels, and remain free of infection. Prescribers and pharmacists work closely with registered dietitians and nurses to monitor the patient for appropriate TPN therapy, and to watch for signs of infection. The nursing staff regularly monitors the patient's weight, vital signs, and blood glucose level to check for changes that may have been caused by TPN therapy. In addition, patients receiving TPN must undergo routine blood draws to determine their electrolyte values and to search for evidence of infection. Such monitoring may be done daily, weekly, or at another interval ordered by the prescriber.

Changes to the TPN solution may be made daily, if necessary, based on lab values or other aspects of patient monitoring. Nursing personnel must also hang a new TPN bag every 24 hours, for the solution provides an ideal medium for bacterial growth due to the complexity of the compounding process.

## Administration Risks of Parenteral Fluids

The administration of parenteral therapy involves potential complications that may lead to injury or, possibly, death for patient recipients. Therefore, all patients receiving parenteral fluids should be monitored for the following complications:

- nosocomial infection
- allergic reaction (including anaphylaxis)
- phlebitis
- tissuing
- embolism
- extravasation
- cellulitis
- Stevens-Johnson syndrome
- nephrotoxicity

***TPN Administration Risks*** The primary risk associated with TPN administration is **nosocomial infection**, also known as *healthcare associated infection (HAI)*. This risk is greater for patient recipients of TPN because these patients are often very ill and, therefore, have compromised immune systems. Their delicate conditions, coupled with the parenteral route used in TPN administration, put patients at risk for dangerous blood infections from incorrect IV insertion or improper care of the access site.

The administration of TPN also carries higher risks for extravasation, tissuing, and phlebitis due to the chemical properties of the solutions. In general, TPN solutions are more acidic, hypertonic, and hyperosmolar than human blood plasma. Consequently, TPN administration into a peripheral vein should be avoided.

Prior to patient administration, it is advisable for nursing personnel to filter the TPN solution for possible particulate matter that may have entered the solution during the compounding process. This complication could stem from multiple injections into the IV bag (which might introduce coring) or from incompatibility issues (specifically, particulate matter due to precipitation). During TPN preparation, visual identification of particulates is difficult because these solutions are often comprised of colored ingredients—e.g., orange for TPNs containing MVI, and milky white for TPNs containing Liposyn. Therefore, most facilities address this issue by employing an in-line filter to remove potential particulate matter from the TPN solution prior to patient administration. An in-line filter is attached near the end of the IV tubing through which the TPN is administered to the patient. In-line TPN filters may have filtration capabilities of 0.2 micron, 0.22 micron, 0.45 micron, or 0.5 micron. Consult your facility's P&P manual to determine the guidelines regarding TPN filtration.

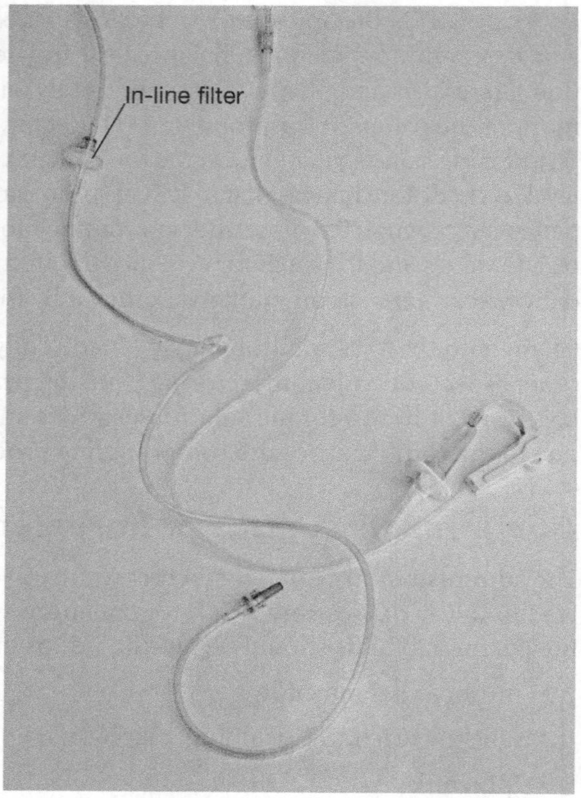

IV tubing with in-line filter.

## Special Considerations for Preparing TPNs

TPN solutions are complex sterile preparations that require special considerations during the compounding process. Before preparing a TPN, IV technicians must carefully consider the compounding method and procedures for prescribing, monitoring, and administering the TPN. Processes for quality assurance, monitoring of compounding equipment, and training of sterile compounding personnel must also be clearly defined. For all of these special considerations, facility protocol must be identified and closely adhered to by pharmacy personnel, prescribers, and nursing staff.

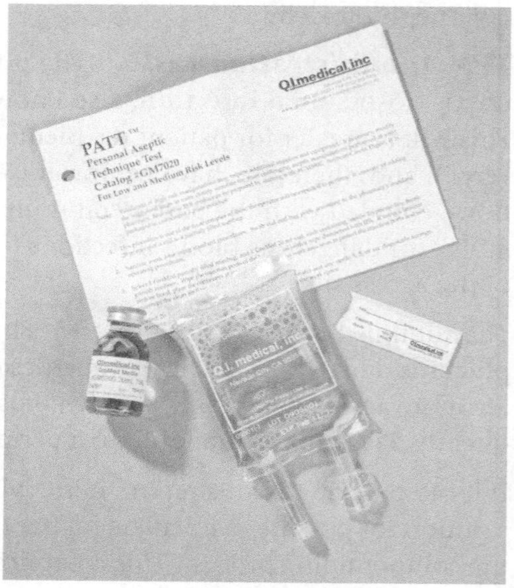

Aseptic technique testing kit (ATTACK kit).

***Training for Sterile Compounding Personnel*** USP Chapter <797> mandates that, at a minimum, sterile compounding personnel must be expertly trained and pass both a written exam and hands-on process validation test, as well as successfully complete a negative-growth ATTACK kit (or similar type of basic media-fill test procedure) at the following intervals: upon completion of training, prior to preparing IVs for patient use (annually thereafter), and upon observance of a **break in aseptic technique**. Sterile compounding personnel must also undergo additional training and testing specific to this complex procedure. This advanced training includes the completion of a negative-growth, media-fill test procedure that is more difficult than the basic media-fill test procedure. The **advanced media-fill test procedure** requires the technician to aseptically perform manipulations from multiple containers. If applicable, those who prepare TPN solutions must also receive special training in cleaning, calibrating, and operating the ACD. Additionally, TPN preparers must receive training in procedures regarding the identification of equipment malfunction, particulate matter, and incompatibility. It is considered best practice for sterile compounding personnel who prepare TPN solutions to complete TPN-specific training labs and process validation upon completion of initial training, and annually thereafter.

## USP Chapter <797> Guidelines for TPN Preparation

In addition to the sterile compounding preparatory procedures discussed in this chapter, the related procedures and overarching principles are presented in USP Chapter <797> and in each facility's P&P manual. Sterile compounding personnel must pay strict attention to aseptic technique protocols both in the anteroom and clean room. Any breach in these protocols may result in medication errors, sepsis, or, possibly, death for patient recipients. Therefore, as a TPN compounding technician, you bear primary responsibility for the preparation and integrity of the CSPs. With that in mind, only those personnel who have been specially trained, process validated, and certified in aseptic technique and sterile product preparation should be allowed to compound sterile products. In addition, personnel who prepare TPN solutions must undergo TPN-specific training, testing, and process validation and successfully complete an advanced media-fill test procedure prior to preparing TPNs for patient administration. Part 2 of this chapter guides you through the discovery and demonstration of proper aseptic technique in TPN preparation.

# Concepts Self-Check

## Check Your Understanding

*Write your answers on a separate sheet of paper, as modeled in these examples: 1d; 2c; 3b; etc. Check your answers using the Answer Key in Appendix A.*

**1.** Which type of feeding method did Hippocrates and Galen employ?

a. force feeding
b. rectal feeding
c. nasogastric tube feeding
d. J tube feeding

**2.** Which of the following scientists is credited with inventing modern-day TPN therapy?

a. Galen
b. Robert Elman
c. Arvid Wretlind
d. Jonathan Rhoads

**3.** What does the abbreviation TPN stand for?

a. the patient's nutrition
b. the parenteral nutrition
c. total patient nutrition
d. total parenteral nutrition

**4.** Which of the following conditions may necessitate TPN therapy?

a. gastrectomy
b. short-bowel syndrome
c. cachexia
d. all of the above
e. only *b* and *c*

**5.** Which list of TPN ingredients reflects the mixing order followed by most facilities?

a. base solution, phosphate, remaining additives, calcium, MVI
b. phosphate, remaining additives, MVI, calcium, base solution
c. calcium, phosphate, remaining additives, base solution, MVI
d. base solution, MVI, phosphate, remaining additives, calcium

## Apply Your Knowledge

*On a separate sheet of paper, write your answers to the questions posed in the paragraph below. Use complete sentences and take time to create a thorough and thoughtful response. Check your answers against the Answer Key in Appendix A.*

In Part 1 of this chapter, you learned that TPN preparation requires IV technicians to undergo additional training, testing, and process validation. In addition, TPN preparers must pass a more complicated and difficult media-fill test procedure than those technicians who do not prepare TPNs. With that in mind, what is the rationale for mandating more advanced training and testing for sterile compounding personnel who prepare TPNs? Do you believe that the preparation of TPNs warrants its designation as a medium-risk activity, a higher level than most other sterile compounding procedures? Why or why not?

# Part 2: Training

*Before performing this lab, review the Sterile Compounding Area Procedures listed on pages 162–163 at the end of the Unit 2 opener, and preview the accompanying process validation checklist in Appendix D.*

## Understand the Resources and Supplies

USP Chapter <797> prescribes a number of special requirements for the preparation of TPNs. This chapter and the corresponding lab provide resources and supplies that are in alignment with the directives set forth in USP Chapter <797>.

### Essential Supplies

Supplies used in the anteroom include a medication order and a CSP label; a standard calculator; a pen; a permanent, felt-tip marker; large and small plastic bags; aseptic garb; a sterile gown; presaturated, aseptic cleaning wipes; sterile, foamed 70% isopropyl alcohol (IPA); a waste container; and a transport vehicle. (Various other compounding supplies, such as those needed for aseptic hand washing and hood cleaning, are necessary supplies, but, for the purposes of this lab, are not included on the Essential Supplies list.) In the clean room, essential supply items include sterile, foamed 70% IPA; sterile, powder-free gloves; sterile 70% IPA swabs; a sharps container; a waste container; and a laminar airflow hood. Additionally, needles, syringes, hemostats, EECs, base components, and additive vials are generally kept in the anteroom and brought into the clean room just prior to use.

### Procedure-Specific Supplies

In addition to the previously listed essential supplies, each sterile compounding procedure requires supply items specific to the procedure being performed. The type, number, and amount of procedure-specific supply items are determined by the IV technician prior to performing the procedure, based on information provided on the TPN order (and corresponding CSP label) and medication additive labels. After reading these labels, the IV technician performs one or more calculations that reveal the number and volume of additives needed to prepare the TPN. This information, in turn, dictates the number, size, and types of syringes needed for the procedure.

In general, teaching environments do not have ready access to ACDs. Therefore, for the purpose of this TPN training lab, instruction will be provided in the proper procedures necessary to perform a manual TPN compounding procedure.

***TPN Supplies*** The process of compounding a TPN involves the manipulation of syringes, regular needles and, in particular, vials and IV base solutions. Familiarity with the appearances of these items as well as any specific handling requirements is essential in sterile compounding procedures.

**POINTER**
If the training environment is such that an ACD is available, and the instructor directs you to use the TPN device during the Chapter 13 procedural lab, refer to the manufacturer's instructions of the ACD for step-by-step procedures related to setup, cleaning, verification, and use of the automix and/or micromix compounder(s).

**EEC** A 1000-mL EEC is used as the final container into which the base components and additives are injected. The EEC contains a relative negative air pressure, which helps to draw the fluid from the base components into the EEC. EECs larger than 100 mL often have a special type of aluminum cap that must be removed prior to use. It is important to remove the cap carefully and in a specific order. Incorrect aluminum-cap removal from an EEC may cause a jagged edge, which may lead to injury for the person preparing the CSP. The step-by-step procedure for proper aluminum-cap removal from an EEC is provided in the *Preview the Lab Procedure* section of this chapter.

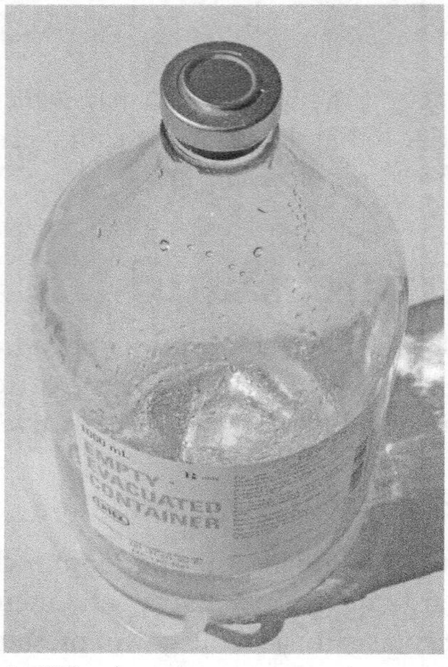

An EEC with an aluminum cap in place.

**IV Tubing** During the TPN compounding process, IV tubing transfers fluid from each of the source containers (base component bags) into the EEC. Prior to using the tubing, the IV technician aseptically removes the cap from the tubing needle adaptor, attaches a regular needle to the adaptor, and temporarily places the unit (needle and attached IV tubing) on the hood surface within the DCA. Next, the tubing port plug is removed from the base component bag, and the cap is removed from the IV tubing spike. The IV technician then inserts the spike into the tubing port of the base component bag. (For reminders on the components and handling of certain supply items, refer to Chapter 3 of this textbook.)

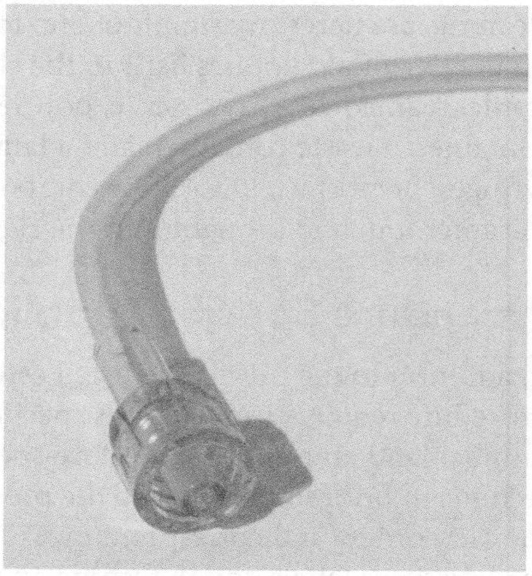
A needle adaptor at the one end of the IV tubing.

On the other end of the tubing, the IV technician removes the needle cap and, using strict aseptic technique, inserts the needle into the top of the EEC. Once the desired volume of the first base component has been drawn into the EEC, a **hemostat** or another type of medical clamp is used to clamp the tail of the base component bag so that it does not leak when the tubing is removed.

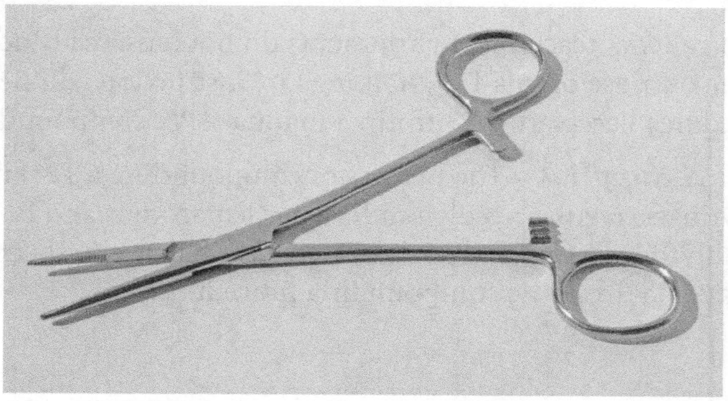
A hemostat used in sterile compounding to temporarily clamp tubing or the tail of an IV bag.

The IV tubing spike is then removed from the first base component bag and aseptically inserted into the next base component bag. The required volume of the second base component is then run into the EEC, and the procedure is repeated with the third base component.

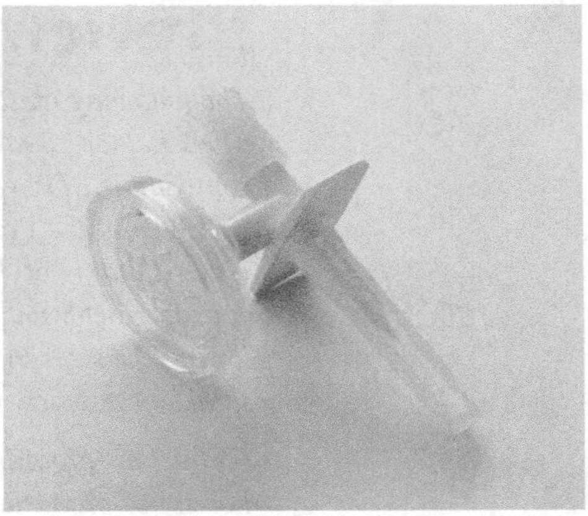

A dispensing pin used in TPN preparation.

**TPN Additive Preparation Supply Items** The additives needed for this TPN solution are provided in vials. Refer to Chapter 8 of this textbook for standard vial techniques. Syringes of appropriate size to correctly withdraw the necessary ingredient volumes are required to separately draw up each of the additives. Once the TPN base solution has been prepared, the additives have been drawn up, and both the base solution and additives have been checked, then the additives are injected into the EEC.

In practice, several TPNs may use the same additive vials. To reduce the likelihood of coring, use a **vented dispensing pin** (a small, sterile plastic spike with a Luer-lock syringe tip adaptor at one end). Insert the spike into the additive vial; then twist the syringe onto the dispensing pin. Once the syringe is filled to the desired volume, remove it from the dispensing pin and attach a needle. The procedure may be repeated, as necessary, to draw up multiple doses of the additive for numerous TPNs, without inserting multiple needles into the vial. Consequently, coring is less likely to occur. ***Note:*** Due to the high cost of providing separate dispensing pins for each additive and the fact that the lab procedure only requires one withdrawal from each additive vial, the procedural lab requires you to use a regular needle and syringe to draw up each additive.

**POINTER**

Some dispensing pins have a filter component (the plastic disc-shaped structure located at the side of the item), whereas others do not. This component varies according to the manufacturer and to the procedure for which the dispensing pin is used.

## Critical Sites of TPN Supplies

Before beginning preparatory procedures in the anteroom or clean room, the IV technician must recall the critical sites of the supplies. Identifying the critical site of each supply item helps you to determine the proper procedure for handling the item once you have entered the clean room and begin to work in the hood.

In addition to the syringe tip and needle, the critical sites of the procedure-specific supplies used in the Chapter 13 procedural lab include the IV tubing spike, the needle adaptor, and the base component tubing port. These critical sites are provided in sterile form and, therefore, should never be swabbed, shadowed, or touched by anything other than the sterile device to which they are attached. Care must be taken to keep the critical sites within the direct compounding area (DCA) of the hood so that they receive uninterrupted airflow from the HEPA filter.

**USP Chapter <797>**

Because manufacturers supply the syringe tip and all parts of the needle in sterile form, you must not swab them with IPA. Doing so may contaminate these critical sites.

Critical sites such as vial tops, base solution injection ports, and the rubber top of the EEC must be swabbed with sterile, 70% IPA prior to needle insertion. Once they have been swabbed, care must be taken to keep the critical sites within the DCA so that they receive uninterrupted airflow from the HEPA filter.

# Preview the Lab Procedure

*The following material provides a brief overview of the lab procedure that you will perform. The Chapter 13 lab procedure will walk you through the process of preparing a manually compounded TPN solution. First, read the* Preview the Lab Procedure *section. Then read each step of the* Procedural Lab *section carefully, visualizing every action. Next, reinforce your understanding of the process by watching the demonstration video. Once you are in the lab, your instructor will demonstrate the procedure, and then you will perform the procedure by following the steps in the* Procedural Lab *section. Practice the lab procedure multiple times. After sufficient practice, you will complete the lab procedure for process validation by your instructor.*

***Note:*** *This procedural lab requires the use of a basic, open-sided, horizontal laminar airflow hood. For pharmacies that do not have this type of hood, IV technicians should consult the* Instruction Guide *provided by the hood's manufacturer or their facility's P&P manual to determine which procedures may need to be adjusted to suit their hood.*

**POINTER**

Sterile compounding personnel must comply with certain restrictions when working in the anteroom and clean room areas. These restrictions include no gum chewing, horseplay, or food or drink in both the anteroom and clean room, and no hair spray, perfume, makeup, artificial or polished nails, or jewelry in the sterile compounding environment.

## Anteroom Preparatory Procedures

Because preparation for the sterile compounding process begins in the anteroom, that transition area provides a space for implementing the standard pharmacy protocols discussed in Chapters 3–6 of this textbook, including:

- verifying the CSP label (TPN label) against the medication order (TPN order)
- performing correct pharmacy calculations to determine type, size, and number of supply items needed
- gathering and cleaning of supplies
- performing aseptic garbing and hand washing
- donning a sterile gown

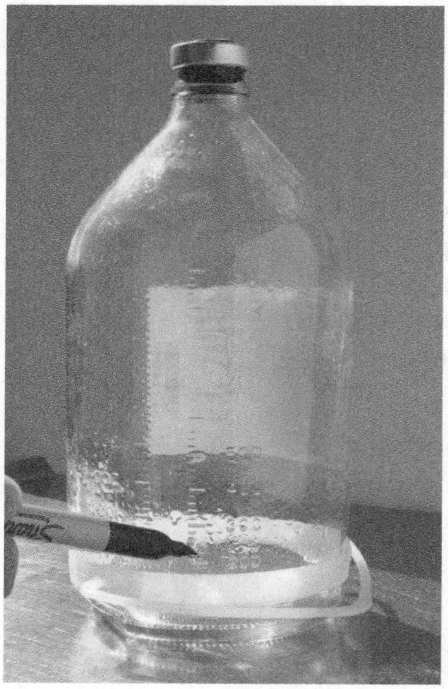


An IV technician drawing a line on the EEC to show the volume of dextrose needed for the TPN preparation.

***Verifying the CSP Label*** Compare the TPN order form to the CSP label to verify that all of the information on the CSP label matches the TPN order form exactly. Read the CSP label to determine the desired concentration and total final volume of each of the base solution components. Then read the CSP label to determine the additives that must be used to prepare the TPN solution. Read the label on the first additive vial to determine its concentration; then repeat for each additive to be used in this procedure.

***Performing Pharmacy Calculations*** Read the manufacturer's solution identification information on the face of each base solution component to determine concentrations. Perform a separate calculation to determine the volume of each base solution component needed to prepare the TPN solution. In order to easily measure the amount of each base solution component, use a permanent marker to draw a line on the EEC to signify the dextrose volume. Draw separate lines on the EEC to indicate the volume of Aminosyn and the volume of sterile water to be added to the EEC.

Using information gleaned from the CSP label and each additive vial label, calculate the desired volume of each additive to be used in this procedure. The desired volume is the volume that you must withdraw from the vial to deliver the dose ordered by the prescriber. (For additional assistance on performing calculations, refer to Chapter 5 of this textbook.)

***Gathering and Cleaning Supplies*** After performing the calculations, place the CSP label into a small plastic bag, place the TPN order form into a large plastic bag, and seal both bags. You should then gather all of the necessary compounding supplies needed for the procedure, and wipe down all of the supply items.

***Donning PPE*** Don the appropriate personal protective equipment (PPE), including aseptic garb and a sterile gown. (To review the step-by-step preparatory procedures performed in the anteroom, refer to Chapter 8 of this textbook.)

Due to time constraints, you will not perform aseptic hand-washing procedures during this procedural lab. Keep in mind that, in sterile compounding practice, aseptic hand-washing procedures are mandatory and must be performed prior to donning a sterile gown.

## Clean Room Preparatory Procedures

When preparing TPNs for patient administration, sterile compounding personnel must diligently follow established pharmacy clean room protocols as well. These protocols, discussed in Chapters 6 and 7, include:

- cleansing hands with sterile, foamed 70% IPA
- donning sterile gloves
- cleaning the hood

Once the preparatory steps have been completed, TPN compounding procedures may begin.

Upon entering the clean room, place the transport basket or tray onto a clean shelf, table, or countertop. If the transport vehicle used is a cart, wheel it so that it is positioned away from the hood prefilter. Cleanse your hands and forearms with sterile, foamed 70% IPA and allow them to dry thoroughly. Don sterile gloves according to standard aseptic technique procedures. (For additional assistance on the procedure for donning sterile gloves, refer to Chapter 6 of this textbook.)

Due to time constraints, you will not perform hood-cleaning procedures during this procedural lab. Keep in mind that, in sterile compounding practice, hood-cleaning procedures are mandatory and must be performed prior to sterile compounding and at the intervals prescribed by USP Chapter <797>.

***Arranging and Preparing Supplies in the Hood*** Due to the large number of supplies used in the Chapter 13 procedural lab, bring supply items into the hood in stages in the order they are needed in the procedural lab. Once the hood has been cleaned, place small supply items—such as the vials, EEC, needles, syringes, and alcohol swabs—in the outer six-inch zone of the hood. Keep the large supply items in the transport vehicle until you are instructed to bring the items into the hood. (For additional assistance on arranging and preparing supplies in the hood, refer to Chapter 8.)

## TPN Compounding Procedure

When compounding a TPN solution, you must follow a specific order for mixing the ingredients. As mentioned earlier, you begin with the base solution components: dextrose first, followed by the amino acids (in this case, Aminosyn), and then the sterile water. You will add the additives last.

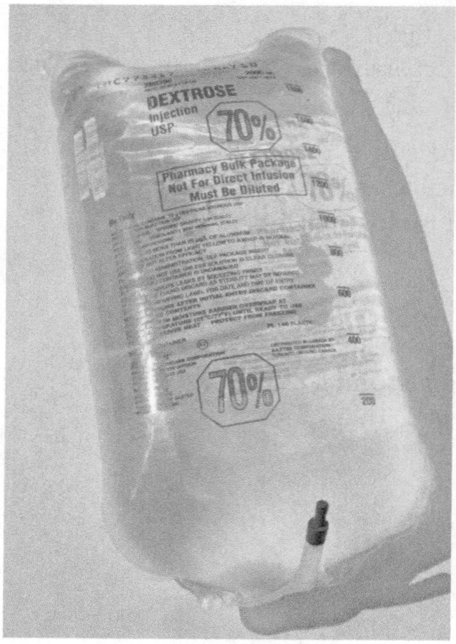

A $D_{70}W$ bag used in TPN preparation.

***Adding the First Base Component to the EEC*** With the small supply items arranged in the outer six-inch zone of the hood, you are ready to begin the TPN compounding procedure. Remove the outer dust cover from the first base component (in this lab, dextrose 70% in water [$D_{70}W$]); then place the dust cover into the waste container. Temporarily place the $D_{70}W$ bag onto the hood's work surface within the DCA. Place the IV tubing, regular needle, and an IPA swab into the DCA of the hood.

Remove the IV tubing from its outer wrapping. Shut the tubing clamp by rolling it downward. At one end of the tubing there is a needle adaptor. Remove the cap from this tubing needle adaptor and place it into the discard pile. While still holding the needle adaptor, carefully remove the outer wrapper from a regular needle. Aseptically attach the needle to the needle adaptor. Place the needle wrapper into the discard pile. Temporarily place the tubing—with the attached, capped needle—onto the hood's work surface within the DCA.

Grasp the pull tag on the tubing port plug of the $D_{70}W$ bag. Pull down on the pull tag to remove it from the tubing port. Grasp the drip chamber of the IV tubing with the thumb and forefinger of your dominant hand, so that the tip of the IV tubing spike is pointing toward your nondominant hand, and the thumb and forefinger rest against the plastic crossbar. Remove the cap from the IV tubing spike and carefully insert the spike into the bag's tubing port. Hang the $D_{70}W$ bag, with attached IV tubing, on a hook on the hood's hang bar.

Bring the EEC into the DCA of the hood and carefully remove the aluminum cap by gently lifting up the small pull tab on the top of the cap; then grasp the pull tab and pull it down toward the bottom of the EEC, pulling the tab all the way down and removing it. Take care not to twist the tab, so that it does not break in two. Once the entire tab has been removed, use it as a tool for prying off the aluminum ring that encircles the rubber stopper and EEC top. Lift off and then discard the coin-like aluminum circle resting atop the EEC's rubber stopper. This technique is illustrated in Figure 13.6.

Position the EEC within the DCA so that the top of the EEC receives uninterrupted airflow from the HEPA filter. Swab the rubber top of the EEC with sterile IPA. Place the used swab onto the hood's work surface within the DCA. Place the wrapper from the swab into the discard pile. Pick up the IV tubing at the capped needle end, holding the tube at the adaptor. Remove the needle cap and use proper needle insertion procedures to insert the needle—with attached tubing—into the top of the EEC.

FIGURE 13.6

**Cap Removal from an EEC**

To correctly remove the aluminum cap from an EEC, follow the same technique as removing the cap from a bulk vial.

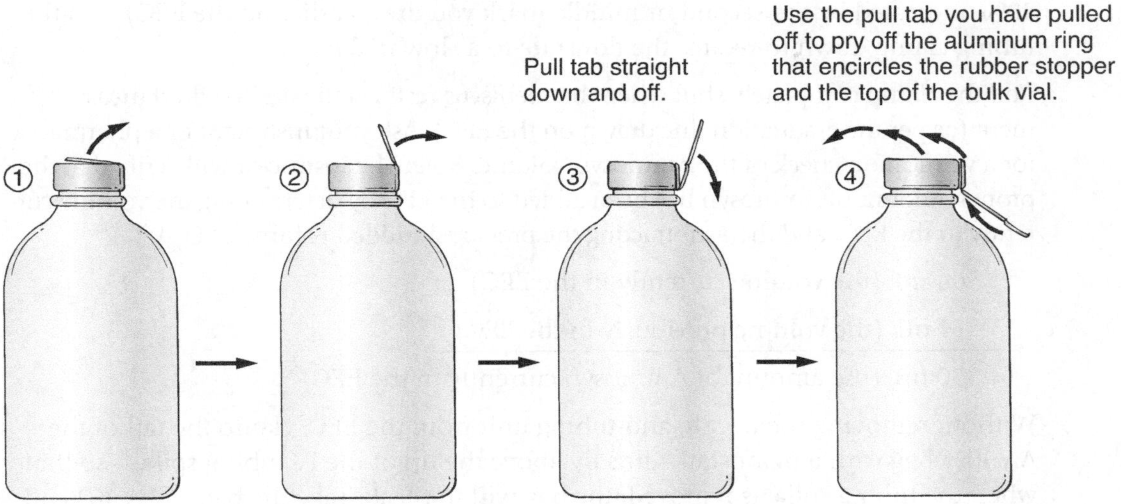

Use the pull tab you have pulled off to pry off the aluminum ring that encircles the rubber stopper and the top of the bulk vial.
Pull tab straight down and off.
①
②
③
④


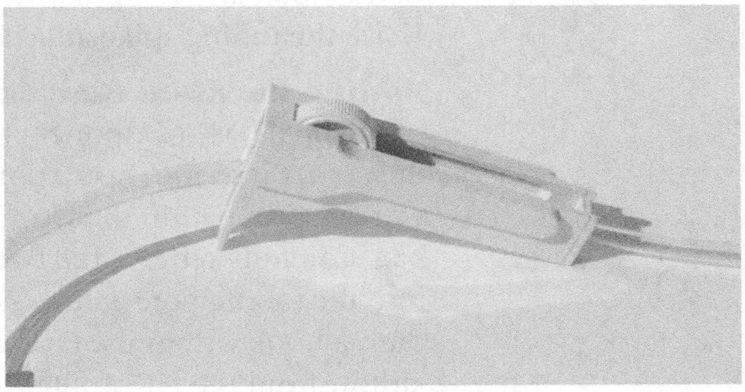

The IV tubing clamp rolls up and down to control the flow rate of the solution.

Begin the flow of $D_{70}W$ into the EEC by rolling up the IV tubing clamp. Monitor the flow of dextrose into the EEC. When the volume of fluid in the EEC reaches approximately 20 mL less than the desired volume of $D_{70}W$ (in this case, the desired volume of $D_{70}W$ is equivalent to the first, or lowest mark you made on the EEC bottle), roll the tubing clamp down to restrict the flow rate to a slow trickle. Roll the clamp completely shut when the **meniscus** rests on the desired fluid measurement (as per the graduation line drawn on the EEC). Ask your instructor or a pharmacist for a verification check of the $D_{70}W$ volume before continuing with the lab procedure.

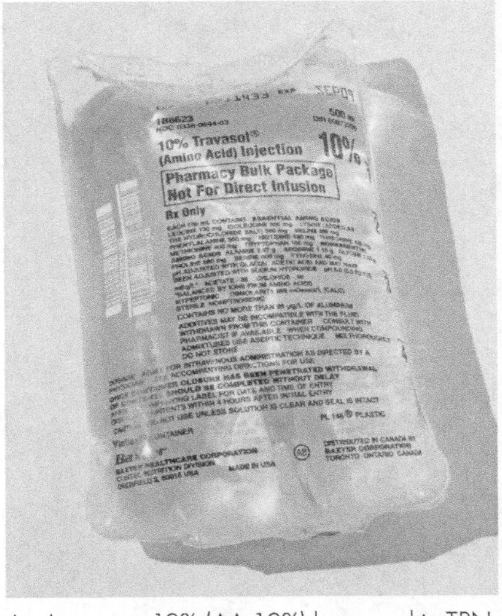


An Aminosyn 10% (AA 10%) bag used in TPN preparation.

Without removing the needle-and-tubing unit from the EEC, clamp the tail of the $D_{70}W$ bag with a hemostat—directly above the tip of the IV tubing spike—so that when the tubing spike is removed, the bag will not leak. Take the bag of $D_{70}W$ off the hook and temporarily lay it on the hood's work surface within the DCA. ***Note:*** Leave the tubing spike attached to the bag.

***Adding the Second Base Component to the EEC*** Remove the outer dust cover from the second base component (in this lab, Aminosyn 10% [AA 10%]), and then place the dust cover into the waste container. Temporarily place the AA 10% bag onto the hood's work surface within the DCA, and then pull down on the pull tag to remove it from the tubing port. Carefully remove the IV tubing spike from the $D_{70}W$ and immediately insert it into the tubing port on the AA 10% bag. Move the $D_{70}W$ bag, with hemostat still attached, back onto a hook within the DCA.

Place the bag of AA 10% onto another hook within the DCA. Begin the flow of AA 10% into the EEC by rolling the tubing clamp up. Monitor the flow of AA 10% into the EEC. When the volume of fluid in the EEC reaches approximately 20 mL less than the desired combined volume (or the volume of $D_{70}W$ plus the volume of AA 10%, indicated by the second or middle mark you drew earlier on the EEC), roll the tubing clamp down to reduce the flow rate to a slow trickle.

Roll the clamp completely shut when the meniscus rests on the desired fluid measurement (as per the graduation line drawn on the EEC). Ask your instructor or a pharmacist for a verification check of the Aminosyn volume. ***Note:*** The instructor will verify that the proper amount of Aminosyn has been added to the EEC by determining the volume currently in the EEC, and then subtracting the previously added volume of $D_{70}W$:

564 mL (the volume currently in the EEC)

– 214 mL (the volume previously in the EEC)

= 350 mL (the amount of Aminosyn currently in the EEC)

Without removing the needle-and-tubing unit from the EEC, clamp the tail of the AA 10% bag with a hemostat—directly above the tip of the IV tubing spike—so that when the tubing spike is removed, the bag will not leak. Take the bag of AA 10% off of the hook and temporarily lay it on the hood's work surface within the DCA. ***Note:*** Leave the tubing spike attached to the bag.

***Adding the Final Base Component to the EEC*** Remove the outer dust cover of the final base component bag (in this lab, sterile water [SW]), and then place the dust cover into the waste container. Temporarily place the SW bag onto the hood's work surface within the DCA. Remove the pull tag from the tubing port on the SW bag. Carefully remove the IV tubing spike from the AA 10%, and immediately insert it into the tubing port on the SW bag. Move the bag of AA 10% with attached hemostat onto a hook within the DCA (next to the bag of $D_{70}W$), so that it does not interrupt airflow from the HEPA filter.

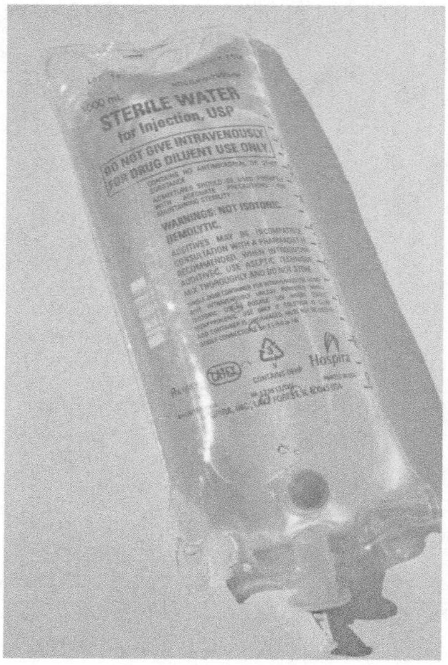


A 1000-mL bag of sterile water used in TPN preparation.

Hang the SW bag on another hook within the DCA. Begin the flow of SW into the EEC by rolling the tubing clamp up. Closely monitor the flow of SW into the EEC. When the volume of fluid in the EEC reaches approximately 20 mL less than the desired total volume (or the volume of $D_{70}W$ plus the volume of AA 10% plus the volume of SW, indicated by the third or uppermost line that you drew earlier on the EEC), roll the clamp down to reduce the flow rate to a slow trickle.

Roll the clamp completely shut when the meniscus rests on the desired fluid measurement (as per the graduation line drawn on the EEC). Ask your instructor or a pharmacist for a verification check of the SW bag. Using a third hemostat, clamp the tail of the SW bag just above the IV tubing spike. The hemostat prevents fluid from leaking out of the bag once the IV tubing spike has been removed from the SW bag.

Temporarily lay the SW bag on the hood's work surface within the DCA. Carefully remove the tubing spike from the SW bag and place it temporarily on the hood within the DCA. Grasp the opposite end of the IV tubing—on the hard plastic of the needle adaptor, just above the connection to the needle. Carefully remove the needle-and-tubing unit from the EEC.

Immediately place the needle-and-tubing unit into the sharps container. Hang the SW bag, with attached hemostat, on a hook within the DCA. Leave the EEC on the hood within the DCA.

***Preparing the TPN Additives*** Place all of the remaining supply items into the staging area of the hood. Review the CSP label to determine the first additive listed on the label; this additive is listed immediately below the base solution components, near the top of the CSP label. Bring the first additive vial into the DCA, remove the flip-top cap, and disinfect the vial's rubber top with an IPA swab. Assemble the appropriate-sized syringe and capped needle in such a way as to avoid touch contamination and shadowing of the syringe tip and needle hub. After removing the needle cap, use aseptic technique to insert the needle into the additive vial. Then use the milking technique to withdraw the appropriate volume of the first additive into the syringe. Place the filled-and-capped additive syringe next to the additive vial on the hood's work surface within the DCA. ***Note:*** For the purposes of this lab procedure, place each additive syringe to the immediate left of the vial from which it was withdrawn.

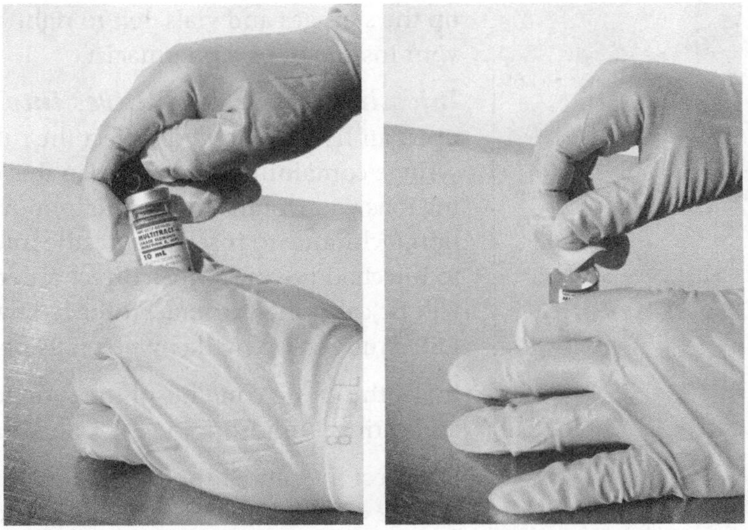

An IV technician removing an additive vial's flip-top cap and then swabbing the vial's rubber top.

Then bring the second additive vial into the DCA, remove the flip-top cap, and disinfect the vial's rubber top with an IPA swab. Aseptically assemble the appropriate syringe and capped needle. After removing the needle cap, use aseptic technique to insert the needle into the vial. Then use the milking technique to withdraw the appropriate volume of the additive into the syringe. Place the filled-and-capped additive syringe next to the additive vial on the hood's work surface within the DCA. ***Note:*** For the purposes of this lab procedure, place each additive syringe to the immediate left of the vial from which it was withdrawn.

**POINTER**

Policies regarding the placement of TPN syringes and vials may vary among facilities. Refer to your facility's P&P manual to determine whether additive syringes should be placed to the immediate left or immediate right of each vial. Regardless of the placement of the syringe, follow a consistent pattern when arranging supplies for a verification check.

Repeat this procedure with each of the remaining additive vials. As the additives are withdrawn from each vial, place the syringe on the hood, to the immediate left of the vial from which it was withdrawn (so that it lays immediately adjacent to the vial). Because several syringes and vials are needed for this procedure, place each syringe on the same side (the left side) of each vial after it is withdrawn from that vial.

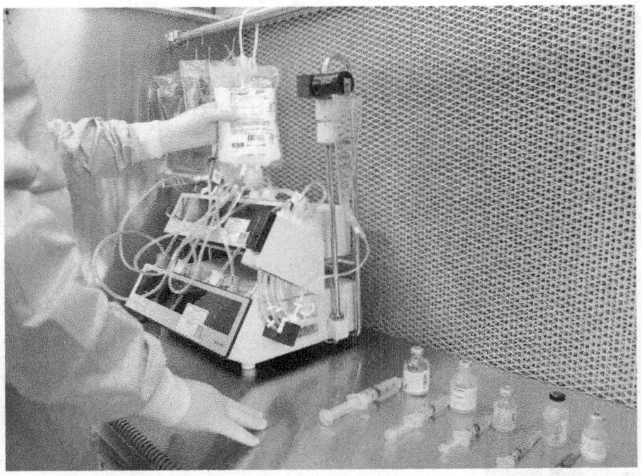

An IV technician awaiting a verification check on additives drawn up for the TPN preparation.

After you have placed each of the additives to the immediate left of the vials from which they were withdrawn and lined

**POINTER**
To avoid coring, do not inject needles immediately adjacent to holes made by previous needle insertions in the EEC's rubber top. Coring the top of the EEC causes contamination of the TPN solution and requires you to repeat the entire procedure from the beginning, using new supply items.

**POINTER**
Some facilities use a special supply item called a *male adaptor plug*, or *port saver*. The small injection plug attaches to the needles, and the additives are then injected into the EEC. The plug allows multiple additives to be injected into the EEC through one needle (via the male adaptor plug), thereby reducing the likelihood of coring the top of the EEC due to multiple needle insertions.

up the syringes and vials, left to right, within the DCA, await a verification check by your instructor or a pharmacist.

***Injecting the TPN Additives into the EEC*** After the verification check, open an IPA swab and disinfect the rubber top of the EEC. Pick up the first additive syringe containing phosphate (in this case, the potassium phosphate syringe), holding it as you would a dart. After removing the needle cap, use proper needle insertion technique to insert the needle into the rubber top of the EEC. As you continue to inject additives (in the correct order and remembering that the final two additives will be calcium gluconate, followed by MVI), take care to avoid the holes in the EEC's rubber top made by previous needle insertions.

Inject the entire contents of the syringe into the EEC. Carefully remove the needle-and-syringe unit from the EEC, and place it into the sharps container.

Disinfect the rubber top of the EEC with a new sterile, 70% IPA swab. Pick up the syringe containing the next additive from the hood surface. Using proper needle insertion, carefully insert the needle into the top of the EEC. ***Note:*** The vacuum within the EEC may pull the fluid out of the syringe and into the EEC without you having to push down on the plunger's flat knob.

Inject the syringe contents into the EEC. Place the empty needle-and-syringe unit into the sharps container. Repeat the procedure with each of the remaining additives, until all of the additives have been injected into the EEC.

Examine the filled EEC for solution clarity, particulate matter, or evidence of incompatibility. Label the EEC containing the compounded TPN solution with the CSP label, and cover the EEC's rubber top with an IVA seal.

***Performing Clean-up Procedures*** Upon completion of the TPN compounding procedure, dispose of used vials and supply items in the appropriate waste container. Return the TPN, the clamped base component bags, and any unused supply items to the transport vehicle, and then return them to the anteroom.

Destroy the base component bags by cutting off the bags' tails with a pair of scissors, draining their contents down the sink, and then disposing of the empty bags in a waste receptacle. Wipe off the hemostats and scissors with a damp paper towel, and then return them to their storage locations in the anteroom.

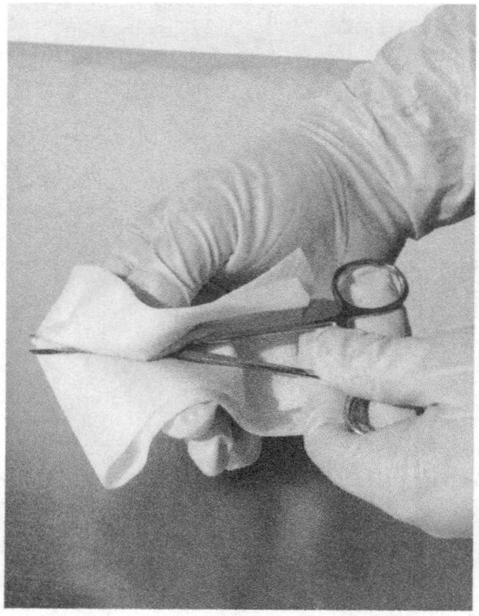
Cleaning the hemostats at the completion of a TPN compounding procedure.

Record the date and your initials on the CSP label. Remove PPE in the order and manner described in Chapter 6 of this textbook.

# Watch the Demonstration Video

*Watch the Chapter 13 Demonstration Video, which shows the step-by-step aseptic procedures for manually compounding TPN solutions. For the purposes of the Chapter 13 Demonstration Video, neither aseptic hand washing nor hood cleaning is demonstrated. Refer to the Chapter 6 video for a demonstration of aseptic hand-washing procedures, and to the Chapter 7 video for a demonstration of correct hood-cleaning procedures.*

Training Videos DVD

# Procedural Lab

*This lab walks you through the step-by-step actions that you must follow to properly prepare a 2-in-1 TPN solution using the manual compounding method. Take your time. Work through each step methodically and with close attention to detail.*

**Note:** *For the purposes of this procedural lab, you will not perform aseptic hand-washing or hood-cleaning procedures unless directed to do so by your instructor. Should your instructor ask you to perform these procedures, refer to Chapter 6 for instructions on aseptic hand washing and to Chapter 7 for directions on correct hood cleaning.*

**Note:** *For step 1 below, please refer to Chapter 4 for a reminder of the step-by-step procedures required for medication order and CSP label verification. For steps 2–14, refer to Chapter 5 for pharmacy calculation procedures. For steps 15–18, refer to Chapter 3 for a reminder of the process for gathering and cleaning supplies. For steps 19–25, refer to Chapter 6 for step-by-step aseptic garbing, hand-washing, and gloving procedures. You should perform steps 1–22 and steps 64–67 in the anteroom. Perform steps 23–63 in the clean room.*

## Supplies

### *Essential Supplies*

To complete the Unit 2 procedural labs, you will need to ensure that various essential anteroom and clean room supplies such as those listed in Table 13.3 are available for your use.

**Table 13.3 Essential Anteroom and Clean Room Supplies for Sterile Compounding**

| Anteroom Supplies |
|---|
| medication order form (TPN order form) and CSP label (TPN label)<br>calculator<br>pen<br>permanent, felt-tip marker<br>plastic bags (small and large)<br>aseptic garb, including shoe covers, hair cover, face mask, and beard cover (if appropriate)<br>sterile gown<br>presaturated, aseptic cleaning wipes<br>sterile, foamed 70% IPA<br>waste container<br>transport vehicle (optional) |
| **Clean Room Supplies** |
| sterile, foamed 70% IPA<br>sterile, powder-free gloves<br>sterile, 70% IPA swabs, individually packaged × 9<br>sharps container<br>waste container<br>laminar airflow hood |

### *Procedure-Specific Supplies*

In addition to the supplies listed in Table 13.3, gather the following items specific to the Chapter 13 TPN procedural lab:

- regular needles (nonfilter, nonvented needles, either 18 or 19 gauge) × 8
- dextrose 70% in water ($D_{70}W$), 2000 mL (may substitute any volume bag size ≥ 500 mL)

- Aminosyn 10% (AA 10%), 500 mL (may substitute any volume bag size ≥ 500 mL)
- sterile water (SW), 1000 mL (may substitute any volume bag size ≥ 500 mL)
- 1000-mL EEC
- potassium phosphate ($KP0_4$), 3 Mm/mL vial
- sodium chloride (NaCl), 4 mEq/mL vial
- potassium chloride (KCl), 2 mEq/mL vial
- trace minerals, 5-mL vial
- MVI, 10-mL vial
- Humulin R (regular) insulin, 100 units/mL vial
- calcium gluconate, 0.48 mEq/mL vial
- 1-mL Luer-lock syringe
- 5-mL Luer-lock syringe × 2
- 10-mL Luer-lock syringe × 3
- 30-mL Luer-lock syringe
- hemostats × 3
- IV tubing
- IVA seal
- scissors (used during disposal of base component fluids)
- paper towels (used to clean hemostats and scissors)
- access to sink appropriate for base component fluid disposal

## Procedure

### *Verifying the Label*

1. Review the CSP label to verify that all of the information on the label matches the TPN medication order. To help you with this task, compare the CSP label (see Figure 13.7) to the medication order (see Figure 13.8).

**FIGURE 13.7**

**CSP Label for TPN**

****Total Parenteral Nutrition****

Memorial Hospital

**Pt. Name:** Sarah Mansfield **Room:** TCU-07

**Pt. ID#:** 66734 **Rx#:** 126981

**Base Solution Concentration:**
**Dextrose 15%**
**Aminosyn 3.5%**
**Sterile Water qs to 1000 mL TV**
**Rate: 40 mL/hr**

**Additives:**
**Sodium chloride 40 mEq**
**Potassium chloride 20 mEq**
**Potassium phosphate 12 mM**
**Calcium gluconate 10 mEq**
**Multiple vitamins 10 mL**
**Trace minerals 5 mL**
**Regular insulin 60 units**

Keep refrigerated – warm to room temperature before administration.

Expiration Day/Time: __________ Tech ______ RPh ______

**FIGURE 13.8**

**TPN Medication Order**

**Memorial Hospital Pharmacy**

**Pt. Name:** Sarah Mansfield **Pt. ID#:** 66734
**Room:** TCU-07 **Rx#:** 126981

## Physician Orders

## TOTAL PARENTERAL NUTRITION (TPN) ADULT

**Primary Diagnosis:** Multiple Trauma – post MVA **Ht:** 181 cm Dosing Wt: 80 kg

**DOB:** 2/11/80 **Allergies:** NKDA

**Instructions:** This form must be completed for a new order or continuation of PN and faxed to the pharmacy by 2 pm to receive same-day preparation. TPN administration begins at 6 pm daily.

**Administration Route:** ☒ CVC or PICC *Note: Proper tip placement of the CVC or PICC must be confirmed prior to PN infusion.*
❑ Peripheral IV (PIV) (*Final PN Osmolarity ≤ ____ mOsm/L*)

**Monitoring:** Daily weights; strict input & output; bedside glucose monitoring every 8 hours
☒ Na, K, Cl, $CO_2$, Glucose, BUN, Scr, Mg, $PO_4$ every Day
☒ T. Billi, Alk Phos, AST, ALT, Albumin, Triglycerides, Calcium every Week

**Base Solution:** *Total parenteral nutrition **MUST** be administered through a dedicated infusion port and filtered with a 1.2-micron in-line filter at all times. Discard any unused volume after 24 hours.*
*Select one*

| ❑ PERIPHERAL 2-in-1 | ☒ CENTRAL 2-in-1 | ❑ CENTRAL 3-in-1 |
|---|---|---|
| Dextrose ____ g | Dextrose 15% | Dextrose ____ g |
| Amino Acids (*Brand* ____) ____ g | Amino Acids (*Brand* Aminosyn) 3.5% | Amino Acids (*Brand* ____) ____ g |
| | | Fat Emulsion (*Brand* ____) ____ g |
| *For patients with PIV and established glucose tolerance; provides ____ kcal; maximum rate not to exceed ____ mL/hour.* | *For patients with CVC or PICC and established glucose tolerance; provides ____ kcal; maximum rate not to exceed ____ mL/hour.* | *For patients with CVC or PICC and established glucose/fat emulsion tolerance; provides ____ kcal; maximum rate not to exceed ____ mL/hour.* *Use of additional fat emulsion not required with 3-in-1 base solution.* |

**RATE & VOLUME:** 40 mL/hour for 24 hours = 960 mL/day
***Must specify***
*or* CYCLIC INFUSION: ____ mL/hour for ____ hours, then ____ mL/hour for ____ hours = ____ mL/day

**Fat Emulsion (Brand 0) – via PIV or CVC with 2-in-1 base solutions (select caloric density & volume)**

❑ 10% ❑ 20% Infuse at ____ mL/hour over ____ hours. Frequency ____
❑ 250 mL ❑ 500 mL *(Note: Infusions < 4 or > 12 hours not recommended)* *Discard any unused volume after 12 hours.*

| **Additives:** (per liter) | | *Normal Dosages* |
|---|---|---|
| **Sodium** Chloride | 40 mEq | *1–2 mEq sodium/kg/day* |
| as Acetate | ____ mEq | *pH or $CO_2$ dependent* |
| as Phosphate | ____ mmol of $PO_4$ | *Consider if hyperkalemic* |
| **Potassium** Chloride | 20 mEq | *1–2 mEq potassium/kg/day* |
| as Acetate | ____ mEq | *pH or $CO_2$ dependent* |
| as Phosphate | 12 mmol of $PO_4$ | *20-40 mmol/day (1 mmol Phos = 1.5 mEq K)* |
| **Calcium Gluconate** | 10 mEq | *5–15 mEq/day* |
| Magnesium **Sulfate** | ____ mEq | *8–24 mEq/day* |
| Adult **Multivitamins** | 10 mL/day | *Contains vitamin K 160 mcg* |
| Adult **Trace Elements** | 5 mL/day | *Zn __ mg, Cu __ mg, Mn __ mg, Cr __ mcg, Se __ mcg (with normal hepatic function)* |
| **$H_2$ Antagonist** | ____ mg | *____ mg/day with normal renal function* |
| **Other:** | | |

**Additives:** (per liter)
**Regular Insulin** 60 units
*Recommended if hyperglycemic; start with 1 unit for every 10 g of dextrose.*

**Pharmacy Use Only:** Ca/$PO_4$
**Limit Checked** MKing, RPh
*(Note: Some brands of amino acids contain phosphate.)*

Physician's Signature Kumar Singh, MD Pager Number: 6-5411 Date/time: 8/14/2016

Orders transcribed by: RMcManus Date/time: 8/14/16 11:30 am Orders verified by: MKing, RPh Date/time: 8 14 16 2:45 pm

### *Calculating the Desired Volume of Dextrose*

2. Read the TPN order (and corresponding CSP label) to determine the desired concentration (DC) of dextrose and the desired total volume (TV) of the TPN solution. Then look at the dextrose base component (BC) to determine its concentration.

3. Assuming that the TPN order calls for a desired dextrose concentration of 15%, and a total volume of 1000 mL, and the dextrose base component ($D_{70}W$) has a concentration of 70%, perform a calculation to determine the amount of $D_{70}W$ in milliliters ($x$ mL) needed to prepare the TPN. Use the formula: (TV / BC) × DC = $x$ mL.

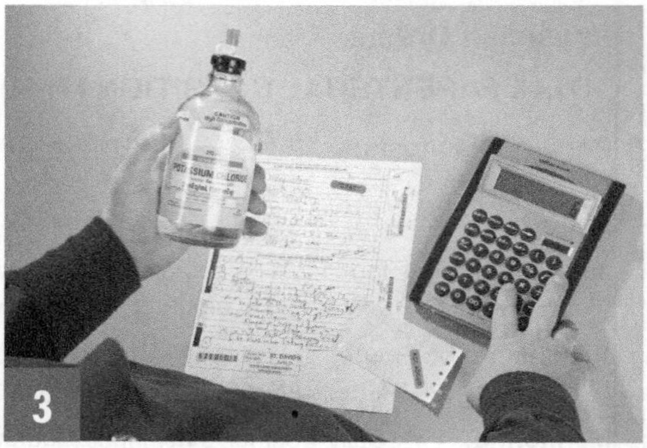

   (1000 / 70) × 15 = $x$ mL

   (1000 / 70 = 14.29) × 15 = 214.29 or 214 mL (rounded to the nearest mL)

4. Use a permanent marker to record the approximate volume of 214 mL on the EEC.

   ***Note:*** Because each graduation mark on a 1000-mL EEC indicates a 20-mL change in volume, it is impossible to accurately measure a volume of 214 mL. Therefore, you should mark the EEC at/or just slightly below the 220-mL graduation indicator on the EEC.

### *Calculating the Desired Volume of Aminosyn*

5. Read the TPN order to determine the desired concentration (DC) of Aminosyn, and the desired total volume (TV) of the TPN solution. Look at the Aminosyn base component (BC) to determine its concentration.

6. Assuming that the TPN order calls for a desired Aminosyn concentration of 3.5% and a total volume of 1000 mL, and the Aminosyn base component (AA 10%) has a concentration of 10%, perform a calculation to determine the amount of AA in milliliters needed to prepare the TPN. Use the formula: TV / BC × DC = $x$ mL.

   (1000 / 10) × 3.5 = $x$ mL

   (1000 / 10 = 100) × 3.5 = 350 mL

7. Calculate the volume of dextrose plus the volume of Aminosyn:

   214 mL + 350 mL = 564 mL

   Use a permanent marker to record the approximate volume of 564 mL on the EEC. ***Note:*** Since each graduation mark on a 1000-mL EEC indicates a 20-mL change in volume, it is impossible to accurately measure a volume of 564 mL. Therefore, you should mark the EEC at/or slightly above the 560-mL graduation indicator.

### *Calculating the Desired Volumes of Additives*

**8.** Look at the TPN order to determine the desired dose of the first additive, and then look at the vial label on the corresponding additive (the sodium chloride label). Perform a calculation to determine the volume of sodium chloride needed for the TPN. Assuming that the desired dosage is 40 mEq and the concentration on the sodium chloride label indicates that it has a concentration of 4 mEq/mL, use the basic formula calculation to determine the volume needed for this dose.

40 mEq / 4 mEq = $x$ mL

40 / 4 = 10 mL

Therefore, 10 mL must be drawn up for this TPN.

**9.** Using a ballpoint pen, neatly record the amount you determined in step 8, in parentheses, on the TPN order, immediately following the sodium chloride dosage. For this lab, record *(10 mL)*.

**10.** Look at the TPN order to determine the desired dose of the second additive, and then look at the vial label on the corresponding additive. For this lab, look at the potassium chloride label. Perform a calculation to determine the volume of potassium chloride needed for the TPN. Assuming that the desired dosage is 20 mEq and the concentration on the potassium chloride label indicates that it has a concentration of 2 mEq/mL, use the basic formula calculation to determine the volume needed for this dose.

20 mEq / 2 mEq = $x$ mL

20 / 2 = 10 mL

Therefore, 10 mL must be drawn up for this TPN.

**11.** Using a ballpoint pen, neatly record the amount you determined in step 10, in parenthesis, on the TPN order (in this case, *10 mL*), immediately following the potassium chloride dosage.

**12.** Repeat steps 10 and 11 for each of the remaining additives, except for the trace minerals (TM) and MVI additives on the TPN order. ***Note:*** The trace mineral and MVI dose ordered by the prescriber is already in milliliters. Therefore, you simply draw up the volume indicated on the TPN order for these two additives.

**POINTER**

Remember that the basic formula is D / H = $x$ mL. *D* represents the desired dose (the dose ordered by the prescriber on the TPN order); *H* represents the concentration on hand (the concentration strength of the drug *per milliliter*); and $x$ represents the unknown volume of the additive needed to be drawn up for the preparation of the TPN.

### *Calculating the Desired Volume of Sterile Water*

**13.** To calculate the desired volume of sterile water (SW), add together the volume of each of the additives. You determined the volume of each additive in steps 8–12. Then, determine the volume of sterile water needed for the TPN by subtracting the volume of dextrose, Aminosyn, and all of the additives (determined in steps 2–12 above) from the desired total volume (TV) of the TPN solution.

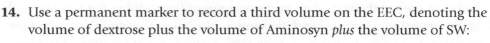

10 mL sodium chloride
10 mL potassium chloride
4 mL potassium phosphate
20.83 mL calcium gluconate
5 mL trace minerals
10 mL MVI
+ 0.6 mL regular insulin

= 60.43 or approximately 60 mL (rounded to the nearest mL); the total volume of additives

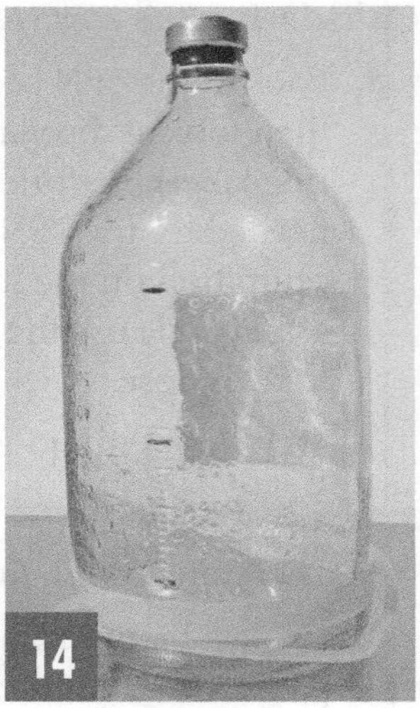


Now, starting with 1000 mL, *subtract* 214 mL (the volume of $D_{70}W$), *subtract* 350 mL (the volume of AA 10%), and then *subtract* 60 mL (the volume of all the additives) = *x* mL of SW

1000 – 214 – 350 – 60 = 376 mL of SW

**POINTER**
Once the additives have been injected into the TPN base solution, the total volume will be 1000 mL. You can check this by adding the following volumes: 214 mL ($D_{70}W$) + 350 mL (AA 10%) + 376 mL (SW) + 60 mL (additives) = 1000 mL (TV)

**14.** Use a permanent marker to record a third volume on the EEC, denoting the volume of dextrose plus the volume of Aminosyn *plus* the volume of SW:

214 mL + 350 mL + 376 mL = 940 mL

Mark the approximate volume of 940 mL on the EEC. The three marks on the EEC make it easier for you to measure the proper base component volumes.

### *Gathering and Cleaning Supplies*

**15.** Gather all of the remaining items on the Chapter 13 supply list.

**16.** Open the package of aseptic cleaning wipes. Remove one or, if necessary, more wipes, and thoroughly wipe down the entire transport vehicle.

**17.** Place used wipes in the waste receptacle.

**18.** Remove a new aseptic cleaning wipe and wipe down the exterior surface of each of the supply items. Place the cleaned supply items into the transport vehicle. Place the used wipes into the waste receptacle. Place the CSP label and TPN order form into plastic bags.

### *Garbing*

**POINTER**
During aseptic garbing, best practice is to reapply sterile, foamed 70% IPA to your hands after donning shoe covers and again after donning a hair cover.

**19.** Don shoe covers.

**20.** Put on a hair cover.

**21.** Don a face mask and beard cover (if appropriate).

*Note:* For the purposes of this training lab, you will skip the mandatory aseptic hand-washing procedure.

**22.** Don a sterile gown.

**23.** Bring all supply items, including an unopened package of sterile, powder-free gloves, into the clean room.

**24.** Place the transport vehicle onto a clean surface or countertop within the clean room. If a cart is used, position it so that it does not interrupt airflow into the hood prefilter.

25. Apply sterile, foamed 70% IPA to your hands. Allow them to air-dry and then don sterile gloves.

*Note:* For the purposes of this training lab, you will skip the mandatory hood-cleaning procedure.

### *Preparing the TPN Base Solution: Adding $D_{70}W$ to the EEC*

26. Remove the bag of $D_{70}W$ from the dust cover. Place the dust cover into the waste container. Place the $D_{70}W$ bag temporarily onto the hood's work surface within the DCA. Place the IV tubing, regular needle, and IPA swabs into the outer six-inch staging area of the hood.
27. Remove the outer wrapping from the IV tubing. Place the IV tubing onto the hood's work surface, within the DCA. Place the tubing's outer wrapper into the waste container. Roll the tubing clamp shut by using your thumb and forefinger to roll the clamp down, toward the tubing needle adaptor.
28. Manipulate the needle adaptor at the end of the tubing, opposite the spike, so that it receives uninterrupted airflow from the HEPA filter. Hold the tubing between the thumb and forefinger of your dominant hand, approximately one inch back from the cap covering the needle adaptor on the end of the tubing. Use your nondominant hand to remove the cap from the needle adaptor. Place the cap from the needle adaptor into the discard pile. Take care not to touch or shadow the uncapped needle adaptor at any time.
29. While holding the tubing needle adaptor, carefully remove the outer wrapper from a regular needle. Aseptically attach the needle to the adaptor. Place the needle package into the discard pile. Temporarily place the tubing—with attached, capped needle—onto the hood's work surface within the DCA.
30. Position the pull tag on the $D_{70}W$ bag so that it receives uninterrupted airflow from the HEPA filter. Grasp the pull tag on the bag's tubing port and pull it down and off, thereby removing the tubing port plug from the bag.
31. Grasp the drip chamber of the IV tubing with the thumb and forefinger of your dominant hand, such that the tip of the tubing spike is pointing toward your nondominant hand and the thumb and forefinger rest against the plastic crossbar.
32. Keeping the tubing within the DCA, use your nondominant hand to remove the spike cap. Place the spike cap into the discard pile.
33. Grasp the tail of the tubing port on the $D_{70}W$ with the thumb and forefinger of your nondominant hand. Aseptically insert the IV tubing spike into the bag's tubing port. Use a gentle back-and-forth, twisting motion to ensure that the spike is completely inserted into the port. Hang the $D_{70}W$ bag, with attached tubing-and-needle unit, onto a hook on the hang bar within the hood so that it does not impede HEPA filter airflow to any of the other supply items.
34. Bring the EEC into the hood and carefully remove the aluminum cap by gently lifting up the small pull tab on the top of the cap. Grasp the pull tab and pull it down toward the bottom of the EEC, pulling the tab all the way down and removing it. Take care not

**POINTER**

If you are using IV tubing that has a pinch clamp instead of a roll clamp, pinch the clamp firmly onto the tubing to shut it.

**POINTER**

Be sure not to touch or shadow the IV tubing spike or the tubing port of the $D_{70}W$ bag at any time during the procedure. These areas are critical sites and are supplied from the manufacturer in sterile form. Therefore, they should not be swabbed with alcohol.

**BE AWARE**

Take care when removing an EEC's aluminum cap. Using a twisting motion to remove the cap creates a sharp, jagged edge and may lead to injury. To remove the cap safely, pull down on the tab.

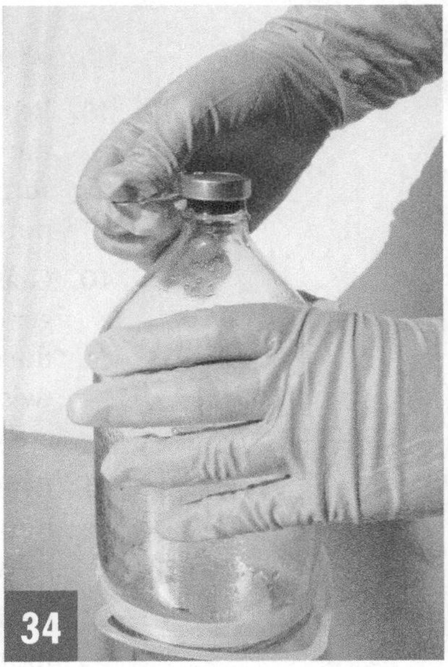

34

to twist the tab, so that it does not break in two. Once the entire tab has been removed, use it as a tool for prying off the aluminum ring that encircles the rubber stopper and EEC top. Lift off and discard the coin-like aluminum cap resting atop the EEC's rubber stopper.

35. Position the EEC within the DCA so that the top of the EEC receives uninterrupted airflow from the HEPA filter. Open an IPA swab and disinfect the rubber top of the EEC. Place the used swab onto the hood's work surface within the DCA. Place the wrapper from the swab into the discard pile.

36. Pick up the tubing at the end with the capped needle. Holding the tubing adaptor, carefully remove the needle cap and place it onto the IPA swab. Using proper needle insertion technique, insert the needle—with attached tubing—into the top of the EEC.

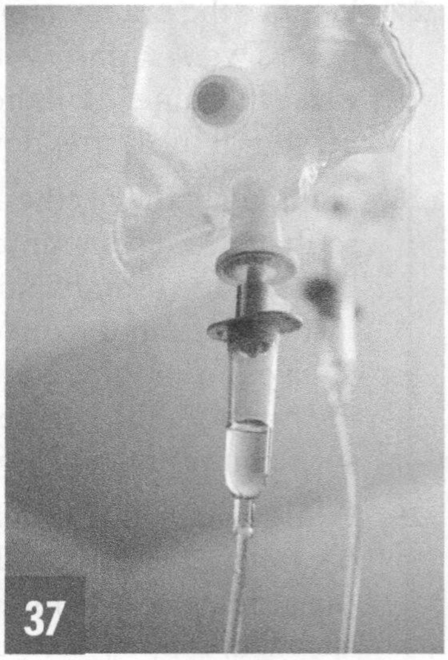
37

37. Begin the flow of $D_{70}W$ into the EEC by rolling the tubing clamp up. Closely monitor the flow of dextrose into the EEC. When the volume of fluid in the EEC reaches approximately 200 mL (or approximately 20 mL less than the desired volume of $D_{70}W$), roll the clamp down to restrict the flow rate to a slow trickle. Roll the clamp completely shut when the meniscus of the fluid rests on your first mark on the EEC (i.e., the mark that indicates a volume of approximately 214 mL). Ask for a verification check by your instructor or a pharmacist of the $D_{70}W$ volume in the EEC.

38. After the base component verification check, and without removing the needle-and-tubing unit from the EEC, clamp the tail of the tubing port of the $D_{70}W$ bag with a hemostat, directly above the tip of the tubing spike. Take the bag of $D_{70}W$ off the hook and temporarily lay it on the hood's work surface within the DCA.

### *Adding Aminosyn to the EEC*

39. Remove the outer dust cover from the AA 10% bag. Place the dust cover into the waste container. Place the AA 10% bag temporarily onto the hood's work surface within the DCA. Pull down on the pull tag to remove it from the tubing port on the AA 10% bag.

40. Grasp the tail of the tubing port of the $D_{70}W$ bag between the thumb and forefinger of your nondominant hand. Grasp the drip chamber of the tubing between the thumb and forefinger of your dominant hand. Use a gentle back-and-forth, twisting motion to pull the IV tubing spike out of the bag's tubing port. Immediately insert the tubing spike into the tubing port of the AA 10% bag.

**POINTER**
When placing items on the hang bar, be sure that they do not interrupt airflow to the other supply items in the hood.

41. Return the $D_{70}W$ bag, with the hemostat still attached, back onto the hang bar hook. Place the bag of AA 10% onto another hook on the hood's hang bar, next to the bag of $D_{70}W$.

42. Begin the flow of AA 10% into the EEC by rolling the tubing clamp up. Closely monitor the flow of AA 10% into the EEC. When the volume of fluid in the EEC reaches approximately 540 mL (or approximately 20 mL less than the

desired combined volume of dextrose and Aminosyn), roll the clamp down to reduce the flow rate to a slow trickle. Roll the clamp completely shut when the meniscus of the fluid rests on your second mark on the EEC (i.e., the mark that indicates a volume of approximately 564 mL). Ask for a verification check by your instructor or a pharmacist of the Aminosyn volume in the EEC.

**43.** Without removing the needle-and-tubing unit from the EEC, clamp the tail of the AA 10% bag with a new hemostat, directly above the tip of the IV tubing spike, so that when the tubing spike is removed, the bag will not leak. Take the bag of AA 10% off of the hook and temporarily lay it on the hood's work surface within the DCA.

### *Adding Sterile Water to the EEC*

**44.** After the pharmacist's or instructor's base component verification check, repeat steps 39–41 using the SW bag.

**45.** Begin the flow of SW into the EEC by rolling the tubing clamp up. Closely monitor the flow of SW into the EEC. When the volume of fluid in the EEC reaches approximately 920 mL (or approximately 20 mL less than the desired total volume), roll the clamp down to reduce the flow rate to a slow trickle. Roll the clamp completely shut when the meniscus rests on the third mark you made on the EEC (i.e., the mark that indicates a volume of approximately 940 mL).

**46.** Clamp the third hemostat to the tail of the SW bag, just above the tubing spike. The hemostat in this location prevents fluid from leaking out of the bag once the IV tubing has been removed from the SW bag.

**47.** Temporarily lay the SW bag on the hood's work surface within the DCA. Carefully remove the IV tubing spike from the SW bag and temporarily place the tubing on the hood within the DCA. Grasp the opposite end of the IV tubing—on the hard plastic of the needle adaptor, just above the connection point to the needle. Carefully remove the needle-and-tubing unit from the EEC. Immediately place the needle-and-tubing unit into the sharps container. Hang the SW bag with attached hemostat on a hook within the DCA. Leave the EEC—which contains the three base solution components, but no longer has attached IV tubing—on the hood's work surface within the DCA.

### *Preparing the TPN Additives*

**48.** Place all of the remaining supply items into the outer six-inch staging area of the hood. Bring the sodium chloride into the DCA and remove the flip-top cap. Open an IPA swab and disinfect the vial's rubber top. Place the used swab onto the hood's work surface within the DCA.

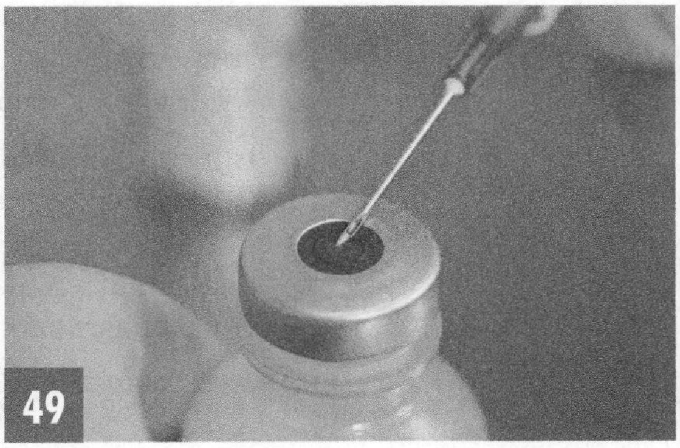


**49.** Aseptically attach a regular needle to a 10-mL syringe. Pull down on the flat knob of the plunger to draw approximately 10 mL of air into the empty syringe. Remove the needle cap and place it on the alcohol swab. Use proper needle insertion technique to insert the needle into the sodium chloride vial.

50. Use a clockwise motion (counterclockwise if you are left-handed) to invert the vial above the attached needle-and-syringe unit. Use the milking technique to withdraw the appropriate volume of sodium chloride into the syringe.

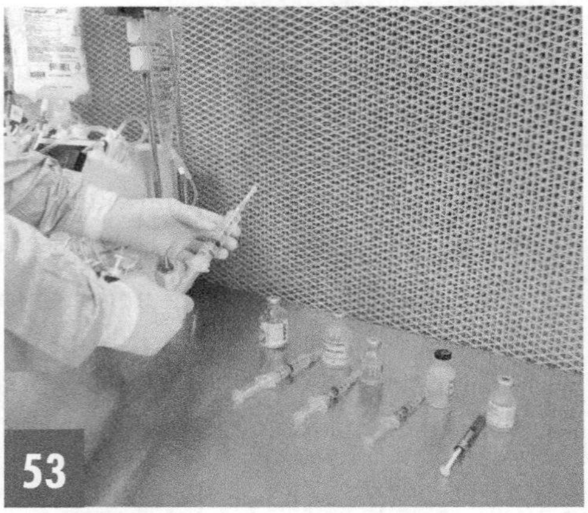

53

51. Use a counterclockwise motion (clockwise if you are left-handed) to return the vial with attached needle-and-syringe unit to its original position, with the vial upright on the hood's work surface.

52. Holding only the barrel of the syringe, carefully remove the needle-and-syringe unit from the vial. Carefully recap the needle of the filled syringe. Set the filled syringe and vial to the far left of the staging area within the DCA, placing the syringe on the left side of the vial.

53. Repeat steps 48–52 with each of the other additives. Draw the correct volume of each additive into the appropriate-sized syringe and then place it immediately adjacent and to the left of the vial from which it was withdrawn. Line up the syringes and vials left to right within the DCA.

54. Ask for a verification check by your instructor or a pharmacist of the filled syringes and vials, as well as the base solution EEC.

**POINTER**

In order to inject the additives into the EEC in the proper order (i.e., phosphate first, followed by all of the other additives, then the calcium, and lastly, the MVI), you may find it helpful to rearrange the syringes on the hood from the original order in which they were drawn up to the order in which they must be added.

**BE AWARE**

Remember that potassium phosphate and calcium gluconate should not be injected consecutively into a TPN because a precipitate will form. Separate the two additives by injecting the potassium phosphate first, followed by all of the other TPN additives, then the calcium gluconate, and, finally, the MVI.

### *Injecting the TPN Additives into the EEC*

55. After the verification check, open a new IPA swab and disinfect the top of the EEC. Place the used swab on the hood's work surface within the DCA.

56. Pick up the potassium phosphate syringe, holding the syringe as you would a dart. Remove the needle cap and place the cap onto the IPA swab on the hood's work surface. Using proper needle insertion technique, insert the needle into the EEC's rubber top.

57. Push down on the flat knob of the plunger until all of the potassium phosphate has been injected into the EEC. Holding the syringe at the barrel, carefully remove the needle-and-syringe unit from the EEC and place it into the sharps container.

58. Open a new IPA swab and reswab the rubber top of the EEC. Pick up the syringe containing the next additive—in this case, sodium chloride—holding it as you would a dart. Remove the needle cap and place it onto an alcohol swab.

59. Using proper needle insertion technique, insert the needle into the rubber top of the EEC. Push down on the flat knob of the plunger to inject the sodium chloride into the EEC. Holding only the barrel of the syringe, remove the needle-and-syringe unit from the EEC. Place the empty needle-and-syringe unit into the sharps container.

60. Repeat steps 55–59 to inject all of the remaining additives.

61. Examine the EEC—which now contains TPN base solution and all of the additives—to verify that the solution is free of particulate matter or other evidence of incompatibility.

62. Remove the CSP label from the plastic bag and affix the label to the EEC containing the compounded TPN solution. Be sure that the label does not cover any of the graduation markings on the EEC. Then cover the EEC's rubber top with an IVA seal.

***Cleaning Up After the Procedure***

63. Upon completion of the TPN compounding procedure, dispose of used vials and supply items in the appropriate waste container.

64. Return the TPN and any unused supply items to the transport vehicle, and then return the vehicle to the anteroom.

65. In the anteroom, complete the compounding procedure by using a ballpoint pen to record the date and your initials on the CSP label. Return any unused supply items to their proper storage locations. Remove PPE according to standard procedures, as described in Chapter 6 of this textbook.

66. Place the base component bags into the sink. Remove the hemostats. Destroy each of the base component bags by cutting a hole through the PVC with a pair of scissors. Dump the remaining fluid from each of the bags down the sink. Place the empty PVC bags into a waste container. Wipe off the hemostats and scissors with a damp paper towel, and then return them to their storage locations in the anteroom.

67. Ask for a final verification check from your instructor or a pharmacist.

# Process Validation by Instructor

*Your instructor will use the process validation checklist provided in Appendix D to evaluate your technique for this lab. In order to receive ACPE certification, and prior to making TPN CSPs for patient use, you must correctly perform each component of the lab procedure. Review the Chapter 13 lab and thoroughly practice each of the steps prior to your evaluation.*

# Part 3: Assessment

## Chapter Summary

- Theories regarding the impact of nutrition on wellness have existed for thousands of years.
- Rectal feedings were commonly used in early civilizations to treat diseases, supplement fluid loss, and improve the overall well-being of patients.
- Twelfth-century Muslim physician Avenzoar was the first practitioner to attempt parenteral nutrition.
- Gastric feedings were common treatments in the sixteenth and seventeenth centuries.
- Total parenteral nutrition emerged in the twentieth century.
- In the 1960s, hospital pharmacies started to compound IV solutions that combined sterile water, dextrose, amino acids, and Liposyn, as well as an assortment of electrolytes, vitamins, and minerals, thus setting the stage for modern TPN therapy.
- TPN is often prescribed for patients who need long-term nutritional therapy but are, because of illness, treatment, or injury, unable to tolerate oral or enteral feedings.
- TPN solutions have chemical properties that make them more acidic, hypertonic, and hyperosmotic than human blood plasma.
- Nutritional administration into a peripheral vein may lead to extravasation or tissue destruction; therefore, the use of this administration route should be avoided. TPN solutions are generally administered continuously through a CVC.
- TPN preparation is considered a medium-risk compounding activity because multiple additives are injected into a nutrient-rich base solution, which provides an ideal medium for bacteria growth.
- The most common TPN formula is the 3-in-1 TPN solution. The solution provides all of the nutrients needed for a 24-hour period, including fatty acids in the form of Liposyn.
- The most common TPN additives are electrolytes, vitamins, and minerals.
- Manual TPN compounding requires the IV technician to gravity drain the TPN base components into an EEC or IV bag and then draw up and inject each individual additive into the final container.
- Manual TPN compounding and TPN compounding using the underfill method are often used in facilities that prepare a small number of TPNs.
- Partially automated TPN compounding utilizes an ACD to pump the base solution(s) from the source container(s) into the final container. The technician then draws up each additive and injects each one into the TPN bag.
- The partially automated TPN compounding method is frequently used in hospital and home infusion pharmacies that prepare a moderate number of TPN solutions each day.
- Fully automated TPN compounding uses an automix compounder to prepare the base and a micromix compounder to prepare the additives. Fully automated TPN compounding is used in facilities that prepare a large number of TPNs.
- Special considerations for TPN preparations include solution compatibility, order of ingredient mixing, storage and BUD, and filtration requirements.
- Therapeutic, chemical, or physical incompatibility may occur from incorrect mixing of TPN ingredients and may result in solution decomposition, layering, precipitation, or other problems that render the solution unsuitable for administration.
- The order of mixing TPNs is dextrose, amino acids, sterile water, fatty acids, and then additives.
- Additives containing phosphate should be separated from additives containing calcium. Some facilities require additives with color to be added last so that potential precipitates may be more easily identified.

- Because TPNs are a medium-risk compounding activity, the maximum BUD for TPNs is as follows: ≤ 30 hours at room temperature; ≤ 9 days when refrigerated; ≤ 45 days when frozen.
- Many facilities filter the TPN solution using an in-line filter connected to the administration tubing, which removes potential particulate matter from the solution.
- TPNs are administered into a large vein such as the subclavian, femoral, or umbilical vein, usually through the use of a CVC.
- ACDs must be cleaned and calibrated daily.
- The IV technician must record the cleaning and calibration of ACDs on the ACD Cleaning and Verification Log Sheet.

## Key Terms

**ACD Cleaning and Verification Log Sheet** a written record of the cleaning and calibration of the ACD; this log sheet is located in the anteroom and must be kept on file within the pharmacy for the lifetime of the equipment

**acquired immune deficiency syndrome (AIDS)** an epidemic, transmittable, retroviral disease due to infection by the human immunodeficiency virus (HIV); HIV attacks certain types of lymphocytes, severely impairing cell-mediated immunity in sufferers of the disease

**additive** a vitamin, trace element, electrolyte, or similar substance, as well as an occasional medication (such as heparin); most TPN solutions have at least 5 additives, and some may be comprised of as many as 50 additives

**advanced media-fill test procedure** a test of aseptic technique involving drawing up doses of a growth medium, such as soy broth, injecting them into an IV bag containing another test medium component, and allowing the bag to incubate for a certain number of days or hours; an *advanced* media-fill test procedure requires the technician to aseptically perform manipulations from multiple containers

**anorexia** the symptom of poor appetite; not to be confused with the eating disorder *Anorexia nervosa*

**automated compounding device (ACD)** a machine composed of pump stations, each of which is fitted with tubing (a "lead"); one end of each lead spikes into a container holding a TPN component, and the other end merges into the centralized TPN pump station tubing, which automatically delivers fluid into the final container; also known as an *automated TPN compounder*, *automix*, or, simply, a *compounder*

**automated TPN compounding** the use of an automated compounding device to prepare TPNs

**basic media-fill test procedure** a test of aseptic technique involving drawing up doses of a growth medium, such as soy broth, injecting them into an IV bag containing another test medium component, and allowing the bag to incubate for a certain number of days or hours; a *basic* media-fill test typically requires the technician to aseptically draw up from one container and inject into one bag

**beyond-use date (BUD)** the expiration date of a CSP (a mandatory designation) determined by the temperature conditions under which the CSP is stored in comparison to the maximum storage period guidelines provided by a facility; under no circumstances may the BUD exceed the USP Chapter <797> guidelines for maximum storage period

**break in aseptic technique** a step in a compounding process that deviates from a facility's P&P manual and/or USP Chapter <797> guidelines

**cachexia** profound general ill health and malnutrition, typically accompanied by weakness, emaciation, and muscle wasting

**central venous catheter (CVC)** a catheter inserted into a large vein, such as the internal jugular (or subclavian), and leading into the superior vena cava or right atrium; catheter used to administer TPNs or medications; also called a *central line*

**chemical incompatibility** a type of incompatibility that occurs when two substances are mixed, producing a chemical change (such as decomposition or a destructive alteration to the pH of the solution)

**clyster** a crude syringe-like device used to inject fluid into the rectum for the purposes of disease treatment, cleansing, or fluid restoration

**colectomy** excision of part or all of the colon

**congenital disorder** a physical condition present at birth

**Crohn's disease** a chronic inflammatory disease involving any part of the GI tract, but most commonly affecting the distal portion of the small intestine; disease leads to scarring and thickening of the bowel wall, intestinal obstruction, and abscess formation

**end-product testing** tests for prepared TPN solutions to identify chemical and other incompatibilities that are difficult to see

**enteral nutrition therapy** the delivery of nutrients either naturally via the mouth and esophagus, or in a liquid form through a feeding tube directly into the stomach, duodenum, or jejunum; also called *enteral feeding*

**extravasation** the discharge or escape of blood or some other fluid (such as an IV medication) from a vessel into the surrounding tissues, where it may cause irritation or necrosis

**feeding funnel** a hollow cone used to administer oral feedings to a patient unable to move the lips or masticate

**final container** the container into which the TPN base solutions and additives are injected; the empty TPN bag or EEC, once filled with TPN solution, is called the final container

**force feeding** a method of providing nutritional support for a person who cannot or will not eat; feeding via the NG tube, G tube, J tube, or via TPN

**fully automated TPN compounding** a compounding procedure in which the TPN base solution is prepared using an ACD; then the electrolytes and most other additives are drawn up using an automated micronutrient compounder, which attaches to the final container through special tubing

**gastrectomy** excision of part or all of the stomach

**gastric feeding** administration of a liquid nutritional supplement such as Ensure into a G tube, J tube, or PEG tube placed into a patient's stomach; a method of providing "oral" nutrition to patients who are unable to tolerate oral feedings

**gastric (G) tube** a type of tubing inserted through the skin directly into a patient's stomach; serves as a conduit for TPN administration

**gastrointestinal (GI) tract** the tubular passage of mucous membrane extending from the mouth to the anus

**gravimetric** pertaining to measurement by weight; ACDs operating by the gravimetric method calculate the amount of each TPN component to be added based on the component's weight

**gravity draining method** a method of manually compounding a TPN; the technician runs the base solution components through IV transfer tubing into an EEC or empty IV bag; also called the *gravity drainage method* or the *empty bag method*

**hemostat** a stainless steel, snap-lock clamp used in pharmacy sterile compounding to temporarily clamp tubing or the tail of an IV bag

**home infusion pharmacy** a pharmacy that prepares and delivers IVs (including TPNs) and IV supplies directly to patients receiving treatment in their homes

**hyperalimentation** a type of IV solution that provides a 24-hour supply of nutrients for a patient receiving long-term nutritional therapy; administration of greater-than-normal amounts of nutrients; *parenteral hyperalimentation* is another name for TPN

**incompatibility** the quality of being incompatible—that is, not suitable for combination or simultaneous administration

**in-line filter** a type of filter attached near the end of a patient's IV tubing to remove potential particulate matter from a TPN solution prior to administration

**ischemic bowel disease** a condition in which there is an acute insufficiency in the blood supply to the colon, often leading to ulceration of the colon; also known as *ischemic colitis*

**IV tubing** tubing that transfers fluid from each of the source containers (base component bags) into the EEC

**IV tubing spike** a color-coded attachment ("spike") at one end of the source tubing that connects to a source container filled with base solution; the opposite end of the tubing connects to a larger, centralized TPN pump-station tube on an ACD; several source-tubing lines combine into the centralized tube, thus mixing several base components together and sending the combined mixture through the centralized tube into the final container

**jejunum (J) tube** a type of tubing inserted through the skin directly into a patient's stomach; serves as a conduit for TPN administration

**Levin tube** a type of NG tube that is used for tube feeding

**manual compounding** a method of TPN compounding in which the base solution is gravity drained into an EEC or empty TPN bag and the additives are drawn up by hand; also known as *nonautomated TPN compounding*

**marasmus** a form of malnutrition due to prolonged and severe caloric deficit, usually during the first year of life; results in growth retardation and muscular wasting

**meniscus** the curved upper surface of a column of liquid

**micromix compounder** a special type of automated compounding device for use in fully automated TPN compounding; used to measure TPN additives such as MVIs, trace elements, electrolytes, and similar substances; is attached to the final container through special micromix tubing

**multiple-channel TPN solution** a premixed TPN solution manufactured in such a way that nothing may be injected into the bag; primarily used in home healthcare situations in which the patient requires long-term TPN therapy and has consistently stable lab values (so that no variations in TPN base components or additives are required)

**nasogastric (NG) tube** a soft rubber or plastic enteral feeding tube that is inserted through a nostril and threaded down the esophagus to the stomach

**nontunneled catheter insertion** a procedure that provides an IV access point by inserting a short, sterile catheter directly into a vein, allowing IV access through an injection port at the opposite end of the catheter

**nosocomial infection** healthcare associated infection; also known as *hospital-acquired infection (HAI)*

**parenteral nutrition** IV administration of a 24-hour supply of a sterile nutritional supplement such as total parenteral nutrition; also known as *IV nutrition therapy*

**partially automated TPN compounding** a compounding procedure in which the TPN base solution is prepared using an ACD; an IV technician draws up any TPN additives (MVIs, trace elements, electrolytes, etc.) in individual syringes and, following a check by a pharmacist, injects them into the final container

**partial parenteral nutrition (PPN)** parenteral nutrition solutions that are less concentrated than TPN solutions and are administered through a peripheral vein; also known as *peripheral parenteral nutrition*

**peripherally inserted central catheter (PICC)** a long, slender, flexible tube inserted into a peripheral vein, typically in the upper arm, and advanced until the catheter tip terminates in a large vessel near the heart; catheter provides IV access

**physical incompatibility** a type of incompatibility in which a chemical interaction between additives in a TPN solution or between the base solution components themselves results in a physical change to the end product, such as a change in color, a separation or layering of the various components, or the appearance of a precipitate

**precipitation** the formation of a precipitate, or a substance that settles to the bottom of a solution in solid particles; in TPN preparation, adding calcium gluconate and potassium phosphate sequentially will create calcium phosphate, which precipitates out of solution

**pump station** a component of an ACD; refers to one of the "stations" where a TPN ingredient is hung, its container is spiked, and the required amount of the ingredient is deployed into the final container

**rectal feeding** an archaic method of administering parenteral nutrition by enema

**short-bowel syndrome** a malabsorption condition that results from drastic resection of the small bowel; characterized by diarrhea and malnutrition; also known as *short-gut syndrome*

**source container** a container or bag containing the individual components of a TPN, such as amino acid solution, lipid, $D_{70}W$, etc.

**source solution** an individual component of a TPN base solution such as $D_{70}W$, AA, or SW

**subclavian vein** a main vein in the upper arm that joins with the internal jugular vein to form the brachiocephalic vein

**superior vena cava** the second-largest vein in the human body, located in the upper chest; the superior vena cava returns deoxygenated blood from the body to the heart

**therapeutic incompatibility** a type of incompatibility that occurs when two or more combined drugs result in a change in the effectiveness of one or more of the drugs upon administration

**3-in-1 TPN solution** a TPN formula that provides all of the nutrients needed for a 24-hour period, including fatty acids in the form of Liposyn; also known as a *total nutrient admixture* (TNA)

**total parenteral nutrition (TPN)** IV administration of total nutrient requirements to patients who require a long-term alternative to enteral feeding

**TPN flow rate** the rate at which the TPN is administered to the patient, as ordered by the prescriber on the TPN order form

**tunneled catheter insertion** a procedure that provides an IV access point by inserting a flexible catheter into a vein and tunneling its short tubing under the skin for a few inches; the end of the tubing has an attached injection port for IV fluid administration

**2-in-1 TPN solution** a total parenteral solution that provides a 24-hour supply of all nutrients except fatty acids, which are administered separately and are not included in the compounded TPN bag

**ulcerative colitis** chronic, recurrent ulceration in the colon

**underfill method** a method of manually compounding a TPN; amino acids and other base components are added (via gravity drainage) to a commercially available, partially filled bag of dextrose solution; additives are then injected into the solution prior to patient administration

**vented dispensing pin** a small, sterile plastic spike with a Luer-lock syringe tip adaptor at one end; allows the IV technician to draw up multiple doses of the additive without inserting multiple needles into the vial, thereby reducing the likelihood of coring

**volumetric** pertaining to measurement by volume; ACDs operating by the volumetric method calculate the amount of each TPN component to be added based on the component's volume

## Check the Basics

*On a separate sheet of paper, write your answers as modeled in these examples:* 1d; 2c; 3b; *etc.*

**1.** What does the abbreviation ACD mean?

a. automated containment device
b. automated compounding device
c. aseptic containment device
d. aseptic compounding device

**2.** Which of the following sterile compounding procedures might require the use of a hemostat?

a. clamping IV tubing or the tail of a base component bag
b. injecting multiple additives into an EEC through one needle
c. destroying base component bags at the end of the procedure
d. both *a* and *c*

**3.** Which of the following critical sites should never be disinfected with an IPA swab?

a. needle, syringe tip, tubing spike
b. needle adaptor, base component tubing port
c. injection port, EEC top
d. all of the above
e. only *a* and *b*

**4.** Which of the following best describes the type of clamp used to control the flow of fluid from the base component into the EEC?

a. hemostat
b. roll clamp
c. pinch clamp
d. all of the above
e. only *b* and *c*

**5.** Which of the following best describes a TPN solution prepared without fatty acids?

a. 1-in-1 TPN solution
b. 2-in-1 TPN solution
c. 3-in-1 TPN solution
d. 4-in-1 TPN solution

**6.** Which of the following formulas describes the basic formula calculation (where *D* is the desired dose; *H* is the concentration on hand; and *x* is the unknown volume)?

a. $D \times H = x$ mL
b. $H \times D = x$ mL
c. $D / H = x$ mL
d. $H / D = x$ mL

7. Which of the following statements is true regarding the method of determining the amount of SW needed for the TPN solution?
   a. subtract the total mL of $D_{70}W$, AA 10%, and additives from the TV = amount of SW
   b. add the total mL of $D_{70}W$, AA 10%, and additives to the TV = amount of SW
   c. subtract the total mL of $D_{70}W$ and AA 10% from the TV = amount of SW
   d. add the total mL of $D_{70}W$ and AA 10% to the TV = amount of SW
8. When removing the aluminum cap from the top of the EEC, which of the following statements is true?
   a. The tab should be twisted back-and-forth until it comes off; the tab should then be used to pry off the aluminum ring.
   b. The tab should be carefully pulled down and off; the tab should then be used to pry off the aluminum ring.
   c. The tab should be carefully pulled down and off, so that the spike may be inserted in the tubing port.
   d. The tab should be twisted back-and-forth until it comes off, so that the spike may be inserted into the tubing port.
9. At what point(s) in the procedure should you get a verification check from your instructor or a pharmacist?
   a. after adding the necessary volume of $D_{70}W$ to the EEC
   b. after adding the necessary volume of AA 10% to the EEC
   c. after adding the necessary volume of SW to the EEC
   d. after drawing up all of the additives
   e. all of the above
10. Which of the following describes the proper disposal of the used base solution components?
   a. Cut the PVC bags with scissors and pour the solutions into the clean room sink.
   b. Cut the PVC bags with a hemostat and pour the solutions into the clean room sink.
   c. Cut the PVC bags with scissors and pour the solutions into the anteroom sink.
   d. Cut the PVC bags with a hemostat and pour the solutions into the anteroom sink.

# Make Connections

*On a separate sheet of paper, write your answers to the following three questions, using complete sentences and making sure your answers are thorough and thoughtful. Note that the third question requires Internet access.*

1. On a TPN order form, prescribers order TPN electrolyte dose amounts *per liter* and indicate the TPN flow rate of the solution. If the prescriber orders the TPN to be administered at a flow rate of 125 mL per hour, the pharmacy, in turn, needs to supply a 3000-mL bag for each 24-hour period. With that in mind, would an IV technician adjust the desired volume of electrolyte additives when preparing a 3000-mL TPN bag rather than a 1-L bag? Explain your reasoning.
2. In general, the trace minerals and MVI additives are the only two additives that are not affected by the TPN flow rate. No matter what size TPN is prepared by the pharmacy, there will always be 5 mL of trace minerals and 10 mL of MVI in the TPN. What is the rationale for handling these two additives differently than the other TPN additives, which are adjusted based on the TPN flow rate/TPN bag volume?
3. Go to the website of the Food and Drug Administration (www.fda.gov) and perform a search for *Alabama TPN Recall 2011*. Read about the TPN recall from March 2011. Nine patients died and at least ten others were sickened after receiving TPNs contaminated with bacteria. What is the name of this deadly bacteria? Type the name of this bacteria into your Internet search bar. What information do you find about the connection between nosocomial infections and this bacteria? Based on what you have read, and what you have learned about the importance of aseptic technique, do you believe that poor aseptic technique may have been a factor in the TPN contamination? Why or why not?

## Meet the Challenge

***Scenario*** This "precipitating" activity will give you the opportunity to discover physical incompatibilities within a TPN solution.

***Challenge*** Your instructor has a handout outlining the supplies and steps for an activity centered around the physical incompatibility between phosphate and calcium. This procedure takes your understanding of the importance of mixing order in a TPN preparation to a deeper level. To meet this challenge, ask your instructor for the handout and give it a try, either individually, in small groups, or as a class.

### ADDITIONAL RESOURCES

*Go to the Paradigm Internet Resources Center at* www.paradigmcollege.net/sterilecomp *to access live links related to these Chapter 13 topics:*

+ Sterile compounding and BUD for TPNs
+ Information and support for consumers of home TPN therapy
+ TPN therapy for healthcare professionals (according to *The Merck Manual*)
+ Information on parenteral and enteral nutrition therapy for researchers, healthcare professionals, patients, and caregivers

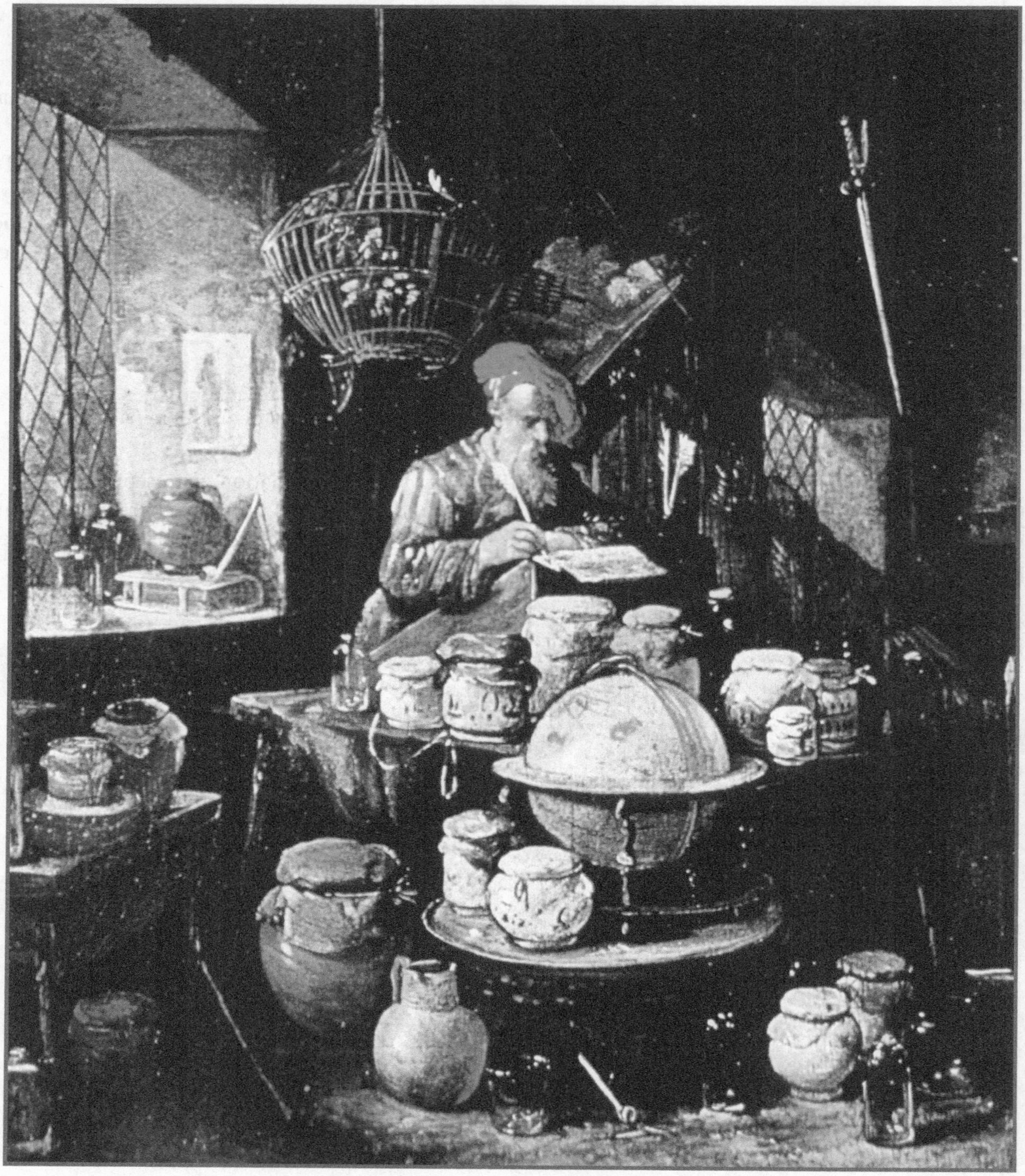

# Chapter 14

# Chemotherapy Products and Procedures

## Learning Objectives

- Gain an awareness of the historical roots of using chemotherapy to treat cancer.
- Identify the special situations and actions that must be considered when preparing chemotherapy.
- Identify the USP Chapter <797> procedures that must be performed when compounding chemotherapy.
- Demonstrate correct technique in preparing chemotherapy CSPs.

Cancer, the second-leading cause of death in the United States, is not a modern-day affliction. In fact, the disease is as old as the beginnings of humankind. Archaeologists have uncovered melanoma lesions in the skeletal remains of Peruvian Incas (2400 BCE) and cancerous growths in the skull of a female who lived during the Bronze Age (1900–1600 BCE). Cancer was also found in the mummified remains of early Egyptians. These ancient Egyptian civilizations believed that the appearance of a **tumor**, or swelling, on an individual's body was a form of punishment from the gods or the mark of an evil curse placed on the victim. To appease the goddess Sekhmet, who was thought to be responsible for curses and threats, early Egyptians would perform elaborate rituals to rid the victim of this deadly disease.

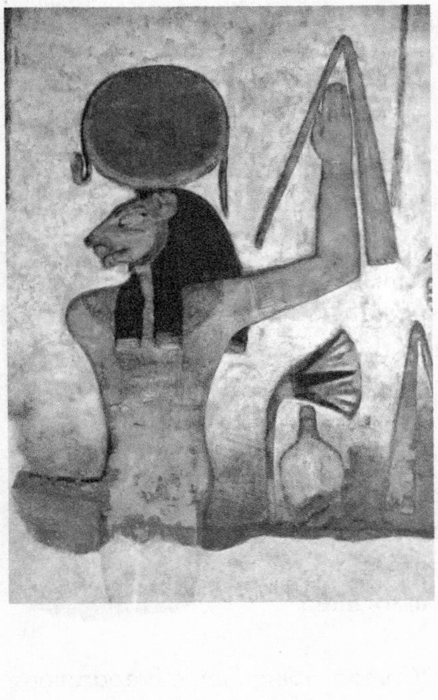

## Primitive Cancer Treatments

Recognition of cancerous tumors can be found in ancient Egyptian writings as well. The **Edwin Smith Papyrus**, a hieroglyphic inscription dating back to around 3000 BCE, discusses eight cases of breast tumors that were treated with a tool called a "fire drill." This instrument, most likely a burning stick, was used to sear the tumor and surrounding tissue (an early form of cauterization). Other treatments used by early Egyptian cultures included poultices of barley, pig's ear, and various natural remedies that were placed on tumors to provide a small measure of comfort for the

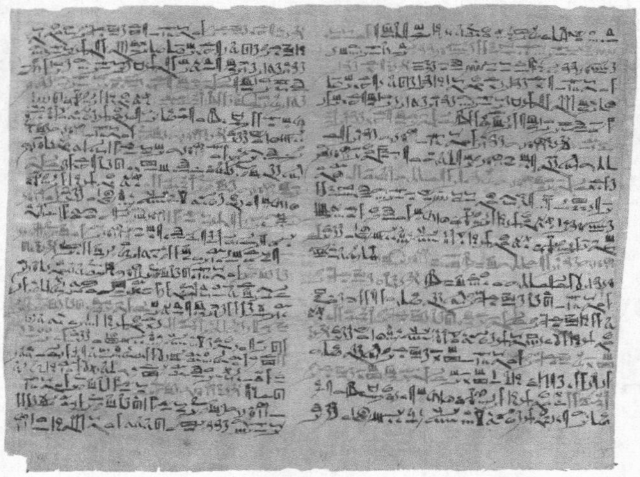

sufferer. Even then, with virtually no knowledge of the **pathophysiology** of cancer, these early practitioners recognized that cancer was a formidable opponent, acknowledging in their writings that no cure existed for the disease.

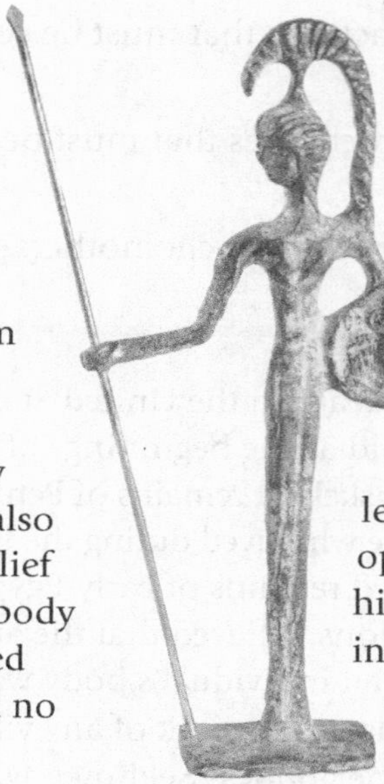

Early Greek cultures also used a combination of spiritual healing and medicinal remedies to treat cancer. Individuals afflicted with the disease would pray to Athena, the Greek goddess of healing, to banish the tumors from their bodies. Practitioners would compound pastes and ointments from natural substances and apply the salves to tumors. They would also perform rectal cleansing, in the belief that this procedure would rid the body of toxins. Both procedures provided some relief to the patients but had no effect on the disease.

## Humoral Imbalance and Cancer

Notable Greek physician Hippocrates studied the disease, seeking an understanding of its origins and growth. In fact, the source of the word *cancer* is attributed to Hippocrates, who used the Greek word *karkinos* (meaning "crab") to describe a fast-growing tumor. Hippocrates thought that the blood vessels projecting from the tumor resembled the tentacle-like projections of a crab. He was also the first practitioner to classify the tumors as **malignant** or **benign**. According to Hippocrates, cancer was caused by an excess of black bile, one of the four humors of the body. The result of this condition was a physical state he called *melancholy*. His humoral theory was built upon the observation that an untreated tumor turned black and eventually erupted through the skin, leaking black fluids.

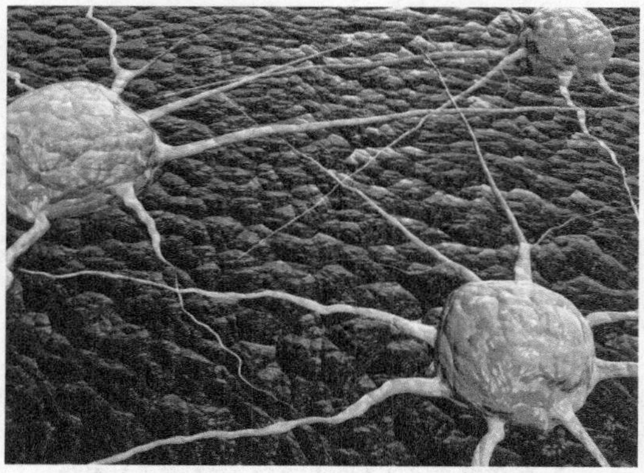

By the second century, Greek physician Galen made a distinction between the terms *tumor* and *cancer*, referring to benign tumors as *oncos*, the Greek word for swelling, and to malignant or cancerous tumors as *carcino*. The terms **oncology** and *carcinoma*—still part of the medical lexicon among cancer specialists— stem from Galen's coinage. Like his predecessor, Galen also believed that the disease was a result of the imbalance of the body's humors, and he experimented with a wide range of treatments, including bloodletting and the application of poultices made of opium and licorice. However, Galen realized that his efforts were palliative and that patients suffering from malignant cancers were incurable—a medical belief that would continue for centuries to come.

## Caustic Cures for Cancer

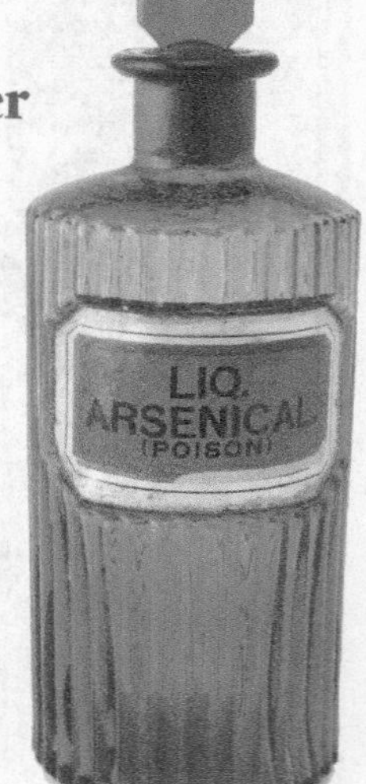


In the ensuing years, many different remedies were used to treat cancerous tumors. Practitioners turned to **caustic** substances to control the spread of the disease. Pastes were compounded from metals such as arsenic and mercury and applied to tumors. **Arsenic**, a highly poisonous substance, was thought to halt the growth of the tumor; **mercury**, a metal long associated

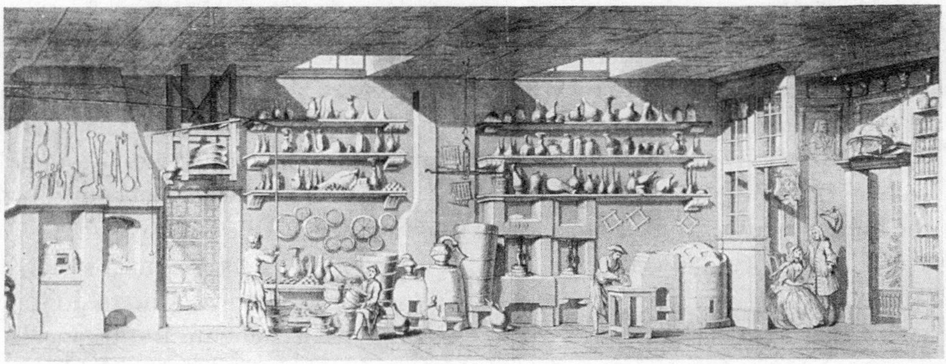

with mystical properties and a common treatment for skin disorders, was thought to curb the swelling caused by the underlying tumor. Arsenic later became a key ingredient in Plunkett's powder, a remedy compounded from sulfur, white arsenic, egg yolk, and the plants crowfoot and dog-fennel; this remedy was applied as a poultice to tumors. Today, ironically, both arsenic and mercury are considered possible human carcinogens.

Poisonous plants, such as **hemlock** and **belladonna** (deadly nightshade), were also used to treat cancer. Roman practitioners would crush the herbs and mix the residue with fluid before using the extract in poultices. Centuries later, Austrian physician Anton von Störck conducted studies with hemlock extract (conium), administering the liquid to patients suffering from breast cancer. His results were seemingly favorable, and word quickly spread that the ingestion of Storck's Extract of Hemlock (its dispensing pot shown below) could cure the disease. However, the extract would prove to be an ineffective cancer treatment.

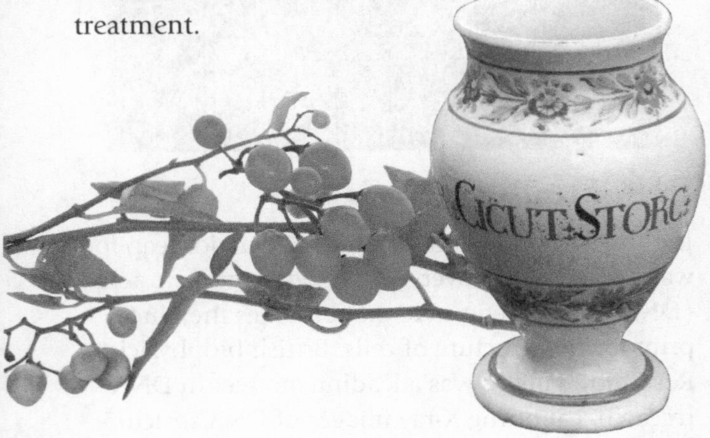


## Emerging Cancer Theories

By the beginnings of the Renaissance, medical practitioners began to have a better understanding of human anatomy and physiology. With the discovery of the circulatory and lymphatic systems, scientists and practitioners refuted the existence of black bile and investigated other origins of cancer by conducting laboratory experiments.

In the 1660s, Dutch scientist François de la Boe Sylvius challenged the humoral theory of cancer, establishing his theory that cancer was caused by excessively acidic lymph. Other scientists believed cancer was an infectious disease that was spread through physical contact and that infected individuals should be sent away from their homes and communities to live in isolation. Still others thought that the disease was caused by external toxins, viruses, bacteria, or even trauma. In fact, in 1779, the first cancer hospital in France was forced to move out of the city of Reims due to a fear that cancer was caused by a contagious parasite.

Investigations into the different causes of cancer began with the conduction of the first human **autopsy** by Italian practitioner Giovanni Morgagni in 1791. The dissection of the human body—up to this point, a procedure prohibited by religious doctrines—led to vast improvements in the understanding of human anatomy and physiology and the pathophysiology of the disease process. Consequently, several new theories about the cause of cancer emerged, paving the way for the study of oncology.

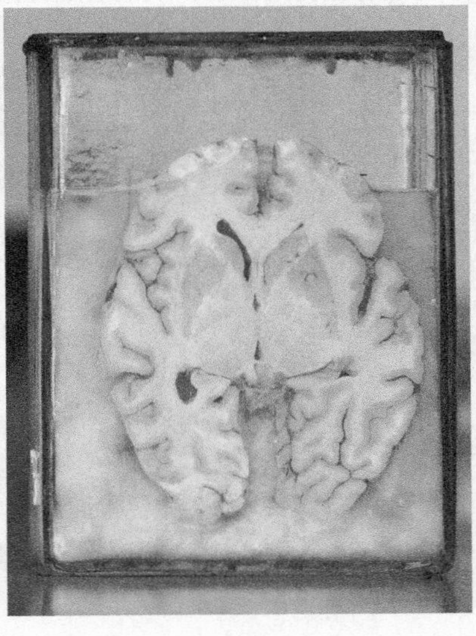

New methods of treating cancer were also explored. Instead of applying medicinal poultices or ingesting liquid remedies, surgery became a viable treatment option. One of the proponents for surgery was eminent Scottish physician John Hunter (1728–1793), who suggested that a patient with no evidence of **metastasis** could have the tumor removed to prevent the progression of the disease. Hunter surmised that cancer moved through the body's blood supply via the lymphatic system. His **lymph theory** built upon the idea that the human body's fluid system was the key to understanding the spread of cancer.

In 1838, German pathologist Johannes Müller advanced his theory, called the **blastema theory**, which was based on his belief that cancer cells arose from connective tissue (blastema). His student, German pathologist Rudolph Virchow, theorized that chronic irritation of tissues caused cancer and that cancer spread throughout the body like liquid saturating a sponge. Even though these early theories regarding the cause and spread of cancer were eventually disproven, they were valuable stepping stones that led to a greater understanding of the human body and the mechanism by which cancer forms and spreads.

## Advances in Cancer Diagnosis and Treatment

By 1865, German surgeon Karl Thiersch had demonstrated that cancer originates in **epithelial** cells and metastasizes by the spread of malignant cells. Microscopic cell studies continued into the late nineteenth century when German bacteriologist Paul Ehrlich used methylene blue stain to demonstrate cell pathology. His research in immunology and tissue- and cell-staining techniques paved the way for genetic studies in cancer research and drugs that interfere with the cellular process. In fact,

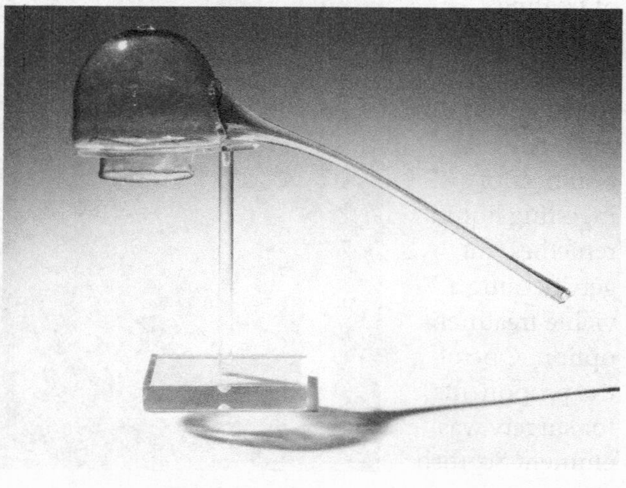

Ehrlich is credited with coining the word **chemotherapy**, a term derived from the words *chemical* and *therapy* that was originally used to refer to any chemical or drug used to treat any type of disease. Ehrlich won a Nobel Prize in 1908 for pioneering the use of chemical compounds to treat diseases. He famously said, "We must search for magic bullets. We must strike the parasites and the parasites only… and to do this we must learn to aim with chemical substances." For his pioneering work, Ehrlich is considered the "Father of Chemotherapy."

By the close of the nineteenth century, advances in surgical techniques, infection control, and anesthesia made excision of tumors a viable option for cancer patients. The invention of X-rays in 1896 made diagnosis of the disease easier, and the discovery of radium in 1898 made **radiation therapy**, or the use of radiation to harness or kill cancer cells, a treatment option. Both technological advances improved patient prognosis.

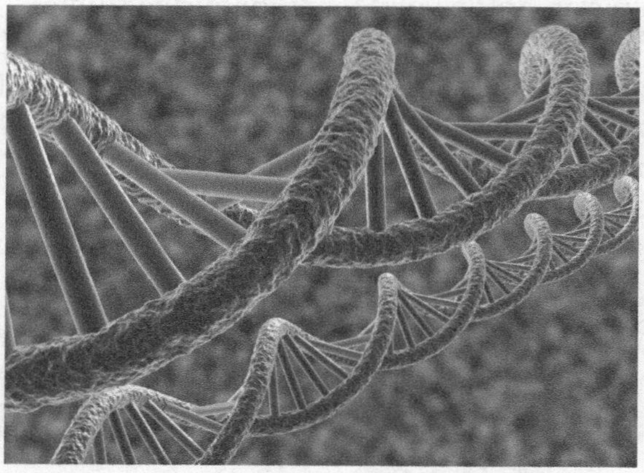

## DNA Studies and Cancer

In the 1940s, cancer research took a major leap forward with the discovery of **deoxyribonucleic acid (DNA)**, the genetic code that provides the blueprint for the structure of cells. British biophysicist Rosalind Franklin was a leading pioneer in DNA research, capturing X-ray images of DNA structure that proved essential in understanding DNA make-up. In 1953, American biologist James Watson and British biologist Francis Crick published a scientific paper that identified the structure of DNA as a double helix—resembling a continuously twisting ladder—containing all of the sugars and base molecules that determine physical characteristics. Cracking this genetic code allowed scientists to understand the functions of genes and the role of defective genes in the development of cancer. They concluded that cancer cells with defective DNA did not die like normal cells did; rather, the cancer cells continued to grow and divide uncontrollably. The pathophysiology of cancer was finally understood by the medical community. To acknowledge this breakthrough discovery, Watson and Crick, along with British molecular biophysicist Maurice Wilkins, were awarded the Nobel Prize in Physiology or Medicine in 1962.

Many researchers and historians believe that Franklin should have been included as a Nobel Prize recipient, as the noted accomplishment was based upon much of her early research. However, at that time in history, women's contributions to science were often overlooked. Although it is clear that Franklin played a crucial role in the discovery of DNA, the debate over how much credit she should receive for those contributions continues to this day. What is clear is that the work of Thiersch, as well as each of these early DNA researchers, paved the way for the modern understanding of the origin, metastasis, and treatment of cancer.

## The Beginnings of Chemotherapy

The first effective cancer chemotherapy treatment was not developed until 1946. American pharmacologists Dr. Alfred Gilman and Dr. Louis Goodman were commissioned by the U.S. Department of Defense to study agents that might be used in chemical warfare and discovered that **nitrogen mustard** (when injected intravenously into cancerous mice) caused a reduction in the size and number of cancer tumors. Nitrogen mustard is an alkylating agent. As a cytotoxic drug, it binds to nucleic acids and inhibits cell division by damaging the cell's DNA. Nitrogen mustard was subsequently administered intravenously to several patients with advanced lymphoma and had limited results. However, its use ushered in a class of chemotherapeutic agents still utilized today.

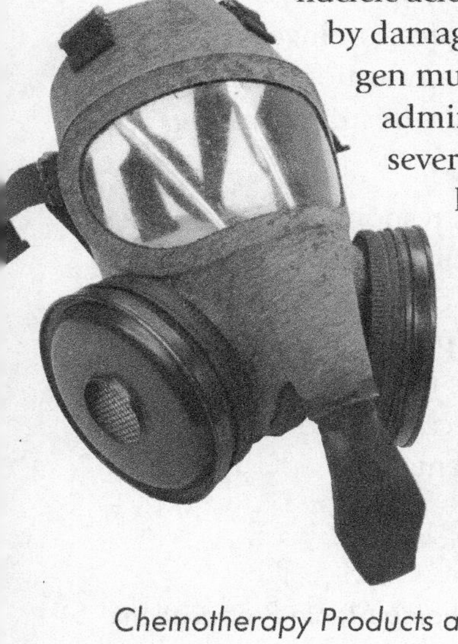

By the second half of the twentieth century, several chemotherapy drugs had been developed, including oral, injectable, and intravenous forms. These drugs decrease tumor size, control tumor growth, or destroy cancerous cells by targeting specific parts of the cell or cell cycle.

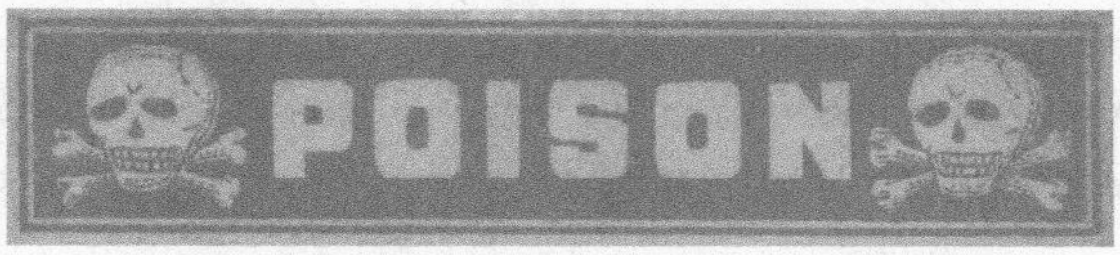


## Cancer Therapy Today

*Cancer* is a term used today to describe a class of diseases characterized by the presence of abnormal cells that divide and multiply uncontrollably and invade nearby tissue. Cancer cells can spread to other parts of the body through the lymphatic system and, therefore, the blood. Cancer that has spread from one part of the body to another is said to have *metastasized*. Certain chemicals, viruses, and exposure to radiation can cause cancer. In addition, some forms of cancer are caused by **genetic mutations**. Cancer may develop in almost any organ or body system; some of the most common cancers originate in the breast, lung, colon, skin, prostate, and ovary. Other common forms of cancer are **leukemia**, which originates in the blood, and **lymphoma**, which originates in the lymph system.

Today, dramatic improvements in cancer treatment have led to greatly improved survival rates. In general, if cancer is detected and treated before it metastasizes to another part of the body, the patient has a much greater chance of being cured, or at least experiencing long-term **remission**. Modern cancer therapy may involve surgery, radiation, hormone therapy, chemotherapy, **immunotherapy**, or a combination of these treatments. Because detection is key to the prevention, diagnosis, and treatment of cancer, the National Cancer Institute and the

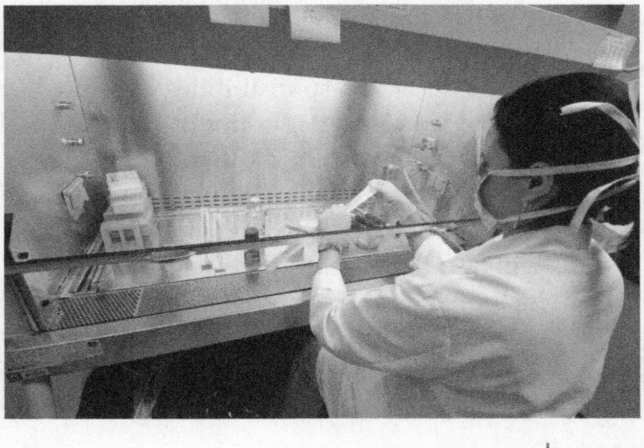

National Human Genome Research Institute began The Cancer Genome Atlas Pilot Project in 2006. The project's goal is twofold: 1) to map the genomic (genetic) changes in brain, lung, and ovarian cancers to determine the feasibility of exploring the genomic changes in every type of cancer, and 2) to develop new methods for the prevention, diagnosis, and treatment of the disease.

## Responsibilities of the IV Technician in Chemotherapy Preparation

There are multiple steps to follow to properly compound chemotherapy preparations. Proper procedures and strict aseptic protocol must be followed, regardless of the sterile compounding scenario. The preparation of chemotherapy products also requires additional education and training in calculations and compounding procedures, as well as knowledge of the special equipment and ingredients used in the compounding process. Chapter 14 provides the background information, aseptic technique details, and specific sequence of sterile compounding procedures used in chemotherapy preparation.

## Future of Sterile Compounding

Now that you have learned the history of sterile compounding and aseptic technique, what does the future hold for sterile compounding personnel? In the future, pharmacies and sterile compounding facilities will see many changes as educational and training requirements, job responsibilities, and new technologies continue to evolve.

***Educational and Training Requirements*** Training, testing, and certification for pharmacy technicians will become more standardized in the coming years. This is driven, in part, by the National Association of Boards of Pharmacy (NABP) directive that all students who take the Pharmacy Technician Certification Exam (PTCE) should have first graduated from an ASHP-accredited pharmacy technician training program. The NABP has set a goal of 2015 for this requirement.

***Job Responsibilities*** Many of the tasks that were traditionally performed by pharmacists will be designated as job responsibilities of future pharmacy technicians. For example, specially trained technicians will be required to perform "tech-check-tech" duties, including the verification of compounded sterile preparations. Technicians will also have areas of greater specialization, including neonatology, chemotherapy, and total parenteral nutrition compounding—as well as roles in the training and supervision of sterile compounding technicians.

***New Technologies*** In the future, automated sterile compounding machines will likely be used more frequently, and technicians will need to know how to operate these devices. There will also be a developing market for technicians who are specially trained to assemble and service these automated compounding devices.

Advances in computer technology will also allow more pharmacists to move off-site to perform order entry via scanner or computer, and to check compounded sterile preparations via video chat programs. The adoption of electronic medication administration records (eMars) by healthcare facilities will change the practice of dispensing medication as barcode technology will assist personnel in the tracking of medication inventory, the verification of patient identification, and the monitoring of medication administration at the patient's bedside.

Despite changes in the roles, responsibilities, and working environments of pharmacy technicians, one principle will not change: Pharmacy technicians will continue to place the utmost importance on following the protocol of sterile compounding and aseptic technique to ensure the health and safety of patients.

# Part 1: Concepts

Chemotherapy is primarily used to treat cancer. However, there are a limited number of other conditions for which chemotherapy may be prescribed, including **autoimmune disorders** such as lupus and rheumatoid arthritis. For these conditions, low doses of chemotherapy may be administered to suppress the overactive immune system response, which is a characteristic of autoimmune diseases.

Cancer chemotherapy is classified as primary, adjuvant, or palliative, depending on the patient's condition and the goal of treatment. **Primary chemotherapy** is prescribed with the intention of curing the patient. Most patients diagnosed with a type of inoperable cancer—due to the size or location of the tumor—receive primary chemotherapy. Examples of such cancers include leukemia and lymphoma. **Adjuvant chemotherapy** is prescribed as a follow-up treatment to the removal or reduction of a tumor by surgery and is commonly prescribed after surgical procedures, such as a **mastectomy** in breast cancer, or an **oopharectomy** in ovarian cancer. **Palliative chemotherapy** is sometimes prescribed as a treatment for incurable cancers. The purpose of palliative chemotherapy is to reduce the size of the tumor in order to improve the patient's quality of life.

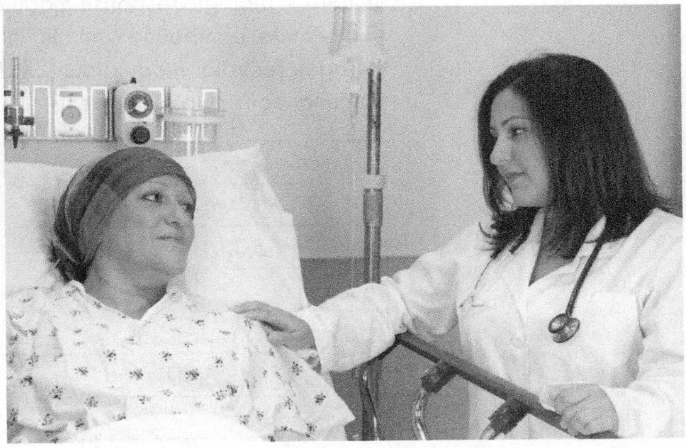

Cancer patient being comforted by a healthcare professional.

## Common Chemotherapy Drug Categories

There are several categories of chemotherapy drugs used in the treatment of cancer. These categories include alkylating agents, antimetabolites, antimicrotubule agents, chemotherapeutic antibiotics, hormone therapies, mitotic inhibitors, targeted therapies, and topoisomerase inhibitors. The prescriber orders the chemotherapy treatment proven to be most effective against the patient's specific type, location, and **stage of cancer**. Other factors such as the patient's age, kidney function, liver function, and ability to tolerate the side effects of the specific chemotherapy treatment are considered when choosing the most appropriate chemotherapy.

**Alkylating agents** are drugs that bind to specific DNA cells and stop their replication. **Antimetabolite medications** are drugs that block the use of nutrients essential to the growth of cancer cells. **Antimicrotubule agents** are drugs that interfere with cell formation and growth. **Chemotherapeutic antibiotics**, also known as *antitumor antibiotics*, are special types of antibiotics formulated to inhibit **RNA synthesis** as well as slow down or prevent cell **mitosis**. Unlike other antibiotics, chemotherapeutic antibiotics are not used for the treatment of infections.

**Hormone therapy** employs drugs that interfere with the growth of certain proteins within cancer cells, thereby inhibiting their growth or replication. The use of hormones or their **antagonists** slows the growth of hormone-dependent tumors. This kind of therapy is used to treat hormone-sensitive cancers of the breast and prostate. **Mitotic inhibitors** are drugs that inhibit the process of cell mitosis. **Targeted therapy** is a sophisticated type of chemotherapy that targets the specific molecular features of certain cancer cells to inhibit their growth. **Topoisomerase inhibitors** disrupt DNA repair functions within the cell, thereby inhibiting the growth and replication of cancer cells. Many cancer treatment regimens incorporate treatment with a combination of chemical agents, hormone therapies, surgery, and radiation. Table 14.1 lists these common chemotherapy drug categories and their corresponding parenteral medications.

### Table 14.1 Common Parenteral Chemotherapy Medications

Most chemotherapy agents are classified into one of the several categories listed below. Some chemotherapy agents may be further classified into more specific categories, including aromatase inhibitors, biologic response modifiers, cycle-phase specific agents, cycle-phase nonspecific agents, heavy metal compounds, mitotic inhibitors, monoclonal antibodies, nitrosoureas, retinoids, selective estrogen receptor modulators (SERMs), taxanes, tyrosine kinase inhibitors, vinca alkaloids, and miscellaneous cytotoxic agents.

| Generic Name | Brand Name |
|---|---|
| **Alkylating Agents** | |
| Arsenic trioxide | Trisenox |
| Busulfan | Busulfex, Myleran |
| Carboplatin | Paraplatin |
| Carmustine (BCNU) | BiCNU |
| Chlorambucil | Leukeran |
| Cisplatin | Platinol-AQ |
| Cyclophosphamide | Cytoxan |
| Dacarbazine | DTIC-Dome |
| Docetaxel | Taxotere |
| Ifosfamide | Ifex |
| Mechlorethamine | Mustargen |
| Melphalan | Alkeran |
| Oxaliplatin | Eloxatin |
| Thiotepa | Thioplex |
| **Antimetabolites** | |
| Capecitabine | Xeloda |
| Cladribine | Litak, Movectro |
| Clofarabine | Clolar |
| Cytarabine | Ara-C, Cytosar-U, DepoCyt |
| Floxuridine | FUDR |
| Fludarabine | Fludara |
| Fluorouracil | Adrucil |
| Gemcitabine | Gemzar |
| Mercaptopurine | Purinethol |
| Methotrexate | Trexall, Folex |
| Pemetrexed | Alimta |

| Generic Name | Brand Name |
|---|---|
| **Antimicrotubules** | |
| Asparaginase | Elspar |
| Docetaxel | Taxotere |
| Paclitaxel | Abraxane, Taxol |
| Vinblastine | Velban |
| Vincristine | Oncovin, Vincasar |
| Vinorelbine | Navelbine |
| **Chemotherapeutic Antibiotics** | |
| Bleomycin | Blenoxane |
| Dactinomycin | Cosmegen |
| Daunorubicin | Cerubidine, DaunoXome |
| Doxorubicin | Adriamycin, Doxil |
| Idarubicin | Idamycin |
| Mitomycin | Mutamycin |
| Mitoxantrone | Novantrone |
| Plicamycin | Mithracin |
| Streptozocin | Zanosar |
| **Hormone Therapies** | |
| Diethylstilbestrol | Stilphostrol |
| Flutamide | Eulexin |
| Leuprolide | Lupron, Eligard |
| Medroxyprogesterone | Provera |
| Megestrol Acetate | Megace |
| Tamoxifen | Nolvadex |
| Testolactone | Teslac |
| **Targeted Therapies** | |
| Azacitidine | Vidaza |
| Bevacizumab | Avastin |
| Bortezomib | Velcade |
| Cetuximab | Erbitux |
| Rituximab | Rituxan |
| Trastuzumab | Herceptin |
| **Topoisomerase Inhibitors** | |
| Epirubicin | Ellence |
| Etoposide | VePesid, VP-16 |
| Idarubicin | Idamycin |
| Irinotecan | Camptosar |
| Mitoxantrone | Novantrone |
| Teniposide | Vumon, VM-26 |
| Topotecan | Hycamtin |

## Properties of Chemotherapy CSPs

Chemotherapy compounded sterile preparations (CSPs) are typically large-volume parenteral (LVP) solutions made from a standard, premade intravenous (IV) base solution, such as normal saline (NS) or dextrose 5% in water ($D_5W$), into which a chemotherapeutic medication is injected during sterile compounding procedures. Medications used in chemotherapy treatment are generally described as cytotoxic or antineoplastic. **Cytotoxic medications** are drugs that poison or otherwise destroy cancer cells so that they are not able to grow or reproduce. Cytotoxic agents are capable of killing healthy cells. **Antineoplastic medications** are drugs that reduce or prevent the growth of cancer cells. The terms *cytotoxic* and *antineoplastic* are often used interchangeably to describe the various drugs used in chemotherapy treatment.

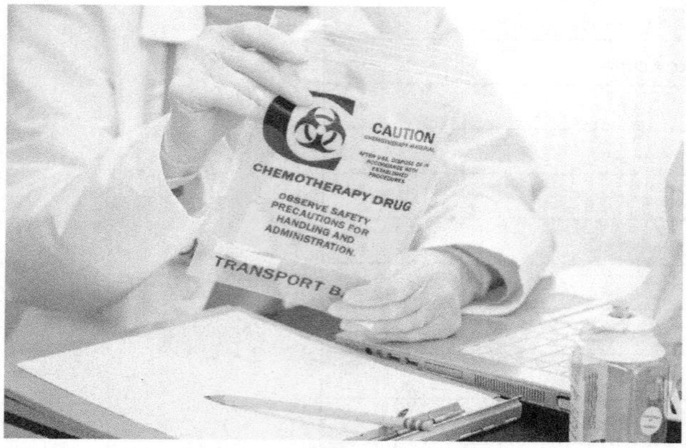

A physician checking a chemotherapy CSP.

In addition to killing cancer cells, many chemotherapeutic agents are also toxic to healthy cells. Chemotherapy medications may have properties that make them **carcinogenic**, **teratogenic**, **mutagenic**, or **immunosuppressive**. Chemotherapy medications may also have numerous side effects. Typical chemotherapy side effects include nausea, vomiting, and hair loss. More serious side effects may include infertility, damage to the kidneys or liver, or bone marrow suppression. **Bone marrow suppression** is a potentially dangerous type of toxicity that may lead to an increased risk of bleeding or infections, such as **septicemia**.

**BE AWARE**

Because of the potential teratogenic effects of chemotherapeutic agents, pregnant health-care workers should not prepare or administer these medications.

In general, chemotherapy solutions have chemical properties that make them more acidic, hypertonic, or hypersosmolar than human blood plasma. Some chemotherapy drugs are **vesicants**, which may cause blisters or tissue necrosis. Due to the properties of these powerful medications, chemotherapy is typically administered as a continuous infusion into a large vein in the chest, rather than a smaller, peripheral vein.

## Compounding of Chemotherapy CSPs

Because there is a limited selection of oral chemotherapy medications readily available, most chemotherapy medications require sterile compounding. As with all CSPs, IV technicians must follow strict aseptic technique in the preparation of chemotherapy to avoid the introduction of pathogens during the sterile compounding process. Due to the dangerous nature of these **hazardous drugs**, many facilities take special precautions prior to the compounding process to avoid chemotherapy-related medication errors. These precautions include the use of a preprinted chemotherapy medication order and the implementation of a standardized dosage calculation method.

***Chemotherapy Medication Orders*** Many facilities use preprinted chemotherapy medication order forms (see Figure 14.1) that provide the medication name, dosage range, and administration rate or interval. The prescriber uses the preprinted medication order to prescribe chemotherapy medications based on body surface area or weight. The use of these preprinted forms helps to prevent medication errors from the misinterpretation of handwriting, signa, abbreviations, or dose.

Typically, the chemotherapy medication order specifies the chemotherapy drug(s), the IV base solution, and the volume of the base solution. If the IV base solution and volume are not provided by the prescriber on the chemotherapy medication order, the pharmacist must determine the most appropriate IV base solution by consulting various pharmacy reference sources.

In addition to the chemotherapy CSP, chemotherapy medication orders generally prescribe a number of other CSPs that are not hazardous drugs. The orders for these CSPs are often called **chemotherapy support orders**, or *chemotherapy comfort orders*. This often includes orders for LVP hydration preparations, intravenous piggyback (IVPB) **antiemetics**, and medications for pain and anxiety.

FIGURE 14.1

**Chemotherapy Medication Order**

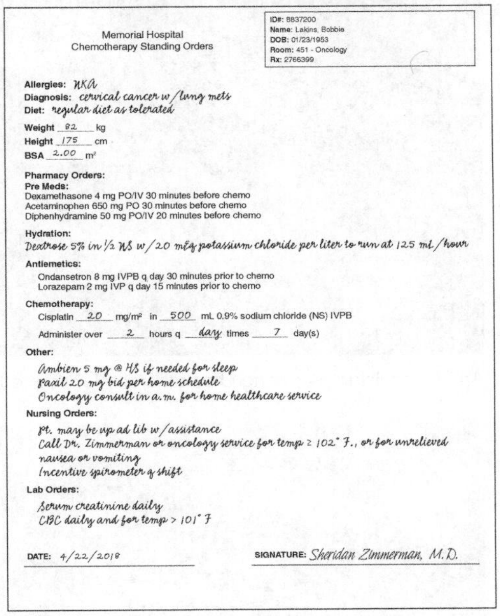
Memorial Hospital
Chemotherapy Standing Orders

ID#: 8837200
Name: Lakins, Bobbie
DOB: 01/23/1953
Room: 451 - Oncology
Rx: 2766399

**Allergies:** NKA
**Diagnosis:** cervical cancer w/lung mets
**Diet:** regular diet as tolerated

**Weight** 82 kg
**Height** 175 cm
**BSA** 2.00 $m^2$

**Pharmacy Orders:**
**Pre Meds:**
Dexamethasone 4 mg PO/IV 30 minutes before chemo
Acetaminophen 650 mg PO 30 minutes before chemo
Diphenhydramine 50 mg PO/IV 20 minutes before chemo

**Hydration:**
Dextrose 5% in ½ NS w/20 mEq potassium chloride per liter to run at 125 mL/hour

**Antiemetics:**
Ondansetron 8 mg IVPB q day 30 minutes prior to chemo
Lorazepam 2 mg IVP q day 15 minutes prior to chemo

**Chemotherapy:**
Cisplatin 20 $mg/m^2$ in 500 mL 0.9% sodium chloride (NS) IVPB
Administer over 2 hours q day times 7 day(s)

**Other:**
Ambien 5 mg @ HS if needed for sleep
Paxil 20 mg bid per home schedule
Oncology consult in a.m. for home healthcare service

**Nursing Orders:**
Pt. may be up ad lib w/assistance
Call Dr. Zimmerman or oncology service for temp ≥ 102° F., or for unrelieved nausea or vomiting
Incentive spirometer q shift

**Lab Orders:**
Serum creatinine daily
CBC daily and for temp > 101° F

**DATE:** 4/22/2018 **SIGNATURE:** Sheridan Zimmerman, M.D.

***Dosage Calculations Methods*** In order to provide the most accurate dosage, chemotherapy medications are often dosed based on a patient's body surface area. **Body surface area (BSA)** is an estimated measurement of the human body based on the patient's height and weight and is expressed in meters squared ($m^2$). The prescriber determines a patient's BSA using a **nomogram**. The prescriber's dosage calculation is then confirmed by a pharmacist. For IV technicians, a familiarity with the BSA dosage calculation method aids in understanding how chemotherapy is prescribed and how BSA affects preparatory compounding procedures, such as CSP label verification and subsequent pharmacy calculations. Tables 1 and 2 of Appendix C provide the steps for using a nomogram to estimate a patient's BSA, as well as sample nomograms for estimating BSA for children and adults.

Refer to Tables 1 and 2 in

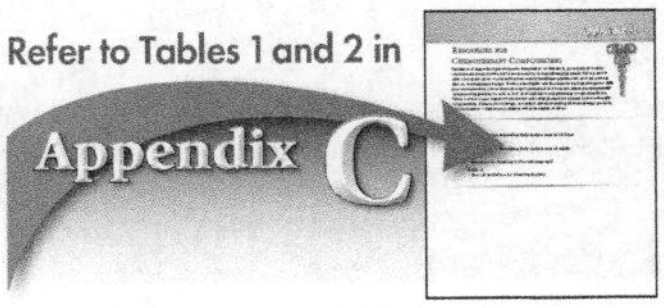


In general, chemotherapy drugs are ordered in milligrams per meter squared ($mg/m^2$). The prescriber first determines the patient's BSA and provides it on the chemotherapy medication order. Either the prescriber or pharmacist then determines the dose based on the patient's BSA, using dimensional analysis. Once the desired dose has been determined, additional dosage calculations—using **dimensional analysis** and either the **basic formula calculation** or the **ratio and proportion calculation**—are required to determine the amount of medication to draw up for the CSP. (For more detailed information on these three different pharmacy calculation formulas, refer to Chapter 5 of this textbook.)

***Chemotherapy Compounding Environment*** Hazardous drug chemotherapy should be prepared in a **vertical laminar airflow hood**, a type of hood that offers added protection to the worker and the environment when working with these toxic chemicals. Nonhazardous CSPs, such as antiemetic and antianxiety medications, may also be included as part of a chemotherapy medication order and should be prepared in a horizontal laminar airflow hood.

There are several types of vertical laminar airflow hoods that may be used in chemotherapy preparation. Two of the most common types are the biological safety cabinet and the compounding aseptic containment isolator. Both of these hoods allow for vertical airflow, ensuring that any potential contaminants are drawn back into the cabinet in order to prevent hazardous material from entering the clean room environment and endangering sterile compounding personnel.

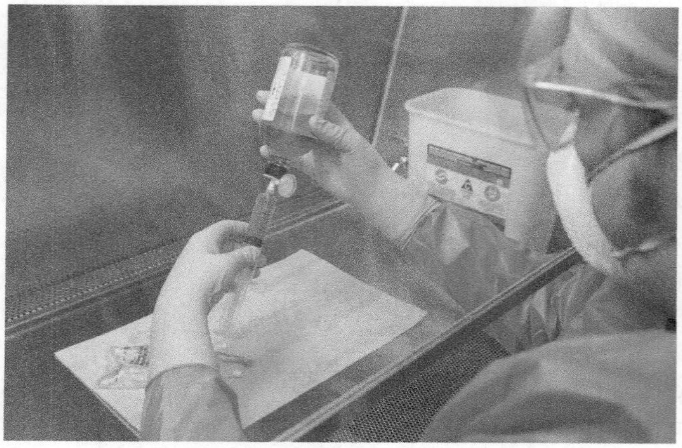

An IV technician preparing chemotherapy CSPs in a BSC.

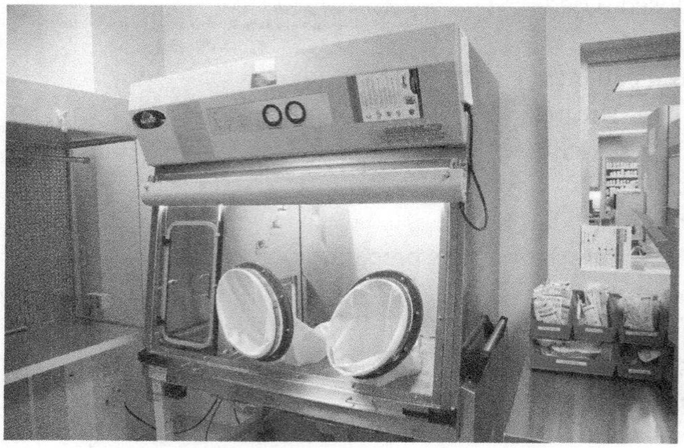

Compounding aseptic containment isolator (CACI).

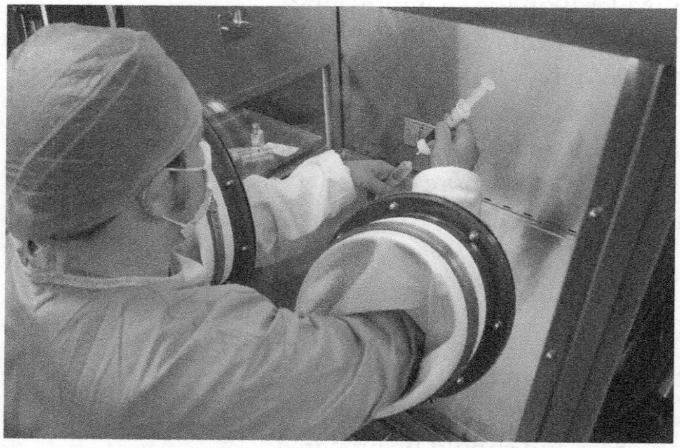

Pharmacy technician preparing chemotherapy within a CACI.

**Biological Safety Cabinet** A **biological safety cabinet (BSC)** is a special hood that has several features specifically designed to protect sterile compounding personnel. Aside from the vertical airflow pattern, a Plexiglas shield at the front of the cabinet protects the IV technician from the hazardous chemicals.

The BSC should be located in a negative-pressure clean room. A **negative-pressure clean room** is one in which the air pressure within the room is less than the air pressure of the room most adjacent to it. The negative pressure within the clean room causes the direction of airflow to flow *into the room* whenever the door to the clean room is opened. This negative-pressure environment helps to prevent hazardous air from being drawn out of the BSC and into the surrounding area. The negative-pressure clean room is different from a standard, positive-pressure clean room in which the positive pressure within the clean room causes the direction of airflow to flow *out of the room* whenever the door to the clean room is opened.

**Compounding Aseptic Containment Isolator** Another type of hood used to prepare chemotherapy is the compounding aseptic containment isolator (CACI). The CACI is a completely enclosed system accessed through the use of a fixed pair of gloves at the front of the hood. The IV technician places his or her hands inside the gloves to manipulate the chemotherapy supplies. In addition to this physical barrier, the CACI also vents contaminated air through a specially dedicated pharmacy ventilation system. More information about the CACI and the BSC can be found in Chapter 2 of this textbook.

In addition to the use of a BSC or CACI, chemotherapy compounding requires special procedures, equipment, and techniques to protect the preparer. The safety features of the BSC and such specialized procedures, equipment, and techniques will be detailed in Part 2 of this chapter.

***Surface Sampling of BSC or CACI*** No matter which type of primary engineering control (PEC) is used during the compounding of chemotherapy CSPs, quality control measures must be implemented to ensure that the hood offers adequate containment for the toxic chemicals. To this end, the work area surrounding the BSC or CACI must undergo surface sampling at least every six months. This type of sampling includes the countertops and compounder chair as well as the nearby floor, walls, and ceiling surfaces. IV technicians should consult their facility's P&P manual to determine appropriate procedures for surface sampling, assay-processing sampling, and assay-finding responses.

## Handling Risks for Chemotherapy

Due to their carcinogenic, mutagenic, teratogenic, or immunosuppressive properties, chemotherapy agents require special handling and preparation prior to patient administration. Taking these precautionary measures protects sterile compounding personnel, nursing personnel, other members of the health-care team, and the patient recipient from potential consequences of long-term exposure.

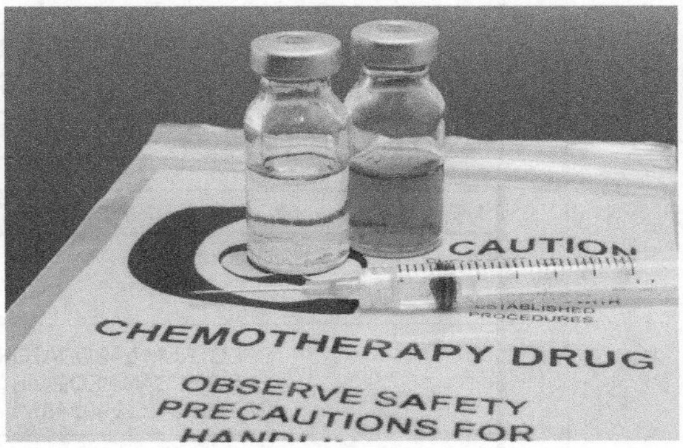

Chemotherapy drug safety warning.

***Safety Regulations*** Safety procedures regarding the preparation and administration of chemotherapy CSPs are defined by USP Chapter <797> and each facility's P&P manual, as well as by several regulatory organizations. These organizations include the National Institute for Occupational Safety and Health (NIOSH), the American Society of Health-Systems Pharmacists (ASHP), and the Occupational Safety and Health Administration (OSHA). In particular, the ASHP technical assistance bulletin *Guidelines on Handling Hazardous Drugs* provides valuable information on the safe handling of chemotherapy drugs, and the OSHA regulations provide guidelines for chemotherapy spills and their subsequent clean-up.

**MSDSs** OSHA regulations require maintenance and easy access to **material safety data sheets (MSDSs)** for all chemotherapy drugs. MSDSs are available from manufacturers for all potentially hazardous drugs and chemical products. These sheets provide detailed information about the storage and handling of hazardous drugs, including safety and cleanup guidelines for an inadvertent chemotherapy spill (see Figure 14.2).

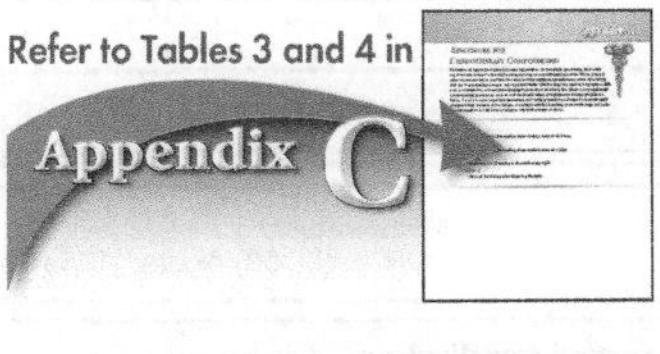


**Chemotherapy Spill Kits** OSHA recommends facilities have a **chemotherapy spill kit** readily available in areas where chemotherapy is compounded or administered. The chemotherapy spill kit contains all of the necessary items required to safely clean powdered or liquid spills, which are classified as small (≤ 5 grams or 5 mL) or large (> 5 grams or 5 mL). Refer to Tables 3 and 4 of Appendix C for the procedures for cleaning a chemotherapy spill, as well as the general guidelines for cleaning the BSC.

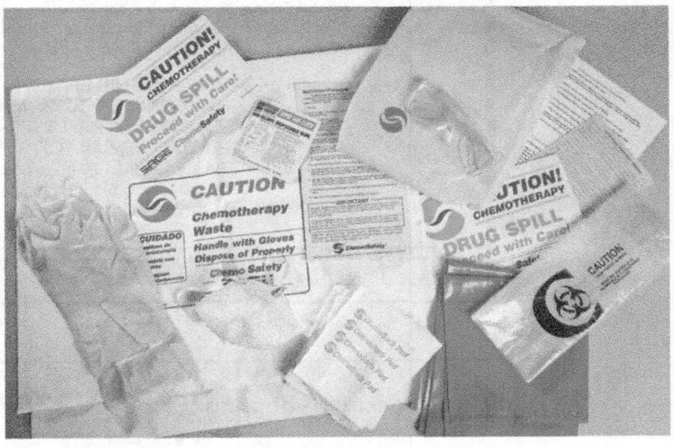

Contents of a chemotherapy spill kit.

***Storage and Labeling of Chemotherapeutic Agents*** All personnel handling chemotherapy must be trained in the proper procedures for the storage and labeling of hazardous drugs such as chemotherapy. Guidelines for this training are defined by several organizations, including OSHA, the Environmental Protection Agency

**FIGURE 14.2**

**MSDS Form**

SPECTRUM®

GARDENA, CA
NEW BRUNSWICK, NJ

ISO 9002 CERTIFIED

# Material Safety Data Sheet

| NFPA | HMIS | Personal Protective Equipment |
|---|---|---|
| 1 (top), 2 (left), 0 (right) | Health Hazard 2<br>Fire Hazard 1<br>Reactivity 0 | See Section 15. |

**Section 1. Chemical Product and Company Identification** — **Page Number: 1**

| | |
|---|---|
| Common Name/ Trade Name | **Methotrexate** |
| Manufacturer | SPECTRUM LABORATORY PRODUCTS INC.<br>14422 S. SAN PEDRO STREET<br>GARDENA, CA 90248 |
| Commercial Name(s) | Amethopterin, Amethopterine, Antifolin, Methotrexat, Methylaminopterin, Methylaminopterium, Ledertrexate |
| Synonym | 4-Amino-4-deoxy-N(sup10)-methylpteroylglutamate;<br>4-Amino-4-deoxy-N(sup10)-methylpteroylglutamic acid;<br>4-Amino-N(sup10)-methylpteroylglutamic acid |
| Chemical Name | N-[4-[[(2,4-Diamino-6-pteridinyl)methyl]methylamino]benzoyl]-L-glutamic acid |
| Chemical Family | Not available. |
| Chemical Formula | C20-H22-N8-O5 |
| Supplier | SPECTRUM LABORATORY PRODUCTS INC.<br>14422 S. SAN PEDRO STREET<br>GARDENA, CA 90248 |

| | |
|---|---|
| Catalog Number(s). | ME131, M1435 |
| CAS# | 59-05-2 |
| RTECS | MA1225000 |
| TSCA | TSCA 8(b) inventory: Methotrexate |
| CI# | Not available. |

IN CASE OF EMERGENCY
CHEMTREC (24hr) 800-424-9300

CALL (310) 516-8000

**Section 2.Composition and Information on Ingredients**

| Name | CAS # | TWA (mg/m³) | STEL (mg/m³) | CEIL (mg/m³) | % by Weight |
|---|---|---|---|---|---|
| | | *Exposure Limits* | | | |
| 1) Methotrexate | 59-05-2 | | | | 100 |

| | |
|---|---|
| Toxicological Data on Ingredients | Methotrexate:<br>ORAL (LD50):Acute: 135 mg/kg [Rat]. 146 mg/kg [Mouse]. |

**Section 3. Hazards Identification**

| | |
|---|---|
| Potential Acute Health Effects | Hazardous in case of ingestion. Slightly hazardous in case of skin contact (irritant), of eye contact (irritant), of inhalation. Severe over-exposure can result in death. |
| Potential Chronic Health Effects | **CARCINOGENIC EFFECTS:** 3 (Not classifiable for human.) by IARC.<br>**MUTAGENIC EFFECTS:** Mutagenic for mammalian somatic cells. Mutagenic for bacteria and/or yeast.<br>**TERATOGENIC EFFECTS:** Not available.<br>**DEVELOPMENTAL TOXICITY:** Not available.<br>The substance may be toxic to blood, kidneys, lungs, liver, gastrointestinal tract, immune system, bone marrow. Repeated or prolonged exposure to the substance can produce target organs damage. Repeated exposure to a highly toxic material may produce general deterioration of health by an accumulation in one or many human organs. |

**Continued on Next Page**

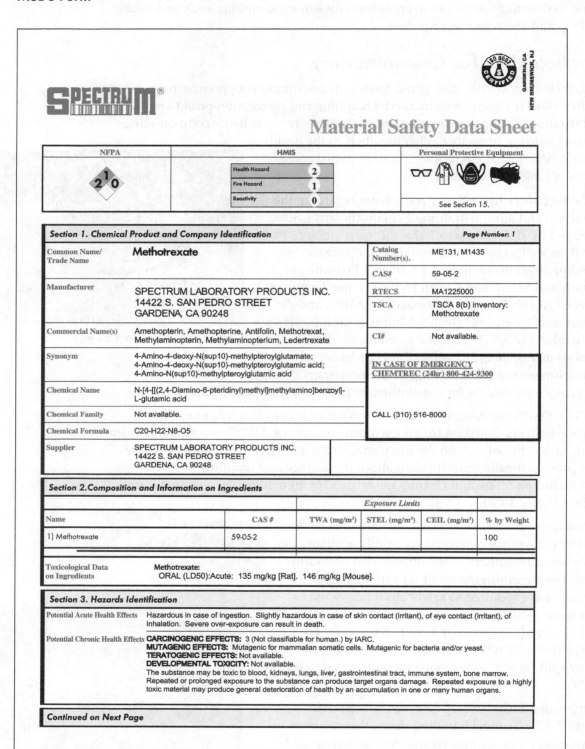

Courtesy of Spectrum Laboratory Products Inc., 2011.

(EPA), and the Department of Transportation (DOT) and are designed to protect personnel from exposure to the dangerous effects of chemotherapeutic medications.

**Storage** Chemotherapy drug manufacturers, cytotoxic drug storage companies, and pharmacies must follow all safety regulations concerning the storage of chemotherapeutic agents. With regard to pharmacies, chemotherapy drugs must be stored separately from other pharmacy inventory. The pharmacy shelves or bins that store chemotherapy drugs should be clearly marked as containing hazardous drugs, and the medications themselves require auxiliary labeling identifying their toxic properties.

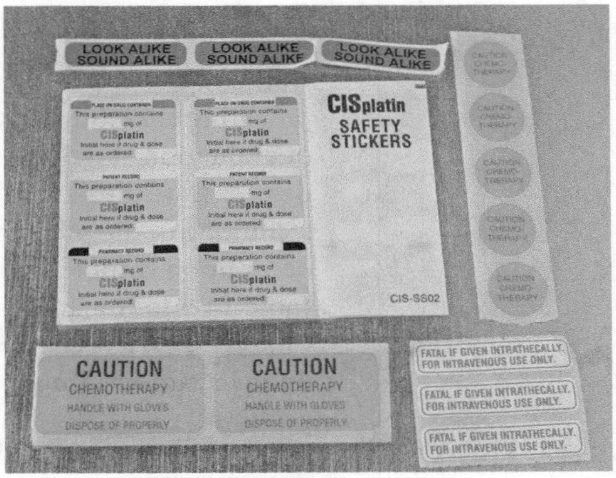

Sample auxiliary chemotherapy warning labels.

**Labeling** Special consideration is also given to the labeling of chemotherapy drugs and CSPs. Some chemotherapy drug manufacturers utilize **tall-man lettering**, also known as *mixed-case lettering*, to draw attention to chemotherapy drug names that look or sound similar. For example, the chemotherapy drugs vinCRIStine and vinBLAStine are often printed in tall-man lettering on manufacturer-labeled vials, with the tall-man lettering emphasizing the differing parts of two similar words. Using this labeling device reduces the likelihood of the two medications being interchanged due to their similar drug names.

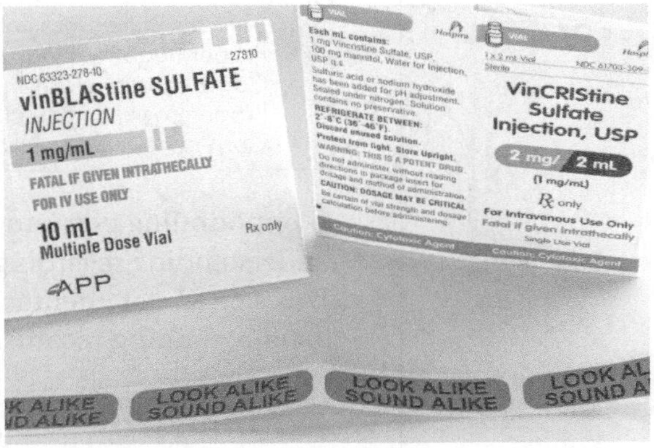

Tall-man lettering on the label of vinBLAStine and vinCRIStine.

***Transport and Disposal of Chemotherapeutic Agents*** All personnel handling chemotherapy medications must also be trained in the proper transport and disposal of chemotherapy agents. Guidelines for these procedures are outlined by several regulatory agencies, including OSHA, EPA, and DOT.

**Transport** Transport companies must follow procedures designed to properly package and transport chemotherapy drugs to protect handlers from breakage or spillage of the containers. In addition, those personnel who stock pharmacy shelves must wear special, extra-thick chemotherapy gloves when handling drug vials.

> **POINTER**
> Even transportation and storage companies must adhere to strict hazardous drug regulations.

**Disposal** Chemotherapy waste containers must be affixed with hazardous drug warning labels. These labels serve to warn all healthcare personnel handling chemotherapy agents to follow hazardous drug precautions. Healthcare personnel handling chemotherapy waste outside of the sterile compounding environment, such as those workers who remove waste containers from a facility, must wear chemotherapy gloves to perform this task.

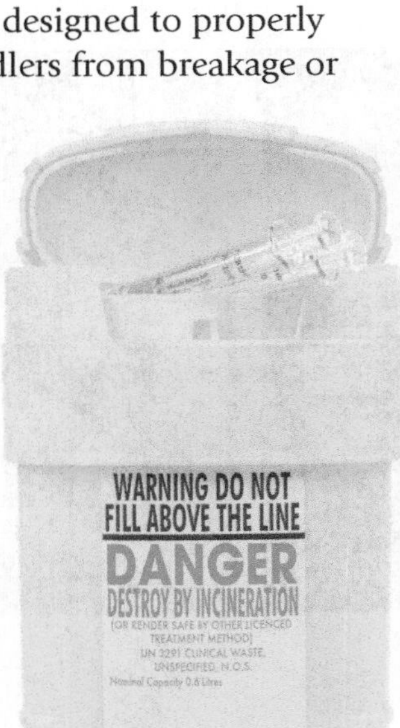
WARNING DO NOT
FILL ABOVE THE LINE
DANGER
DESTROY BY INCINERATION
Chemotherapy waste container marked for incineration.

Although medical waste is typically disposed of in a landfill, chemotherapy waste must be incinerated at a high temperature to avoid human and environmental contamination.

## Training for Chemotherapy Preparers

USP Chapter <797> mandates that, at a minimum, sterile compounding personnel preparing chemotherapy CSPs must be expertly trained and must undergo two types of evaluation: a written exam and a laboratory procedure exam. Both exams must demonstrate the worker's mastery of sterile compounding procedures and aseptic technique in the preparation of chemotherapy medications. These evaluations must occur upon completion of training and, at a minimum, annually thereafter. See Table 14.2 for the USP Chapter <797> hazardous drug guidelines. Refer to the USP Chapter <797> section *Hazardous Drugs as CSPs* for additional information on handling hazardous drugs.

**Table 14.2 USP Chapter <797> Training Guidelines for Hazardous Drug Preparation**

| |
|---|
| USP Chapter <797> hazardous drug guidelines specify the following areas must be addressed during initial and annual training:<br>• Safe aseptic manipulation practices<br>• Proper negative-pressure techniques when using a BSC or CACI<br>• Correct use of closed-system transfer devices<br>• Proper containment, clean-up, and disposal procedures for breakages and spills<br>• Correct treatment of personnel in the event of chemotherapy contact and inhalation exposure |

Compounding personnel with reproductive capabilities should sign a statement of understanding regarding the potential teratogenic risks of handling hazardous drugs. This signed statement is kept in each individual's personnel file along with chemotherapy training records.

## Administration of Chemotherapy CSPs

Most chemotherapy is administered in a hospital or clinic setting by a nurse who is specially trained in the parenteral administration of hazardous drugs. This training includes implementing special precautions to minimize inadvertent exposure to the CSP and to prevent chemotherapy spills.

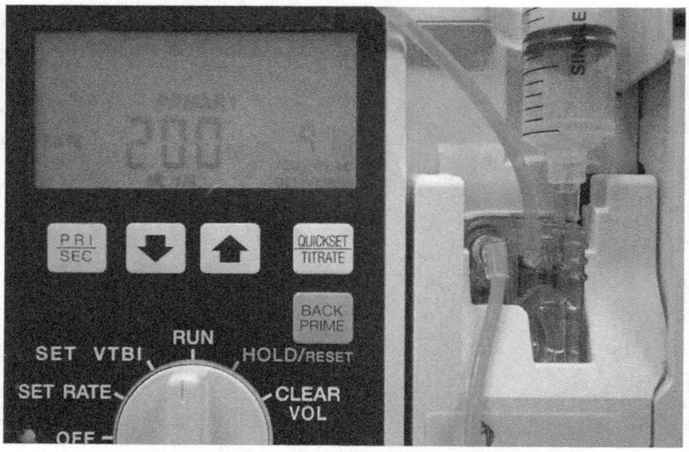

A chemotherapy infusion pump.

Chemotherapy medications are administered intravenously via an IV pump programmed to administer the medication at a controlled IV flow rate specified by the prescriber or pharmacist. Administration time for one session typically requires a minimum of several hours, and chemotherapy treatment may last for a year or more, with monthly cycles lasting approximately one week. The length and number of cycles vary, depending on the type of cancer and the patient's response to treatment.

Due to the caustic, hypertonic, or hyperosmolar nature of most chemotherapy drugs, chemotherapy CSPs are generally administered into a large vein in the chest, most often the **subclavian vein**. IV access into the subclavian vein is accomplished by placing a **central venous catheter (CVC)** into the vein during a minor surgical procedure. Some common CVCs used for chemotherapy administration include the HICKMAN, BROVIAC, and triple-lumen catheters. Because the catheter is placed directly into a major blood vessel and may remain in place for several weeks or longer, proper care of the catheter is essential. The patient or nursing staff must cleanse the catheter site, flush the catheter appropriately, and check the catheter site for swelling, heat, discharge, redness, or other signs of infection.

## Administration Risks of Chemotherapy

The chemotherapy nurse should be vigilant in monitoring patient recipients for potential complications from parenteral therapy. These complications may include:

- nosocomial infection
- allergic reaction (including anaphylaxis)
- phlebitis
- tissuing
- embolism
- extravasation
- cellulitis
- Stevens-Johnson syndrome
- nephrotoxicity

For chemotherapy CSPs, there is a heightened risk of phlebitis, tissuing, extravasation, and nephrotoxicity due to their chemical properties.

Chemotherapy medications may also produce a number of **adverse reactions** and side effects for the patient recipient, including nausea and vomiting, infertility, hair loss, bone marrow suppression, and septicemia. Healthcare personnel must discuss these potential side effects with the patient recipient prior to chemotherapy administration and take appropriate action to treat the patient in response to any of these undesired events.

Patients on chemotherapy must be closely monitored to ensure that the medication is not creating unexpected damage to the patient's vital organs. Therefore, patients' kidney and liver functions are frequently checked while receiving chemotherapy. In addition, patients undergo regular laboratory testing and physical evaluation to detect any sign of infection. Even a minor infection could lead to serious consequences in a cancer patient whose immune system has been suppressed by chemotherapy.

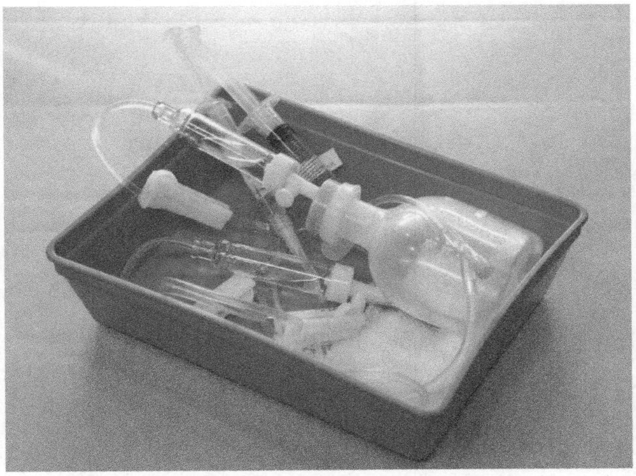

A chemotherapy infusion set.

## USP Chapter <797> Guidelines for Chemotherapy Preparation

USP Chapter <797> outlines several special considerations for the preparation of hazardous drug CSPs. As well as defining the appropriate environment in which chemotherapy CSPs should be prepared, USP Chapter <797> also details the type of equipment that must be used by sterile compounders and the special training requirements for healthcare personnel who compound chemotherapy CSPs. These procedures are reinforced in each facility's P&P manual.

Sterile compounding personnel must pay strict attention to aseptic technique procedures and follow USP Chapter <797> and facility guidelines at all times to ensure patient safety. Only those personnel who have been specially trained, process validated, and certified in aseptic technique and sterile product preparation should be allowed to compound sterile products. In addition, personnel who prepare chemotherapy CSPs must undergo hazardous drug training and testing prior to preparing chemotherapy for patient administration. Part 2 of this chapter guides you through the discovery and demonstration of proper aseptic technique in chemotherapy CSP preparation.

# Concepts Self-Check

## Check Your Understanding

*Write your answers on a separate sheet of paper, as modeled in these examples: 1d; 2c; 3b; etc. Check your answers using the Answer Key in Appendix A.*

**1.** Which of the following scientists demonstrated the spread of cancer via malignant cells?
   a. Hippocrates
   b. John Hunter
   c. Johannes Müller
   d. Karl Thiersch

**2.** Which of the following terms refers to cancer that has spread from the organ in which it originated?
   a. mutation
   b. mitosis
   c. metastasis
   d. malignant

**3.** In general, which type of chemotherapy is given as a follow-up to the surgical removal of a tumor?
   a. primary chemotherapy
   b. adjuvant chemotherapy
   c. palliative chemotherapy
   d. targeted chemotherapy

**4.** Which of the following conditions may result from the administration of chemotherapy drugs?
   a. skin irritation, blisters, or tissue necrosis
   b. other types of cancer
   c. birth defects
   d. immunosuppression
   e. all of the above

**5.** In order to provide the most accurate dosing, most chemotherapy is prescribed based on the patient's_______.
   a. weight
   b. height
   c. DNA
   d. BSA

## Apply Your Knowledge

*On a separate sheet of paper, write your answers to the questions posed in the paragraph below. Use complete sentences and take time to create a thorough and thoughtful response. Check your answers against the Answer Key in Appendix A.*

In Part 1 of this chapter, you learned that chemotherapy requires the IV technician to undergo additional training and testing to properly handle and dispose of hazardous drugs. In addition, sterile compounding personnel who prepare chemotherapy CSPs must demonstrate competency in the use of specialized equipment and techniques used during the compounding procedures. With that in mind, do you believe that these extra safety procedures are warranted? Why or why not? Do you believe that the procedures provide adequate protection for the IV technician? Why or why not?

# Part 2: Training

*Before performing this lab, review the Sterile Compounding Area Procedures listed on pages 162–163 at the end of the Unit 2 opener, and preview the accompanying process validation checklist in Appendix D.*

## Understand the Resources and Supplies

USP Chapter <797> prescribes a number of special requirements for the preparation of chemotherapy. This chapter and the corresponding lab provide equipment, supplies, and procedures that are in alignment with the directives set forth in USP Chapter <797>.

### Essential Supplies

Most chemotherapy sterile compounding procedures require the same essential supply items to be available for use in both the anteroom and the clean room. For the anteroom, these supplies include a chemotherapy medication order and a CSP label; a standard calculator; a pen; a permanent, felt-tip marker; large and small plastic bags; aseptic garb; a sterile gown; presaturated, aseptic cleaning wipes; sterile, foamed 70% isopropyl alcohol (IPA); a waste container; and a transport vehicle. (Various other compounding supplies, such as those necessary for aseptic hand washing and hood cleaning, are necessary supplies, but, for the purposes of this lab, are not included on the Essential Supplies list.) In the clean room, essential supply items include sterile, foamed 70% IPA; sterile, powder-free gloves; sterile 70% IPA swabs; regular needles and syringes; a waste container; and a vertical laminar airflow biological safety cabinet.

### Procedure-Specific Supplies

In addition to the essential supplies listed above, each sterile compounding procedure requires supply items specific to the procedure being performed. The type, number, and amount of procedure-specific supply items are determined by the IV technician prior to performing the procedure, based on information provided on the CSP label and the chemotherapy medication drug label. The CSP label identifies the IV base solution type, strength, and volume. After reading these labels, the IV technician performs one or more calculations that reveal the volume of the drug needed to prepare the CSP. This information, in turn, dictates the number, size, and type of syringes needed for the procedure (to accommodate the volume of the chemotherapy medication and, if applicable, the diluent needed to reconstitute the chemotherapy medication, if the medication is supplied in a powdered form).

**POINTER**
Read the manufacturer's package insert for each chemotherapy drug or ingredient *prior to compounding*. The package insert clearly identifies special precautions, supplies, and/or procedures to follow. For example, certain chemotherapy drugs require the use of glass syringes or specialized needles due to incompatibility with one or more components of the standard compounding supply items.

***Chemotherapy Equipment, Supplies, and Special Procedures*** The process of compounding chemotherapy CSPs involves the manipulation of regular needles and, in particular, vials and IV base solutions. Additionally, chemotherapy procedures require specialized supplies, including a chemotherapy gown, chemotherapy gloves, chemotherapy safety glasses, a compounding mat, a chemotherapy dispensing pin or CSTD, IVA seal, IV tubing, chemotherapy warning labels, chemotherapy transport bag, chemotherapy waste container(s), yellow chemotherapy sharps container, sterile 70% IPA in a pour bottle, and sterile, lint-free gauze. The Chapter 14 procedural lab also requires the use of a BSC with a vertical airflow. Familiarity with the appearances of these items as well as specific handling requirements is essential to chemotherapy sterile compounding procedures.

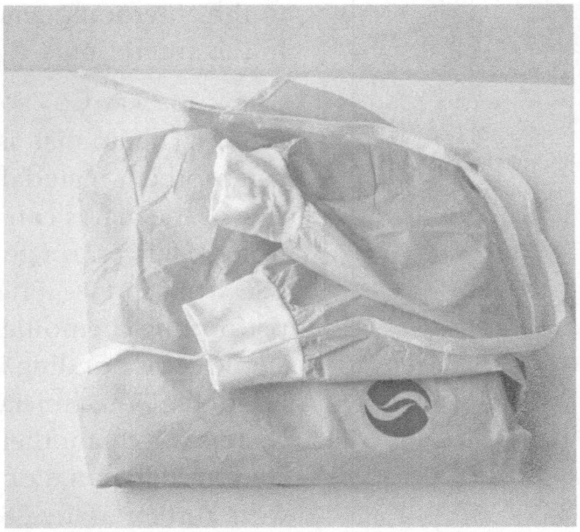
A chemotherapy gown made of thick, woven material.

**Chemotherapy Gown** A chemotherapy gown is a sterile, single-use gown made of a thick, woven material that repels fluid. The gown has neck and waist Velcro closures at the back of the garment and knit cuffs at the wrists to ensure a snug fit. This specialized gown must be worn for all chemotherapy compounding procedures.

In practice, don the chemotherapy gown immediately after completing aseptic hand-washing procedures. Upon completion of the compounding procedures, remove the chemotherapy gown by rolling it down off the shoulders, turning the sleeves and gown inside out as the gown is removed. Take care not to touch the exterior surface of the gown's sleeves or torso. Dispose of the gown in a chemotherapy sharps container immediately upon the completion of chemotherapy sterile compounding (while still in the clean room).

**BE AWARE**

One type of chemotherapy gown is a smock, which only covers the front of the IV technician. If a chemotherapy smock is worn, the technician must first don a regular sterile gown. Upon completion of chemotherapy compounding, the smock must be discarded in the clean room chemotherapy sharps container, and the regular gown must be discarded in the anteroom chemotherapy sharps container.

**Chemotherapy Gloves** Chemotherapy gloves are sterile nitrile gloves that are thicker than regular sterile gloves. Worn over standard, sterile gloves, chemotherapy gloves offer an added layer of protection for handling hazardous drugs.

To perform this double-gloving procedure, sterile compounding personnel must first follow the standard, aseptic gloving procedures outlined in Chapter 6. After donning gloves, the IV technician must ensure that the cuffs of the gloves are tucked under the wrist cuffs of the chemotherapy gown. Next, the technician dons a pair of chemotherapy gloves, following the same gloving procedures. Once the gloves are on, the cuffs of the gloves should be pulled over the wrist cuffs of the chemotherapy gown.

Upon completion of chemotherapy compounding, the IV technician removes each chemotherapy glove by rolling it down from the wrist cuff, turning it inside out in the process. She or he must avoid touching the fingers of the chemotherapy gloves during this removal procedure. The used chemotherapy gloves should then be disposed of in the chemotherapy sharps container in the clean room.

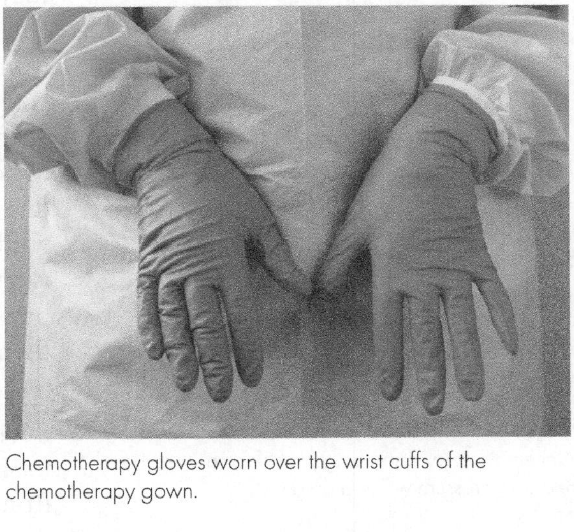
Chemotherapy gloves worn over the wrist cuffs of the chemotherapy gown.

**Chemotherapy Safety Glasses** To prevent serious eye injury from inadvertent splashing or aspiration of hazardous drugs during compounding procedures, chemotherapy preparation requires the use of special eye protection. Chemotherapy safety glasses are constructed of plastic or polyvinyl chloride and are commonly worn by workers in laboratory settings. Before donning the safety glasses, sterile compounding personnel must wipe them with sterile 70% IPA while still in the anteroom. After completing the compounding procedure and returning

**POINTER**
Generally, chemotherapy safety glasses are reusable if they are thoroughly cleaned after each use. Performing this task prevents the possibility of contamination.

to the anteroom, personnel must wipe the safety glasses again and then store them in the anteroom.

**Chemotherapy Compounding Mat** A **chemotherapy compounding mat**, often called a chemo mat, is a thin mat, approximately 12″ × 18″. One side of the mat has an absorbent material to soak up potential liquid spills within the BSC. The other side of the mat is constructed of a material with a low permeability to prevent liquid from soaking through to the BSC work surface. Prior to performing chemotherapy sterile compounding in the hood, the IV technician centers the chemotherapy compounding mat on the work surface of the BSC and leaves it there throughout the compounding procedure. Upon completion of the compounding process, the technician then places the chemotherapy compounding mat into the chemotherapy sharps container within the clean room.

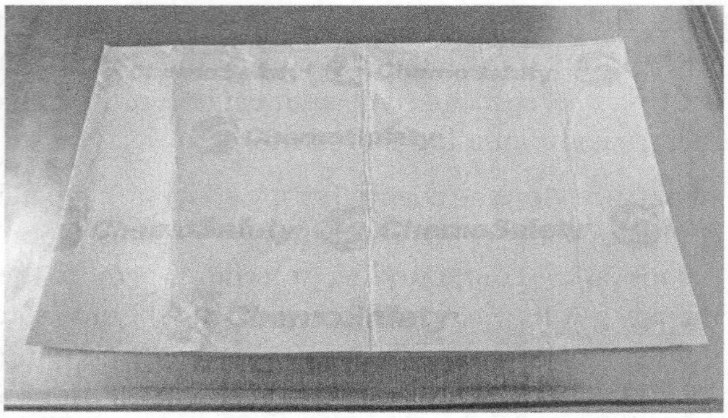

The chemotherapy compounding mat centered on the work surface of the cabinet.

**Chemotherapy Dispensing Pin** A **chemotherapy dispensing pin** is a small plastic device with a spike at one end and a Luer-lock syringe adaptor at the other end. In between the spike and the Luer-lock is a small vent with a 0.22-micron HEPA filter. The spike of the chemotherapy dispensing pin is inserted into the top of a chemotherapy drug vial. The Luer-lock adaptor of the chemotherapy dispensing pin is attached to a syringe. Fluid is then either injected into or withdrawn from the vial into the syringe through the chemotherapy dispensing pin.

The chemotherapy dispensing pin provides a way to relieve negative pressure within the drug vial by venting air into and out of the vial via the dispensing pin's vent. Air may be safely vented from the chemotherapy drug vial without fear of **aerosolization** because any drug particle or fluid escaping from the vial is trapped by the 0.22-micron HEPA filter on the chemotherapy dispensing pin. The chemotherapy dispensing pin is an important supply item in chemotherapy sterile compounding due to its ability to equalize air pressure and facilitate withdrawal from a vial without the need to create positive pressure within the vial. In addition, the chemotherapy dispensing pin is an important safety tool used to protect sterile compounding personnel from exposure to potentially toxic aerosolized chemotherapy solution.

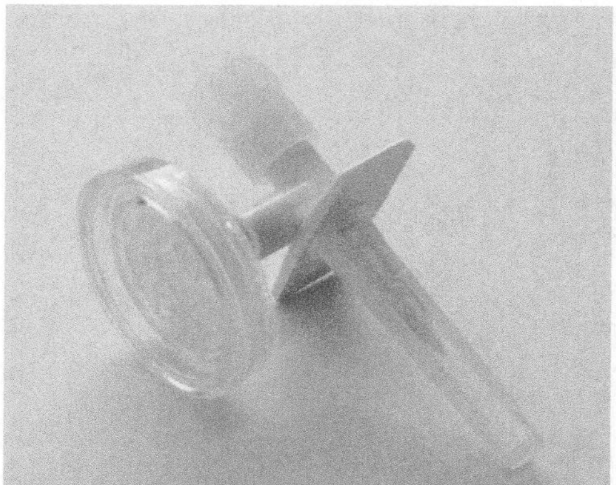

A chemotherapy dispensing pin safely relieves the negative pressure within a drug vial.

**Closed-System Transfer Device** A **closed-system transfer device (CSTD)** is a small, disposable device that may be used to safely draw fluid from a vial into a syringe, or to inject fluid from a syringe into an IV or IVPB. This type of transfer device provides a sealed pathway so that hazardous drugs can be drawn up with less risk to the preparer. There are two types of CSTDs: the injector Luer-lock expansion chamber device and the protector device.

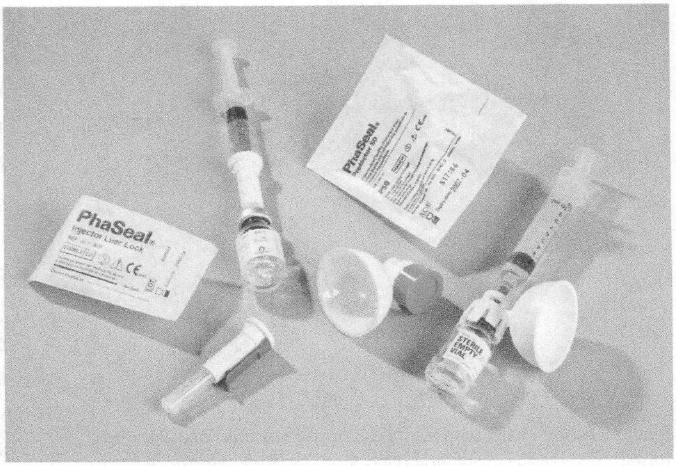

CSTDs used in the preparation of chemotherapy CSPs.

The **injector Luer-lock expansion chamber device** is a CSTD consisting of a small plastic device with a spike at one end and a Luer-lock syringe adaptor at the other end. Between the spike and Luer-lock adaptor, and slightly to the side, is a double-membrane expansion chamber. The expansion chamber expands or contracts to equalize air pressure within a vial during drug withdrawal procedures. The injector Luer-lock expansion chamber device is sometimes used instead of a chemotherapy dispensing pin.

> **POINTER**
> Although CSTDs are often used in chemotherapy sterile compounding, the associated costs make them prohibitive to use in the classroom. Therefore, these devices are not used in the procedural lab of this chapter. IV technicians, however, are taught how to properly use CSTDs during on-the-job training in their sterile compounding facility.

The **protector device** is a small plastic device with a Luer-lock syringe adaptor at one end and a recessed needle at the other end. This device also contains a double-membrane expansion chamber to equalize pressure. The protector device is used to inject medication into an IV or IVPB.

**IV Base Solution Bag** The IV base solution bag is the same type of bag used for other LVPs: a bag with a tail injection port. When inserting a needle into the tail injection port of an IV bag, the needle should be inserted directly into the injection port without regard to the position of the needle bevel, and without creating any bend to the needle, as is done when inserting a needle into a vial.

**IV Tubing and Compounding Completion Supplies** Sterile, nonvented IV tubing is attached to the LVP bag to administer the chemotherapy CSP to the patient. To prevent unintended exposure to the CSP fluid, the IV technician should attach the IV tubing to the LVP and then **prime the tubing** before injecting the chemotherapy medication into the LVP. To "prime the tubing" means to run fluid from the IV base solution through the tubing until the entire tubing has been purged of air. Consequently, fluid fills the entire fluid pathway within the tubing.

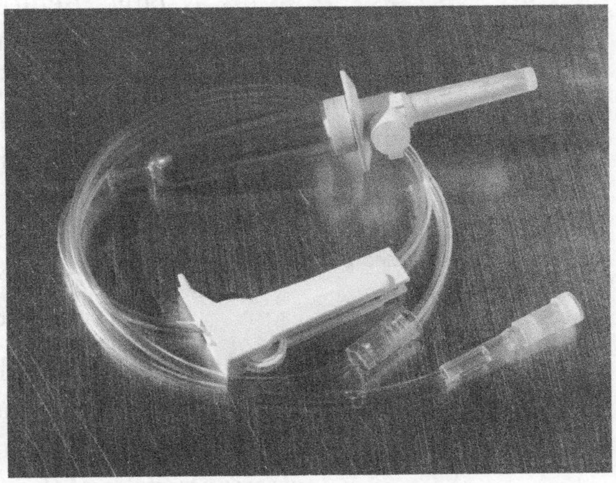
Secondary IV tubing used in chemotherapy administration.

**Chemotherapy Auxiliary Warning Labels and Transport Bags** Due to their toxic nature, chemotherapy CSPs require auxiliary warning labels alerting anyone coming into contact with the medications of their potential harm. Some drugs require additional warning labels due to the potential for patient injury caused by incorrect administration of the medication. For instance, the chemotherapy drugs vincristine and vinblastine can be fatal if administered intrathecally. Such warning labels ensure healthcare personnel take appropriate precautions in regard to storage, handling, administration, cleanup, and disposal of the chemotherapy CSP and related supplies. Chemotherapy auxiliary warning labels should be applied to all CSPs and to chemotherapy

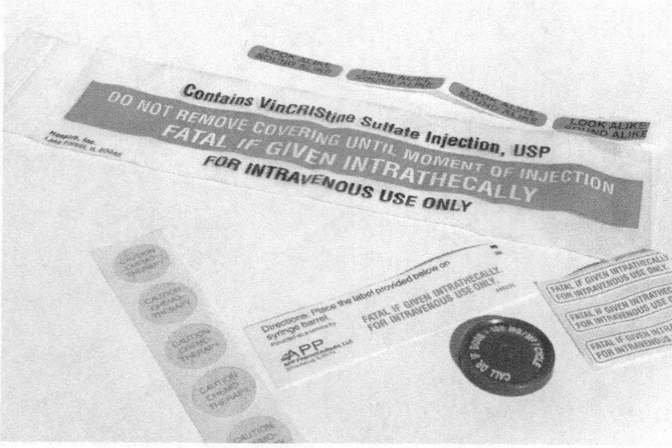


Vincristine and vinblastine medications require auxiliary warning labels, including a label indicating that the medications cannot be administered intrathecally.

transport and storage bins. Most chemotherapy sharps containers are stamped with a chemotherapy warning label; if not, a chemotherapy warning label should be affixed to them as well.

**Chemotherapy Sharps Container** Chemotherapy sharps containers are similar to regular sharps containers in shape and function. They are rigid, plastic buckets that have snap-lock plastic lids. In general, chemotherapy sharps containers are bright yellow in color. All chemotherapy sharps containers should be labeled with a chemotherapy warning label. Keep a small yellow chemotherapy sharps container in the clean room within the BSC on the work surface and/or next to the BSC in an area that does not obstruct traffic or impede airflow into the cabinet. Keep a large chemotherapy sharps container in a designated area in the anteroom.

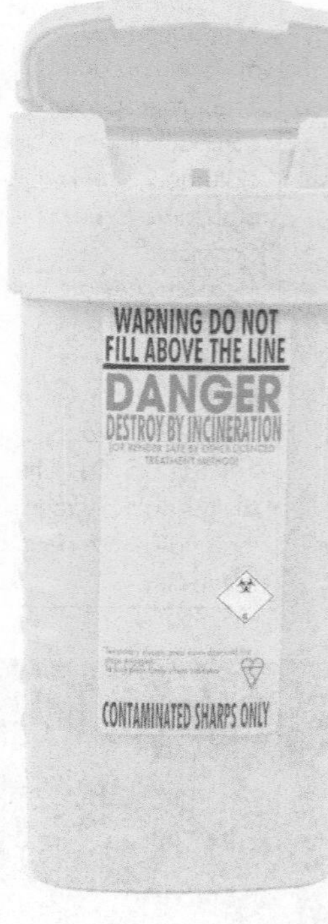


Large chemotherapy sharps container used in the anteroom.

In contrast to regular sharps containers—used solely for the disposal of needles, syringes, broken glass, and blood products—a chemotherapy sharps container is used to dispose all waste and supply items used in chemotherapy sterile compounding. Upon completion of the sterile compounding procedure, the IV technician places the used chemotherapy compounding mat, other chemotherapy-specific supplies (such as needles, syringes, and vials), the chemotherapy gloves and gown, and the chemotherapy waste products (such as IPA swabs) into the chemotherapy sharps container in the clean room. Once in the anteroom, the technician disposes of the regular sterile gloves, face mask, beard cover (if appropriate), hair cover, and shoe covers into the large yellow chemotherapy sharps container in the anteroom.

Facilities that prepare large numbers of chemotherapy CSPs often place a large chemotherapy sharps container on the floor in the clean room and an additional small chemotherapy sharps container on the work surface inside the BSC so that needles and syringes may be easily disposed of during the chemotherapy sterile compounding process. This prevents hazardous chemicals, which may have accumulated on the needle or syringe, from contaminating clean room air if, for example, they were to be brought out of the BSC to be placed into the chemotherapy sharps container on the clean room floor. The large chemotherapy sharps container is used to dispose of items such as the chemotherapy gown and gloves.

Procedures related to the disposal of chemotherapy sharps containers vary among facilities. In general, the small chemotherapy sharps container within the BSC is removed upon the completion of chemotherapy compounding procedures. The exterior surface of the small sharps container is then wiped down with lint-free gauze saturated with sterile 70% IPA. The used gauze is placed in the small chemotherapy sharps container and the lid is snapped shut. The small chemotherapy sharps container is then brought into the anteroom and placed inside of the large chemotherapy sharps container. Once the large chemotherapy sharps container is full, the plastic lid is applied and snapped shut in preparation for transport to off-site hazardous waste disposal. Sterile compounding personnel should refer to their facility's P&P manual to determine appropriate procedures for disposal of chemotherapy sharps containers.

Filled, sealed chemotherapy sharps containers are removed from compounding facilities by companies specially trained in hazardous waste transportation and disposal. The hazardous waste is then transported to a specialized, off-site facility for high-temperature incineration. This method of hazardous waste disposal, which is monitored by the EPA and individual state DOTs, offers the greatest level of protection to the public and the environment.

***BSC*** As mentioned earlier, chemotherapy CSPs must be prepared in a special type of hood known as a BSC. There are three classes of BSCs. The primary differences among the three classes of BSCs are the hoods' venting methods and the level of protection provided for workers.

**Class I BSC** A **Class I BSC** provides protection for the worker but does not provide a suitable HEPA-filtered, ISO Class 5 environment to prepare CSPs. This type of BSC is used for chemical manufacturing and is not appropriate for sterile product preparation.

**Class II BSC** A **Class II BSC** provides protection for the worker and an ISO Class 5 environment suitable for chemotherapy sterile compounding. This type of BSC is the most commonly used hood for chemotherapy sterile compounding. Within Class II are two distinct types: Type A and Type B. A *Class II, Type A BSC* recirculates a percentage of the airflow from the BSC back into the clean room or surrounding environment after it has been filtered through an exhaust HEPA filter located within the BSC. A *Class II, Type B BSC* sends air from within the BSC through a dedicated exhaust ventilation system and into the environment outside of the building after it has been filtered through an exhaust HEPA filter located within the BSC.

The Class II, Type B BSC offers the greatest level of protection for sterile compounding personnel; however, the cost associated with building or modifying a facility to provide a dedicated and properly filtered exhaust ventilation system makes this type of BSC somewhat prohibitive. Therefore, a Class II, Type A BSC is most commonly used for chemotherapy sterile compounding.

**Class III BSC** A Class III BSC is designed for the manufacture of microbiological agents and provides maximum worker protection. Generally, this type of **gas-tight BSC** is not used for chemotherapy sterile compounding due to the exorbitant cost and labor associated with its use.

***Components of the BSC*** The BSC is comprised of seven major components, including the air intake grills, blower, glass shield, exhaust HEPA filter, hood HEPA filter, prefilter, and the work surface (see Figure 14.3).

**Air Intake Grills** The **air intake grills**, located along the interior sides of the BSC work surface, draw contaminated air from within the BSC work space away from the worker and then force the contaminated air from the cabinet into the exhaust HEPA filter.

**Blower** The **blower** serves to draw air into the cabinet, force the air through the hood HEPA filter—thereby creating an ISO Class 5 environment—and then circulate the air out of the cabinet through the exhaust HEPA filter.

**POINTER**
The glass shield at the front of the BSC is adjustable, allowing IV technicians to raise the shield during hood-cleaning procedures.

**Glass Shield** The **glass shield** located at the front of the BSC offers additional protection for the worker. The shield blocks the technician's face and upper torso from inadvertent exposure to the chemotherapy medications and prevents aspiration of the toxic chemicals. The glass shield aperture should be maintained at a height of eight inches during chemotherapy sterile compounding procedures, to provide maximum protection for the technician.

**Exhaust HEPA Filter** The **exhaust HEPA filter** is an important feature of the BSC because it removes hazardous drug contaminants—generated during chemotherapy sterile compounding procedures—from the air within the BSC before the air leaves the cabinet. This filter must be recertified by an independent laminar airflow hood recertification company every six months or whenever the cabinet is moved. Recertification records must be kept on hand in the pharmacy for the life of the BSC.

**Hood HEPA Filter** The **hood HEPA filter** has the same function as the HEPA filter in a standard (non-BSC) laminar airflow hood: The filter provides a source of sterile air for the preparation of CSPs, thus establishing an ISO Class 5 environment within the BSC. However, unlike a standard horizontal laminar airflow hood in which the

**FIGURE 14.3**

**Cross section of Vertical Laminar Airflow Hood (Side View)**

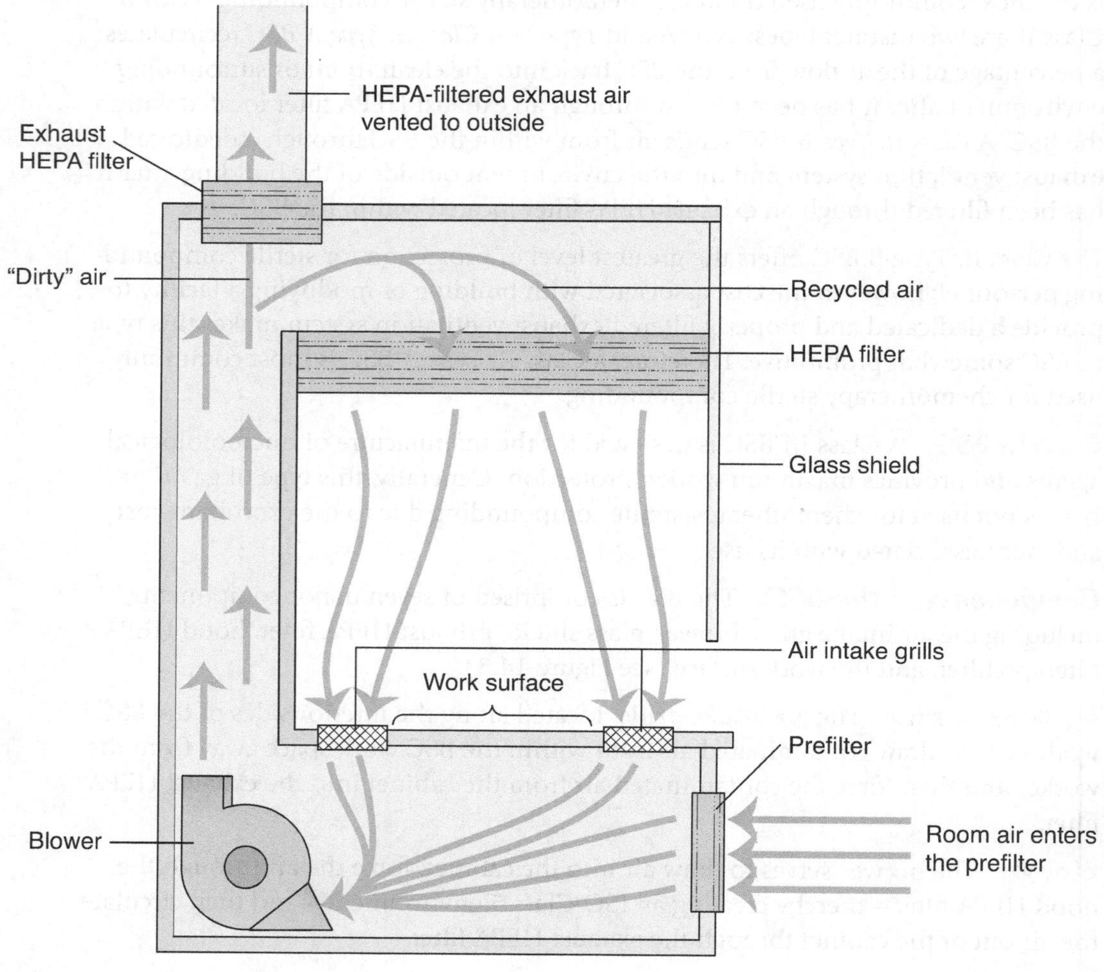

HEPA filter is located at the back wall of the cabinet, the BSC's HEPA filter is typically located in the ceiling of the hood. The position of the hood's HEPA filter means that the airflow within a BSC blows *downward* or *vertically* from the ceiling toward the work surface. Once the HEPA-filtered air reaches the work surface, it is immediately sucked into the air intake grills and drawn away from the worker. Like the exhaust HEPA filter, this filter must be recertified by an independent laminar hood recertification company every six months or whenever the cabinet is moved, and the recertification records must remain in the pharmacy for the life of the cabinet.

**PREFILTER** The BSC's **prefilter** is the same in design and function as the prefilter on a standard horizontal laminar airflow hood. The prefilter must be replaced every 30 days, with the task recorded on a prefilter-replacement checklist that must be kept on file for the life of the BSC. The used prefilter is then placed into a large plastic bag, sealed shut, and labeled with a chemotherapy warning sticker. The bagged prefilter is subsequently transported to off-site hazardous waste disposal to be incinerated along with other chemotherapy waste.

**WORK SURFACE** The BSC **work surface** has the same function and location as the work surface of a horizontal laminar airflow hood.

***Cleaning the BSC*** Cleaning procedures for the BSC are significantly different from those procedures used for cleaning a standard horizontal laminar airflow hood. The variances are due to the different components as well as the airflow movement within the hood. The vertical airflow dictates the cleaning order and direction and requires the worker to move from the area closest to the HEPA filter—in this case, the ceiling of the BSC—toward the parts of the BSC farthest away from the HEPA filter. Because hazardous drugs are prepared within the BSC, additional precautions must be taken in order to clean the hood in a manner that protects the worker. Please reference the ASHP website (www.ASHP.org) for general guidelines for cleaning the BSC.

**POINTER**

The BSC and CACI hoods require special step-by-step cleaning procedures. The steps may vary depending on the type and design of the hood, but they are generally different from the procedures used to clean a horizontal laminar airflow hood. Some of the basic guidelines for cleaning the BSC are provided in Table 4 of Appendix C. Consult USP Chapter <797> for information about procedures specific to the use of a BSC. Always refer to the manufacturer's Instruction Guide for specific BSC or CACI hood-cleaning procedures.

Class II, Type A BSC hoods may be manufactured in several different configurations. For example, in some BSCs, the prefilter is located at the top of the BSC, whereas in others it is located near the bottom, under the work surface. Some BSCs have removable work surfaces to allow for cleaning under the intake grills or alarm systems that alert workers to high contaminant levels in the hood. In light of these variables, it is vital that all sterile compounding personnel understand the operation, use, and cleaning procedures of the BSC. Guidelines for specific BSC operation and hood-cleaning information can be found in the manufacturers' instruction manuals.

***Special Considerations for Supplies*** Unlike other sterile compounding procedures, the compounding of chemotherapy CSPs has unique requirements for the placement, selection, and handling of supply items. For example, unlike a horizontal laminar airflow hood, the outer six-inch zone of the BSC is not considered to be an area of insufficient HEPA-filtered airflow. However, it is advisable for IV technicians to work closer to the back of the BSC (away from the opening in the glass shield) when compounding chemotherapy CSPs. Doing so avoids the air turbulence created as room air enters the cabinet through the glass shield aperture and offers the worker greater protection from exposure to potential contaminants.

When selecting supplies for chemotherapy compounding procedures, sterile compounding personnel must use Luer-lock syringes. Using slip-tip syringes during withdrawal and injection procedures poses an exposure danger should the needle slip off of the syringe tip. The Luer-lock syringes should not be more than three-quarters (¾) full, to prevent accidental leakage should the plunger become separated from the syringe barrel due to overfilling. To prevent such leakage, choose larger syringes than those typically used for nonchemotherapy sterile compounding procedures. For example, when drawing up a chemotherapy drug volume of 19 mL, use a 35-mL syringe. In a nonchemotherapy compounding scenario, a 20-mL syringe would be used to draw up this same volume.

Chemotherapy sterile compounding also requires special handling of supplies. For example, chemotherapy vials must be handled differently than nonchemotherapy vials. IV technicians should never use positive pressure, the milking technique, or vented needles for chemotherapy compounding procedures, as these techniques pose the risk of hazardous drug aspiration. Instead, technicians should use negative-pressure supply items, such as a chemotherapy dispensing pin or a CSTD, to relieve air pressure during chemotherapy sterile compounding.

## Critical Sites of Essential Supplies and Chemotherapy Supplies

Before beginning preparatory procedures in the anteroom or clean room, the IV technician must recall the critical sites of the supplies. Identifying the critical site of each supply item helps you to determine the proper procedure for handling the supply item once you have entered the clean room and begin to work in the hood.

The critical sites of essential supply items include sterile 70% IPA swabs, the syringe tip, the piston plunger and inner plunger shaft of the syringe, and the needle. The critical sites of the procedure-specific supply items include the chemotherapy dispensing pin spike and Luer-lock syringe adaptor, the IV tubing spike, and the IV tubing port. The critical sites of all of these items are supplied from their manufacturers in a sterile form and should, therefore, never be swabbed with alcohol prior to use.

The critical sites of other supplies used for the Chapter 14 procedural lab include the injection port of the IV base solution and the medication vial's rubber top. These critical sites must be swabbed with sterile 70% IPA prior to insertion with a needle or chemotherapy dispensing pin spike.

Use care in all compounding procedures to avoid touch contamination, shadowing, or incorrect placement of the critical sites of any supply item within the hood. In general, the direction of HEPA-filtered air within the BSC flows from the cabinet ceiling downward toward the work surface. The direction of airflow must be considered when working within a vertical airflow BSC so that the critical sites of all supply items receive uninterrupted airflow from the hood's HEPA filter. Adjust aseptic technique procedures as necessary so that items are positioned and manipulated in such a way that nothing passes between the BSC ceiling (where the HEPA filter is located) and the critical sites of the supplies. For example, when handling a vial within a BSC, sterile compounding personnel must tip the vial sideways when inserting a chemotherapy dispensing pin or needle-and-syringe unit into the vial. Turning the vial to the side ensures that neither hand nor supply item interrupts airflow to the top of the vial at any time (for example, when entering the vial top with the spike or needle).

# Preview the Lab Procedure

*The following material provides a brief overview of the lab procedure that you will perform. First, read the* Preview the Lab Procedure *section. Then read each step of the* Procedural Lab *section carefully, visualizing every action. Next, reinforce your understanding of the process by watching the demonstration video. Once you are in the lab, your instructor will demonstrate the procedure, and then you will perform the procedure by following the steps in the* Procedural Lab *section. Practice the lab procedure multiple times. After sufficient practice, you will complete the lab procedure for process validation by your instructor.*

***Note:*** *This procedural lab requires the use of a BSC. For pharmacies that do not have this type of hood, IV technicians should consult the* Instruction Guide *provided by the hood's manufacturer or their facility's P&P manual to determine which procedures may need to be adjusted to suit their hood.*

**POINTER**
Sterile compounding personnel must comply with certain restrictions when working in the anteroom and clean room areas. These restrictions include no gum chewing, horseplay, or food or drink in both the anteroom and clean room, and no hair spray, perfume, makeup, artificial or polished nails, or jewelry in the sterile compounding environment.

## Anteroom Preparatory Procedures

Because preparation for the sterile compounding process begins in the anteroom, that transition area provides a space for implementing the standard pharmacy protocols discussed in Chapters 3–6 of this textbook, including:

- verifying the CSP label against the chemotherapy medication order
- performing correct pharmacy calculations to determine type, size, and number of supply items needed
- gathering and cleaning of supplies
- performing aseptic garbing and hand washing
- donning a sterile chemotherapy gown
- donning chemotherapy safety glasses

***Verifying the CSP Label*** The first step in the preparation of a chemotherapy CSP is verification of the CSP label. Compare the chemotherapy medication order to the CSP label to verify that all of the information on the CSP label matches the chemotherapy medication order exactly. Then read the CSP label to determine the desired dose of the chemotherapy medication. Finally, read the CSP label to determine the correct type of IV base solution.

**POINTER**
It is considered best practice to have a minimum of three pharmacy staff members review the chemotherapy medication order and CSP label. Typically, one pharmacist enters the order into the computer and generates a CSP label; a second pharmacist double-checks all calculations and verifies the accuracy of the CSP label; and an IV technician then repeats the process by double-checking the calculations and verifying the accuracy of the CSP label.

***Performing Pharmacy Calculations*** To confirm that the chemotherapy medication dosage on the CSP label was calculated properly by the pharmacist (or another IV technician) and was based on the chemotherapy medication order for the drug (mg/m$^2$) and the patient's BSA, you must perform a series of calculations. Your calculations determine the volume of drug that must be withdrawn from the reconstituted vial to prepare the desired CSP dose.

***Gathering and Cleaning Supplies*** After performing the necessary calculations, place the chemotherapy medication order and the CSP label into the appropriate-sized plastic bags. Then gather all necessary compounding supplies and obtain a transport vehicle—such as a stainless-steel cart, basket, or tray—to facilitate an easy transfer of supplies into and out of the clean room.

Use a presaturated aseptic cleaning wipe to disinfect the transport vehicle and the exterior surface of every supply item. Then place the cleaned supply items into the

**POINTER**

If you are using a chemotherapy gown that only covers the front of your body (i.e., a smock-type gown), you must first don a regular, sterile gown, and then don a chemotherapy gown on top of the regular gown.

transport vehicle. (*Note:* You will need to disinfect the chemotherapy safety glasses as well, but you will use sterile 70% IPA poured onto sterile, lint-free gauze. This task should be done prior to placing the safety glasses in the transport vehicle.)

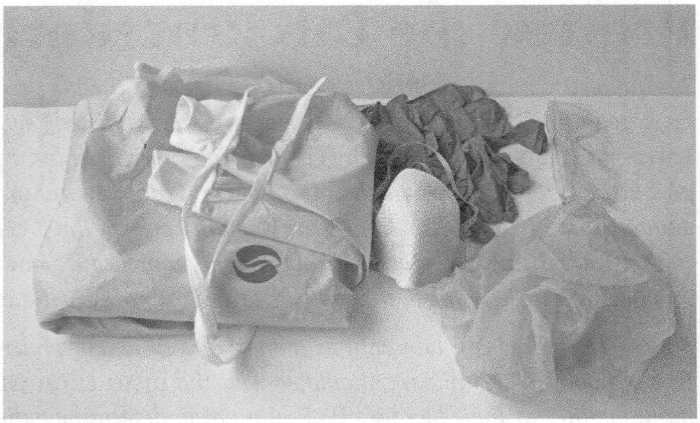

Aseptic garb for chemotherapy compounding.

***Donning PPE*** Now that you have assembled your clean supplies, you must put on personal protective equipment (PPE), a requirement for working in the clean room. Before donning the appropriate aseptic garb, be sure that you are wearing close-toed shoes and either scrub uniforms or another approved lightweight, nonshedding clothing. Then put on aseptic shoe covers, a hair cover, a face mask, and, if appropriate, a beard cover. Lastly, don a sterile chemotherapy gown.

## Clean Room Preparatory Procedures

Refer to Tables 3 and 4 in Appendix C

When preparing chemotherapy CSPs for patient administration, sterile compounding personnel must diligently follow established pharmacy clean room protocols. These protocols are discussed in Chapter 6 and Tables 3 and 4 of Appendix C, with additional chemotherapy-specific regulations discussed throughout this chapter.

Once the preparatory steps have been completed, chemotherapy CSP compounding procedures may begin.

Upon entering the clean room, place the transport basket or cart onto a clean shelf, table, or countertop. If the transport vehicle used is a cart, wheel it so that it is positioned away from the hood prefilter. Cleanse your hands and forearms with sterile, foamed 70% IPA and allow them to dry thoroughly. Don regular sterile gloves. Position the cuffs of the gloves on the forearms, *under* the knit wrist cuffs of the chemotherapy gown. Don sterile chemotherapy gloves by pulling them over the regular sterile gloves. The cuffs of the chemotherapy gloves should be positioned *over* the wrist cuffs of the chemotherapy gown. Lastly, don chemotherapy safety glasses.

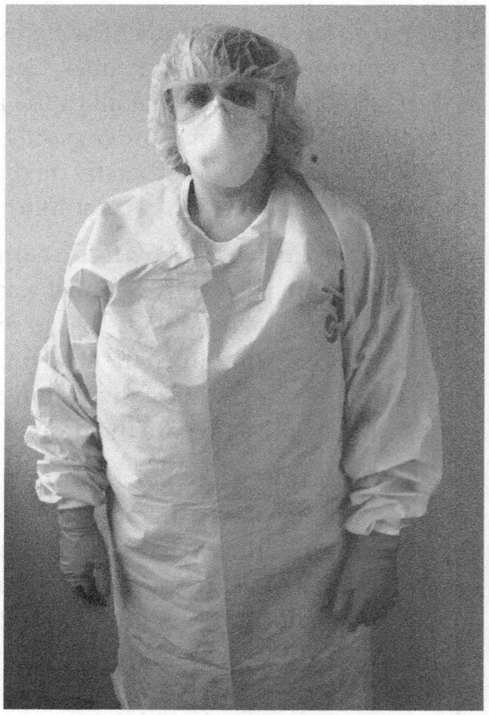

An IV technician wearing chemotherapy aseptic garb.

Due to time constraints, you will not perform BSC-cleaning procedures during this procedural lab. Keep in mind that, in sterile compounding practice, BSC-cleaning procedures are mandatory and must be performed prior to sterile compounding and at intervals prescribed by USP Chapter <797>.

> **POINTER**
> In practice, the small ("interior") yellow chemotherapy sharps container is usually left inside the BSC and used for the disposal of waste from multiple CSPs. The large ("exterior") yellow chemotherapy sharps container remains in the clean room next to (but outside of) the BSC. When both containers are filled within 1" to 2" from their tops, the buckets must be removed for proper disposal.

***Arranging and Preparing Supplies in the BSC*** Once the BSC has been cleaned, you must transfer the clean supplies from the transport vehicle or clean countertop to certain areas within the BSC. Place the small chemotherapy sharps container toward the back of the cabinet's work surface and off to the side. This positioning allows for uninterrupted airflow during compounding operations within the cabinet. (*Note:* For this procedural lab, you will not use a second clean room chemotherapy sharps container, typically positioned on the floor of the clean room next to the BSC; in practice, refer to your facility's P&P manual for protocol.)

Next, center the chemotherapy compounding mat onto the work surface of the BSC. Also on the BSC work surface, opposite from the sharps container, place the IV tubing, drug vial, IPA swabs, syringe, needle, chemotherapy dispensing pin, and one-third of a 3" stack of sterile, lint-free 4 × 4 gauze pads. Remove the outer dust cover from the LVP and place it into the chemotherapy sharps container. Then place the LVP onto the chemotherapy compounding mat. Keep the other supply items temporarily in the transport vehicle.

## Chemotherapy CSP Compounding Procedure

With the chemotherapy sharps container placed to one side of the interior work surface of the BSC, the small compounding items positioned along the other side of the interior work surface of the BSC, and the IV bag centered onto the chemotherapy compounding mat on the BSC work surface, you are ready to begin the compounding procedure. Keep in mind that, during the procedure, only the supplies being used in a particular step should be placed on the chemotherapy compounding mat. Other supply items should remain on the work surface of the BSC until needed.

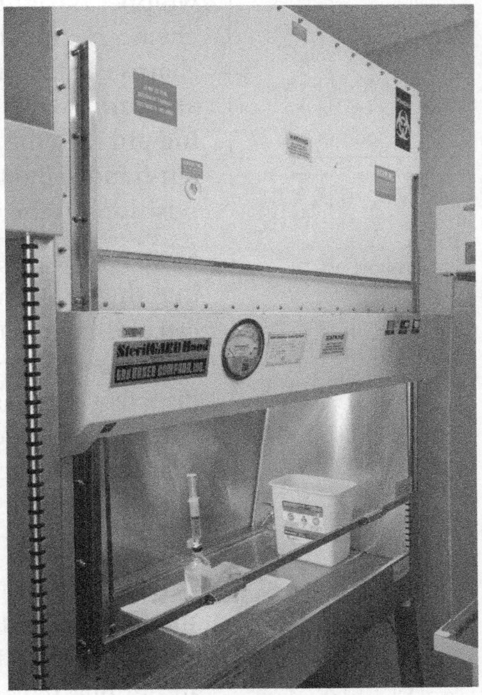

Correct placement of the chemotherapy sharps container and chemotherapy compounding mat within a BSC.

***Priming the IV tubing*** Remove the outer wrapping from the IV tubing, and place the wrapper into the small chemotherapy sharps container in the BSC. Close the roll clamp on the IV tubing, and temporarily place the IV tubing onto the work surface. Next, remove the plastic cap from the tubing needle adaptor, place the plastic cap into the small chemotherapy sharps container, and aseptically attach a regular needle to the adaptor. Remove the pull tag to expose the LVP tubing port and dispose of the removed tag into the small chemotherapy sharps container. Then remove the cap from the tubing spike and place it into the small chemotherapy sharps container as well. Aseptically insert the tubing spike into the LVP port. Take care to avoid touch contamination and shadowing when inserting the spike into the port. Pinch and release the tubing drip chamber once or twice to draw a small amount of fluid from the IV bag into the drip chamber.

Open an IPA swab and place it onto the chemotherapy compounding mat next to the gauze pads. Dispose of the wrapper from the IPA swab into the small chemotherapy sharps container. Remove the needle cap (attached to the IV tubing needle adaptor on the IV tubing), and place the cap onto the IPA swab. Without setting down, touching, or shadowing the needle and attached tubing adaptor, begin the flow of IV fluid by slightly rolling up the clamp. Allow a few drops of IV fluid to drip onto the sterile, lint-free gauze placed on the chemotherapy compounding mat. Roll the tubing clamp shut to stop the flow of fluid. Recap the needle. Temporarily place the LVP with attached, filled tubing and recapped needle onto the work surface within the BSC.

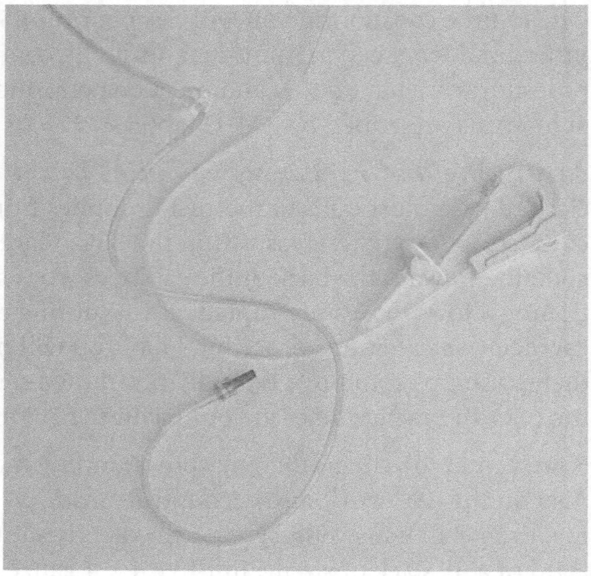

IV tubing with a roll clamp for adjusting the flow of solution.

**POINTER**

Some facilities prefer to have the CSP with attached, primed tubing delivered to the nursing unit without an attached needle. In this case, the tubing needle adaptor is recapped with an attached plastic cap provided by the tubing manufacturer (instead of a needle). The nurse then removes the plastic cap and attaches a regular needle to the adaptor just prior to administering the CSP. Refer to your facility's P&P manual for the established protocol.

***Preparing the Chemotherapy Vial*** Remove the flip-top cap from the drug vial and swab the vial's rubber top with a new IPA swab. Dispose of the flip-top cap and swab wrapper into the small chemotherapy sharps container. Remove the outer wrapper from the chemotherapy dispensing pin and dispose of the outer wrapper into the small chemotherapy sharps container. Remove the cap from the chemotherapy dispensing pin spike. Place the cap into the small chemotherapy sharps container. Without touching or shadowing the spike, pick up the drug vial and turn it slightly sideways; then insert the spike of the chemotherapy dispensing pin into the vial top. With a counterclockwise motion (clockwise if you are left-handed), return the vial (with attached dispensing pin) to its original, upright position on the work surface.

**BE AWARE**

Never draw up and inject air into a chemotherapy vial, as this may create drug aspiration. Avoid using the milking technique to rapidly force fluid into a chemotherapy vial. All manipulations of chemotherapy fluid into or out of containment vessels, such as a vial, should be done slowly and carefully. Also, never use a vented needle for chemotherapy since the air vented from the chemotherapy vial is hazardous.

Next, remove the syringe from its outer wrapper and then dispose of the wrapper into the small chemotherapy sharps container. If applicable, remove the syringe tip cap and then place it into the small chemotherapy sharps container. Without setting the syringe down, remove the Luer-lock syringe adaptor cap on the chemotherapy dispensing pin and place it onto the IPA swab. Still without setting down the syringe, and without touching or shadowing the syringe tip or chemotherapy dispensing pin adaptor, turn the vial (with attached, uncapped syringe adaptor on the dispensing pin) slightly sideways and attach the syringe tip to the Luer-lock adaptor (located on top of the chemotherapy dispensing pin).

Carefully invert the vial (with chemotherapy dispensing pin and syringe still attached) so that the syringe is below the vial. Pull down on the flat knob of the plunger to draw fluid from the vial into the syringe. Gently tap the syringe to force air bubbles toward the tip of the syringe. When all bubbles have risen to the syringe tip, gently push up on the flat knob of the plunger to expel remaining air and unnecessary fluid back into the vial.

Once the proper amount of fluid has been drawn from the vial through the chemotherapy dispensing pin and into the syringe, return the syringe (attached to the dispensing pin, which is attached to the vial) to the original starting position with the vial resting upright on the chemotherapy compounding mat. Turn the chemotherapy dispensing pin-and-syringe unit slightly sideways and then remove the syringe from the dispensing pin by twisting it off the Luer-lock adaptor. Aseptically attach a regular needle to the filled syringe and temporarily place the filled syringe with attached, capped regular needle onto the chemotherapy compounding mat. Recap the Luer-lock adaptor (on top of the dispensing pin) with the cap you earlier placed onto the IPA swab. Arrange the drug vial with attached, filled chemotherapy dispensing pin next to the filled syringe on the chemotherapy compounding mat. Place the LVP (with filled tubing) next to the filled syringe on the chemotherapy mat within the BSC. Ask for a verification check by a pharmacist or your instructor.

**BE AWARE**

Do not draw up any air into the syringe in order to inject positive pressure into the vial, as this may cause dangerous aerosolization of the chemotherapy drug. The chemotherapy dispensing pin equalizes negative air pressure so that fluid may be safely withdrawn from the vial. This negative-pressure technique is required whenever performing chemotherapy sterile compounding procedures.

***Preparing the Chemotherapy CSP*** After the verification check has been completed, open an IPA swab and place the wrapper into the small chemotherapy sharps container. Disinfect the injection port of the IV bag with the swab and then place the used swab under the injection port to absorb any medication that may drip from the port. Carefully remove the needle cap from the filled needle-and-syringe unit. Dispose of the cap into the small chemotherapy sharps container. Then insert the needle into the IV bag injection port, taking care not to puncture the sidewall of the port. Push up on the flat knob of the plunger to inject the medication from the syringe into the IV bag. Once all of the medication has been injected into the IV bag, grasp the barrel of the syringe and remove the needle-and-syringe unit from the IV bag. Without recapping the needle, place the empty needle-and-syringe unit into the small chemotherapy sharps container.

***Cleaning and Compounding Completion Procedures*** Upon completion of the chemotherapy compounding procedures, dispose of the used vial with attached chemotherapy dispensing pin, caps, IPA swabs, used gauze pads, chemotherapy compounding mat, and any remaining supply items into the small chemotherapy sharps container. Gently squeeze the CSP to check the bag for leakage, and then inspect the solution for precipitate matter. If neither issue is present, cover the LVP injection port with an IVA seal. The IVA seal prevents exposure to minute drops of fluid that may leak from the CSP injection port due to needle punctures made during compounding.

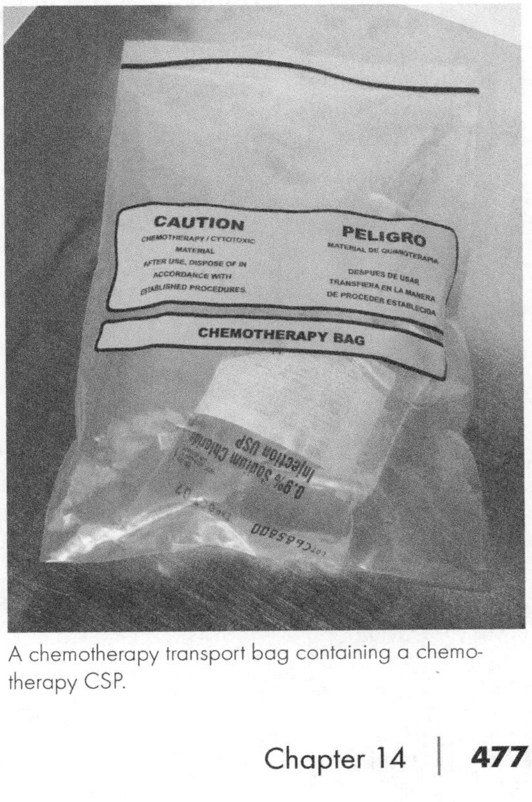

A chemotherapy transport bag containing a chemotherapy CSP.

Outside of the BSC, lightly saturate another one-third stack of the sterile, lint-free gauze with sterile 70% IPA. Bring the CSP and attached, filled tubing out of the BSC, and clean the entire exterior surface of the CSP and the entire attached-and-filled tubing. This action helps to remove any hazardous drug that may have accumulated on the exterior of the supply items during sterile compounding procedures.

Affix the CSP label and a chemotherapy auxiliary warning label to the prepared CSP. Then place the labeled CSP with attached-and-filled tubing into a plastic bag and seal the bag.

**BE AWARE**

To reuse supply items such as the pour bottle of sterile 70% IPA, you must remove any potential contaminants from the exterior of the bottle prior to returning it to the anteroom. This is accomplished by wiping down the exterior surface of the supply item with sterile, lint-free gauze pads saturated with sterile 70% IPA.

Affix a chemotherapy warning label on the plastic transport bag and place the chemotherapy transport bag with labeled CSP into the transport vehicle.

Remove your chemotherapy gloves by pulling them down from the wrist, turning each glove inside out as it is pulled off. Place the used gloves into the small chemotherapy sharps container. Remove the chemotherapy gown by pulling it down off of the shoulders, turning the gown inside out as it is removed. Place the used gown into the small chemotherapy sharps container.

Lightly saturate the remaining one-third stack of sterile, lint-free gauze pads with sterile 70% IPA from the pour bottle. Then, using the saturated gauze pads, disinfect the exterior surface of the IPA pour bottle and the exterior surfaces of other potentially contaminated items that must be returned to the anteroom.

Place the disinfected pour bottle of IPA next to the CSP in the transport vehicle and return them to the anteroom. Remove remaining PPE in the order described in Chapter 6 of this textbook. Dispose of the removed PPE (including the regular gloves) into the anteroom chemotherapy sharps container. Remove the chemotherapy safety glasses and wipe them down with an aseptic cleaning wipe or a stack of lint-free gauze pads saturated with sterile 70% IPA. Record the date and your initials on the CSP label. Ask for a final verification check from a pharmacist or your instructor.

# Watch the Demonstration Video

*Watch the Chapter 14 Demonstration Video, which shows the step-by-step aseptic procedures for compounding a chemotherapy preparation. For the purposes of the Chapter 14 Demonstration Video, neither aseptic hand washing nor hood cleaning is demonstrated. Refer to the Chapter 6 video for a demonstration of aseptic hand-washing procedures, and to Table 4 of Appendix C for general instructions regarding the cleaning of the BSC.*

**Training Videos DVD**

# Procedural Lab

*This lab walks you through the step-by-step actions that you must follow to properly prepare a chemotherapy CSP using a vertical airflow BSC. Take your time. Work through each step methodically and with close attention to detail.*

***Note:*** *For the purposes of this procedural lab, you will not perform aseptic hand-washing or BSC-cleaning procedures unless directed to do so by your instructor. Should your instructor ask you to perform these procedures, refer to Chapter 6 for instructions on aseptic hand washing and to Table 4 of Appendix C for general guidelines related to cleaning the BSC.*

***Note:*** *For steps 1–3, refer to Chapter 4 for a reminder of the step-by-step procedures required for medication order and CSP label verification, and to Chapter 5 for pharmacy calculation procedures. For steps 4–7, refer to Chapter 3 for a reminder of the process for gathering and cleaning supplies. For steps 8–15, refer to Chapter 6 for step-by-step aseptic garbing, hand-washing, and gloving procedures. You should perform steps 1–11 and steps 66–69 in the anteroom. You should perform steps 12–65 in the clean room.*

## Supplies

### *Essential Supplies*

To complete the Unit 2 procedural labs, you will need to ensure that various essential anteroom and clean room supplies such as those listed in Table 14.3 are available for your use.

**Table 14.3 Essential Anteroom and Clean Room Supplies for Sterile Compounding**

| |
|---|
| **Anteroom Supplies** |
| chemotherapy medication order and CSP label<br>calculator<br>pen<br>permanent, felt-tip marker<br>plastic bags (small and large)<br>aseptic garb, including shoe covers, hair cover, face mask, and beard cover (if appropriate)<br>sterile gown (if applicable)<br>presaturated, aseptic cleaning wipes<br>sterile, foamed 70% IPA<br>waste container<br>transport vehicle (optional) |
| **Clean Room Supplies** |
| sterile, foamed 70% IPA<br>sterile, powder-free gloves<br>sterile 70% IPA swabs individually packaged × 5<br>waste container |

### *Procedure-Specific Supplies*

In addition to the supplies listed in Table 14.3, gather the following items specific to the Chapter 14 chemotherapy procedural lab:

- sterile chemotherapy gown or smock
- chemotherapy safety glasses
- sterile chemotherapy gloves
- 100-mg/100-mL vial cisplatin
- 500-mL 0.9% NS IV base solution (with tail injection port)
- chemotherapy compounding mat
- IV tubing
- 4 × 4 sterile, lint-free gauze pads, approximately a 3" stack (a few additional pads are needed in the anteroom as well)
- 60-mL Luer-lock syringe
- chemotherapy dispensing pin
- regular, 19-gauge needles × 2
- IVA seal
- small chemotherapy sharps container (for inside the BSC)
- vertical airflow BSC
- chemotherapy warning auxiliary labels × 2
- chemotherapy transport bag (to place the CSP into for transport)
- large chemotherapy sharps container (for the anteroom)

## Procedure

### *Verifying the Label*

1. Review the CSP label (see Figure 14.4) to verify that all of the information on the label matches the chemotherapy medication order exactly (see Figure 14.6). Then read the CSP label to determine the desired dose of cisplatin (40 mg). Finally, read the CSP label to determine the correct type of IV base solution (0.9% NS IV base solution).

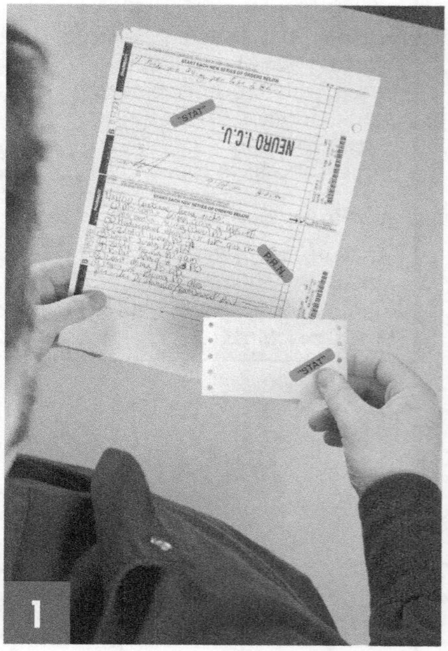

**Chemotherapy IVPB **
Memorial Hospital

**Pt. Name:** Lakins, Bobbie **Room:** 451-Oncology
**Pt. ID#:** 8837200 **Rx#:** 2766399

**Cisplatin 40 mg**
**NS 500 mL**
**Rate: administer IV over 2 hours (250 mL/hour)**
**Frequency: daily at 2 pm × 7 days**

Expires ______
Tech ______
RPh ______

Do Not Refrigerate

****Caution Antineoplastic Agent – Dispose of Hazardous Material According to Chemo Protocol****

**FIGURE 14.4**

**CSP Label for Cisplatin**

### *Calculating Desired Volume*

2. Review the chemotherapy medication order and the CSP label to confirm that the desired dose prescribed on the medication order is accurate, based on the prescriber's order for the drug and the patient's BSA.

   The patient's BSA is 2.00 $m^2$.

   The prescriber ordered cisplatin 20 $mg/m^2$.

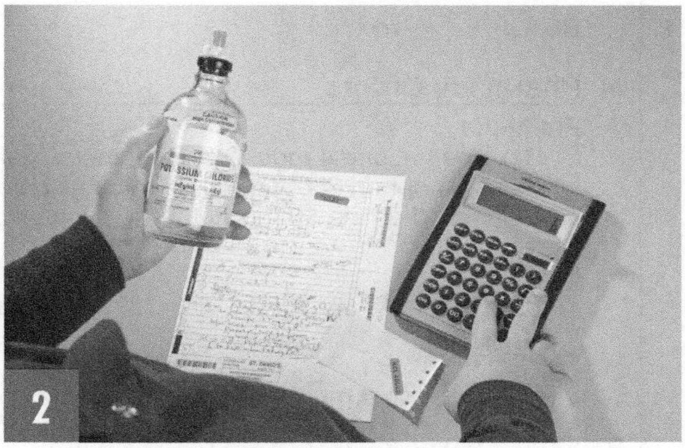


$$2.00 \cancel{m^2} \times \frac{20 \text{ mg}}{\cancel{m^2}} = 2.00 \times 20 = 40 \text{ mg (desired dose)}$$

3. Read the cisplatin medication label (see Figure 14.5). Perform a ratio and proportion calculation to determine how many milliliters ($x$ mL) of cisplatin are needed to prepare the desired CSP dose. (*Note:* For additional assistance on performing ratio and proportion calculations, refer to Chapter 5.)

   The cisplatin drug vial states the concentration is 100 mg/100 mL.

   The cisplatin dose is 40 mg.

$$\frac{100 \text{ mg}}{100 \text{ mL}} = \frac{40 \text{ mg}}{x \text{ mL}}$$

   100 × 40 = 4000 / 100 = 40

   $x$ = 40 mL (volume of cisplatin needed to prepare the CSP)

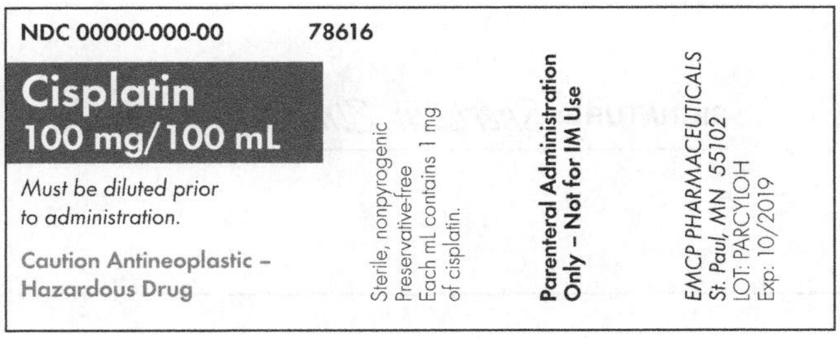
NDC 00000-000-00
78616
Cisplatin
100 mg/100 mL
Must be diluted prior to administration.
Caution Antineoplastic – Hazardous Drug
Sterile, nonpyrogenic
Preservative-free
Each mL contains 1 mg of cisplatin.
Parenteral Administration Only – Not for IM Use
EMCP PHARMACEUTICALS
St. Paul, MN 55102
LOT: PARCYLOH
Exp: 10/2019

**FIGURE 14.5**

**Cisplatin Vial Label**

FIGURE 14.6

**Chemotherapy Standing Orders**

Memorial Hospital
Chemotherapy Standing Orders

**ID#:** 8837200
**Name:** Lakins, Bobbie
**DOB:** 01/23/1953
**Room:** 451 - Oncology
**Rx:** 2766399

**Allergies:** NKA
**Diagnosis:** cervical cancer w/lung mets
**Diet:** regular diet as tolerated

**Weight** 82 kg
**Height** 175 cm
**BSA** 2.00 $m^2$

**Pharmacy Orders**

**Pre Meds**

Dexamethasone 4 mg PO/IV 30 minutes before chemo
Acetaminophen 650 mg PO 30 minutes before chemo
Diphenhydramine 50 mg PO/IV 20 minutes before chemo

**Hydration**

Dextrose 5% in 1/2 NS w/20 mEq potassium chloride per liter to run at 125 mL/hour

**Antiemetics**

Ondansetron 8 mg IVPB q day 30 minutes prior to chemo
Lorazepam 2 mg IVP q day 15 minutes prior to chemo

**Chemotherapy**

Cisplatin 20 mg/$m^2$ in 500 mL 0.9% sodium chloride (NS) IVPB
Administer over 2 hours q day times 7 day(s)

**Other**

Ambien 5 mg @ HS if needed for sleep
Paxil 20 mg bid per home schedule
Oncology consult in a.m. for home healthcare service

**Nursing Orders**

Pt. may be up ad lib w/assistance
Call Dr. Zimmerman or oncology service for temp ≥ 102° F., or for unrelieved nausea or vomiting
Incentive spirometer q shift

**Lab Orders**

Serum creatinine daily
CBC daily and for temp > 101° F

**DATE:** 4/22/2018 **SIGNATURE:** Sheridan Zimmerman, M.D.

### *Gathering and Cleaning Supplies*

4. Place the chemotherapy medication order and the CSP label into the appropriate-sized plastic bags. Gather all the supply items listed in the supply section of the procedural lab.
5. Open the package of aseptic cleaning wipes. Remove one or, if necessary, more wipes, and thoroughly wipe down the entire transport vehicle. Place the used wipes in the waste container.
6. Remove a new aseptic cleaning wipe and wipe down the exterior outer packaging of each supply item. Place the used wipes in the waste container. ***Note:*** Chemotherapy safety glasses should be wiped with sterile 70% IPA prior to placing them in the transport vehicle.
7. Place the cleaned supply items into the transport vehicle.

### *Garbing*

8. Don shoe covers.
9. Put on a hair cover.
10. Don a face mask and beard cover (if appropriate).

    *Note:* For the purposes of this training lab, you will skip the mandatory aseptic hand-washing procedure.

11. Don a sterile chemotherapy gown. ***Note:*** If a chemotherapy smock is used, you must first don a regular sterile gown before donning the smock.
12. Bring all supply items, including an unopened package of sterile chemotherapy gloves, into the clean room. Place the transport vehicle onto a clean surface or countertop within the clean room. If a cart is used, position it so that it does not interrupt airflow into the hood prefilter.
13. Apply sterile, foamed 70% IPA to your hands. Allow them to air-dry and then don sterile gloves. Position the cuffs of the gloves on the forearms, *under* the knit wrist cuffs of the chemotherapy gown.
14. Don sterile chemotherapy gloves by pulling the gloves over the regular gloves. Pull the cuffs of the chemotherapy gloves up onto the forearms, *over* the knit wrist cuffs of the chemotherapy gown.
15. Don chemotherapy safety glasses.

    *Note:* For the purposes of this training lab, you will skip the mandatory BSC-cleaning procedure.

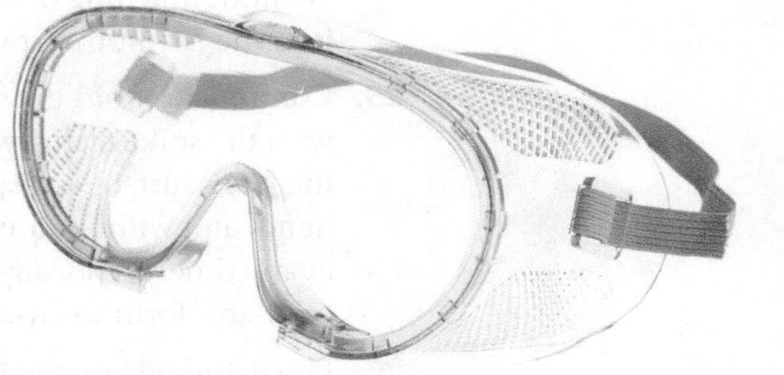

**POINTER**

During aseptic garbing, best practice is to reapply sterile, foamed 70% IPA to your hands after donning shoe covers and again after donning a hair cover.

### *Arranging and Preparing Supplies in the BSC*

16. Place the small chemotherapy sharps container on the work surface within the BSC. Position it on the work surface to the back and side of the cabinet so that it does not obstruct compounding operations within the cabinet.
17. Center the chemotherapy compounding mat onto the work surface of the BSC.

**18.** Along the other side of the BSC work surface (opposite of the sharps container), place the IV tubing, drug vial, IPA swabs, syringe, needle, chemotherapy dispensing pin, and one-third of the stack of the sterile, lint-free 4 × 4 gauze pads.

**19.** Remove the outer dust cover from the LVP. Place the dust cover into the chemotherapy sharps container. Place the LVP onto the chemotherapy compounding mat centered on the BSC work surface. Keep the other supply items temporarily in the transport vehicle.

### *Priming the IV Tubing*

**20.** Remove the outer wrapping from the IV tubing. Dispose of the IV tubing wrapper into the small chemotherapy sharps container.

20

**21.** Using your thumb and forefinger, close the clamp on the IV tubing by rolling it downward.

**22.** Temporarily place the IV tubing onto the work surface. Remove the plastic cap from the tubing needle adaptor. Dispose of the plastic cap in the chemotherapy sharps container. Without setting down or touching the tubing needle adaptor, aseptically attach a regular needle to the adaptor.

**23.** Remove the pull tag that covers the LVP tubing port. Place the removed tag into the chemotherapy sharps container.

**24.** Grasp the drip chamber of the IV tubing with your dominant hand. Hold the tubing so that the tubing spike is pointing toward your nondominant hand. Remove the cap that covers the tubing spike with your nondominant hand. Without touching or setting down the tubing spike, dispose of the spike cap into the chemotherapy sharps container.

**25.** Continue to hold the drip chamber of the IV tubing with your dominant hand, with the spike facing your nondominant hand. Do not set the IV tubing onto the work surface. Grasp the tubing port of the LVP with your nondominant hand, and without touching or shadowing the tubing spike or LVP tubing port at any time, aseptically insert the tubing spike into the LVP port. Twist the spike back-and-forth to ensure that it is firmly seated inside the LVP port.

**26.** Pinch and release the tubing drip chamber once or twice to draw a small amount of fluid from the IV bag into the drip chamber.

**27.** Open a sterile 70% IPA swab and place it onto the chemotherapy compounding mat (next to the gauze pads).

**28.** Discard the IPA swab's wrapper into the small chemotherapy sharps container.

**29.** Hold the IV tubing needle adaptor between the thumb and forefinger of your dominant hand, approximately one inch behind the attached needle cap. Remove the plastic needle cap (attached to the IV tubing needle adaptor on the IV tubing). Place the cap onto the IPA swab.

30. Continue to hold the IV tubing needle adaptor about one inch behind the uncapped needle. Without setting down, touching, or shadowing the tubing needle adaptor, position your hand so that the needle tip is held a few inches above the stack of gauze pads. Gradually roll up the IV tubing clamp with your nondominant hand, beginning a slow flow of fluid from the IV bag through the IV tubing.
31. As soon as the fluid fills the IV tubing and begins to drip onto the gauze pads, stop the flow of fluid by rolling the clamp shut with the thumb and forefinger of your nondominant hand.
32. Using your nondominant hand, pick up the needle cap from its position on the IPA swab, and reattach it to the needle-and-attached-tubing unit.
33. Temporarily place the IV bag with attached, filled tubing (and capped needle) onto the BSC work surface. ***Note:*** Position these supply items toward one side of the work surface, leaving as much room as possible on the chemotherapy compounding mat.

### *Preparing the Chemotherapy Vial*

34. Remove the flip-top cap from the vial of cisplatin and place the cap into the chemotherapy sharps container.
35. Open a new sterile 70% IPA swab and clean the vial's rubber top. Dispose of the swab's outer wrapper into the chemotherapy sharps container.
36. Remove the outer wrapper from the chemotherapy dispensing pin and place the wrapper into the chemotherapy sharps container.
37. Hold the top of the chemotherapy dispensing pin between the thumb and forefinger of your dominant hand and, with the other hand, remove the cap from the chemotherapy dispensing pin spike. Continue to hold the dispensing pin with your dominant hand and place the cap into the chemotherapy sharps container.
38. Without setting the chemotherapy dispensing pin onto the work surface, and without touching or shadowing the dispensing pin spike at any time, move your hand so that the spike points toward the palm of your nondominant hand. Grasp the cisplatin vial with your nondominant hand and then use a clockwise motion to turn the vial on its side, or approximately 90 degrees to the right. Hold the vial in this position, about three inches above the work surface.
39. While maintaining the 90-degree angle of the vial and the position of the chemotherapy dispensing pin, carefully insert the spike of the dispensing pin into the cisplatin vial top.
40. Using a counterclockwise motion, return the vial (with attached chemotherapy dispensing pin) to its original, upright position on the work surface.
41. Remove the syringe from its outer wrapper and then place the wrapper into the small chemotherapy sharps container.
42. Grasp the barrel of the syringe and hold it as you would a pencil or dart. If a plastic cap covers the syringe tip, then remove the cap with your nondominant hand and place it into the chemotherapy sharps container.

**USP Chapter <797>**

Because of the vertical airflow in a BSC, the chemotherapy dispensing pin must be inserted into the vial while both items are at an angle that allows for uninterrupted HEPA-filtered air to pass over the critical sites.

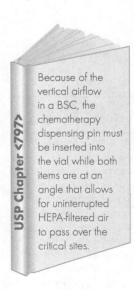

**BE AWARE**

Do not turn the vial too far onto its side, as this may cause the drug to spill onto the work surface. While the syringe is being attached to the dispensing pin, the vial-and-dispensing-pin unit must be turned to the side as much as possible without creating leakage from the pin, so that uninterrupted HEPA-filtered air flows across the Luer-lock syringe adaptor and syringe tip.

**43.** Without setting the syringe onto the work surface, and without touching or shadowing the syringe tip, continue to grasp the barrel of the syringe with your dominant hand while using your nondominant hand to remove the plastic cap that covers the Luer-lock adaptor (on the top of the chemotherapy dispensing pin). Place the plastic cap onto the IPA swab.

**44.** Grasp the vial—with attached, uncapped chemotherapy dispensing pin—with your nondominant hand, and carefully turn it clockwise approximately 75 degrees. Carefully attach the syringe tip to the Luer-lock adaptor (located on the top of the chemotherapy dispensing pin). Securely, but not too tightly, twist the syringe onto the dispensing pin.

**45.** Grasp the vial with your nondominant hand, and the barrel of the syringe with your dominant hand. With a clockwise motion, invert the vial approximately 120 degrees from the original, starting position. The syringe should be below the vial.

**46.** Holding the cisplatin vial with your nondominant hand, pull down on the flat knob of the syringe plunger with your dominant hand until the fluid reaches approximately the 41-mL mark on the syringe. Take care to maintain proper airflow from the hood's HEPA filter (located in the BSC ceiling) to the critical areas—from the tip of the syringe to the neck of the vial, including the entire chemotherapy dispensing pin and the vial's rubber top.

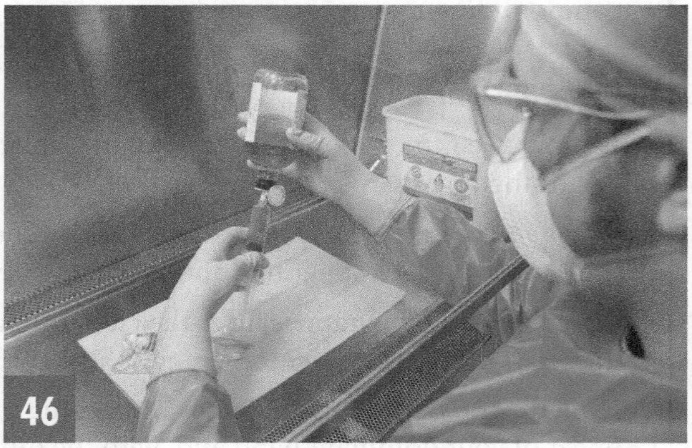
46

**47.** Stabilize the syringe (with chemotherapy dispensing pin and vial attached) against the palm of your nondominant hand and gently tap the syringe with your fingers to force any air bubbles that may have inadvertently transferred from the vial into the syringe toward the tip of the syringe.

**BE AWARE**

To avoid potentially dangerous fluid aspiration, apply a slow, gentle pressure to the flat knob of the syringe when returning excess fluid or residual air to the vial. In fact, all manipulations of chemotherapy fluid into or out of containment vessels, such as a vial, should be done slowly and carefully.

**48.** When all air bubbles have risen to the syringe tip, gently push up on the flat knob of the syringe plunger to expel the remaining air and unnecessary fluid back into the vial. Continue gently pushing up on the syringe flat knob until the exact 40-mL dose is reached.

**49.** With a counterclockwise motion, turn the vial so that it is approximately 45 degrees from its original, upright position on the chemotherapy compounding mat. Grasping only the barrel of the syringe, use your dominant hand to remove the syringe from the chemotherapy dispensing pin (i.e., twist the syringe off the Luer-lock adaptor).

**50.** Without setting down the filled syringe and without shadowing or touching the syringe tip, aseptically attach a regular needle (with attached needle cap) to the filled syringe.

51. Temporarily place the filled syringe with attached, capped regular needle onto the chemotherapy compounding mat. Recap the Luer-lock adaptor (on top of the chemotherapy dispensing pin) with the cap you placed onto the IPA swab earlier. Place the cisplatin vial with attached, capped dispensing pin next to the filled syringe on the chemotherapy compounding mat. Place the LVP (with attached and filled tubing-and-capped-needle unit) next to the filled syringe and vial on the chemotherapy compounding mat within the BSC.
52. Ask for a verification check by a pharmacist or your instructor.

### *Preparing the Chemotherapy CSP*

53. After the verification check has been completed, open a new sterile 70% IPA swab and disinfect the injection port of the IV bag. Place the used swab on the chemotherapy compounding mat directly under the injection port of the IV bag. (The swab will absorb any medication that may drip from the injection port.) Discard the swab's outer wrapper into the small chemotherapy sharps container.
54. Grasp the barrel of the filled syringe with your dominant hand, as you would a dart. Carefully remove the needle cap with your nondominant hand. Place the cap into the small chemotherapy sharps container.
55. Hold the IV bag injection port steady between the thumb and forefinger of your nondominant hand. Carefully insert the needle straight into the bag's injection port.
56. Inject the medication from the syringe into the IV bag by pressing up on the flat knob of the plunger with the thumb of your dominant hand.
57. Once all of the medication has been injected into the bag, reposition your dominant hand so that it grasps only the barrel of the syringe, as you would a dart. Carefully remove the empty needle-and-syringe unit from the IV bag. Without recapping the needle, dispose of the needle-and-syringe unit into the small chemotherapy sharps container.

> **BE AWARE**
>
> The needle insertion into the injection port of the IV bag should be smooth. If you encounter any resistance, the needle has likely entered the sidewall of the injection port stem, which is potentially dangerous. If this occurs, back out and repeat the insertion process with the same needle.

### *Clean-up and Compounding Completion Procedures*

58. Upon completion of the chemotherapy compounding procedures, dispose of the used vial with attached chemotherapy dispensing pin, caps, IPA swabs, used gauze, chemotherapy compounding mat, and remaining supply items into the chemotherapy sharps container.
59. Gently squeeze the CSP, checking for leakage and precipitate matter within the CSP solution. Then cover the LVP injection port with an IVA seal.
60. While holding a one-third stack of sterile, lint-free gauze pads outside of the BSC, lightly saturate the gauze pads with sterile 70% IPA from a pour bottle. Bring the CSP and attached, filled tubing out of the BSC, and clean the entire exterior surface of the CSP and the entire attached-and-filled IV tubing.
61. Affix the CSP label to the prepared IV bag. Affix a chemotherapy warning label to the CSP.

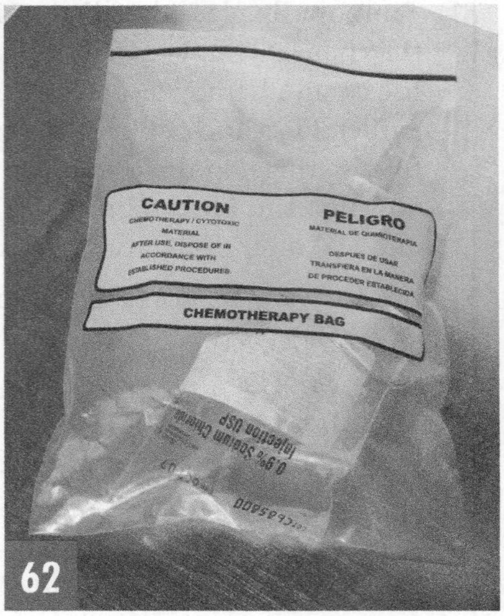


62. Place the labeled CSP with attached-and-filled tubing into a plastic bag, and affix a chemotherapy warning label to the bag. Place the bag into a chemotherapy transport bag and seal the bag. Place the bag with labeled CSP into the transport vehicle.

63. Remove your chemotherapy gloves by pulling them down from the wrist, turning each glove inside out as it is pulled off. Dispose of the used gloves into the small chemotherapy sharps container.

64. Remove your chemotherapy gown by pulling it down off of the shoulders, turning the gown inside out as it is removed. Dispose of the used gown into the small chemotherapy sharps container.

65. Lightly saturate the remaining one-third stack of the sterile, lint-free gauze pads with sterile 70% IPA. Disinfect the sterile 70% IPA pour bottle and any other potentially contaminated items that you must return to the anteroom with the saturated gauze pads. Place the pour bottle of 70% IPA next to the CSP in the transport vehicle, as well as any other supplies, and return them to the anteroom.

66. Remove your sterile gloves, face mask, hair cover, and shoe covers according to standard procedures, and dispose of them in the anteroom chemotherapy sharps container.

67. Remove your chemotherapy safety glasses and wipe them down with an aseptic cleaning wipe or a stack of lint-free gauze pads saturated with sterile 70% IPA. Store the cleaned safety glasses in the appropriate place, per your facility's guidelines.

68. Record the date and your initials on the CSP label.

69. Ask for a final check from the pharmacist or your instructor.

# Process Validation Checklist

*Your instructor will use the process validation checklist provided in Appendix D to evaluate your technique for this lab. In order to receive ACPE certification, and prior to making CSPs for patient use, you must correctly perform each component of the lab procedure. Review the Chapter 14 lab and thoroughly practice each of the steps prior to your evaluation.*

# Part 3: Assessment

## Chapter Summary

- Early philosophers and physicians believed that cancer was caused by an imbalance in the body's four humors.
- The term *carcinoma*, meaning "cancerous tumor," originated from the Greek words for cancer (*karkinos*) and swelling (*oncos*).
- Scottish surgeon John Hunter scientifically researched the theory that cancer moves throughout the body's blood supply via the lymphatic system.
- German surgeon Karl Thiersch demonstrated that cancer originates in epithelial cells and metastasizes by the spread of malignant cells.
- Watson, Crick, and Wilkins, building on the work of Rosalind Franklin, identified the molecular structure of DNA, giving rise to advancement in cancer treatments that target specific DNA strands.
- *Cancer* is a term used to describe a class of diseases characterized by the presence of abnormal cells that divide and multiply uncontrollably and invade nearby tissue. Cancer cells can spread to other parts of the body through the blood or lymphatic systems.
- Modern cancer therapy may involve treatment with surgery, radiation, hormone therapy, immunotherapy, chemotherapy, or a combination of these treatments.
- Cancer chemotherapy is often classified as primary, adjuvant, or palliative. Primary chemotherapy is prescribed with the intention of curing the patient. Adjuvant chemotherapy is prescribed as a follow-up treatment to the removal or reduction of a tumor by surgery. Palliative chemotherapy is sometimes prescribed to improve the patient's quality of life when cancer is deemed incurable.
- The categories of chemotherapy drugs include alkylating agents, antimetabolites, antimicrotubule agents, chemotherapeutic antibiotics, hormone therapy, mitotic inhibitors, targeted therapy, and topoisomerase inhibitors. Chemotherapeutic agents are prescribed based on proven effectiveness against the patient's specific type, location, and stage of cancer.
- Cytotoxic agents are capable of killing living cells. Antineoplastic medications are drugs that reduce or prevent the growth of cancer cells.
- Chemotherapy medications may be carcinogenic, teratogenic, mutagenic, or immunosuppressive. These hazardous drugs require special handling—including special preparation, storage, labeling, transportation, and administration—to protect anyone who might come into contact with them.
- Chemotherapy CSPs must be prepared in a special type of laminar airflow hood called a biological safety cabinet (BSC). A BSC is specifically designed to protect sterile compounding personnel from exposure to cytotoxic drugs during the compounding process.
- Facilities that prepare a small number of chemotherapy CSPs may use a compounding aseptic containment isolator (CACI). Like a BSC, the CACI is designed to protect personnel from exposure to cytotoxic agents during sterile compounding.
- The BSC should be located in a negative-pressure clean room, which helps to prevent hazardous air from being drawn out of the BSC and into the surrounding area.
- A chemotherapy spill kit should be kept wherever chemotherapy is compounded or administered. Spills are classified as small (≤ 5 grams or 5 mL) or large (> 5 grams or 5 mL).
- Chemotherapy is often dosed as $mg/m^2$ based on the patient's BSA, which the prescriber determines using a nomogram.

- In addition to standard aseptic garb, IV technicians who compound chemotherapy should don a sterile chemotherapy gown, chemotherapy safety glasses, and a pair of sterile chemotherapy gloves, the latter of which are applied over a pair of standard sterile gloves.
- IV technicians compounding chemotherapy CSPs use negative-pressure withdrawal methods as well as a chemotherapy compounding mat, chemotherapy dispensing pin, and a CSTD to minimize exposure to chemotherapy agents.
- The primary components of the BSC include the air intake grills, blower, glass shield, exhaust HEPA filter, hood HEPA filter, prefilter, and the work surface.
- All supplies used in the preparation of chemotherapy, including PPE, must be disposed of in a yellow chemotherapy sharps container. The exterior of chemotherapy CSPs must be wiped down with sterile 70% IPA prior to labeling.
- The direction of HEPA-filtered air within the BSC flows downward from the cabinet ceiling toward the work surface. Aseptic technique procedures must be adjusted so that items are positioned and manipulated in such a way that nothing passes between the BSC ceiling (where the HEPA filter is located) and the critical sites.
- Refer to the BSC manufacturer's instruction manual for the proper procedure for cleaning the BSC; likewise, refer to the manufacturer's instruction manual for a CACI.
- In addition to demonstrating consistent, proper technique in sterile product preparation, personnel preparing chemotherapy CSPs must receive a minimum of 20 hours of additional, experiential training specific to chemotherapy preparation prior to making chemotherapy for patient administration.

## Key Terms

**adjuvant chemotherapy** a type of chemotherapy employed after surgical removal or reduction of the primary tumor or tumors

**adverse reaction** an unexpected, undesirable effect caused by a drug

**aerosolization** the undesired release of small particles or spray into the air from a vial or CSP; a fine mist released from a chemotherapy vial due to incorrect use of air pressure during compounding, which results in dangerous contamination of the BSC

**air intake grills** the grills that run along the interior sides of the BSC work surface; these grills pull contaminated air from within the work space away from the worker and into the exhaust HEPA filter

**alkylating agent** a cytotoxic drug that acts by binding to nucleic acids and inhibiting cell division

**antagonist** a substance that interferes with or inhibits the physiological action of another; for example, a hormone antagonist slows the growth of a hormone-dependent tumor

**antiemetic** a drug that suppresses or relieves nausea and vomiting

**antimetabolite medication** a cytotoxic drug that disrupts metabolic pathways, thus preventing target cancer cells from synthesizing components essential for their growth and replication

**antimicrotubule agent** a cytotoxic drug that disrupts the formation of cellular components required for mitosis, thus interfering with cell division and inhibiting growth; also called a *mitotic inhibitor*

**antineoplastic medication** an agent that retards or prevents the growth of cancer cells; the terms *cytotoxic* and *antineoplastic* are often used interchangeably to describe chemotherapy drugs

**arsenic** a chemical element with a high degree of toxicity; subtoxic doses of arsenic are sometimes used in the treatment of cancer; a chemical that was once stockpiled by the United States for use as a chemical weapon

**autoimmune disorder** any disorder characterized by an immune response directed against the body's own tissues

**autopsy** a postmortem examination and dissection performed by a pathologist to determine the cause of death

**basic formula calculation** a pharmaceutical dosage calculation method that uses the formula D / H = *x* mL; refer to Chapter 5 for more information on the basic formula

**belladonna** a potentially toxic substance used as a basis for some traditional and homeopathic medicines; also known as *deadly nightshade*

**benign** a growth of nonmalignant cells; a harmless medical condition

**biological safety cabinet (BSC)** a special type of laminar airflow hood designed for the preparation of chemotherapy CSPs; a BSC is designed to protect the worker from exposure to antineoplastics

**blastema theory** a theory of cancer causation developed in the nineteenth century by the German pathologist Johannes Müller; this theory argued that cancer cells arose from "budding elements" (called *blastema*) in connective tissue

**blower** a component of the BSC that draws air into the cabinet, forces the air through the hood HEPA filter (thus creating an ISO Class 5 environment), and then pushes the air out of the cabinet through the exhaust HEPA filter

**body surface area (BSA)** an estimated measurement of the human body based on a patient's height and weight and expressed in meters squared ($m^2$)

**bone marrow suppression** the decreased ability of the bone marrow to manufacture blood cells; a common side effect of chemotherapy

**cancer** a class of diseases characterized by the presence of abnormal cells that divide and multiply uncontrollably and invade nearby tissues; the natural course of cancer is fatal

**carcinogenic** giving rise to cancer; cancer-causing

**carcinoma** a cancerous tumor; malignant cells

**caustic** a substance that causes blistering or irritation to the skin or other tissues

**central venous catheter (CVC)** a catheter inserted into a large vein, such as the internal jugular vein or the subclavian vein, and leading into the superior vena cava or right atrium; catheter used to administer medications or TPN; also called a *central line*

**chemotherapeutic antibiotic** an antibiotic that is more toxic than traditional antibiotics because it has the ability to kill cancer cells by interacting with DNA; also called an *antitumor antibiotic*

**chemotherapy** the treatment of a disease, usually cancer, by chemical agents

**chemotherapy compounding mat** a thin mat placed on the work surface within the BSC during the preparation of chemotherapy CSPs; the top side of the mat is covered with absorbent material to soak up any liquid spills within the BSC, and the bottom side is made from a low-permeability material that prevents liquid from soaking through to the BSC work surface

**chemotherapy dispensing pin** a small plastic device with a spike at one end, a Luer-lock adaptor at the other end, and—in between—a small vent to which a 0.22-micron HEPA filter is attached; this device is used to relieve the negative pressure within a drug vial safely, while its built-in HEPA filter traps any drug particles or escaping fluid from the vial

**chemotherapy spill kit** a kit for safely cleaning up chemotherapy spills that have occurred outside of the BSC; chemotherapy spill kits typically include protective garb, a disposable dustpan and hand broom, absorbent pads, chemotherapy disposal bags, warning signs, and documentation forms

**chemotherapy support order** a medication order for various nonhazardous drugs intended to make chemotherapy easier or more tolerable for the patient; this order may include LVPs for hydration, antiemetics, and medications for pain or anxiety; also referred to as a *chemotherapy comfort order*

**Class I BSC** a vertical airflow biological safety cabinet used in chemical manufacturing but unsuitable for chemotherapy preparation because it does not provide a HEPA-filtered, ISO Class 5 environment

**Class II BSC** a vertical airflow biological safety cabinet used for chemotherapy preparation; a *Class II, Type A BSC* recirculates a percentage of the BSC airflow back into the clean room after it has been filtered through the exhaust HEPA filter; a *Class II, Type B BSC* forces air through the exhaust HEPA filter and then sends the air through a dedicated exhaust ventilation system to the outside environment

**closed-system transfer device (CSTD)** a small, disposable device that safely draws fluid from a vial into a syringe or injects fluid from a syringe into an IV or IV piggyback; this device protects the worker from exposure to cytotoxic drugs during chemotherapy preparation

**cycles** chemotherapy treatment that is administered in phases, usually over several months, according to a predetermined treatment protocol; cycling chemotherapy allows healthy cells time to recover between treatments

**cytotoxic medication** a drug that poisons or otherwise destroys cancer cells so that they are not able to grow or reproduce

**deoxyribonucleic acid (DNA)** a nucleic acid containing the genetic instructions for all living things (the building blocks of life); new chemotherapy methods work by targeting specific strands of DNA

**dimensional analysis** a pharmaceutical calculation based on the principle that any number can be multiplied by one without changing its value; refer to Chapter 5 for more information on dimensional analysis

**Edwin Smith Papyrus** an ancient Egyptian papyrus that discusses treatments for injuries as well as several types of surgery, including the use of cauterization for breast tumors

**epithelial** pertaining to the epithelium, or the covering of the external and internal surfaces of the body, including the lining of blood vessels

**exhaust HEPA filter** a BSC filter that removes air contaminants generated during chemotherapy sterile compounding before the air leaves the cabinet

**gas-tight BSC** a completely sealed BSC that is impermeable to air or other gases

**genetic mutation** a permanent change in an organism's genetic material, typically occurring in a single gene

**glass shield** the BSC component located at the front of the cabinet that prevents drug aspirate from coming into contact with the technician's face or body

**hazardous drug** a drug that may be genetically harmful to a patient due to its carcinogenic, immunosuppressive, mutagenic, teratogenic, or vesicant properties

**hemlock** a toxic substance derived from the plant species *Conium maculatum*; also known as poison hemlock; used in ancient Greece as a medicinal treatment for various ailments

**hood HEPA filter** a filter typically located in the ceiling of the BSC that provides sterile air for the preparation of chemotherapy CSPs

**hormone therapy** the use of hormones or their antagonists to slow the growth of hormone-dependent tumors; this kind of therapy is used to treat hormone-sensitive cancers of the breast and prostate

**immunosuppressive** a medication or treatment that causes the patient recipient's immune system to be suppressed or weakened; a common side effect of many chemotherapeutic agents

**immunotherapy** a treatment that uses the immune system to fight diseases, including cancer, either by stimulating the patient's own immune system to work harder or by administering certain immune system components, such as manmade antibodies; in cancer therapy, immunotherapy is often used along with or after another type of treatment

**injector Luer-lock expansion chamber device** a device designed to protect sterile compounding personnel from aspiration of toxic chemicals during chemotherapy compounding

**leukemia** cancer of the blood-forming organs that is characterized by abnormal development and proliferation of white blood cells in the blood and bone marrow

**lymphoma** any cancer of the lymphatic system

**lymph theory** a theory of cancer causation and metastasis that was developed in the early eighteenth century; this theory argued that cancer formed from fermenting and degenerating lymphatic fluid and was spread throughout the body via the lymphatic system

**malignant** cancerous; having the properties of invasion and metastasis; tending to become progressively worse and resulting in death

**mastectomy** excision of all or part of the breast

**material safety data sheet (MSDS)** a document providing information about the characteristics, chemical properties, and hazards of a chemical, and identifying the precautions for handling, use, cleanup, and disposal of the chemical

**mercury** a toxic chemical compound that was once used as a medical treatment prior to being banned in most countries in the early twentieth century

**metastasis** the spread of cancer via the transfer of cells from one organ or body part to another not directly connected to it; the capacity to metastasize is characteristic of all malignant tumors

**mitosis** a type of cell division typical of ordinary tissue growth; the cell division results in two daughter cells, each with a nucleus and genetic material identical to that of the parent cell

**mitotic inhibitor** a cytotoxic drug that disrupts the formation of cellular components required for mitosis, thus interfering with cell division and inhibiting growth; also called an *antimicrotubule agent*

**mutagenic** giving rise to mutations

**negative-pressure clean room** a type of clean room that maintains a negative pressure relative to the surrounding rooms or environment; a type of clean room in which a BSC is located for the safe preparation of chemotherapy CSPs

**nitrogen mustard** the first alkylating agent, originally developed as a chemical warfare agent

**nomogram** a chart used by prescribers to calculate the body surface area (BSA) of a patient in order to prescribe a medication dosage

**oncology** the study and treatment of cancer and related medical conditions

**oopharectomy** excision of one or both ovaries

**palliative chemotherapy** a type of chemotherapy that is intended to relieve symptoms and ease pain but is not aimed at curing the cancer

**pathophysiology** a branch of medicine devoted to the study of the biological and physical causes of disease

**prefilter** a BSC component that has the same design and function as the prefilter on a standard, horizontal laminar airflow hood; that is, room air is passed through the prefilter to remove large contaminants and then is compressed and channeled through the hood HEPA filter

**primary chemotherapy** a type of chemotherapy that is prescribed with the intention of curing the patient, particularly in cases in which the cancer cannot be surgically removed

**prime the tubing** to fill the IV tubing with fluid from the IV base solution prior to injecting chemotherapy medications into a CSP; performing this task reduces the likelihood of exposure to the hazardous drug within the CSP during patient administration

**protector device** a device designed to reduce or eliminate aspiration of chemotherapy medication, thereby protecting sterile compounding personnel during chemotherapy preparation

**radiation therapy** a form of medical treatment used by oncologists that employs ionizing radiation to shrink or control the growth of malignant cells; also known as *radiation oncology*

**ratio and proportion calculation** a pharmaceutical dosage calculation method that uses the formula H mg/Y mL = D mg/*x* mL; this method is used whenever three of the four values in a proportion are known

**remission** abatement of the symptoms of a disease; also, the period in which this abatement occurs

**RNA synthesis** the effects of ribonucleic acid (RNA) on protein synthesis during cell growth and development

**septicemia** systemic disease associated with the presence of pathogens in the blood; also called *blood poisoning*

**stage of cancer** a categorization of cancer based on the size and number of tumors and the extent to which the cancer has spread or metastasized; categories range from stage 0 to stage IV, with stage 0 being a small, localized cancer with no evidence of spread and stage IV being indicative of cancer that has spread throughout the lymph system and invaded other organs

**subclavian vein** a large vein in the chest into which hypertonic solutions such as chemotherapy CSPs are often administered

**tall-man lettering** the practice of writing part of a drug's name in uppercase letters and part in lowercase letters to help distinguish sound-alike, look-alike drugs and thus prevent medication errors; also called *mixed-case lettering*

**targeted therapy** a type of chemotherapy targeting specific molecular features of certain cancer cells to inhibit their growth

**teratogenic** giving rise to birth defects

**topoisomerase inhibitor** a cytotoxic drug that blocks the enzyme topoisomerase, which helps repair DNA damage

**tumor** any abnormal new growth of tissue, either benign or malignant, that has no physiological function and arises from uncontrolled, usually rapid cellular proliferation

**vertical laminar airflow hood** a type of hood that employs vertical airflow so that HEPA-filtered air flows down toward the work surface and then is drawn into intake grills located at the sides of the hood; a hood or BSC designed to protect sterile compounding personnel from exposure to cytotoxic medications

**vesicant** a drug that causes blistering

**work surface** the surface within the BSC upon which chemotherapy preparation takes place

## Check the Basics

*On a separate sheet of paper, write your answers as modeled in these examples: 1d; 2c; 3b; etc.*

1. Which of the following procedures or supply items should not be used during chemotherapy sterile compounding?
   a. regular needle, chemotherapy dispensing pin
   b. sterile gloves, sterile 70% IPA
   c. vented needle, milking technique
   d. CSTD, negative pressure
2. With regard to chemotherapy sterile compounding, which of the following statements is true?
   a. Chemotherapy CSPs should be prepared at least two inches inside of the hood.
   b. Chemotherapy CSPs should be prepared in a BSC or a CACI.
   c. Chemotherapy CSPs should be prepared at least eight inches inside of the hood.
   d. Chemotherapy CSPs should be prepared in a CSTD or an OSHA.
3. Which of the following critical sites should never be cleaned with a sterile 70% IPA swab?
   a. chemotherapy dispensing pin spike and Luer-lock adaptor
   b. injection port and vial top
   c. tubing spike and needle adaptor
   d. all of the above
   e. only *a* and *c*
4. Which term describes the process of filling the IV tubing with fluid from the IV bag?
   a. preparing the tubing
   b. priming the tubing
   c. pinching the tubing
   d. placing the tubing
5. What is the primary function of the chemotherapy compounding mat?
   a. to clean up spills outside of the BSC
   b. to absorb spills outside of the BSC
   c. to clean up spills inside of the BSC
   d. to absorb spills inside of the BSC
6. Which of the following safety precautions must be taken when preparing chemotherapy CSPs?
   a. double gloves, safety glasses
   b. chemotherapy mat, chemotherapy dispensing pin
   c. priming the tubing, negative pressure
   d. all of the above
7. With regard to chemotherapy sterile compounding, which of the following statements is true?
   a. HEPA-filtered air flows vertically; therefore, to avoid shadowing, nothing should be placed above the critical site of a supply item.
   b. HEPA-filtered air flows horizontally; therefore, to avoid shadowing, nothing should be placed in front of the critical site of a supply item.
   c. HEPA-filtered air flows vertically; therefore, to avoid shadowing, nothing should be placed in front of the critical site of a supply item.
   d. HEPA-filtered air flows horizontally; therefore, to avoid shadowing, nothing should be placed above the critical site of a supply item.
8. With regard to the procedure for inserting a spike or needle into a vial during chemotherapy sterile compounding, which of the following statements is true?
   a. The vial should remain upright on the work surface during spike or needle insertion.
   b. The vial should be turned clockwise, approximately 90 degrees.
   c. The vial should be turned clockwise, approximately 180 degrees.
   d. none of the above

9. With regard to withdrawing fluid from a vial during chemotherapy sterile compounding, which of the following statements is true?
   a. A volume of air equal to or slightly less than the desired dose volume should be injected into the vial.
   b. No air should be injected into the vial.
   c. A volume of air that is 1 mL greater than the desired dose volume should be injected into the vial.
   d. none of the above

10. Which of the following describes the proper disposal of chemotherapy gowns and gloves?
    a. Place these used PPE items into the chemotherapy sharps container immediately after the completion of compounding procedures.
    b. Place these used PPE items into the chemotherapy sharps container upon completion of your shift.
    c. Place these used PPE items into the regular sharps container immediately after the completion of compounding procedures.
    d. Place these used PPE items into the regular sharps container upon completion of your shift.

## Make Connections

*On a separate sheet of paper, write your answers to the following three questions, using complete sentences and making sure your answers are thorough and thoughtful. Note that the third question requires Internet access.*

1. It is considered best practice to have a minimum of three checks by three pharmacy staff members of the chemotherapy medication order and CSP label. In general, one pharmacist enters the order into the computer and generates a CSP label; a second pharmacist double-checks all of the calculations and verifies the accuracy of the CSP label; and one IV technician then repeats the process by double-checking the calculations and verifying the accuracy of the CSP label. What is the rationale for having three people check chemotherapy medication orders? If workload is particularly heavy, would it be acceptable to skip the IV technician check to save time? Why or why not?

2. A nurse returns a chemotherapy CSP to the pharmacy and reports that the CSP is not leaking. Upon inspection, however, you discover that the CSP does have a small leak, as evidenced by a few drops of fluid that have accumulated inside of the sealed plastic bag. In light of your findings, what is the best course of action to take? Would you take a different course of action if you noticed the leak while the CSP was still inside of the BSC?

3. Go to the website of the National Cancer Institute at www.cancer.gov and then click on the Clinical Trials tab. According to this website, how many clinical trials are currently ongoing? What does the number of available clinical trials indicate about cancer research?

## Meet the Challenge

***Scenario*** This "contaminating" activity will give you the opportunity to use a chemotherapy spill kit to clean up a mock chemotherapy spill.

***Challenge*** Your instructor has a handout outlining the supplies and steps for an activity centered around a mock chemotherapy spill. This procedure takes your understanding of how to use a chemotherapy spill kit to a deeper level. To meet this challenge, ask your instructor for the handout and give it a try, either individually, in small groups, or as a class.

## ADDITIONAL RESOURCES

*Go to the Paradigm Internet Resources Center at* www.paradigmcollege.net/sterilecomp *to access live links related to these Chapter 14 topics:*

- Information on handling hazardous drugs, including chemotherapy
- Guidelines from ASHP's Technical Assistance Bulletin on Handling of Cytotoxic and Hazardous Drugs
- The history of cancer treatment, insight on ongoing research, and various cancer-related resources for healthcare personnel, caregivers, and patients
- Information for protection of workers who compound hazardous drugs as well as MSDS information
- Regulations related to the disposal of hazardous chemicals and waste
- Regulations related to the transportation of hazardous chemicals and waste

# Appendix A

# Student Answer Key for Concepts Self-Check

Use the Concepts Self-Check Answer Key to verify your understanding of the information presented in the Part 1: Concepts section of each chapter. For any incorrect response in the Check Your Understanding section, scan the specific chapter's Concepts section for the text passage that reveals the correct answer. For the Apply Your Knowledge section, compare your written responses to the critical-thinking questions with the modeled responses presented here.

## Chapter 1

### Check Your Understanding

1. d
2. c
3. a
4. b
5. b

### Apply Your Knowledge

A contaminated CSP has the potential to cause serious harm to a patient. Therefore, a CSP that might be contaminated must be immediately discarded. In addition, if you ever experience any confusion as to the ingredients, concentration, or strength of any product that you have compounded, you must dispose of the compound and start over. Never take a chance with something that could harm a patient. The motto of the IV technician should always be "when in doubt, throw it out."

## Chapter 2

### Check Your Understanding

1. c
2. a
3. d
4. d
5. a

### Apply Your Knowledge

Because there is a high potential for contamination of the CSP due to airborne contaminants, any IV technician who is coughing or displaying flu symptoms should not be allowed into the sterile compounding environment. Personnel with any type of transmittable infection must not prepare CSPs.

## Chapter 3

### Check Your Understanding

1. b
2. d
3. a
4. b
5. c

### Apply Your Knowledge

The critical site must receive uninterrupted airflow from the HEPA filter; therefore, the vial should be repositioned so that the airflow is not blocked. Once the airflow is sufficient, the vial top should be swabbed with IPA and then the sterile compound may be prepared. A different course of action would be required if the improper positioning was noted after preparing the compound. Because the product was compounded with insufficient airflow, it is considered contaminated and must be discarded.

## Chapter 4

### Check Your Understanding

1. d
2. c
3. c
4. d
5. a

### Apply Your Knowledge

For healthcare providers, the advantages of using abbreviations, acronyms, and symbols in the healthcare setting are twofold: convenience and expedience. However, the disadvantage of using this shorthand type of communication is the potential risk for serious medical and/or medication errors. Many abbreviations have multiple meanings and may be easily misinterpreted.

## Chapter 5

### Check Your Understanding

1. d
2. d
3. a
4. a
5. a

## Apply Your Knowledge

Yes. You must always check the medication label to determine and/or verify the medication's concentration. Different manufacturers may supply a medication in varying concentrations. Failure to verify the concentration of a drug may lead to a medication error. The concentration must always be determined and/or verified to ensure patient safety.

# Chapter 6

## Check Your Understanding

1. a
2. d
3. d
4. b
5. d

## Apply Your Knowledge

The appropriate course of action is to inform the co-worker of the break in technique so that he or she can repeat the procedure using a new surgical scrub sponge/brush. There should be no difference in the course of action. The co-worker must repeat the procedure, and it is incumbent upon the person who witnessed the contamination to point it out and, if necessary, follow up to ensure that the procedure is done correctly to maintain patient health and safety.

# Chapter 7

## Check Your Understanding

1. a
2. c
3. d
4. d
5. d

## Apply Your Knowledge

USP Chapter <797> regulations require that the hood be cleaned often. Setting standards for the frequency and circumstances of the hood-cleaning process acknowledges the potential for contamination that may occur during the compounding process, as well as the importance of cleaning to reducing this risk factor. USP Chapter <797> regulations also recognize the importance of hood cleaning to the health and safety of patients.

# Chapter 8

## Check Your Understanding

1. d
2. c
3. d
4. d
5. a

## Apply Your Knowledge

The high mortality rates that resulted from the use of contaminated ingredients and supplies became a catalyst for change in the preparation of LVPs and other parenteral solutions. Today, the adherence to high standards of purity, sterility, and quality and the use of medical-grade containers and ingredients provide quality controls in the compounding process. Implementing these safeguards, as well as maintaining proper aseptic technique during sterile compounding, helps to ensure the health and safety of patient recipients.

# Chapter 9

## Check Your Understanding

1. a
2. b
3. c
4. a
5. c

## Apply Your Knowledge

The prevalence of superbugs, as well as the fact that they spread so quickly and are so difficult to treat, indicates that they are powerful organisms with a remarkable ability to effectively and rapidly evolve to avoid destruction by antimicrobial medications. The urgency of the WHO statement indicates that discovering and developing effective treatments for superbugs is a difficult, complex, and extensive process that is currently being outpaced by these fast-evolving pathogenic organisms.

# Chapter 10

## Check Your Understanding

1. e
2. a
3. b
4. a
5. c

## Apply Your Knowledge

The breaking of an ampule creates razor-sharp edges that pose a serious risk to sterile compounding personnel. These edges can easily cut the fingers of the IV technician while handling the ampule. The breaking action can also result in glass shards being scattered on the hood's work surface, creating a hazardous situation for both the worker performing procedures in the hood and to the hood itself. Blood can contaminate the hood's work surface or HEPA filter.

The incorrect breaking and handling of an ampule can also result in serious harm to a patient. If the ampule solution is not properly filtered, glass shards may be inadvertently transferred into the CSP, causing potential injury to the patient recipient.

# Chapter 11

## Check Your Understanding

1. c
2. e
3. a
4. d
5. b

## Apply Your Knowledge

The rationale for handling controlled substances differently from other drugs is that controlled substances have a high potential for addiction and abuse. In addition, there is a market for the illegal sale of narcotics, so drug diversion is a concern. For these reasons, strict regulations surround controlled substances. The rationale for handling C–II drugs differently from C–III through C–V drugs is that C–II drugs have the greatest potential for abuse; therefore, C–II drugs require a higher level of security and regulation than the other classes of drugs.

# Chapter 12

## Check Your Understanding

1. d
2. c
3. d
4. b
5. c

## Apply Your Knowledge

The rationale for handling pediatric CSPs in a different manner is that the pediatric patient is small and fragile. Even minor dosage errors could result in serious injury or death. Given the additional requirements and considerations for pediatric CSPs, it is best practice to require advanced training and certification for those who prepare pediatric CSPs.

# Chapter 13

## Check Your Understanding

1. b
2. d
3. d
4. d
5. a

## Apply Your Knowledge

The rationale for requiring additional training, testing, and process validation for those who prepare TPNs is based on the complexity of the sterile compounding process. Because a TPN solution is comprised of multiple solution components, the risk of contamination from multiple injections is high. In addition, the presence of particulates in the solution or incompatibility of the solution's components can result in infection or other complications for the patient recipient. The TPN line itself leaves the patient at risk for nosocomial infection as well.

The more complicated media-fill test procedure kit is warranted for those who prepare TPNs because the advanced kit requires manipulation of several vials, which is similar to the procedures required during TPN preparation.

Yes, the medium-risk level designation is warranted. TPN solutions are complex CSPs that require multiple manipulations. Also, the TPN solution is nutrient-rich and, therefore, provides an excellent medium for bacterial growth. The medium-risk designation helps to ensure patient health and safety.

# Chapter 14

## Check Your Understanding

1. d
2. c
3. b
4. e
5. d

## Apply Your Knowledge

The extra safety procedures associated with chemotherapy compounding are warranted because chemotherapy CSPs are hazardous drugs. Hazardous drugs may be vesicant, carcinogenic, mutagenic, teratogenic, or immunosuppressive. Exposure to these toxic medications may lead to health problems for the IV technician; therefore, special precautions are necessary to protect those who handle these hazardous drugs.

# Appendix B

## Useful Reference Tables

In preparation for your work as a sterile compounding technician, it is essential that you memorize the information provided in the several tables of Appendix B. The tables' contents are not comprehensive but rather list the most frequently used medical terms (plus root words, prefixes, and suffixes), as well as the most common medical and pharmacy abbreviations, acronyms, and symbols. One effective method for learning this crucial information is to create flash cards and use them as a study tool. Check with your instructor and classmates to discover other learning strategies.

**Table 1**
Common Medical Terminology

**Table 2**
Common Medical Root Words

**Table 3**
Common Medical Prefixes

**Table 4**
Common Medical Suffixes

**Table 5**
Common Abbreviations and Acronyms of Hospital Departments, Units, and Locations

**Table 6**
Common Abbreviations and Acronyms of Professional Titles

**Table 7**
Common Medical Abbreviations and Acronyms

**Table 8**
Common Abbreviations for Diagnoses, Conditions, and Diseases

**Table 9**
Common Abbreviations and Acronyms for Laboratory Tests, Diagnostic and Medical Procedures, and Treatments

**Table 10**
Common Pharmacy Abbreviations and Acronyms

**Table 11**
Common Pharmacy Symbols

**Table 12**
Signa Interpretation

**Table 13**
Common Parenteral Medications

**Table 1 Common Medical Terminology**

| Term | Meaning |
|---|---|
| anemia | blood condition in which there is a low number of red blood cells |
| arteriosclerosis | narrowing or hardening of the arteries |
| bradycardia | slow heart rate |
| carcinoma | cancerous tumor |
| cardiomyopathy | disease of the heart muscle |
| cerebrovascular | pertaining to the brain and the vascular system that supplies it with blood |
| cholecystectomy | surgical removal of the gallbladder |
| dermatitis | inflammation of the skin |
| dyspepsia | a condition of difficult digestion; indigestion; stomach upset |
| epidural | pertaining to the area above the dura mater or the area surrounding the spinal cord and brain |
| hematoma | blood-filled tumor; bruise |
| hyperglycemia | a condition of elevated glucose in the blood |
| hyperkalemia | high blood potassium level |
| hypertension | high blood pressure |
| hypokalemia | low blood potassium level |
| hypotension | low blood pressure |
| hysterectomy | surgical removal of the uterus |
| immunocompromised | describes a condition in which the immune system response is weakened or rendered ineffective by illness or disease |
| inhalation | the action of breathing or inspiration; the process of breathing a medication into the lungs |
| intracardiac | into the heart; into the heart muscle; within the heart |
| intramuscular | within or into the muscle |
| intranasal | into the nose or nasal passages; within the nose or nasal passages |
| intraocular | into the eye(s); within the eye(s) |
| intrathecal | within the subarachnoid space; into or within the spinal canal |
| leukopenia | a blood condition in which there is a low number of white blood cells |
| myalgia | muscle pain |
| nephritis | inflammation of the kidney |
| neuralgia | nerve pain |
| pancreatitis | inflammation of the pancreas |
| percutaneous | through the skin |
| septicemia | a systemic bacterial infection of the blood |
| subcutaneous | under the skin; pertaining to the tissue underlying the dermis |
| sublingual | under the tongue |
| tachycardia | fast heart rate |
| topical | applied to the skin |
| tracheotomy | an incision into the trachea; insertion of a breathing tube into the trachea |

**Table 2 Common Medical Root Words**

| Root | Meaning |
|---|---|
| abdomen/o | abdomen; abdominal |
| aden/o | gland |
| angi/o | vessel |
| arteri/o | artery |
| arthr/o | joint |
| aur/o | ear |
| bronch/o | bronchus |
| bucc/o | cheek |
| carcin/o | cancer; cancer-causing |
| cardi/o | heart |
| cephal/o | head |
| colon/o | colon |
| cyst/o | bladder |
| cyt/o | cell |
| derm/o | skin |
| enter/o | intestine |
| esophag/o | esophagus |
| gastr/o | stomach |
| gluc/o | glucose; sugar |
| gyne/o | female reproductive organs |
| hemat/o | blood |
| hepat/o | liver |
| hydr/o | water |
| lip/o | fat |
| lymph/o | lymph; pertaining to lymph node or system |
| mamm/o; mast/o | breast |
| my/o | muscle |
| narc/o | sleep |
| nas/o | nose |
| nephr/o | kidney |
| neur/o | nerve |
| ocul/o; ophthalm/o | eye |
| or/o | mouth |
| oste/o; orth/o | bone |
| ped/i | child; children |
| phleb/o | vein |
| pneum/o | lungs; air |
| psych/o; psych/e | mind; mental |
| pulmon/o | lungs; breathing |
| ren/o | kidney |
| septi | bacteria |
| spir/o | breath |
| thorac/o | chest |
| thyr/o | thyroid |
| vascul/o; vas/o | vein |

Table 3 **Common Medical Prefixes**

| Prefix | Meaning |
|---|---|
| a–; an– | no; not; without |
| ana– | against; upward; back |
| ante– | before; forward |
| anti– | against; opposite |
| bi– | two; both |
| brady– | slow |
| contra– | opposite; against |
| dys– | painful; difficult; bad |
| en–; endo– | inside; within |
| epi– | above |
| ex– | out; outward |
| hyper– | excessive; above |
| hypo– | insufficient; below |
| infra– | under; below |
| inter– | between |
| intra– | within |
| iso– | equal; same |
| micro– | small |
| multi– | many; multiple |
| neo– | new |
| para– | beside; near |
| per– | through |
| peri– | around; about |
| poly– | many; excessive |
| post– | after; behind |
| pre– | before |
| semi– | half; one-half |
| sub– | below; under |
| tachy– | fast |
| trans– | through; across |

**Table 4 Common Medical Suffixes**

| Suffix | Meaning |
|---|---|
| -algia | pain |
| -cyte | cell |
| -ectomy | excision; removal |
| -edema | swelling |
| -emia | blood; blood condition |
| -esthesia | feeling |
| -gram | record; writing |
| -graph | instrument for recording |
| -ia; -ic | pertaining to a pathological state or condition |
| -ism | condition |
| -itis | inflammation |
| -lysis | separation; destruction |
| -meter | instrument for measuring |
| -ology | study of |
| -oma | tumor |
| -osis | condition; abnormal condition |
| -otomy | incision into |
| -pathy | disease |
| -plasty | surgical repair |
| -plegia | paralysis |
| -sclerosis | hardening |
| -scope; -scopy | to view; process of viewing |
| -spasm | involuntary contraction; twitching |
| -stasis | standing still; balance |
| -stenosis | narrowing; stricture |
| -stomy | to form an opening |
| -therapy | treatment; to treat |
| -tomy | incision |
| -uria | urine |

**Table 5 Common Abbreviations and Acronyms of Hospital Departments, Units, and Locations**

| Abbreviation | Meaning |
|---|---|
| CCU | Cardiac Care Unit; Coronary Care Unit |
| ECF | Extended-Care Facility |
| ED; ER | Emergency Department; Emergency Room |
| ICU | Intensive Care Unit |
| Lab; LAB | Laboratory |
| LDR; L&D; LD&R | Labor and Delivery Room; Labor and Delivery; Labor, Delivery, and Recovery |
| LTAC | Long-Term Acute Care |
| LTC | Long-Term Care |
| MICU | Medical Intensive Care Unit |
| NH | Nursing Home |
| NICU | Neonatal Intensive Care Unit |
| OB | Obstetrics |
| OB-GYN; OB-Gyn | Obstetrics and Gynecology |
| OR | Operating Room |
| OT | Occupational Therapy |
| PACU | Post-Anesthesia Care Unit |
| Peds | Pediatric Department |
| PICU | Pediatric Intensive Care Unit |
| PT | Physical Therapy |
| RR | Recovery Room |
| SICU | Surgical Intensive Care Unit |
| SSU | Short-Stay Unit |
| TCU | Trauma Care Unit |
| X-Ray; x-ray | Radiology |

**Table 6 Common Abbreviations and Acronyms of Professional Titles**

| Abbreviation | Meaning |
|---|---|
| CNA | Certified Nursing Assistant |
| CNM | Certified Nurse Midwife |
| CPhT | Certified Pharmacy Technician |
| DO | Doctor of Osteopathy |
| ENT | Ear, Nose, and Throat specialist |
| GP | General Practitioner |
| HO | House Officer |
| LPN | Licensed Practical Nurse |
| LVN | Licensed Vocational Nurse |
| MD | Medical Doctor |
| NP | Nurse Practitioner |
| PA | Physician Assistant |
| PharmD | Doctor of Pharmacy |
| PhTR | Pharmacy Technician Registered; Registered Pharmacy Technician |
| PIC | Pharmacist-In-Charge |
| RN | Registered Nurse |
| RPh | Registered Pharmacist |
| Rx Mgr | Pharmacy Manager |

**Table 7 Common Medical Abbreviations and Acronyms**

| Abbreviation | Meaning |
|---|---|
| AD; a.d. | right ear |
| ADA | American Dietetic Association (diet) |
| ad lib | at liberty; freely; as desired |
| AS; a.s. | left ear |
| ASAP | as soon as possible |
| ATC | around the clock |
| AU; a.u. | both ears |
| BM | bowel movement |
| BP | blood pressure |
| BSA | body surface area |
| Bx | biopsy |
| cc* | cubic centimeters; milliliters |
| cm | centimeter |
| CNS | central nervous system |
| CPR | cardiopulmonary resuscitation |
| DNI | do not intubate |
| DNR | do not resuscitate |
| DOB | date of birth |
| Dx | diagnosis |
| F/U | follow-up |
| Fx | fracture |
| GI | gastrointestinal |
| GT | gastrostomy tube |
| GU | genitourinary |
| GYN; Gyn | gynecology |
| HAI | healthcare associated infection; hospital acquired infection: nosocomial infection |
| HOB; H.O.B. | head of bed |
| HR | heart rate |
| Hx | history |
| I/O; I&O | intake and output |
| Ⓛ; lt | left |
| LMP | last menstrual period |
| $m^2$ | meter squared; square meter |
| NG | nasogastric |
| NGT; ngt | nasogastric tube |
| NKA | no known allergies |
| NKDA | no known drug allergies |
| NSA | no salt added (diet) |
| NV; N&V | nausea and vomiting |

**Table 7 Common Medical Abbreviations and Acronyms** *(continued)*

| Abbreviation | Meaning |
|---|---|
| OD; o.d. | right eye |
| OOB | out of bed |
| ORTH; Ortho | orthopedic |
| OS; o.s. | left eye |
| OU; o.u. | both eyes |
| P | pulse |
| $\bar{p}$ | post; after |
| pp | postprandial; after meals |
| Ⓡ; rt | right |
| RE: | concerning |
| R/O | rule out |
| RR | respiratory rate |
| S/P | status post; condition after |
| Sx | symptom; signs |
| T; temp | temperature |
| Tx | treatment |
| UGI | upper gastrointestinal |
| VS; v.s. | vital signs (temperature, pulse, respiratory rate, blood pressure) |
| YO; y/o | year old |

* Please note that this abbreviation is being considered for possible future inclusion in the Joint Commission's Official "Do Not Use" List of Abbreviations.

**Table 8 Common Abbreviations for Diagnoses, Conditions, and Diseases**

| Abbreviation | Meaning |
|---|---|
| AAA | abdominal aortic aneurysm |
| AF | atrial fibrillation |
| AIDS | acquired immunodeficiency syndrome |
| ALL | acute lymphocytic leukemia |
| ALS | amyotrophic lateral sclerosis |
| AMI | acute myocardial infarction |
| ARDS | acute respiratory distress syndrome |
| BKA | below-knee amputation |
| BPH | benign prostatic hypertrophy |
| BRP | bathroom privileges |
| Ca | cancer |
| CABG | coronary artery bypass graft |
| CAD | coronary artery disease |
| CHF | congestive heart failure; chronic heart failure |
| CMV | cytomegalovirus |
| COPD | chronic obstructive pulmonary disease |
| CVA | cerebrovascular accident (stroke) |
| DKA | diabetic ketoacidosis |
| DM | diabetes mellitus |
| DT | delirium tremens |
| DVT | deep vein thrombosis |
| EBV | Epstein-Barr virus |
| ESRD | end-stage renal disease |
| GERD | gastroesophageal reflux disease |
| GSW | gunshot wound |
| HA | headache |
| HIV | human immunodeficiency virus |
| HPV | human papillomavirus |
| HTN | hypertension |
| IBS | irritable bowel syndrome |
| JRA | juvenile rheumatoid arthritis |
| MD | muscular dystrophy |
| MI | myocardial infarction (heart attack) |
| MRSA | methicillin-resistant *Staphylococcus aureus* |
| MS | multiple sclerosis |
| MVA | motor vehicle accident |
| OA | osteoarthritis |

**Table 8 Common Abbreviations for Diagnoses, Conditions, and Diseases** *(continued)*

| Abbreviation | Meaning |
|---|---|
| PID | pelvic inflammatory disease |
| PVD | peripheral vascular disease |
| RA | rheumatoid arthritis |
| SCA | sickle-cell anemia |
| SCT | sickle-cell trait |
| SLE | systemic lupus erythematosus |
| SOB | shortness of breath |
| STD | sexually transmitted disease |
| SVT | supraventricular tachycardia |
| TB | tuberculosis |
| TIA | transient ischemic attack |
| TMJ | temporomandibular joint |
| TSS | toxic shock syndrome |
| URI | upper respiratory infection |
| UTI | urinary tract infection |

**Table 9 Common Abbreviations and Acronyms for Laboratory Tests, Diagnostic and Medical Procedures, and Treatments**

| Abbreviation | Meaning |
|---|---|
| ABGs | arterial blood gases |
| Alb | albumin |
| BG | blood glucose |
| BS | blood sugar |
| BUN | blood urea nitrogen |
| Ca | calcium |
| C&S | culture and sensitivity |
| CBC | complete blood count |
| CHOL | cholesterol |
| Cl | chloride |
| $CO_2$ | carbon dioxide |
| CrCl | creatinine clearance |
| CS; C-section | Cesarean section |
| CSF | cerebrospinal fluid |
| CT; CT scan; CAT scan | computer tomography; computer-aided tomography |
| CXR | chest x-ray |
| ECG; EKG | electrocardiogram |
| ECHO | echocardiogram |
| ECT | electroconvulsive therapy |
| EEG | electroencephalogram |
| ENDO | endoscopy |
| ETOH; EtOH | alcohol; ethyl alcohol |
| FBS | fasting blood sugar |
| Fe | iron |
| FFP | fresh frozen plasma |
| Gluc | glucose; blood sugar |
| H&H | hemoglobin and hematocrit |
| HBO | hyperbaric oxygen |
| Hct | hematocrit |
| HDL | high-density lipoprotein |
| HEENT | head, eyes, ears, nose, throat |
| Hgb | hemoglobin |
| $H_2O$ | water |
| INR | international normalized ratio |
| IPPB | intermittent positive-pressure breathing |
| I/S; IS | incentive spirometer |

**Table 9 Common Abbreviations and Acronyms for Laboratory Tests, Diagnostic and Medical Procedures, and Treatments** *(continued)*

| Abbreviation | Meaning |
|---|---|
| IVP | intravenous pyelography |
| JT; J-tube | jejunostomy tube |
| K; K+ | potassium |
| lap chole | laparoscopic cholecystectomy (gallbladder removal) |
| LDL | low-density lipoprotein |
| LP | lumbar puncture |
| lytes | electrolytes |
| Mg; mag | magnesium |
| MRI | magnetic resonance imaging |
| Na | sodium |
| NC | nasal cannula |
| NSA | no salt added (diet) |
| $O_2$ | oxygen |
| $O_2$ per NC | oxygen by nasal cannula |
| OT | occupational therapy |
| P&PD | percussion & postural drainage |
| PCVC | percutaneous central venous catheter |
| PET | positron emission tomography |
| PICC | peripherally inserted central catheter |
| PLTs | platelets |
| Post-op; Postop | postoperatively; after surgery |
| PRBCs | packed red blood cells |
| Pre-op; Preop | preoperatively; before surgery |
| PT | physical therapy |
| RBC | red blood cell |
| RT | respiratory therapy |
| SSE | soapsuds enema |
| TP | total protein |
| trig | triglycerides |
| TSH | thyroid-stimulating hormone |
| UA | urinalysis |
| U/S; sono | ultrasound; sonography |
| WBC | white blood cell |
| WRBCs | washed red blood cells |
| X-ray | radiographic image or film |

**Table 10 Common Pharmacy Abbreviations and Acronyms**

| Abbreviation | Meaning |
|---|---|
| **A-B-C** | |
| AA | amino acid; Aminosyn |
| aaa | apply to affected area |
| ABX; ABx | antibiotic |
| ac; a.c.; AC | before meals |
| ACD | automated compounding device |
| ACE | angiotensin-converting enzyme |
| ad; a.d.; AD | right ear |
| AHF | antihemophilic factor |
| AM; a.m. | morning |
| amp | ampule |
| APAP | acetaminophen; Tylenol |
| aq | water |
| as; a.s.; AS | left ear |
| ASA | aspirin |
| au; a.u.; AU | both ears; each ear |
| AZT; ZDV | azidothymidine; zidovudine |
| $B_1$ | vitamin $B_1$; thiamin |
| $B_2$ | vitamin $B_2$; riboflavin |
| $B_5$ | vitamin $B_5$; pantothenic acid |
| $B_6$ | vitamin $B_6$; pyridoxine HCl |
| $B_{12}$ | vitamin $B_{12}$; cyanocobalamin |
| b.i.d.; BID | twice daily |
| BSA | body surface area |
| BSC | biological safety cabinet |
| BUD | beyond-use date |
| °C | degrees centigrade; temperature in degrees centigrade |
| Ca | calcium |
| CACI | compounding aseptic containment isolator |
| CaCl; $CaCl_2$ | calcium chloride |
| CaG; CaGluc | calcium gluconate |
| CAI | compounding aseptic isolator |
| Cap | capsule |
| CCB | calcium-channel blocker |
| CHIP | Children's Health Insurance Program |
| Cleo | clindamycin; Cleocin |
| CSP | compounded sterile preparation |
| Cu | copper |

Table 10 **Common Pharmacy Abbreviations and Acronyms** *(continued)*

| Abbreviation | Meaning |
|---|---|
| **D-E-F** | |
| $D_5$; $D_5W$; D5W | dextrose 5% in water |
| $D_5$ ¼; D5 1/4 | dextrose 5% in ¼ normal saline; dextrose 5% in 0.225% sodium chloride |
| $D_5$ ⅓; D5 1/3 | dextrose 5% in ⅓ normal saline; dextrose 5% in 0.33% sodium chloride |
| $D_5$ ½; D5 1/2 | dextrose 5% in ½ normal saline; dextrose 5% in 0.45% sodium chloride |
| $D_5LR$; D5LR | dextrose 5% in lactated Ringer's solution |
| $D_5NS$; D5NS | dextrose 5% in normal saline; dextrose 5% in 0.9% sodium chloride |
| $D_{10}$; $D_{10}W$; D10W | dextrose 10% in water |
| $D_{50}$; $D_{50}W$; D50W | dextrose 50% in water |
| $D_{70}$; $D_{70}W$; D70W | dextrose 70% in water |
| DAW | dispense as written |
| DC; d/c | discontinue |
| D/C | discharge |
| DCA | direct compounding area |
| Dig | digoxin |
| disp | dispense |
| DPT; DTP | diphtheria, pertussis, tetanus (immunization) |
| dtd | dispense this dose; dispense such dose |
| EC | enteric-coated |
| EC ASA | enteric-coated aspirin |
| EEC | empty evacuated container |
| Elix | elixir |
| eMAR | electronic medication administration record |
| E-mycin; Emycin; E.E.S. | erythromycin |
| epi | epinephrine |
| EPO | epoetin alfa; erythropoietin |
| ER; XR; XL | extended-release |
| °F | degrees Fahrenheit; temperature in degrees Fahrenheit |
| FDA | Food and Drug Administration |
| Fen-Phen | fenfluramine/phentermine |
| $FeSO_4$ | ferrous sulfate; iron |
| fl | fluid |
| fl. oz | fluid ounce |
| 5-fu; 5-Fu | fluorouracil |

*(continues)*

**Table 10 Common Pharmacy Abbreviations and Acronyms** *(continued)*

| Abbreviation | Meaning |
|---|---|
| **G-H-I** | |
| g, G | gram |
| Gent | gentamicin |
| gr | grain |
| gtt; gtts | drop; drops |
| h; hr | hour |
| HC | hydrocortisone |
| HCl | hydrochloride |
| HCTZ | hydrochlorothiazide |
| HEPA | high-efficiency particulate air (filter) |
| HIPAA | Health Insurance Portability and Accountability Act |
| HL; heplock; lock | heparin lock; heparin lock flush; saline lock; saline lock flush |
| HMO | Health Maintenance Organization |
| $H_2O_2$ | hydrogen peroxide |
| HRT | hormone replacement therapy |
| h.s.; HS | bedtime |
| Hyperal | hyperalimentation; TPN; total parenteral nutrition |
| i; ṫ | one |
| ii ; ṫṫ | two |
| iii; ṫṫṫ | three |
| IA | intra-arterial |
| IBU | ibuprofen; Motrin |
| IC | intracardiac |
| ID | intradermal |
| Ig | immunoglobulin |
| IgG | immunoglobulin G |
| IM | intramuscular |
| Inj | injection |
| IPA | isopropyl alcohol |
| Irr. | irrigation |
| ISDN | isosorbide dinitrate |
| ISMO | isosorbide mononitrate |
| ISMP | Institute for Safe Medication Practices |
| ISO | International Organization for Standardization |
| IT | intrathecal |
| IV | intravenous |

**Table 10 Common Pharmacy Abbreviations and Acronyms** *(continued)*

| Abbreviation | Meaning |
|---|---|
| IVF | intravenous fluid |
| IVIG; IVIg | intravenous immunoglobulin |
| IVP | intravenous push |
| IVPB | intravenous piggyback |
| **J-K-L** | |
| K; K+ | potassium |
| $K_1$ | vitamin K; phytonadione |
| KCl | potassium chloride |
| KCZ; KTZ | ketokonazole |
| kg | kilogram |
| $KMnO_4$ | potassium permanganate |
| L | liter |
| LAFW | laminar airflow workbench; hood |
| LAH | laminar airflow hood |
| LAX | laxative |
| lb | pound |
| LD | loading dose |
| Lido | lidocaine |
| LOC | laxative of choice |
| LR; RL | lactated Ringer's solution; Ringer's lactate |
| LVP | large-volume parenteral |
| **M-N-O** | |
| Mag; Mg; MAG | magnesium |
| Mag cit; Mg. Citrate; Mg Citrate; MgCitrate; Mag. Citrate; MAG. Citrate | magnesium citrate; citrate of magnesium |
| Mag. Oxide; MAG. Oxide; Mg. Oxide; Mg Oxide; MgOxide | magnesium oxide |
| MAOI | monoamine oxidase inhibitor |
| MAR | medication administration record |
| mcg; µg* | microgram |
| MDI | metered-dose inhaler |
| MDV | multiple-dose vial |
| Med; MED; med; meds | medication; medications |
| mEq | milliequivalent |
| mEq/L | milliequivalents per liter |

*(continues)*

Table 10 **Common Pharmacy Abbreviations and Acronyms** *(continued)*

| Abbreviation | Meaning |
|---|---|
| mEq/min | milliequivalents per minute |
| mEq/mL | milliequivalents per milliliter |
| mg | milligram |
| mg/kg | milligrams per kilogram |
| mg/kg/day; mg/kg/d | milligrams per kilogram per day |
| mg/kg/hr | milligrams per kilogram per hour |
| mg/kg/min | milligrams per kilogram per minute |
| $MgSO_4$† | magnesium sulfate; magnesium |
| mL | milliliter |
| mL/hr | milliliters per hour |
| mL/min | milliliters per minute |
| mm | millimole |
| MMR | measles, mumps, rubella (immunization) |
| Mn | manganese |
| MOM; M.O.M. | milk of magnesia |
| MR | may repeat |
| M.S.† | morphine sulfate |
| MU†; mu | million units |
| MVI; MVI-12 | multiple vitamin injection; multivitamins for parenteral administration |
| Na | sodium |
| NaCl | sodium chloride; salt |
| $NaPhos_3$; $Na_3PO_4$ | sodium phosphate |
| NDC | National Drug Code |
| NF; non-form | nonformulary |
| NOR-EPI | norepinephrine |
| NPO | nothing by mouth |
| NR; d.n.r. | no refills; do not repeat |
| NS | normal saline; 0.9% sodium chloride |
| ½ NS | one-half normal saline; 0.45% sodium chloride |
| ¼ NS | one-quarter normal saline; 0.225% sodium chloride |
| NSAID | nonsteroidal anti-inflammatory drug |
| NTG | nitroglycerin |
| od; o.d.; OD | right eye |
| ODT | orally disintegrating tablet |
| OPTH; OPHTH; Opth | ophthalmic |

Table 10 **Common Pharmacy Abbreviations and Acronyms** *(continued)*

| Abbreviation | Meaning |
|---|---|
| os; o.s.; OS | left eye |
| OTC | over the counter; no prescription required |
| ou; o.u.; OU | both eyes; each eye |
| oz | ounce |
| **P-Q-R** | |
| p.c.; PC | after meals |
| PCA | patient-controlled anesthesia |
| PCN | penicillin |
| PDR | Physicians' Desk Reference |
| PEC | primary engineering control |
| Per | by |
| PF | preservative-free |
| PFS | prefilled syringe |
| PHI | protected health information |
| PM; p.m. | afternoon; evening |
| PO | orally; by mouth |
| $PO_4$ | phosphate |
| PPD | purified protein derivative; TB skin test |
| PPE | personal protective equipment |
| PPI | proton pump inhibitor |
| PPN | partial parenteral nutrition |
| PPO | preferred provider organization |
| PR | per rectum; rectally |
| PRN; p.r.n. | as needed; as occasion requires |
| PV | per vagina; vaginally |
| PVC | polyvinyl chloride |
| q | every |
| q.h.; qhour | every hour |
| q2h | every 2 hours |
| q4h | every 4 hours |
| q6h | every 6 hours |
| q8h | every 8 hours |
| q12h | every 12 hours |
| q24h | every 24 hours |
| q48h | every 48 hours |

*(continues)*

Table 10 **Common Pharmacy Abbreviations and Acronyms** *(continued)*

| Abbreviation | Meaning |
|---|---|
| QA | quality assurance |
| QAM; qam | every morning |
| qDay; QD† | every day |
| q.i.d.; QID | four times daily |
| QOD; Q other day; Q.O. Day | every other day |
| QPM; qpm | every evening |
| qs; qsad | quantity sufficient; a sufficient quantity to make |
| QTY; qty | quantity |
| qwk; qweek | every week |
| Rx | prescription; pharmacy; medication; drug; recipe; take |
| **S-T** | |
| SDV | single-dose vial |
| sig | write on label; signa; directions |
| SL; sub-L | sublingual |
| SMZ-TMP | sulfamethoxazole and trimethoprim; Bactrim |
| $SO_4$ | sulfate |
| sol | solution |
| SR | sustained-release |
| SS; ss | one-half |
| SSI | sliding-scale insulin |
| SSRI | selective serotonin reuptake inhibitor |
| Stat | immediately; now |
| Sub-Q; SC; SQ; sq | subcutaneous |
| SUPP; Supp | suppository |
| susp | suspension |
| SVP | small-volume parenteral |
| SW | sterile water |
| SWFI | sterile water for injection |
| Tab | tablet |
| TAB | triple antibiotic (solution or ointment); bacitracin, neomycin, and polymyxin B |
| TBSP; tbsp | tablespoon; tablespoonful; 15 mL |
| TCN | tetracycline |
| Td | tetanus-diphtheria toxoid |
| TDS | transdermal delivery system |

**Table 10 Common Pharmacy Abbreviations and Acronyms** *(continued)*

| Abbreviation | Meaning |
|---|---|
| t.i.d.; TID | three times daily |
| tinct | tincture |
| t.i.w.; TIW | three times a week |
| TKO; TKVO; KO; KVO | to keep open; to keep vein open; keep open; keep vein open (a slow IV flow rate) |
| TO; T.O. | telephone order |
| Top | topical; applied to the skin |
| TPA | tissue plasminogen activator |
| TPN | total parenteral nutrition |
| TSP; tsp | teaspoon; teaspoonful; 5 mL |
| **U-V-W** | |
| U | unit |
| ung | ointment |
| Units/hr; u†/hr | units per hour |
| ut dict | as directed |
| VAG; vag | vagina; vaginally |
| Vanco | vancomycin |
| VO; V.O.; V/O | verbal order |
| w/ | with |
| WA; w.a. | while awake |
| wk; WK | week |
| w/o | without |
| **X-Y-Z** | |
| Zn | zinc |
| ZnO; ZNO | zinc oxide |
| $ZnSO_4$ | zinc sulfate |
| Z-Pak | azithromycin; Zithromax |

† Please note that this abbreviation is on the Joint Commission's Official "Do Not Use" List of Abbreviations. However, you may occasionally encounter its use in your practice. If you see this abbreviation on a medication order, alert the pharmacist who will, in turn, clarify the order with the prescriber.
* Please note that this abbreviation is being considered for possible future inclusion in the Joint Commission's Official "Do Not Use" List of Abbreviations.

### Table 11 Common Pharmacy Symbols

| Symbol | Meaning |
|---|---|
| + | plus; add; additional; positive; combine; and |
| – | subtract; remove; negative; minus; without |
| ↑ | increase; above |
| ↓ | decrease; below |
| / | per; over |
| ≥ | greater than or equal to |
| ≤ | less than or equal to |
| >* | greater than |
| <* | less than |
| = | equal; equal to |
| @ | at |
| " | inches |
| Δ | change |
| ∅ | no; none; zero |
| ° | hour; degree |
| ā | before |
| āā | of each |
| c̄ | with |
| s̄ | without |
| p̄ | after |
| # | number; pounds |
| % | percent; percent strength |
| & | and; also; with |
| ♏ | minim |
| ʒ | dram |
| f | fluid ounce |
| ℥ | ounce |

* Please note that this symbol is being considered for possible future inclusion in the Joint Commission's Official "Do Not Use" List of Abbreviations.

**Table 12 Signa Interpretation**

Transcribing or interpreting a signa is the process of translating the prescriber's directions for a particular medication. Interpreting the signa correctly will assist you with understanding the medication order, preparing the medication label, and compounding the prescription. The signa provides very specific information that answers the same four or five questions regarding *what, how, where,* and *when* to administer a medication. Each medication ordered by the prescriber has its own signa. Most signas answer the following questions:

| | |
|---|---|
| **1)** | **WHAT is the nurse supposed TO DO?** |
| | The answer to this question will always take the form of a verb because it requires some sort of action. The verb used will depend on what the prescriber wants the nurse to do. The action that the nurse should take depends on the route of administration.<br><br>If the prescribed medication is . . .<br>• an **oral medication** (tablet, capsule, or liquid), then the nurse should "**GIVE**" or "**ADMINISTER**" the medication to the patient.<br>*Note: In the hospital setting, a nurse or other healthcare professional administers the medication to the patient; therefore, the most commonly used verb will be "give." In the retail pharmacy setting, the patient administers the medication to himself or herself; therefore, the word "take" would be used in place of "give."*<br>• an **eye or ear medication**, then the nurse is being directed to "**INSTILL**" the medication.<br>• a **vaginal or rectal medication**, then the nurse is being directed to "**INSERT**" the medication.<br>• a **topical medication** (patch, cream, ointment, etc.), then the nurse is being directed to "**APPLY**" the medication.<br>• an **inhaled medication**, then the nurse is being directed to have the patient "**INHALE**" the medication. |
| **2)** | **HOW MANY __________ is the patient supposed to receive?** |
| | The answer to this question MUST contain two parts: a number and a dosage form (see the examples below).<br>one tablet<br>five milliliters<br>two puffs<br>three capsules<br>one patch |
| **3)** | **WHERE should the medication be PUT?** |
| | The answer to this question will depend on the dosage form or the administration site.<br><br>If the prescribed medication is for . . .<br>• **oral (p.o.) tablets, capsules, or liquids**, the nurse is being directed to administer this medication "**ORALLY**," or "**BY MOUTH**."<br>• **a cream, ointment, or patch**, the nurse is being directed to administer this medication "**TOPICALLY**," or "**TO THE SKIN**."<br>• **a suppository or an intravaginal medication**, the nurse is being directed to administer the medication "**RECTALLY**" or "**VAGINALLY**" (whatever is most appropriate based on the context of the order).<br>• **an eye or ear medication**, the nurse is being directed as to which body part (s) the medication is to be placed–for example, "**RIGHT EYE**," "**LEFT EAR**," "**BOTH EYES**," or "**EACH EAR**." |

*(continues)*

Table 12 **Signa Interpretation** *(continued)*

| | |
|---|---|
| **4)** | **WHEN is the medication to be given?** |
| | The signa will provide very specific directions related to the prescriber's requested dosing interval (see the examples below).<br>every day<br>at bedtime<br>every eight hours<br>twice daily<br>Monday through Friday<br>as needed |
| **5)** | **Is there any ADDITIONAL, SUPPORTING, AUXILIARY, OR MISCELLANEOUS INFORMATION that must be transcribed from the signa onto the label?** |
| | IF the prescriber includes auxiliary information in the signa, those instructions MUST be included on the label and followed by the nurse when administering the medication (see the examples below).<br>for pain<br>rinse<br>with food<br>until gone<br>for 14 days<br>for sleep<br>swish and swallow<br>for itching<br>for nausea and vomiting<br>for infection<br>as directed |
| **EXAMPLE OF CORRECT SIGNA TRANSLATION:** | |
| **signa** | 1 tab q8h prn pain or fever >101 |
| **Translation:** | Give one tablet by mouth every eight hours as needed for pain or for fever above 101 degrees. |

Table 13 **Common Parenteral Medications**

| Generic Name | Brand Name | Class or Common Use |
|---|---|---|
| **A-B-C** | | |
| abatacept | Orencia | antirheumatic |
| acetazolamide | Diamox | diuretic; urinary alkalinizer; antiglaucoma; anticonvulsant |
| acyclovir | Zovirax | antiviral |
| adalimumab | Humira | rheumatoid arthritis treatment |
| alteplase | Activase | thrombolytic agent; catheter occlusion dissolution |
| amikacin | Amikin | anti-infective; antibacterial |
| aminophylline | | bronchodilator; respiratory stimulant |
| amiodarone hydrochloride | Cordarone | antiarrhythmic |
| amphotericin B | Abelcet; Amphotec; AmBisome | antifungal |
| ampicillin | Principen; Omnipen | anti-infective |
| ampicillin sodium/ sulbactam sodium | Unasyn | anti-infective |
| antihemophilic factor (recombinant) | Xyntha | hematological agent; anti-hemorrhagic |
| antithymocyte globulin | Thymoglobulin | immunosuppressant |
| apomorphine | Apokyn | dopamine agonist |
| argatroban | Acova | anticoagulant |
| atenolol | Tenormin | cardiac agent; beta blocker |
| atracurium besylate | Tracrium | skeletal muscle relaxant; paralytic |
| azithromycin | Zithromax; Zmax | anti-infective |
| aztreonam | Azactam | antibiotic |
| baclofen | Lioresal | skeletal muscle relaxant |
| bivalirudin | Angiomax | anticoagulant |
| cefamandole | Mandol | anti-infective |
| cefazolin sodium | Ancef; Kefzol | antibiotic |
| cefepime | Maxipime | anti-infective |
| cefmetazole | Zefazone | antibacterial |
| cefonicid | Monocid | anti-infective |
| cefoperazone | Cefobid | antibiotic |
| cefotaxime sodium | Claforan | antibiotic |
| cefotetan disodium | Cefotan | antibiotic |
| cefoxitin sodium | Mefoxin | antibiotic |
| ceftazidime | Fortaz; Ceptaz | antibiotic |
| ceftizoxime sodium | Cefizox | antibiotic |
| ceftriaxone sodium | Rocephin | antibiotic |
| cefuroxime sodium | Kefurox; Zinacef | antibiotic |

*(continues)*

**Table 13 Common Parenteral Medications** *(continued)*

| Generic Name | Brand Name | Class or Common Use |
|---|---|---|
| cephradine | Velosef | anti-infective |
| chloramphenicol | Chloromycetin | anti-infective |
| cimetidine | Tagamet | gastric acid inhibitor; antiulcer |
| clevidipine butyrate | Cleviprex | antihypertensive; calcium-channel blocker |
| clindamycin | Cleocin | anti-infective; antiprotozoal |
| **D-E-F** | | |
| dalteparin sodium | Fragmin | anticoagulant |
| danaparoid sodium | Orgaran | anticoagulant |
| daptomycin | Cubicin | anti-infective |
| dexamethasone | Decadron | anti-inflammatory; antiemetic; immunosuppressant |
| diazepam | Valium | antianxiety agent; centrally acting muscle relaxant |
| digoxin | Lanoxin | cardiac agent; treats congestive heart failure and atrial fibrillation |
| dobutamine hydrochloride | Dobutrex | cardiac stimulant; inotropic agent |
| dopamine hydrochloride | | cardiac stimulant; vasopressor; inotropic agent |
| doripenem | Doribax | anti-infective |
| doxycycline | Vibramycin | antibacterial; antiprotozoal; antimalarial |
| enalapril | Vasotec | antihypertensive |
| epinephrine HCl | Adrenalin Cl | cardiac stimulant; bronchodilator; antiallergic; vasopressor |
| ertapenem | Invanz | anti-infective |
| erythromycin lactobionate | Erythrocin | anti-infective |
| famotidine | Pepcid | gastric acid inhibitor; antiulcer |
| fentanyl | Sublimaze | narcotic analgesic; analgesia premedicant |
| fluconazole | Diflucan | antifungal |
| fosphenytoin | Cerebyx | anticonvulsant |
| furosemide | Lasix | diuretic |
| **G-H-I** | | |
| gentamicin | Garamycin | antibacterial; aminoglycoside antibiotic |
| heparin sodium | Heparin | anticoagulant |
| hydralazine hydrochloride | Apresoline | antihypertensive |
| hydromorphone HCl | Dilaudid | narcotic analgesic |
| imipenem/cilastatin | Primaxin | antibacterial |
| isoproterenol | Isuprel | cardiac stimulant; antiarrhythmic; bronchodilator |

Table 13 **Common Parenteral Medications** *(continued)*

| Generic Name | Brand Name | Class or Common Use |
|---|---|---|
| **J-K-L** | | |
| kanamycin sulfate | Kantrex | antibacterial |
| labetalol | Normodyne; Trandate | alpha/beta-adrenergic blocking agent; antihypertensive |
| levofloxacin | Levaquin | anti-infective |
| lidocaine | Xylocaine | antiarrhythmic |
| **M-N-O** | | |
| meperidine hydrochloride | Demerol | narcotic analgesic |
| meropenem | Merrem | antibacterial |
| metoclopramide HCl | Reglan | gastrointestinal stimulant; antiemetic |
| metoprolol | Lopressor | antihypertensive; antianginal |
| mezlocillin | Mezlin | anti-infective |
| midazolam hydrochloride | Versed | sedative |
| morphine | Duramorph; Infumorph | narcotic analgesic |
| nafcillin sodium | Nafcil; Nallpen | antibacterial |
| nesiritide citrate | Natrecor | cardiac agent; congestive heart failure treatment |
| nicardipine hydrochloride | Cardene | antihypertensive; antianginal |
| nitroglycerin | Nitro-Bid; Tridil | antihypertensive; antianginal; vasodilator |
| norepinephrine | Levophed | vasopressor |
| ondansetron HCl | Zofran | antiemetic |
| oxacillin sodium | Bactocill; Prostaphlin | antibacterial |
| **P-Q-R** | | |
| pancuronium bromide | Pavulon | neuromuscular blocking agent |
| penicillin G | Pfizerpen | anti-infective |
| pentobarbital sodium | Nembutal Na | barbiturate; sedative; anticonvulsant |
| piperacillin sodium | Pipracil | anti-infective |
| piperacillin/tazobactam | Zosyn | antibacterial |
| prochlorperazine | Compazine | antiemetic; antipsychotic |
| promethazine | Phenergan | antiemetic; sedative; antihistamine |
| propranolol | Inderal | beta-adrenergic blocking agent; antiarrhythmic |
| ranitidine | Zantac | $H_2$ antagonist; gastric acid inhibitor; antiulcer agent |
| reteplase recombinant | Retavase | thrombolytic agent |
| **S-T** | | |
| succinylcholine | Anectine | neuromuscular blocking agent; anesthesia adjunct |
| thiopental sodium | Pentothal | barbiturate; anesthetic; anticonvulsant |

*(continues)*

**Table 13 Common Parenteral Medications** *(continued)*

| Generic Name | Brand Name | Class or Common Use |
|---|---|---|
| ticarcillin | Ticar | anti-infective |
| tigecycline | Tygacil | antibiotic |
| tinzaparin sodium | Innohep | thrombolytic agent |
| tobramycin | Nebcin | anti-infective; aminoglycoside antibiotic |
| tranexamic acid | Cyklokapron | antihemorrhagic; antifibrinolytic |
| trimethoprim/sulfamethoxazole | Bactrim; Septra | antibacterial |
| **U-V-W** | | |
| vancomycin | Vancocin | anti-infective; aminoglycoside antibiotic |
| warfarin | Coumadin | anticoagulant |
| **X-Y-Z** | | |
| zidovudine | Retrovir | antiviral |

# Appendix C

## Resources for Chemotherapy Compounding

The tables of Appendix C provide useful information on standards, procedures, and safety requirements unique to the sterile compounding of chemotherapy products. Tables 1 and 2 offer nomogram tables similar to the ones used by healthcare practitioners when calculating BSA for chemotherapy dosages. Having a familiarity with the steps for reading nomograms aids your understanding of how chemotherapy is prescribed and how BSA affects your preparatory compounding procedures, such as CSP label verification and pharmacy dosage calculations. Tables 3 and 4 discuss important procedures and safety precautions relevant to chemotherapy compounding. Because of the dangers associated with the handling of chemotherapy products, this information is vital to your safety as well as the safety of others.

### Table 1 Nomogram for Estimating Body Surface Area of Children

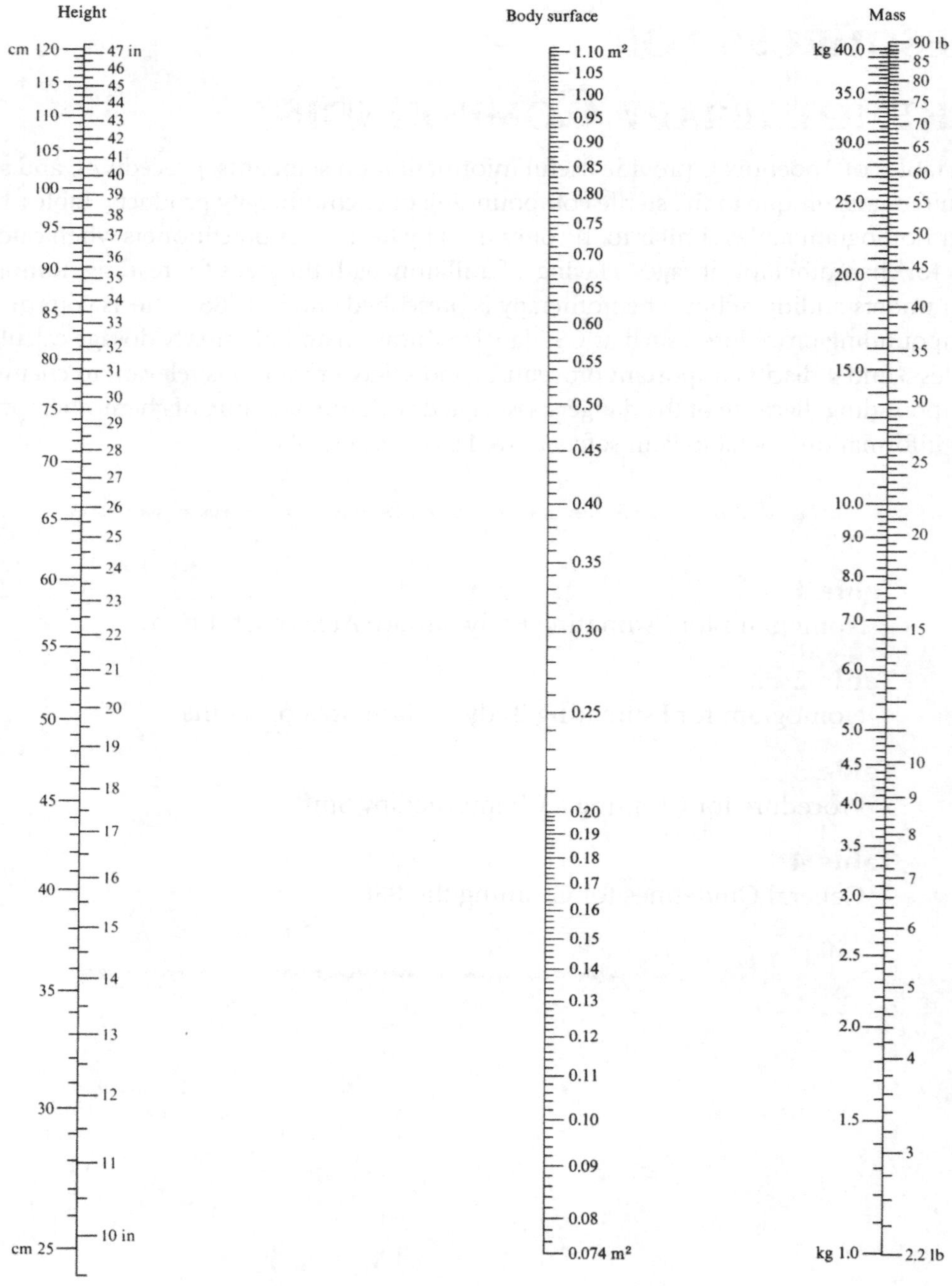




**Steps for Reading a Nomogram for Estimating BSA**

**Step 1.** Mark the patient's height on the left column.

**Step 2.** Mark the patient's weight on the right column.

**Step 3.** Draw a line or place a straight-edge ruler on the two marks.

**Step 4.** Read the BSA by noting where the straight edge crosses the center column. When the straight edge crosses between two numbers, the BSA should be estimated to the nearest one-half unit.

## Table 2 Nomogram for Estimating Body Surface Area of Adults

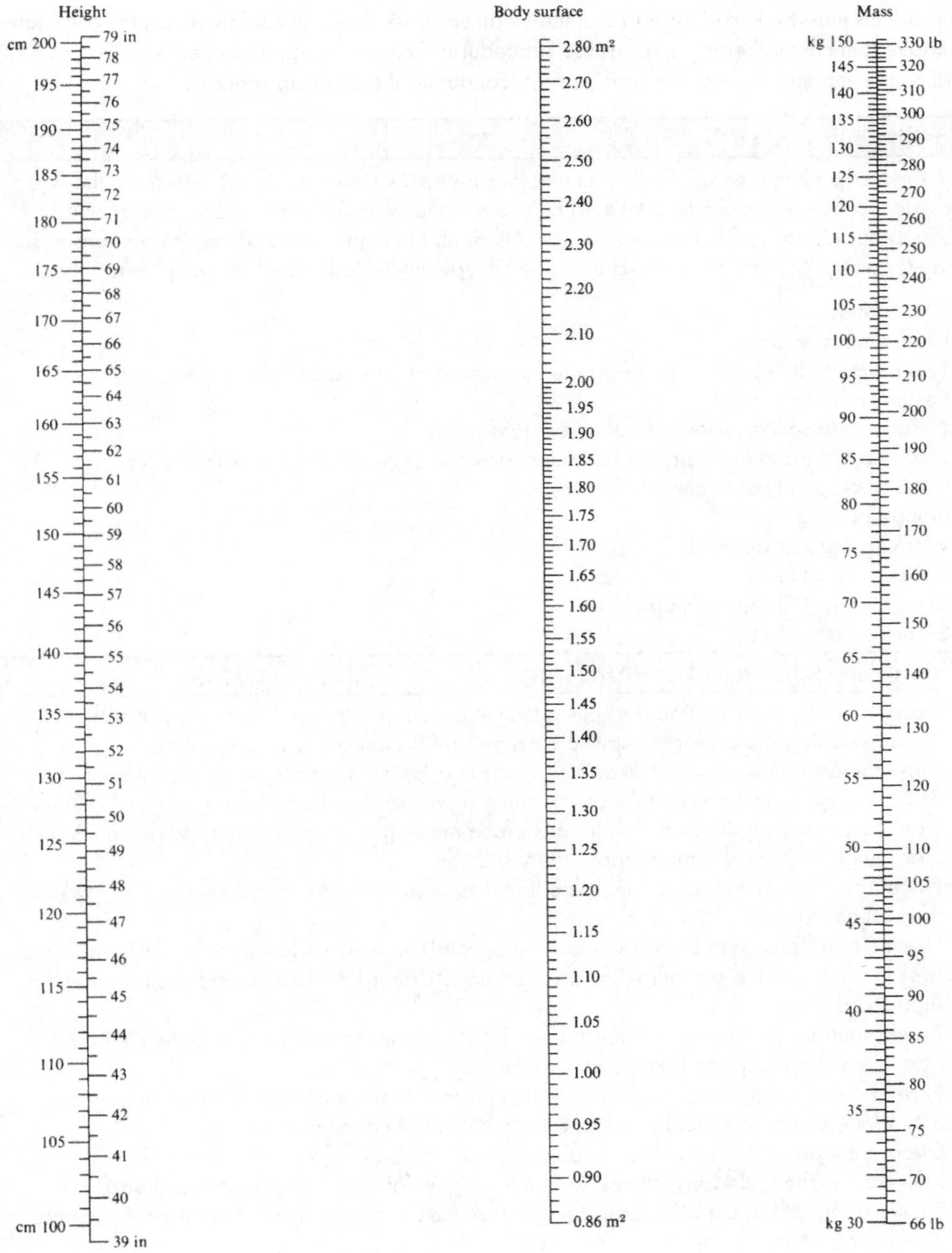




### Steps for Reading a Nomogram for Estimating BSA

**Step 1.** Mark the patient's height on the left column.

**Step 2.** Mark the patient's weight on the right column.

**Step 3.** Draw a line or place a straight-edge ruler on the two marks.

**Step 4.** Read the BSA by noting where the straight edge crosses the center column. When the straight edge crosses between two numbers, the BSA should be estimated to the nearest one-half unit.

## Table 3 Procedure for Cleaning a Chemotherapy Spill

Because chemotherapy agents are considered hazardous drugs, healthcare personnel who handle these products must be knowledgeable of the clean-up procedures and safety measures associated with inadvertent chemotherapy spills. These procedures include the use of a chemotherapy spill kit, as well as the implementation of a specific protocol during the clean-up process.

| Chemotherapy Spill Kit |
|---|
| In the event of a chemotherapy spill, a chemotherapy spill kit must be used to clean up the liquid or powder spills. Consequently, a kit must be readily available for use in every chemotherapy storage, preparation, and administration site. Although the components of the chemotherapy spill kit may vary slightly among manufacturers, the kit typically includes the following items:<br>• Chemotherapy safety glasses<br>• Chemotherapy gown<br>• Two pairs of gloves (one pair of standard gloves and one pair of chemotherapy gloves)<br>• Respirator or face mask<br>• Absorbent towels or pillows (to absorb liquid spills)<br>• Small dustpan and hand broom (to collect powdered medication or broken glass)<br>• Puncture-resistant container<br>• Biohazard bag<br>• Warning signs or placards<br>• Incident report form<br>• Chemotherapy sharps container<br>• Clean-up instructions |
| **Chemotherapy Spill Clean-Up Procedures** |
| 1. Cordon off the area around the spill to limit exposure to other personnel or patients.<br>2. Set up warning signs near the spill to alert people to stay away from the area.<br>3. Grab the chemotherapy spill kit as well as these additional supplies: aseptic, lint-free wipes; SW in a pour bottle; an appropriate cleaning agent; and a chemotherapy sharps container.<br>4. Don shoe covers, hair cover, respirator or face mask, gloves, chemotherapy gown, chemotherapy gloves, and chemotherapy safety glasses.<br>5. Place absorbent towels or pillows onto liquid spills. Discard saturated towels or pillows into the biohazard bag.<br>6. Use the hand broom to brush powdered drug and/or broken glass into the dustpan. Place broken glass into the puncture-resistant container. Discard the broom and dustpan into the biohazard bag.<br>7. Lightly saturate an aseptic, lint-free pad with SW. Clean the spill area with the saturated pad. Place the used pad into the biohazard bag.<br>8. Repeat step 7 using an appropriate cleaning agent; then clean the spill area again using SW. *Note:* The area should be cleaned a minimum of three times.<br>9. Discard the puncture-resistant container into the biohazard bag.<br>10. Remove the chemotherapy gloves, and then dispose of them in the biohazard bag.<br>11. Tie the open end of the biohazard bag, and place the bag into the chemotherapy sharps container.<br>12. Remove PPE and dispose of it into the chemotherapy sharps container.<br>13. Place warning signs, SW, IPA, and any other supplies (except the incident report form) into the chemotherapy sharps container, and seal the container.<br>14. Return the chemotherapy sharps container and any other supplies to the anteroom.<br>15. Perform a basic aseptic hand washing.<br>16. Fill out the incident report form and submit it to the pharmacy supervisor. |
| ***Note:*** In the event of exceptionally large spills (≥ 250 mL), spills containing nuclear or other highly hazardous waste, spills of drugs that are incompatible with alcohol, or spills in a carpeted area, consult the MSDS for clean-up procedures. Contact the facility's hazardous materials (Haz-Mat) response team. Some spills are beyond the scope of pharmacy personnel responsibility. If the Haz-Mat team determines additional precautions are required, they will call for assistance. |

## Table 4 General Guidelines for Cleaning the BSC

The BSC must be cleaned at intervals prescribed by USP Chapter <797>, and a thorough decontamination of the cabinet must be performed at least once a week. Several safety precautions must be in effect prior to cleaning the BSC:

- The cabinet must run continuously during cleaning and contamination procedures.
- The clean room should be empty of sterile compounding personnel. No other compounding procedures should take place during the cleaning of the BSC.
- Sterile compounding personnel must be appropriately garbed for contact with surfaces contaminated with hazardous chemicals. Workers must don aseptic garb, including a sterile, disposable, low-permeability chemotherapy gown and two pairs of gloves (one of which should be chemotherapy gloves, which are thicker and more puncture-resistant than standard sterile gloves).
- BSC-cleaning procedures require the technician to don a NIOSH-approved respirator appropriate for the hazard.
- Aseptic hand-washing procedures should be implemented prior to cleaning the BSC as well as at the completion of the cleaning process.

The design of the BSC, as well as the type of CSPs prepared in the BSC, necessitates special cleaning procedures. The HEPA filter in the BSC is located in the ceiling of the cabinet and, like the HEPA filter in other types of laminar airflow hoods, should never be touched. The order and direction of cleaning the BSC must take into consideration the HEPA-filtered air, which flows down vertically toward the work surface. With that in mind, you clean the hang bar and hooks of the BSC first, followed by the back wall or *panel*. Use overlapping, side-to-side strokes and move from the area closest to the HEPA filter down toward the work surface. Next, clean the side walls and glass shield of the BSC. Again, use overlapping, side-to-side strokes and move from the area closest to the HEPA filter down to the work surface. Then clean the work surface of the BSC using side-to-side strokes, and move from the inner part of the cabinet toward the outer edge of the cabinet.

Most BSCs have a removable work surface (called a *work tray*). Tilt up the tray and rest it against the interior rear wall of the cabinet. Decontaminate the area underneath the work tray (sometimes called the *drain spillage trough* or the *trough*), including the air intake grills. The work tray and drain spillage trough should be cleaned a minimum of two times because it can be heavily contaminated. Clean the BSC at intervals prescribed by USP Chapter <797>. Also perform a more thorough, complete decontamination of the BSC at least once a week.

***Note:*** The procedures below are appropriate for use when cleaning most BSCs; however, it is advisable to refer to the manufacturer's instructions for the BSC model in your facility before initiating cleaning procedures. It is also advisable to consult with the OSHA Technical Manual (OTM) Section VI: Chapter 2, Controlling Occupational Exposure to Hazardous Drugs, prior to cleaning the BSC.

| Cleaning the Biological Safety Cabinet |
|---|
| **Preparatory Procedures in the Anteroom** |
| 1. Gather cleaning supplies, including a stack of aseptic, lint-free wipes; SW in a pour bottle; sterile 70% IPA in a pour bottle; a presaturated aseptic cleaning wipe (which will be used to wipe down eyewear at the end of the procedure); and a chemotherapy sharps container.<br>2. Follow standard preparatory procedures, including donning aseptic garb and performing aseptic hand-washing procedures. Refer to Chapter 6 for procedures related to garbing and hand washing.<br>3. Don protective eyewear.<br>4. Don a sterile, disposable, low-permeability chemotherapy gown.<br>5. Don an NIOSH-approved respirator. |

| Cleaning the Biological Safety Cabinet *(continued)* |
|---|
| **Preparatory Procedures in the Clean Room** |
| 6. Apply sterile, foamed 70% IPA to your hands and allow them to air-dry; then don sterile gloves, tucking them *under* the gown's wrist cuffs.<br>7. Don sterile chemotherapy gloves, pulling them *over* the sterile gloves and over the gown wrist cuffs.<br>8. Temporarily place the cleaning supplies onto a clean countertop or other clean surface within the clean room.<br>9. Remove any extraneous supplies from the BSC and place them into the chemotherapy sharps container. |
| **Cleaning the BSC** |
| 10. Raise the glass shield (or *aperture*) to its full height, creating an approximate 12" to 14" opening (as opposed to the standard 8" opening when the shield is in its lowered position).<br>11. Place half of the stack of aseptic, lint-free wipes onto the work surface within the BSC.<br>12. Lightly saturate the stack of wipes with SW.<br>13. Use one pad from the stack of water-saturated wipes to clean the hang bar and hooks. Dispose of the used pad in the chemotherapy sharps container.<br>14. Use a new pad from the stack of water-saturated wipes and clean the interior back wall of the hood, starting closest to the HEPA filter (located in the ceiling of the BSC) and gradually moving down toward the work surface. Use overlapping, side-to-side strokes. Dispose of the used pad in the chemotherapy sharps container.<br>15. Use a new pad from the stack of water-saturated wipes and clean one interior side wall of the hood, starting closest to the HEPA filter and gradually moving down toward the work surface. Again, use overlapping, side-to-side strokes. Dispose of the used pad in the chemotherapy sharps container.<br>16. Using a new pad, repeat step 14 on the other interior side wall of the hood.<br>17. Take a new pad from the stack of water-saturated wipes to clean the BSC work surface, using overlapping, side-to-side strokes. Move from the innermost corner of the work surface toward the outer edge of the work surface. Dispose of the used pad in the chemotherapy sharps container.<br>18. Tip the work tray up so that it leans against the interior back wall of the BSC. Use the remaining water-saturated pads to clean the trough and air intake grills. Dispose of the used pads in the chemotherapy sharps container.<br>19. Repeat steps 10–17 using the remaining aseptic, lint-free wipes. First, lightly saturate the stack with sterile 70% IPA.<br>20. Return the work tray to its starting position. Lower the glass shield to its starting position. |
| **Clean-Up Procedures and PPE Removal in the Clean Room** |
| 21. Place the bottle of SW and the bottle of IPA into the chemotherapy sharps container.<br>22. Place any extraneous supplies into the chemotherapy sharps container.<br>23. Remove your chemotherapy gloves, turning them inside out as they are pulled off of your hands. Place the gloves into the chemotherapy sharps container.<br>24. Remove your chemotherapy gown, pulling it inside out as you pull it off of your shoulders. Dispose of the chemotherapy gown in the small chemotherapy sharps container. |
| **Completion Procedures in the Anteroom** |
| 25. Return to the anteroom. Remove your sterile gloves and place them into the chemotherapy sharps container.<br>26. Remove your chemotherapy safety glasses. Wipe the glasses down using a presaturated aseptic cleaning wipe. Place the eyewear in the proper storage location.<br>27. Remove remaining regular PPE—face mask, beard cover (if appropriate), hair cover, shoe covers, etc.—and place garb into a chemotherapy sharps container. *Note:* A second chemotherapy sharps container used to contain regular PPE should be kept in the anteroom.<br>28. Wash and dry your hands according to basic hand-washing procedures.<br>29. Record the date, time, and your initials on the BSC cleaning log. |

# Appendix D

## Process Validation Checklists

The process validation checklists correspond with the Chapters 6–14 Procedural Labs. The checklists must be completed by an observing pharmacist or instructor as you perform the sterile compounding procedures of each chapter. Due to time constraints, your instructor may direct you to skip the aseptic hand-washing and hood-cleaning procedures for some of the procedural labs. However, in practice, you are mandated to perform these procedures for process validation.

While your instructor will use these forms to evaluate your compliance with correct procedures and aseptic technique, these process validation checklists are designed for training purposes only. They may be used for pharmacy "in-house" initial and annual training evaluations, provided that only those personnel who achieve 100% compliance be validated as having the necessary skills, technique, and ability to perform sterile compounding and aseptic technique procedures.

The process validation checklists in Appendix D are not suitable for process evaluation and validation in order to achieve ACPE certification. Visit *www.paradigmcollege.net/sterilecomp* for more information on obtaining ACPE certification in sterile compounding and aseptic technique.

### Preliminary Information

- You will be evaluated on your ability to accurately follow the directives of the procedural lab while using correct aseptic technique.
- Although your instructor will be present during the procedure, you must work through the steps as if you were alone. Your instructor will not provide any verbal feedback to you during the procedure.
- Once you begin the lab, you must complete the entire procedure. If at any point during the process you feel that your aseptic technique has been compromised, you must *verbalize the error to your instructor, explain what you would do to fix it, and then continue the process*.
- During your demonstration of the procedure, your instructor will observe your skills and complete a checklist. On the checklist, your instructor will mark "Yes," "No," or "NA" for each step as you perform the step. "No" means that either the required step was not performed, or that it was not performed correctly. Your instructor may write additional comments if necessary.
- After the procedure and process validation checklist have been completed, your instructor will provide you with complete feedback on your demonstrated skills.
- For ACPE certification, you will be required to demonstrate this procedure with 100% compliance before being allowed to prepare sterile products for patient use. However, your instructor may determine a grading system specifically for your training in class.

# Lab Procedure Process Validation Checklist

## Chapter 6: Aseptic Garbing, Hand Washing, and Gloving

### Supplies

- Shoe covers
- Hair cover
- Face mask
- Beard cover (if appropriate)
- Sterile gown
- Presaturated surgical scrub sponge/brush
- Aseptic, lint-free paper towels or sterile gauze
- Sink appropriate for aseptic hand washing
- Sterile, foamed 70% IPA
- Sterile, powder-free gloves
- Waste container

### Basic Instructions

- Gather the necessary supplies from the supply list.
- Once your instructor gives you permission to begin, garb in the proper order to the point that you would prior to washing your hands.
- Then proceed to the sink and complete an aseptic hand washing.
- Finally, don a sterile gown and gloves.

### Lab Procedure Process Validation Checklist

| | Yes | No | NA |
|---|---|---|---|
| **Garbing** | | | |
| Removed all jewelry | ❑ | ❑ | ❑ |
| Dressed in clean scrubs or other, appropriate, nonshedding garments | ❑ | ❑ | ❑ |
| Did not wear makeup, perfume, nail polish, or artificial nails | ❑ | ❑ | ❑ |
| Properly donned shoe covers | ❑ | ❑ | ❑ |
| Properly donned hair cover | ❑ | ❑ | ❑ |
| Properly donned face mask and beard cover (if appropriate) | ❑ | ❑ | ❑ |
| Donned garb in proper order | ❑ | ❑ | ❑ |
| **Aseptic Hand Washing** | | | |
| Squeezed sponge packet before opening to activate soapsuds | ❑ | ❑ | ❑ |
| Added water to the sponge as needed to maintain adequate lather | ❑ | ❑ | ❑ |
| Used pick to clean under all fingernails before washing, and threw away pick after use | ❑ | ❑ | ❑ |
| Used brush to clean under fingernails and around cuticles of each nail | ❑ | ❑ | ❑ |
| Used sponge to clean all four surfaces of each finger | ❑ | ❑ | ❑ |
| Cleaned each finger individually | ❑ | ❑ | ❑ |
| Used sponge to clean the palm of each hand | ❑ | ❑ | ❑ |
| Used sponge to clean the back of each hand | ❑ | ❑ | ❑ |
| Used sponge on forearms, using a circular motion from wrist up to elbow | ❑ | ❑ | ❑ |
| Maintained an appropriate amount of lather during procedure | ❑ | ❑ | ❑ |

| | | | |
|---|---|---|---|
| Did not touch the sink, faucet, or other contaminant during process | ❑ | ❑ | ❑ |
| Rinsed with fingers pointing up and water running down toward the elbow | ❑ | ❑ | ❑ |
| Rinsed all soap residue from fingers, hands, and forearms | ❑ | ❑ | ❑ |
| Completed the hand-washing procedure in the proper order | ❑ | ❑ | ❑ |
| Dried hands with clean, lint-free paper towels or sterile gauze | ❑ | ❑ | ❑ |
| Properly turned off water by either using a foot pedal or, for sinks without a foot pedal, a paper towel to turn off the faucet | ❑ | ❑ | ❑ |
| **Gowning and Gloving** | | | |
| Opened gown package so that gown remained sterile | ❑ | ❑ | ❑ |
| Properly donned sterile gown | ❑ | ❑ | ❑ |
| Used sterile, foamed 70% IPA to clean hands prior to donning gloves | ❑ | ❑ | ❑ |
| Properly donned sterile gloves | ❑ | ❑ | ❑ |
| Did not contaminate garb, clean hands, or gloves during procedure | ❑ | ❑ | ❑ |
| **Removing Personal Protective Equipment** | | | |
| Removed gloves properly | ❑ | ❑ | ❑ |
| Removed gown properly and placed it in the correct location | ❑ | ❑ | ❑ |
| Removed face mask, beard cover (if appropriate), hair cover, and shoe covers in proper order | ❑ | ❑ | ❑ |

## Instructor Feedback

Date

Student/Trainee

Trainer Name

License or Registration Number

Trainer Signature

State Licensed

# Lab Procedure Process Validation Checklist

## Chapter 7: Cleaning the Horizontal Laminar Airflow Hood

### Supplies

- Aseptic, lint-free hood-cleaning wipes
- Sterile water in a pour bottle
- Sterile 70% IPA in a pour bottle
- Shoe covers
- Hair cover
- Face mask
- Beard cover (if appropriate)
- Sterile gown
- Sterile, foamed 70% IPA
- Sterile, powder-free gloves
- Aseptic cleaning wipes presaturated with appropriate cleaning solution
- Horizontal laminar airflow hood
- Hood-cleaning checklist encased in a plastic sheet protector
- Pen
- Permanent, felt-tip marker
- Waste container

### Basic Instructions

- Gather the necessary supplies from the supply list.
- Once your instructor gives you permission to begin, garb in the proper order to the point that you would prior to washing your hands.
- Cleanse your hands and forearms with sterile, foamed 70% IPA and then don a sterile gown.
- Finally, don sterile gloves.

***Note:*** *For the purposes of this process validation, you will not perform hand-washing procedures.*

### Lab Procedure Process Validation Checklist

| | Yes | No | NA |
|---|---|---|---|
| **Garbing** | | | |
| Appropriately attired for work in a clean room | ❑ | ❑ | ❑ |
| Donned garb aseptically and in the proper order | ❑ | ❑ | ❑ |
| Aseptically donned sterile gloves | ❑ | ❑ | ❑ |
| **Horizontal Laminar Airflow Hood Cleaning** | | | |
| Recorded date, time, and initials on sterile water and 70% IPA bottles | ❑ | ❑ | ❑ |
| Wiped exterior of supply bottles with cleaning wipe prior to entering the clean room | ❑ | ❑ | ❑ |
| Brought all necessary supplies into clean room in one trip | ❑ | ❑ | ❑ |
| Removed extraneous supplies from hood prior to cleaning it | ❑ | ❑ | ❑ |
| Used wipes that are appropriate for hood cleaning | ❑ | ❑ | ❑ |
| Used sterile water for preliminary cleaning | ❑ | ❑ | ❑ |
| Used an appropriate amount of sterile water in cleaning | ❑ | ❑ | ❑ |
| Used side-to-side, overlapping motions, moving from back of hood toward outside edge when cleaning ceiling and work surface of hood | ❑ | ❑ | ❑ |

| | | | |
|---|---|---|---|
| Used down-and-up overlapping motions, moving from back of hood toward outside edge when cleaning sides of hood | ❑ | ❑ | ❑ |
| Used sterile 70% IPA as primary cleaning agent | ❑ | ❑ | ❑ |
| Used an appropriate amount of alcohol in cleaning | ❑ | ❑ | ❑ |
| Cleaned the entire hood in the proper order | ❑ | ❑ | ❑ |
| Did not contaminate hood at any time during the procedure | ❑ | ❑ | ❑ |
| **Documentation** | | | |
| Correctly filled out the hood-cleaning checklist | ❑ | ❑ | ❑ |
| **Removal of Personal Protective Equipment** | | | |
| Removed gloves properly | ❑ | ❑ | ❑ |
| Removed gown properly and placed it in the correct location | ❑ | ❑ | ❑ |
| Removed face mask, beard cover (if appropriate), hair cover, and shoe covers in proper order | ❑ | ❑ | ❑ |

## Instructor Feedback

| |
|---|
| |

Date ______________________ Student/Trainee ______________________

Trainer Name ______________________ License or Registration Number ______________________

Trainer Signature ______________________ State Licensed ______________________

# Lab Procedure Process Validation Checklist

## Chapter 8: Large-Volume Parenteral Preparations

### Supplies

- Calculator (basic)
- Pen
- Medication order in large, clear-plastic, resealable bag
- CSP label in small, clear-plastic, resealable bag
- Potassium chloride 2 mEq/mL; 20-mL vial size (or larger)
- 20-mL Luer-lock syringe
- Regular needle (nonfilter, nonvented needle, either 18 or 19 gauge)
- Sterile 70% IPA swabs, individually packaged × 3
- 1000 mL of LR solution in an IV bag with a tail injection port
- IVA seals (optional)
- Aseptic cleaning wipes presaturated with appropriate cleaning solution
- Transport vehicle (optional)
- Shoe covers
- Hair cover
- Face mask
- Beard cover (if appropriate)
- Sterile gown
- Sterile, foamed 70% IPA
- Sterile, powder-free gloves
- Horizontal laminar airflow hood
- Permanent, felt-tip marker
- Waste container
- Sharps container

### Basic Instructions

- Perform any necessary calculations and then gather the supplies from the supply list.
- Once your instructor gives you permission to begin, garb in the proper order to the point that you would prior to washing your hands.
- Cleanse your hands and forearms with sterile, foamed 70% IPA and then don a sterile gown.
- Finally, don sterile gloves.

***Note:*** *For the purposes of this process validation, you will not perform hand-washing or hood-cleaning procedures.*

### Lab Procedure Process Validation Checklist

| | Yes | No | NA |
|---|---|---|---|
| **CSP Label Verification** | | | |
| Compared med order to CSP label to verify patient information | ❑ | ❑ | ❑ |
| Compared med order to CSP label to verify drug information | ❑ | ❑ | ❑ |
| Compared med order to CSP label to verify base solution information | ❑ | ❑ | ❑ |
| **Dosage Calculation and Supply Determination** | | | |
| Reviewed the med order to determine the desired dose | ❑ | ❑ | ❑ |
| Reviewed the vial label to determine the concentration | ❑ | ❑ | ❑ |
| Correctly performed the mathematical dosage calculations | ❑ | ❑ | ❑ |
| Gathered correct supply items | ❑ | ❑ | ❑ |

| | Yes | No | NA |
|---|---|---|---|
| **Anteroom Preparations** | | | |
| Wiped down transport vehicle and all supply items properly | ❑ | ❑ | ❑ |
| Donned aseptic shoe covers, hair cover, face mask, and beard cover (if appropriate) in the proper order | ❑ | ❑ | ❑ |
| Donned sterile gown without contaminating it | ❑ | ❑ | ❑ |
| **Clean Room Procedures and LVP Preparation** | | | |
| Placed supplies in the proper area in the clean room | ❑ | ❑ | ❑ |
| Used sterile, foamed 70% IPA prior to donning sterile gloves | ❑ | ❑ | ❑ |
| Removed the dust cover of the IV bag prior to placing it in DCA of hood | ❑ | ❑ | ❑ |
| Placed small supply items in outer six-inch zone of hood | ❑ | ❑ | ❑ |
| Opened all alcohol swabs within the DCA | ❑ | ❑ | ❑ |
| Made appropriate use of the waste discard pile, or discarded waste into the appropriate container throughout the procedure | ❑ | ❑ | ❑ |
| Cleaned all critical sites of supplies with sterile 70% IPA swabs | ❑ | ❑ | ❑ |
| Maintained uninterrupted airflow to the critical sites of all supply items throughout injection and other preparation procedures | ❑ | ❑ | ❑ |
| Did not touch the critical sites of the needle or syringe | ❑ | ❑ | ❑ |
| Did not place the syringe onto the hood surface without first attaching a capped needle | ❑ | ❑ | ❑ |
| Used proper technique when inserting the needle into the vial | ❑ | ❑ | ❑ |
| Used proper technique when removing the needle from the vial | ❑ | ❑ | ❑ |
| Recapped the needle using proper technique | ❑ | ❑ | ❑ |
| Placed items on the hood properly in preparation for verification check by pharmacist or instructor | ❑ | ❑ | ❑ |
| Repositioned the IV bag so that the injection port received uninterrupted airflow from the HEPA filter | ❑ | ❑ | ❑ |
| Swabbed the injection port of the IV bag prior to needle insertion | ❑ | ❑ | ❑ |
| Used proper technique when inserting the needle into the injection port of the IV bag | ❑ | ❑ | ❑ |
| Used proper technique when removing the needle from the injection port of the IV bag | ❑ | ❑ | ❑ |
| Checked bag for leakage, precipitate, or incompatibility | ❑ | ❑ | ❑ |
| Properly affixed the CSP label to the LVP | ❑ | ❑ | ❑ |
| Applied an IVA seal over the injection port of the IV bag (optional—depending on facility/instructor directions) | ❑ | ❑ | ❑ |
| Disposed of sharps and nonsharps waste in appropriate receptacles | ❑ | ❑ | ❑ |
| **Completion Activities Performed Upon Return to the Anteroom** | | | |
| Initialed the CSP label in the appropriate place | ❑ | ❑ | ❑ |
| Recorded date, time, and initials on the drug label | ❑ | ❑ | ❑ |
| Returned any remaining supplies to their proper locations | ❑ | ❑ | ❑ |
| Removed PPE according to standard procedures | ❑ | ❑ | ❑ |

## Instructor Feedback

Date

Student/Trainee

Trainer Name

License or Registration Number

Trainer Signature

State Licensed

# Lab Procedure Process Validation Checklist

## Chapter 9: Small-Volume Parenteral Preparations

### Supplies

- Calculator (basic)
- Pen
- Medication order in large, clear-plastic, resealable bag
- CSP labels in small, clear-plastic, resealable bags ×2
- Ampicillin 500-mg vials × 2
- Sterile water 10-mL diluent vials × 2
- 10-mL Luer-lock syringes × 3
- 3-mL Luer-lock syringe
- Regular needles (nonfilter, nonvented needles, either 18 or 19 gauge) × 3
- Vented needle
- Sterile 70% IPA swabs, individually packaged × 10
- 0.9% sodium chloride, 100-mL IVPBs × 2
- IVA seals (optional)
- Aseptic cleaning wipes presaturated with appropriate cleaning solution
- Transport vehicle (optional)
- Shoe covers
- Hair cover
- Face mask
- Beard cover (if appropriate)
- Sterile gown
- Sterile, foamed 70% IPA
- Sterile, powder-free gloves
- Horizontal laminar airflow hood
- Permanent, felt-tip marker
- Waste container
- Sharps container

### Basic Instructions

- Perform any necessary calculations and then gather the supplies from the supply list.
- Once your instructor gives you permission to begin, garb in the proper order to the point that you would prior to washing your hands.
- Cleanse your hands and forearms with sterile, foamed 70% IPA and then don a sterile gown.
- Finally, don sterile gloves.

***Note:*** *For the purposes of this process validation, you will not perform hand-washing or hood-cleaning procedures.*

## Lab Procedure Process Validation Checklist

| | Yes | No | NA |
|---|---|---|---|
| **CSP Label Verification** | | | |
| Compared med order to CSP label to verify accuracy of all information | ❑ | ❑ | ❑ |
| **Dosage Calculation and Supply Determination** | | | |
| Reviewed the med order to determine the desired dosages | ❑ | ❑ | ❑ |
| Reviewed each vial label to determine the medication's desired concentration and the diluent volume | ❑ | ❑ | ❑ |
| Correctly performed the mathematical dosage calculations | ❑ | ❑ | ❑ |
| Gathered correct supply items | ❑ | ❑ | ❑ |
| **Anteroom Preparations** | | | |
| Wiped down transport vehicle and all supply items properly | ❑ | ❑ | ❑ |
| Donned aseptic shoe covers, hair cover, face mask, and beard cover (if appropriate) in the proper order | ❑ | ❑ | ❑ |
| Donned sterile gown without contaminating it | ❑ | ❑ | ❑ |
| **Clean Room Procedures and SVP Preparation** | | | |
| Placed supplies in the proper area in the clean room | ❑ | ❑ | ❑ |
| Used sterile, foamed 70% IPA prior to donning sterile gloves | ❑ | ❑ | ❑ |
| Removed the dust cover of the IVPB prior to placing it in DCA of hood | ❑ | ❑ | ❑ |
| Placed small supply items in outer six-inch zone of hood | ❑ | ❑ | ❑ |
| Opened all alcohol swabs within the DCA | ❑ | ❑ | ❑ |
| Made appropriate use of the waste discard pile or discarded waste into the appropriate container throughout the procedure | ❑ | ❑ | ❑ |
| Cleaned all critical sites of supplies with sterile 70% IPA swabs | ❑ | ❑ | ❑ |
| Maintained uninterrupted airflow to the critical sites of all supply items throughout injection, withdrawal, and needle-removal procedures | ❑ | ❑ | ❑ |
| Did not touch the critical sites of the needle or syringe at any time | ❑ | ❑ | ❑ |
| Did not touch critical site of IVPB or vial without first reswabbing the site before needle insertion | ❑ | ❑ | ❑ |
| Did not place any syringe onto the hood surface without first attaching a capped needle | ❑ | ❑ | ❑ |
| Used proper technique when inserting needle into vial | ❑ | ❑ | ❑ |
| Used milking technique to withdraw diluent from vial | ❑ | ❑ | ❑ |
| Used proper technique to remove needle-and-syringe unit from vial | ❑ | ❑ | ❑ |
| Recapped the needle using proper technique | ❑ | ❑ | ❑ |
| Withdrew the proper volume of diluent for CSP Scenario One | ❑ | ❑ | ❑ |
| Used milking technique to reconstitute the powder in Scenario One | ❑ | ❑ | ❑ |
| Drew up the proper volume of drug to prepare CSP #1 | ❑ | ❑ | ❑ |
| Withdrew the proper volume of diluent for CSP Scenario Two | ❑ | ❑ | ❑ |
| Used vented needle to reconstitute the powder in Scenario Two | ❑ | ❑ | ❑ |
| Drew up the proper volume of drug to prepare CSP #2 | ❑ | ❑ | ❑ |
| Placed items on the hood properly in preparation for verification check by pharmacist or instructor | ❑ | ❑ | ❑ |
| Used the correct IVPB base solution for each CSP | ❑ | ❑ | ❑ |

| | | | |
|---|---|---|---|
| Repositioned each SVP so that the injection port received uninterrupted airflow from the HEPA filter | ❑ | ❑ | ❑ |
| Swabbed the injection port of each IVPB bag | ❑ | ❑ | ❑ |
| Used proper technique when inserting the needle into the injection port of each IVPB bag | ❑ | ❑ | ❑ |
| Used proper technique when removing the needle from the injection port of each IVPB bag | ❑ | ❑ | ❑ |
| Checked each bag for leakage, precipitate, or incompatibility | ❑ | ❑ | ❑ |
| Properly affixed the correct CSP label to the back of the corresponding IVPB bag | ❑ | ❑ | ❑ |
| Applied an IVA seal over the injection port of each IVPB bag (optional–depending on facility/ instructor directions) | ❑ | ❑ | ❑ |
| Disposed of sharps and nonsharps waste in appropriate receptacles | ❑ | ❑ | ❑ |
| **Completion Activities Performed Upon Return to the Anteroom** | | | |
| Initialed the CSP labels in the appropriate places | ❑ | ❑ | ❑ |
| Recorded date, time, and initials on the vials' drug labels | ❑ | ❑ | ❑ |
| Returned any remaining supplies to their proper locations | ❑ | ❑ | ❑ |
| Removed PPE according to standard procedures | ❑ | ❑ | ❑ |

## Instructor Feedback

| |
|---|
| |

Date ______________________ Student/Trainee ______________________

Trainer Name ______________________ License or Registration Number ______________________

Trainer Signature ______________________ State Licensed ______________________

# Lab Procedure Process Validation Checklist

## Chapter 10: Ampule-Based Preparations

### Supplies

- Calculator (basic)
- Pen
- Medication order in large, clear-plastic, resealable bag
- CSP label in small, clear-plastic, resealable bag
- Promethazine 50 mg/2-mL ampule
- 3-mL Luer-lock syringe
- Regular needle (nonfilter, nonvented needle, either 18 or 19 gauge)
- Filter needle
- Sterile 70% IPA swabs, individually packaged × 2
- $D_5W$ 100-mL IVPB
- IVA seal (optional)
- Aseptic cleaning wipes presaturated with appropriate cleaning solution
- Transport vehicle (optional)
- Shoe covers
- Hair cover
- Face mask
- Beard cover (if appropriate)
- Sterile gown
- Sterile, foamed 70% IPA
- Sterile, powder-free gloves
- Horizontal laminar airflow hood
- Permanent, felt-tip marker
- Waste container
- Sharps container

### Basic Instructions

- Perform any necessary calculations and then gather the supplies from the supply list.
- Once your instructor gives you permission to begin, garb in the proper order to the point that you would prior to washing your hands.
- Cleanse your hands and forearms with sterile, foamed 70% IPA and then don a sterile gown.
- Finally, don sterile gloves.

***Note:*** *For the purposes of this process validation, you will not perform hand-washing or hood-cleaning procedures.*

# Lab Procedure Process Validation Checklist

| | Yes | No | NA |
|---|---|---|---|
| **CSP Label Verification** | | | |
| Compared med order to CSP label to verify accuracy of all information | ❑ | ❑ | ❑ |
| **Dosage Calculation and Supply Determination** | | | |
| Reviewed the CSP label to determine the desired dosage | ❑ | ❑ | ❑ |
| Reviewed the ampule to determine the medication concentration | ❑ | ❑ | ❑ |
| Correctly performed the mathematical dosage calculations | ❑ | ❑ | ❑ |
| Gathered correct supply items | ❑ | ❑ | ❑ |
| **Anteroom Preparations** | | | |
| Wiped down transport vehicle and all supply items properly | ❑ | ❑ | ❑ |
| Donned aseptic shoe covers, hair cover, face mask, and beard cover (if appropriate) in the proper order | ❑ | ❑ | ❑ |
| Donned sterile gown without contaminating it | ❑ | ❑ | ❑ |
| **Clean Room Procedures and Ampule Preparation** | | | |
| Placed supplies in the proper area in the clean room | ❑ | ❑ | ❑ |
| Used sterile, foamed 70% IPA prior to donning sterile gloves | ❑ | ❑ | ❑ |
| Removed the dust cover of the IVPB prior to placing it in DCA of hood | ❑ | ❑ | ❑ |
| Placed small supply items in outer six-inch zone of hood | ❑ | ❑ | ❑ |
| Opened all alcohol swabs within the DCA | ❑ | ❑ | ❑ |
| Made appropriate use of the waste discard pile, or discarded waste into the appropriate container throughout the procedure | ❑ | ❑ | ❑ |
| Cleaned all critical sites of supplies with sterile 70% IPA swabs | ❑ | ❑ | ❑ |
| Maintained uninterrupted airflow to the critical sites of all supply items throughout injection, withdrawal, and needle-removal procedures | ❑ | ❑ | ❑ |
| Did not touch the critical sites of the needle or syringe | ❑ | ❑ | ❑ |
| Did not touch the critical sites of the IVPB or ampule without then reswabbing the sites before needle insertion or ampule opening | ❑ | ❑ | ❑ |
| Did not place any syringe onto the hood surface without first attaching a capped needle | ❑ | ❑ | ❑ |
| Used two needles–one regular needle, one filter needle–appropriately during the procedure | ❑ | ❑ | ❑ |
| Withdrew the proper volume of drug from the ampule | ❑ | ❑ | ❑ |
| Used proper technique to remove bubbles from syringe | ❑ | ❑ | ❑ |
| Placed items on the hood properly in preparation for verification check by pharmacist or instructor | ❑ | ❑ | ❑ |
| Used correct IVPB base solution and repositioned items in the hood so that the needle-and-syringe unit and injection port of IVPB received uninterrupted airflow from the HEPA filter | ❑ | ❑ | ❑ |
| Swabbed the injection port of the IVPB bag | ❑ | ❑ | ❑ |
| Used proper technique when inserting the needle into the injection port of the IVPB bag | ❑ | ❑ | ❑ |
| Used proper technique when removing the needle from the injection port | ❑ | ❑ | ❑ |
| Checked bag for leakage, precipitates, or incompatibility | ❑ | ❑ | ❑ |
| Properly affixed the CSP label to the back of the IVPB bag | ❑ | ❑ | ❑ |

| | Yes | No | NA |
|---|---|---|---|
| Applied an IVA seal over the injection port of the IVPB bag (optional–depending on facility/instructor directions) | ❑ | ❑ | ❑ |
| Disposed of sharps and nonsharps waste in appropriate receptacles | ❑ | ❑ | ❑ |
| **Completion Activities Performed Upon Return to the Anteroom** | | | |
| Initialed the CSP label in the appropriate place | ❑ | ❑ | ❑ |
| Recorded date, time, and initials on the drug label | ❑ | ❑ | ❑ |
| Returned any remaining supplies to their proper locations | ❑ | ❑ | ❑ |
| Removed PPE according to standard procedures | ❑ | ❑ | ❑ |

## Instructor Feedback

Date

Student/Trainee

Trainer Name

License or Registration Number

Trainer Signature

State Licensed

# Lab Procedure Process Validation Checklist

## Chapter 11: Narcotic Preparations

### Supplies

- Calculator (basic)
- Black ballpoint pen
- Red ballpoint pen
- Medication order in large, clear-plastic, resealable bag
- Narcotic CSP label in small, clear-plastic, resealable bag
- Perpetual inventory record for meperidine 50 mg/mL, 2-mL vials
- Meperidine 50 mg/mL, 2-mL vials × 5
- 10-mL Luer-lock syringe
- 60-mL Luer-lock syringe
- Regular needles × 2
- Luer-to-Luer connector
- 0.9% sodium chloride (NS) IVPB, 50-mL bag
- Sterile 70% IPA swabs, individually packaged × 2
- Syringe cap
- IVA syringe seal (optional)
- Aseptic cleaning wipes presaturated with appropriate cleaning solution
- Transport vehicle (optional)
- Shoe covers
- Hair cover
- Face mask
- Beard cover (if appropriate)
- Sterile gown
- Sterile, foamed 70% IPA
- Sterile, powder-free gloves
- Horizontal laminar airflow hood
- Permanent, felt-tip marker
- Waste container
- Sharps container

### Basic Instructions

- Perform any necessary calculations and then gather the supplies from the supply list.
- Once your instructor gives you permission to begin, garb in the proper order to the point that you would prior to washing your hands.
- Cleanse your hands and forearms with sterile, foamed 70% IPA and then don a sterile gown.
- Finally, don sterile gloves.

***Note:*** *For the purposes of this process validation, you will not perform hand-washing or hood-cleaning procedures.*

## Lab Procedure Process Validation Checklist

| | Yes | No | NA |
|---|---|---|---|
| **CSP Label Verification** | | | |
| Compared med order to CSP label to verify accuracy of all information | ❑ | ❑ | ❑ |
| **Dosage Calculation and Supply Determination** | | | |
| Reviewed the CSP label to determine the desired dosages | ❑ | ❑ | ❑ |
| Performed the proper narcotic sign-out procedures | ❑ | ❑ | ❑ |
| Correctly performed the mathematical dosage calculations | ❑ | ❑ | ❑ |
| Gathered correct supply items | ❑ | ❑ | ❑ |
| **Anteroom Preparations** | | | |
| Wiped down transport vehicle and all supply items properly | ❑ | ❑ | ❑ |
| Donned aseptic shoe covers, hair cover, face mask, and beard cover (if appropriate) in the proper order | ❑ | ❑ | ❑ |
| Donned sterile gown without contaminating it | ❑ | ❑ | ❑ |
| **Clean Room Procedures and PCA Preparation** | | | |
| Placed supplies in the proper area in the clean room | ❑ | ❑ | ❑ |
| Used sterile, foamed 70% IPA prior to donning sterile gloves | ❑ | ❑ | ❑ |
| Removed the dust cover of the IVPB prior to placing it in the DCA of hood | ❑ | ❑ | ❑ |
| Placed supply items in outer six-inch staging zone of hood | ❑ | ❑ | ❑ |
| Opened all alcohol swabs within the DCA | ❑ | ❑ | ❑ |
| Cleaned the vial's rubber top with sterile 70% IPA swab | ❑ | ❑ | ❑ |
| Maintained uninterrupted airflow to the critical sites of all supply items throughout injection, withdrawal, and needle-removal procedures | ❑ | ❑ | ❑ |
| Did not touch the critical sites of the needle, syringe, or Luer-to-Luer connector at any time | ❑ | ❑ | ❑ |
| Did not touch the critical site of the IVPB without reswabbing site prior to needle insertion | ❑ | ❑ | ❑ |
| Did not place any syringe or needle onto the hood surface without first attaching a Luer-to-Luer connector | ❑ | ❑ | ❑ |
| Used proper needle insertion technique into the vial and IVPB | ❑ | ❑ | ❑ |
| Withdrew the proper volume from the vial and IVPB | ❑ | ❑ | ❑ |
| Used proper technique to remove bubbles from syringe | ❑ | ❑ | ❑ |
| Placed items on the hood properly in preparation for verification check by pharmacist or instructor | ❑ | ❑ | ❑ |
| Used correct solutions and repositioned items in the hood so that the syringes and Luer-to-Luer connector received uninterrupted airflow from the HEPA filter at all times | ❑ | ❑ | ❑ |
| Swabbed the injection port of the IVPB bag | ❑ | ❑ | ❑ |
| Used proper technique when removing the needle from the injection port of the IVPB | ❑ | ❑ | ❑ |
| Aseptically attached a syringe cap | ❑ | ❑ | ❑ |
| Properly affixed the CSP label on the PCA syringe | ❑ | ❑ | ❑ |
| Applied an IVA syringe seal over the tip of the syringe | ❑ | ❑ | ❑ |
| Disposed of sharps and nonsharps waste in appropriate receptacles | ❑ | ❑ | ❑ |
| Examined syringe to determine amount of narcotic remaining; used proper narcotic waste disposal techniques if applicable | ❑ | ❑ | ❑ |

| Completion Activities Performed Upon Return to the Anteroom | Yes | No | NA |
|---|---|---|---|
| Initialed the CSP label in the appropriate place | ❑ | ❑ | ❑ |
| Returned any remaining supplies to their proper locations | ❑ | ❑ | ❑ |
| Removed PPE according to standard procedures | ❑ | ❑ | ❑ |

## Instructor Feedback

| |
|---|
| |

Date

Student/Trainee

Trainer Name

License or Registration Number

Trainer Signature

State Licensed

# Lab Procedure Process Validation Checklist

## Chapter 12: Pediatric Preparations

### Supplies

- Calculator (basic)
- Pen
- Medication order in large, clear-plastic resealable bag
- CSP label in small, clear-plastic, resealable bag
- Pediatric gentamicin 10-mg/mL vial (PF)
- 0.9% sodium chloride 10-mL vial (PF)
- 3-mL Luer-lock syringes × 2
- Regular needles (nonfilter, nonvented needles, either 18 or 19 gauge) × 2
- EEC vial (5-mL or 10-mL)
- Sterile 70% IPA swabs, individually packaged × 4
- IVA syringe seal
- Aseptic cleaning wipes presaturated with an appropriate cleaning solution
- Transport vehicle (optional)
- Shoe covers
- Hair cover
- Face mask
- Beard cover (if appropriate)
- Sterile gown
- Sterile, foamed 70% IPA
- Sterile, powder-free gloves
- Horizontal laminar airflow hood
- Permanent, felt-tip marker
- Waste container
- Sharps container

### Basic Instructions

- Perform any necessary calculations and then gather the supplies from the supply list.
- Once your instructor gives you permission to begin, garb in the proper order to the point that you would prior to washing your hands.
- Cleanse your hands and forearms with sterile, foamed 70% IPA and then don a sterile gown.
- Finally, don sterile gloves.

***Note:*** *For the purposes of this process validation, you will not perform hand-washing or hood-cleaning procedures.*

# Lab Procedure Process Validation Checklist

| | Yes | No | NA |
|---|---|---|---|
| **CSP Label Verification** | | | |
| Compared med order to CSP label to verify accuracy of all information | ❑ | ❑ | ❑ |
| **Dosage Calculation and Supply Determination** | | | |
| Reviewed the CSP label to determine the desired concentration and volumes | ❑ | ❑ | ❑ |
| Reviewed the vial labels to determine the drug vial concentration and verify that drug and diluent are PF | ❑ | ❑ | ❑ |
| Correctly performed the mathematical dosage calculations | ❑ | ❑ | ❑ |
| Gathered the correct supply items | ❑ | ❑ | ❑ |
| **Anteroom Preparations** | | | |
| Wiped down transport vehicle and all supply items properly | ❑ | ❑ | ❑ |
| Donned aseptic shoe covers, hair cover, face mask, and beard cover (if appropriate) in the proper order | ❑ | ❑ | ❑ |
| Donned sterile gown without contaminating it | ❑ | ❑ | ❑ |
| **Clean Room Procedures and Preparation of a Pediatric Special Dilution** | | | |
| Placed supplies in the proper area in the clean room | ❑ | ❑ | ❑ |
| Used sterile, foamed 70% IPA prior to donning sterile gloves | ❑ | ❑ | ❑ |
| Placed supply items in outer six-inch staging zone of hood | ❑ | ❑ | ❑ |
| Opened all alcohol swabs within the DCA of hood | ❑ | ❑ | ❑ |
| Swabbed the vials' rubber tops with sterile 70% IPA swab | ❑ | ❑ | ❑ |
| Maintained uninterrupted vertical airflow to the critical sites of all supply items throughout injection, withdrawal, and needle-removal procedures | ❑ | ❑ | ❑ |
| Did not touch the critical sites of the needle or syringe | ❑ | ❑ | ❑ |
| Did not touch the critical sites of vials without then reswabbing the sites before needle insertion | ❑ | ❑ | ❑ |
| Did not place any syringe onto the hood surface without first attaching a capped needle | ❑ | ❑ | ❑ |
| Did not place an unwrapped needle onto the hood surface at any time during procedure | ❑ | ❑ | ❑ |
| Used proper needle insertion technique into the vials | ❑ | ❑ | ❑ |
| Withdrew the proper volume from the vials | ❑ | ❑ | ❑ |
| Used proper technique to remove bubbles from syringe | ❑ | ❑ | ❑ |
| Placed items on the hood properly in preparation for a verification check by pharmacist or instructor | ❑ | ❑ | ❑ |
| Used correct solutions and repositioned items in the hood so that the syringes and EEC received uninterrupted airflow from the HEPA filter at all times during CSP procedures | ❑ | ❑ | ❑ |
| Used proper technique to vent air from EEC | ❑ | ❑ | ❑ |
| Used proper technique when removing the needle-and-syringe unit from vials | ❑ | ❑ | ❑ |
| Properly affixed the CSP label to the EEC | ❑ | ❑ | ❑ |
| Applied an IVA seal over the EEC vial top | ❑ | ❑ | ❑ |
| Disposed of sharps and nonsharps waste in appropriate receptacles | ❑ | ❑ | ❑ |
| Examined filled EEC for solution clarity | ❑ | ❑ | ❑ |

| | Yes | No | NA |
|---|---|---|---|
| **Completion Activities Performed Upon Return to the Anteroom** | | | |
| Dated and initialed the CSP label in the appropriate place | ❑ | ❑ | ❑ |
| Returned any remaining supplies to their proper locations | ❑ | ❑ | ❑ |
| Removed PPE according to standard procedures | ❑ | ❑ | ❑ |

## Instructor Feedback

Date

Student/Trainee

Trainer Name

License or Registration Number

Trainer Signature

State Licensed

# Lab Procedure Process Validation Checklist

## Chapter 13: Total Parenteral Nutrition

### Supplies

- Calculator (basic)
- Pen
- TPN medication order in large, clear-plastic, resealable bag
- TPN label in small, clear-plastic, resealable bag
- $D_{70}W$, 2000 mL (may substitute any volume bag size ≥ 500 mL)
- Aminosyn 10%, (AA 10%), 500 mL (may substitute any volume bag size ≥ 500 mL)
- SW, 1000 mL; may substitute with any volume ≥ 500-ml bag
- 1000-mL EEC
- Regular needles (nonfilter, nonvented needles, either 18 or 19 gauge)
- Sterile, 70% IPA swabs, individually packaged × 9
- Potassium phosphate ($KPO_4$), 3 Mm/mL vial
- Sodium chloride (NaCl), 4 mEq/mL vial
- Potassium chloride (KCl), 2 mEq/mL vial
- Trace minerals (TM), 5-mL vial
- MVI, 10-mL vial
- Humulin R (regular) insulin, 100 units/mL vial
- Calcium gluconate (CaGl), 0.48 mEq/mL vial
- 1-mL Luer-lock syringe
- 5-mL Luer-lock syringes × 2
- 10-mL Luer-lock syringes × 3
- 30-mL Luer-lock syringe
- Hemostats × 3
- IV tubing
- IVA seal
- Aseptic cleaning wipes presaturated with an appropriate cleaning solution
- Transport vehicle (optional)
- Aseptic garb, including shoe covers, hair cover, face mask, and beard cover (if appropriate)
- Sterile gown
- Sterile, foamed 70% IPA
- Sterile, powder-free gloves
- Scissors
- Paper towels
- Access to sink appropriate for base component fluid disposal
- Horizontal laminar airflow hood
- Permanent, felt-tip marker
- Waste container
- Sharps container

### Basic Instructions

- Perform any necessary calculations and then gather the supplies from the supply list.
- Once your instructor gives you permission to begin, garb in the proper order to the point that you would prior to washing your hands.
- Cleanse your hands and forearms with sterile, foamed 70% IPA and then don a sterile gown.
- Finally, don sterile gloves.

***Note:*** *For the purposes of this process validation, you will not perform hand-washing or hood-cleaning procedures.*

## Lab Procedure Process Validation Checklist

| | Yes | No | NA |
|---|---|---|---|
| **TPN Label Verification** | | | |
| Compared TPN order to TPN label to verify accuracy of all information | ❑ | ❑ | ❑ |
| **Dosage Calculation and Supply Determination** | | | |
| Reviewed the TPN label to determine the desired concentration and volumes | ❑ | ❑ | ❑ |
| Correctly performed the mathematical dosage calculations | ❑ | ❑ | ❑ |
| Gathered the correct supply items | ❑ | ❑ | ❑ |
| **Anteroom Preparations** | | | |
| Wiped down transport vehicle and all supply items properly | ❑ | ❑ | ❑ |
| Donned aseptic shoe covers, hair cover, face mask, and beard cover (if appropriate) in the proper order | ❑ | ❑ | ❑ |
| Donned sterile gown without contaminating it | ❑ | ❑ | ❑ |
| **Clean Room Procedures and TPN Preparation** | | | |
| Placed supplies in the proper area in the clean room | ❑ | ❑ | ❑ |
| Used sterile, foamed 70% IPA prior to donning sterile gloves | ❑ | ❑ | ❑ |
| Opened all alcohol swabs within the DCA | ❑ | ❑ | ❑ |
| Swabbed the rubber tops of EEC and vials with sterile 70% IPA swab | ❑ | ❑ | ❑ |
| Prepared the correct volume of each base component and had pharmacist verify base components prior to proceeding | ❑ | ❑ | ❑ |
| Maintained uninterrupted airflow to the critical sites of all supply items throughout injection, withdrawal, and needle-removal procedures | ❑ | ❑ | ❑ |
| Did not touch the critical sites of the needle or syringe at any time | ❑ | ❑ | ❑ |
| Did not touch critical site of each vial without reswabbing site prior to needle insertion | ❑ | ❑ | ❑ |
| Did not place any syringe onto the hood surface without first attaching a capped needle | ❑ | ❑ | ❑ |
| Used proper needle insertion technique into the vials | ❑ | ❑ | ❑ |
| Withdrew the proper volume from each vial | ❑ | ❑ | ❑ |
| Used proper technique to remove bubbles from syringes | ❑ | ❑ | ❑ |
| Placed syringes and vials on the hood properly in preparation for verification check by pharmacist or instructor | ❑ | ❑ | ❑ |
| Used correct solutions and repositioned items in the hood so that the syringes, tubing spike, and EEC received uninterrupted airflow from the HEPA filter at all times | ❑ | ❑ | ❑ |
| Used proper technique to insert tubing spike into bags | ❑ | ❑ | ❑ |
| Used proper technique when removing the needle-and-syringe unit from vials | ❑ | ❑ | ❑ |
| Properly affixed the TPN label to the EEC | ❑ | ❑ | ❑ |
| Applied an IVA seal over the EEC vial top | ❑ | ❑ | ❑ |
| Disposed of sharps and nonsharps waste in proper receptacles | ❑ | ❑ | ❑ |
| Examined EEC for solution clarity at appropriate times | ❑ | ❑ | ❑ |

| | Yes | No | NA |
|---|---|---|---|
| **Completion Activities Performed Upon Return to the Anteroom** | | | |
| Initialed the TPN label in the appropriate place | ❑ | ❑ | ❑ |
| Returned any remaining supplies to their proper locations | ❑ | ❑ | ❑ |
| Destroyed base components according to instructions | ❑ | ❑ | ❑ |
| Removed PPE according to standard procedures | ❑ | ❑ | ❑ |

## Instructor Feedback

| |
|---|
| |

Date

Student/Trainee

Trainer Name

License or Registration Number

Trainer Signature

State Licensed

# Lab Procedure Process Validation Checklist

## Chapter 14: Chemotherapy Products and Procedures

### Supplies

- Calculator (basic)
- Pen
- Chemotherapy medication order in large, clear-plastic, resealable bag
- Chemotherapy CSP label in small, clear-plastic resealable bag
- Cisplatin 100-mg/100-mL vial
- 0.9% NS IV base solution (with tail injection port) 500 mL
- Chemotherapy compounding mat
- IV tubing
- 4 × 4 sterile, lint-free gauze, approximately a 3" stack (a few additional pads are needed in the anteroom as well)
- 60-mL Luer-lock syringe
- Chemotherapy dispensing pin
- Regular, 19-gauge needles × 2
- IVA seal
- Aseptic cleaning wipes presaturated with appropriate cleaning solution
- Transport vehicle (optional)
- Aseptic garb, including shoe covers, hair cover, face mask, and beard cover (if appropriate)
- Sterile gown (if donning a chemotherapy smock)
- Sterile chemotherapy gown or smock
- Sterile, foamed 70% IPA
- Sterile, powder-free gloves
- Sterile chemotherapy gloves
- Chemotherapy safety glasses
- Vertical airflow biological safety cabinet (BSC)
- Chemotherapy transport bag (to place the CSP into for transport)
- Chemotherapy warning auxiliary label
- Permanent felt-tip marker
- Small chemotherapy sharps container (for inside the BSC)
- Large chemotherapy sharps container (for the anteroom)
- Waste container

### Basic Instructions

- Perform any necessary calculations and then gather the supplies from the supply list.
- Once your instructor gives you permission to begin, garb in the proper order to the point that you would prior to washing your hands.
- Cleanse your hands and forearms with sterile, foamed 70% IPA and then don a chemotherapy gown. (If wearing a chemotherapy smock, done a sterile gown prior to putting on the smock.)
- Don sterile gloves followed by chemotherapy gloves.

## Lab Procedure Process Validation Checklist

| | Yes | No | NA |
|---|---|---|---|
| **Chemotherapy CSP Label Verification** | | | |
| Compared chemotherapy med order to CSP label to verify accuracy of all information; verified that the dose matches order per BSA | ❑ | ❑ | ❑ |
| **Dosage Calculation and Supply Determination** | | | |
| Reviewed the CSP label to determine the desired concentration and volumes | ❑ | ❑ | ❑ |
| Correctly performed the mathematical dosage calculations | ❑ | ❑ | ❑ |
| Gathered the correct supply items | ❑ | ❑ | ❑ |
| **Anteroom Preparations** | | | |
| Wiped down transport vehicle and all supply items properly | ❑ | ❑ | ❑ |
| Donned aseptic shoe covers, hair cover, face mask, and beard cover (if appropriate) in the proper order | ❑ | ❑ | ❑ |
| Donned sterile chemotherapy gown without contaminating it | ❑ | ❑ | ❑ |
| **Clean Room Procedures and Chemotherapy Preparation** | | | |
| Placed supplies in the proper area in the clean room | ❑ | ❑ | ❑ |
| Used sterile, foamed 70% IPA prior to donning sterile gloves | ❑ | ❑ | ❑ |
| Opened all alcohol swabs within the DCA | ❑ | ❑ | ❑ |
| Properly donned chemotherapy gloves | ❑ | ❑ | ❑ |
| Prepared the correct volume of drug using a chemotherapy dispensing pin and negative pressure | ❑ | ❑ | ❑ |
| Maintained uninterrupted airflow to the critical sites of all supply items throughout spike insertion, fluid withdrawal, and needle insertion/removal procedures | ❑ | ❑ | ❑ |
| Did not touch the critical sites of the needle, syringe, spike, or Luer-lock adaptor at any time | ❑ | ❑ | ❑ |
| Did not touch critical site of vial or IV bag without reswabbing site prior to needle insertion | ❑ | ❑ | ❑ |
| Did not place any syringe onto the hood surface without first attaching a capped needle | ❑ | ❑ | ❑ |
| Used proper technique to prime the tubing | ❑ | ❑ | ❑ |
| Used proper tubing spike insertion technique | ❑ | ❑ | ❑ |
| Used proper technique to remove bubbles from syringe | ❑ | ❑ | ❑ |
| Placed syringes and vial on the hood properly in preparation for verification check by pharmacist or instructor | ❑ | ❑ | ❑ |
| Used proper technique to inject drug into IV bag | ❑ | ❑ | ❑ |
| Disposed of needle-and-syringe unit without recapping needle | ❑ | ❑ | ❑ |
| Properly disposed of items in small sharps container | ❑ | ❑ | ❑ |
| Properly wiped down the IV bag/tubing | ❑ | ❑ | ❑ |
| Applied an IVA seal over the LVP injection port | ❑ | ❑ | ❑ |
| Properly examined and labeled CSP, placed warning label on CSP and bag, placed CSP into chemotherapy transport bag | ❑ | ❑ | ❑ |
| Placed chemotherapy gown and gloves into chemotherapy sharps container while in the clean room | ❑ | ❑ | ❑ |

| | Yes | No | NA |
|---|---|---|---|
| **Completion Activities Performed Upon Return to the Anteroom** | | | |
| Initialed the CSP label in the appropriate place | ❑ | ❑ | ❑ |
| Returned any remaining supplies to their proper locations | ❑ | ❑ | ❑ |
| Destroyed base components according to instructions | ❑ | ❑ | ❑ |
| Removed PPE according to standard procedures and placed in chemotherapy sharps container | ❑ | ❑ | ❑ |

## Instructor Feedback

| |
|---|
| |

Date ____________________ Student/Trainee ____________________

Trainer Name ____________________ License or Registration Number ____________________

Trainer Signature ____________________ State Licensed ____________________

# Historical Images Index

| Location | Image | Description | Source |
|---|---|---|---|
| Unit 1<br>Page 1 | 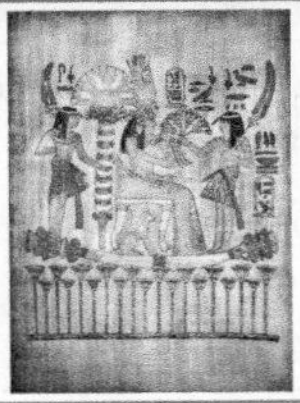 | Egyptian papyrus depicting a scene of royalty; early advanced medical understanding was typically reserved for royalty and the wealthy but often drew from the common knowledge of trial and error and inherited remedies. | Shutterstock |
| Unit 1<br>Page 2 | 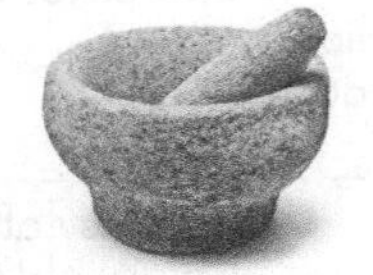 | Stone mortar and pestle; an ancient apothecary symbol. | Shutterstock |
| Unit 1<br>Page 2<br>Page 3 | 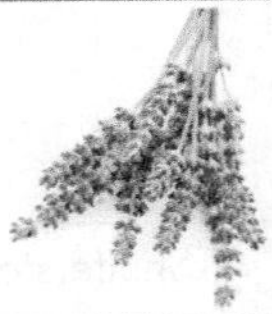 | Freshly picked lavender, a popular aromatic ingredient in ancient remedies; essential oil of lavender has been found to have antiseptic and anti-inflammatory properties. | Shutterstock |
| Unit 1<br>Page 2 | 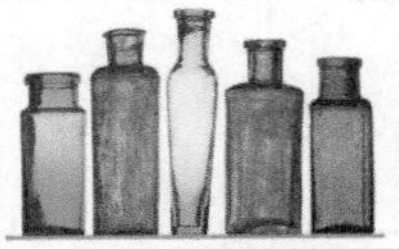 | Old glass storage bottles of the type commonly found on the shelves of apothecary shops; sealed with corks and often wax, bottles like these were not effective preservation for rapidly degrading or sensitive medical substances. | istockphoto.com |
| Unit 1<br>Page 2 | 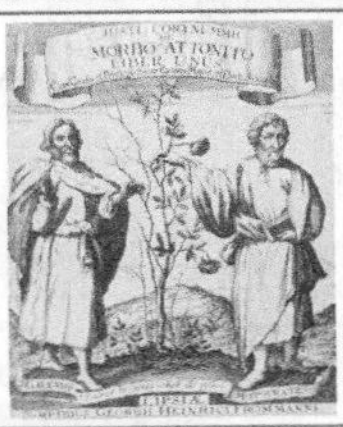 | A 1677 drawing of Galen and Hippocrates by Justus Cortnumm. | Courtesy of the National Library of Medicine |
| Unit 1<br>Page 3 | 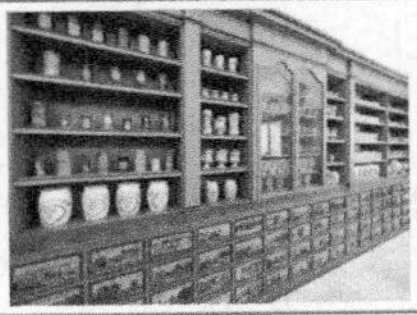 | Recreation of late eighteenth-century pharmacy storage shelves and cabinets, well-organized and filled with supplies. | istockphoto.com |
| Unit 1<br>Page 3 | 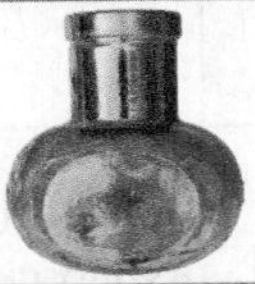 | Ceramic apothecary bottle from an unknown date. | istockphoto.com |
| Chapter 1<br>Page 4 | 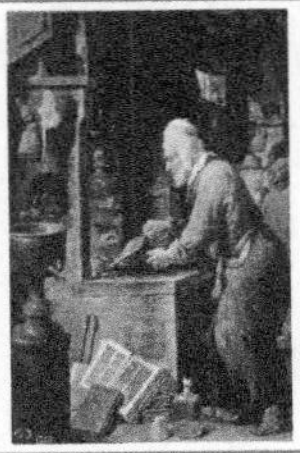 | *The Alchemist* by David Teniers the Younger (1582–1649); its date is unknown, but it is currently displayed at the Museo del Prado in Madrid, Spain. | Courtesy of the National Library of Medicine |
| Chapter 1<br>Page 5 | 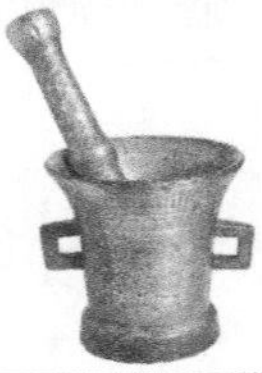 | Aged metal mortar and pestle; relatively modern but from an unknown date. | Shutterstock |

| Location | Image | Description | Source |
|---|---|---|---|
| Chapter 1 Page 6 | 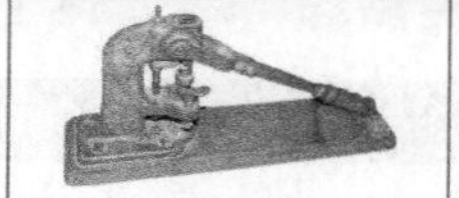 | Vintage nineteenth-century pill-pressing machine typically used by pharmacists to prepare custom medications. | Shutterstock |
| Chapter 1 Page 6 | 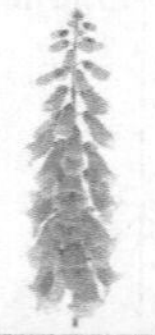 | Foxglove, a popular traditional remedy to relieve heart pain and regulate heart rate; its active chemical ingredients were first isolated in 1785. | Shutterstock |
| Chapter 1 Page 6 | 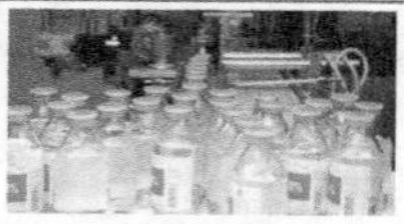 | Assembly line in a modern medical supplies factory; mechanization of many processes has increased production and efficiency, though sterile compounding still requires active personal involvement. | Shutterstock |
| Chapter 2 Page 26 | 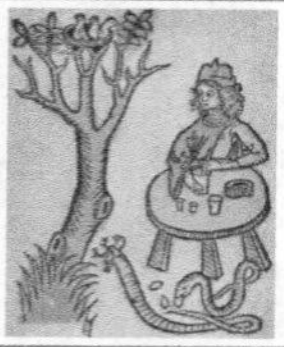 | *An Apothecary Compounding Theriac*, a hand-colored woodcut published in Mainz, Germany, in 1491; Mainz was the site of the first European books printed by mechanical movable type (the printing press), a revolutionary innovation introduced by Johannes Gutenberg in the 1440s. | Courtesy of the National Library of Medicine |
| Chapter 2 Page 27 | 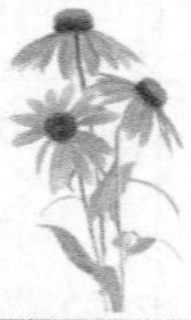 | Echinacea flowers, a popular healing plant used to treat infections and colds and to strengthen the immune system. | Shutterstock |
| Chapter 2 Page 28 | 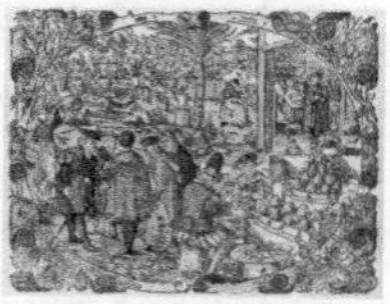 | *Consultation in a 16th Century Herbarium* in a publication by German botanist Adam Lonicer, from 1557; image shows a bedside scene with urine examination in upper right corner; the cultivation, harvesting, and processing of plants for medicinal purposes along the perimeter; and a group of physicians in consultation in the center. | Courtesy of the National Library of Medicine |
| Chapter 2 Page 28 | 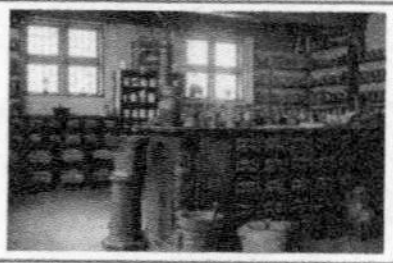 | Recreation of a seventeenth-century apothecary shop; medicines during that period were compounded either in the same area as they were sold, or in a dedicated back room. | istockphoto.com |
| Chapter 2 Page 29 | 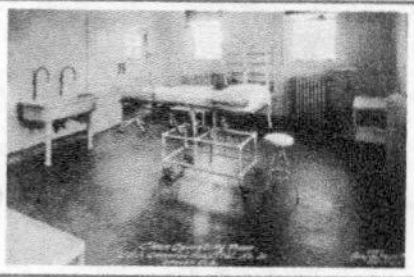 | Clean operating room of U.S. Army Fitzsimons General Hospital in Denver, Colorado, circa 1940; named after Lt. William T. Fitzsimons, the first American medical officer killed in World War I. | Courtesy of the National Library of Medicine |
| Chapter 2 Page 29 | 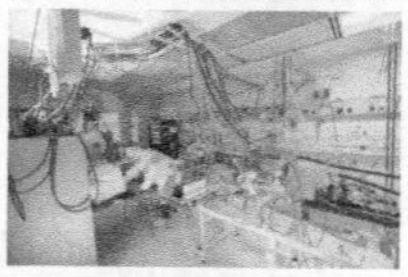 | The Owen Hall Clean Room or Solid State Materials and Devices Lab at Oregon State University in Corvallis, Oregon—a university research clean room, not an industrial manufacturing clean room. | Oregon State University and the Oregon Nanoscience and Microtechnologies Institute |
| Chapter 3 Page 52 | 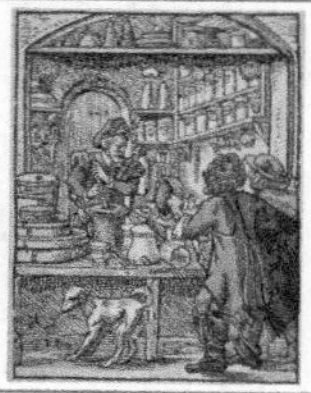 | *Der Apotecker* (The Apothecary) woodcut by Jost Amman (1539–1591); shows a sixteenth-century apothecary open-air shop being visited by two customers. | Courtesy of the National Library of Medicine |

| Location | Image | Description | Source |
|---|---|---|---|
| Chapter 3<br>Page 53 | 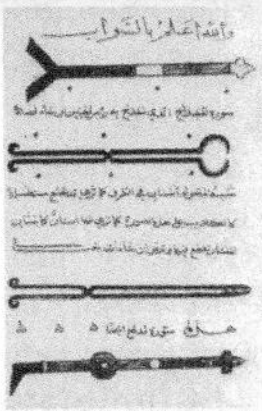 | Illustration of medical instruments from Albucasis's *Kitab al-Tasrif* (The Method of Medicine), circa 1000 CE (from a fifteenth-century copy); includes forceps, spreader, and surgical blades. | Public Domain |
| Chapter 3<br>Page 54 | 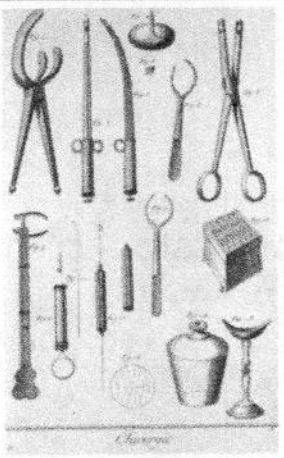 | Medical instruments including a Petit stylet for counteropening, an instrument to address an inflammation of the pharynx, an apparatus designed to fissure the palate, a screw nut, a "speculum oculi," tweezers for polyps, a syringe and a stylet for lachrymal organs, a needle to remove cataracts, scarificators, a cupping glass, and an eye cup to wash the eye. | Courtesy of the National Library of Medicine |
| Chapter 3<br>Page 54 | 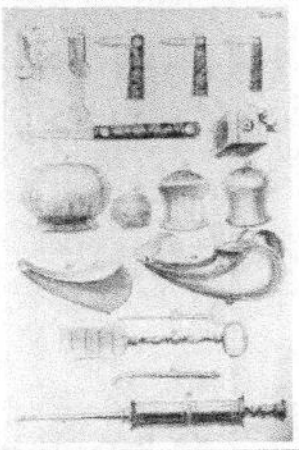 | Blood-letting instruments including cupping bells, lancets, scarificators, and others, from an engraving that appears in *Instrumentarium Chirurgicum Viennense* by the popular military surgeon Brambilla; published in 1772. | Courtesy of the National Library of Medicine |
| Chapter 3<br>Page 55 | 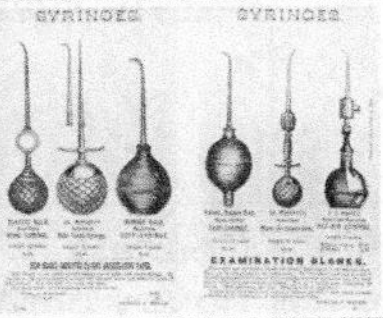 | Various dental bulb syringes from an 1881 advertisement in a Philadelphia medical magazine. | Courtesy of the National Library of Medicine |
| Chapter 3<br>Page 55 | 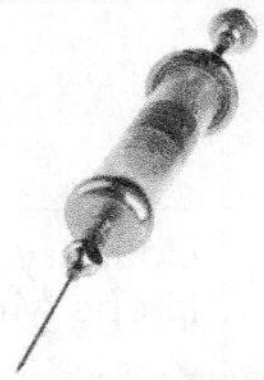 | Early twentieth-century syringe resembling the first mass-produced Luer glass syringes. | istockphoto.com |
| Chapter 3<br>Page 55 | 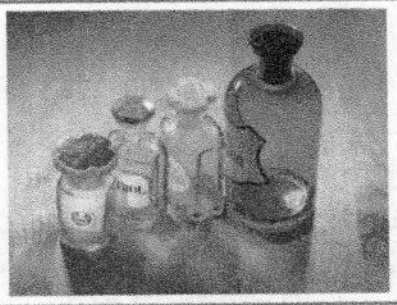 | Various antique vials that once had effective (but not completely airtight) seals for the medications they stored. | Shutterstock |
| Chapter 3<br>Page 56 | 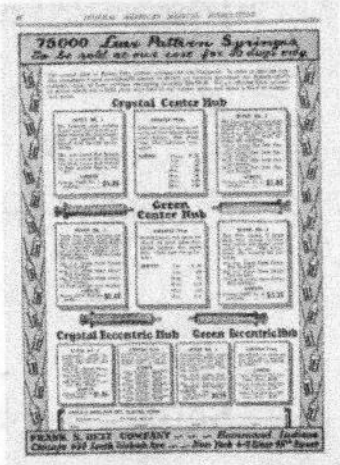 | 1926 advertisement for various Luer-lock syringes, marketed by the Frank S. Betz company in Hammond, Indiana, and published in the *Journal of the American Medical Association*. | © Paradigm Publishing |
| Chapter 4<br>Page 84 | 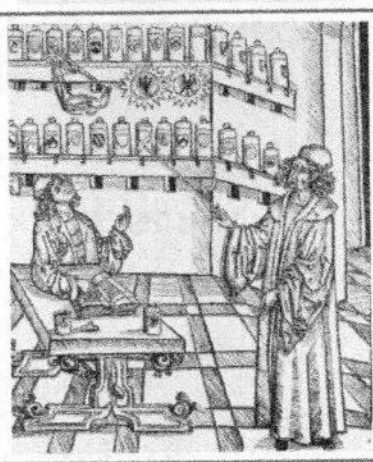 | Woodcut titled *A Pharmaceutical Lesson* by Heironymous Brunschwig, published in 1500; the interior view of a pharmacy shows the master, standing and pointing to shelves of apothecary jars, instructing the novice who is sitting at a table with an open book. | Courtesy of the National Library of Medicine |

| Location | Image | Description | Source |
|---|---|---|---|
| Chapter 4 Page 85 | 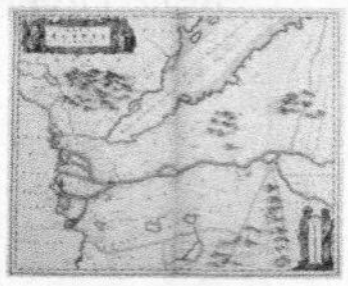 | Map of Egyptian borders in 1635, published by the Dutch cartographer Willem Blaeu in *Atlas Novus;* at this point in history, Egypt had suffered major invasions from the Muslim and Ottoman empires, several disastrous famines, and had lost complete control of its empire, though still functioned as an essential trade route for many nations. | istockphoto.com |
| Chapter 4 Page 86 |  | Clay tablet with Sumerian cuneiform, circa 3000 BCE; tablets like these contain some of the earliest known written examples of prescriptions. | Shutterstock |
| Chapter 4 Page 86 | 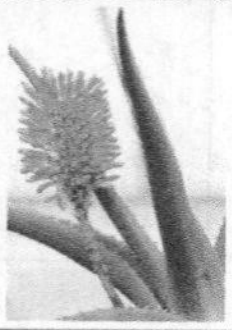 | Flower and leaves of an aloe plant, documented by ancient Egyptians to heal and soothe burns, and still used for that purpose today. | istockphoto.com |
| Chapter 4 Page 86 | 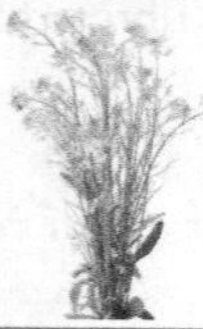 | Flowers of mustard, a plant (along with its seeds) popular in ancient herbal remedies and still used today in topical ointments to induce vomiting and as an antivenom for certain snake and scorpion poisons. | Shutterstock |
| Chapter 4 Page 87 | 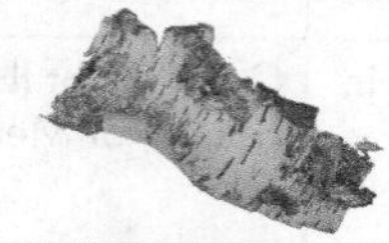 | Piece of birch bark, used extensively for writing and documentation prior to the use of wood pulp to make paper. | © Paradigm Publishing |
| Chapter 4 Page 87 | 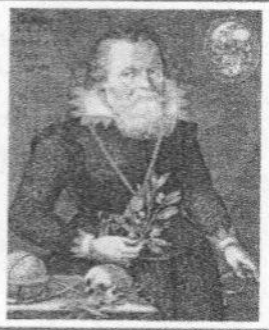 | Portrait of Gregor Horst (1578–1636), a German alchemist, doctor and apothecary; a popular medici of his time. | Courtesy of the National Library of Medicine |
| Chapter 4 Page 87 | 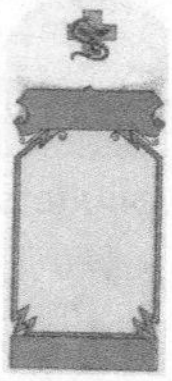 | Vintage medication label, left blank to allow pharmacist to customize prescription information for a patient. | Courtesy of Vintage Image Madness |
| Chapter 4 Page 88 | 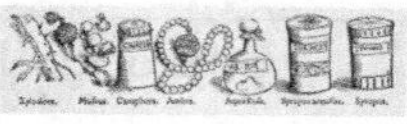 | Latinized copy of *Taqwim al-Sihha* (Maintenance of Health) by Ibn Butlan, from the eleventh century; collection of various medical items and herbs such as aloe, camphor, and an amber amulet. | Courtesy of the National Library of Medicine |
| Chapter 4 Page 88 | 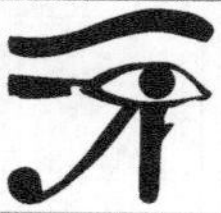 | The Eye of Horus, an ancient Egyptian symbol of protection, royal power, and good health; Horus was the sky god usually depicted as a falcon. | istockphoto.com |
| Chapter 4 Page 88 | 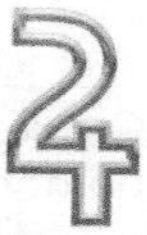 | Ancient symbol for the Roman god of Jupiter, the king of Gods and equivalent to the Greek Pantheon's Zeus; a possible inspiration for the modern-day prescription symbol. | Shutterstock |
| Chapter 4 Page 88 | 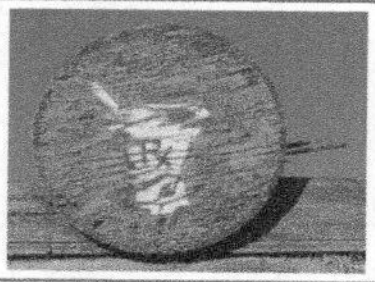 | Aged sign using the Rx symbol and mortar and pestle, signaling the location of a pharmacy. | Shutterstock |

| Location | Image | Description | Source |
|---|---|---|---|
| Chapter 4 Page 89 | 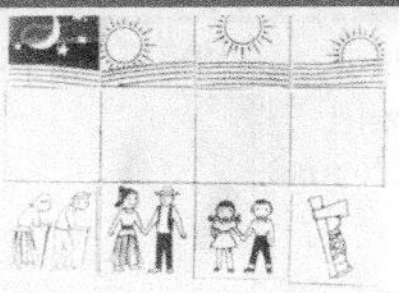 | A label for use on bottles of medications prescribed for those unable to read the directions. It depicts the rising and setting of the sun, a quarter moon, and the human life cycle. | Courtesy of the National Library of Medicine |
| Chapter 4 Page 89 | 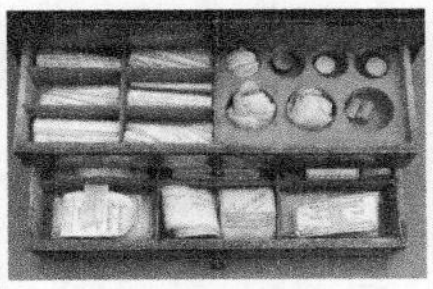 | English pharmacist's label cabinet dating from 1850–1930; before the wide-scale manufacture of chemical medicines, pharmacists created their own labels and stored them in a cabinet such as this one; made of mahogany, the three drawers contain drug labels with dosage instructions, along with the drugs themselves. | Courtesy of Science Museum of London |
| Chapter 5 Page 114 | 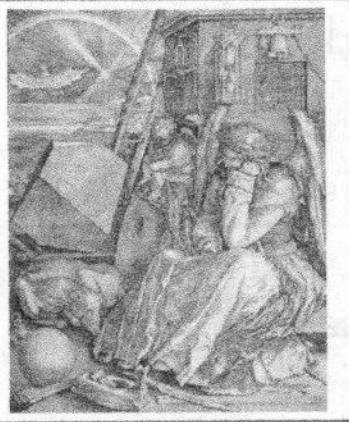 | *Melancolia I*, a drawing of the famous engraving by Albrecht Dürer; the engraving explores the processes of creativity, reasoning, inspiration, and intellectual frustration with its many symbols, including a compass, balance, hourglass, winged figure representing Genius (a reoccurring spiritual inspiration present in Roman mythology), and the mysterious 3-D object known as Dürer's solid. | Courtesy of the National Library of Medicine |
| Chapter 5 Page 115 | 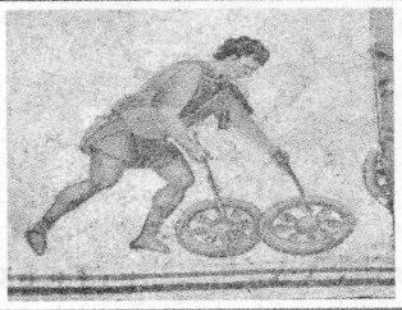 | Ancient Byzantine mosaic depicting a surveyor or architect determining the dimensions of a new building, using an unknown measurement system. | Shutterstock |
| Chapter 5 Page 116 | 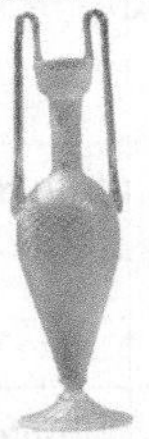 | Blue glass amphora, a copy of the popular clay vessels used in many ancient cultures as liquid storage; the weight of water held inside was used to represent a talent, a common ancient unit of weight, but inconsistencies across civilizations and even nearby cities made accurate measurements for trade difficult. | Shutterstock |
| Chapter 5 Page 116 | 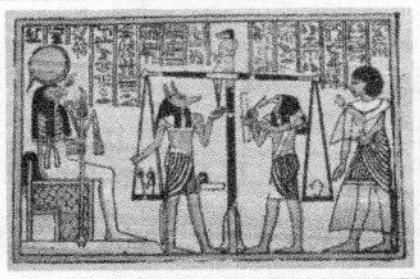 | Egyptian papyrus depicting the use of a balance; the deities Anubis (head of a jackal) and Thoth (head of an ibis) weigh treasures for Horus (sometimes called Ra, with the head of a falcon), who is often considered the supreme god of ancient Egypt and presented here as a pharaoh or ruler. | istockphoto.com |
| Chapter 5 Page 116 | 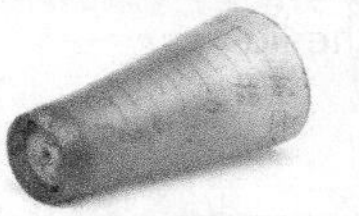 | Eighteenth-century apothecary measure made from a horn; graduated in two scales that have been etched by hand, from 0 to 16 fluid ounces and another from 0 to 2 in a measure that may be equivalent to tablespoons. | Image courtesy of Phisick Medical Antiques (www.phisick.com) |
| Chapter 5 Page 116 | 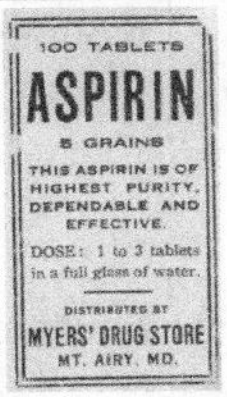 | Antique aspirin label utilizing the obscure and obsolete unit of grains in its administration directions. | Courtesy of Vintage Image Madness |
| Chapter 5 Page 117 | 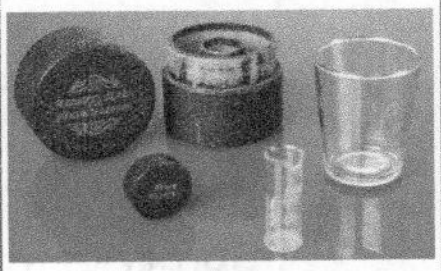 | Medicine glasses and minim measures like these remained standard pieces of equipment throughout the nineteenth century; used for accurately measuring liquid medicine, a minim (equivalent to a drop of water) was used by apothecaries, and the larger glasses (with scales for teaspoon and tablespoon scratched on the side) were for larger quantities; often carried by doctors, found in a nurse's kit, or kept in homes. | Courtesy of Science Museum of London |

| Location | Image | Description | Source |
|---|---|---|---|
| Chapter 5<br>Page 117 | 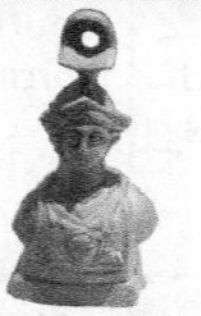 | Decorative ancient weight of unknown mass; the uniformity of ancient weights was highly subjective and regionalized, leading to much confusion as trading among distant nations developed and expanded. | Shutterstock |
| Chapter 5<br>Page 117 | 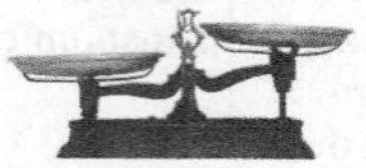 | Antique metal table scale; although too large and insensitive for measuring drug compounds, this scale was likely heavily used in financial transactions. | Shutterstock |
| Chapter 5<br>Page 118 | 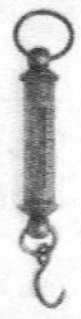 | Late nineteenth-century spring scale; spring scales were popular for large shipping loads, but relatively inaccurate for smaller weights and tended to stretch with prolonged use. | Shutterstock |
| Chapter 5<br>Page 118 | 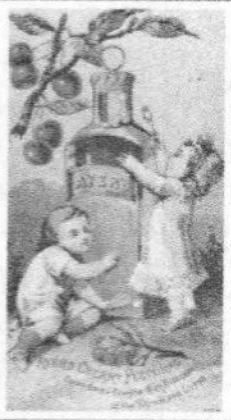 | Late nineteenth-century advertisement for Ayer's Cherry Pectoral, claiming to cure "colds, coughs, and all diseases of the throat and lungs." | Courtesy of the National Library of Medicine |
| Chapter 5<br>Page 119 | 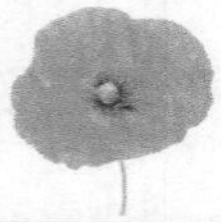 | Flower of the poppy plant; opium, a powerful and popular compound, has been an essential ingredient of medicine for thousands of years. | Shutterstock |
| Chapter 5<br>Page 120 | 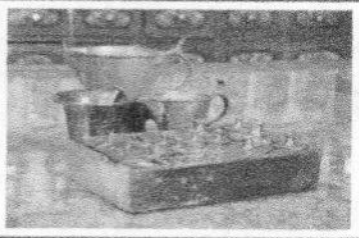 | Traditional apothecary weights, measuring cups, and a mortar and pestle. | Shutterstock |
| Chapter 5<br>Page 120 | 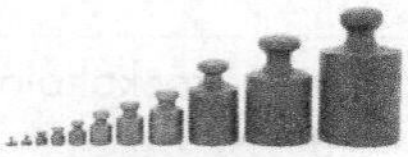 | Vintage brass and iron weights from 1 gram to 2 kilograms, typical of a set used by many apothecaries. | Shutterstock |
| Unit 2<br>Page 156 | 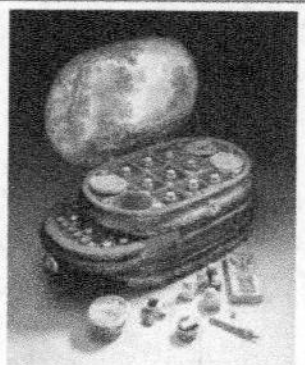 | Sixteenth-century medicine chest, originally belonging to the last Genoese governor of the island of Chios in the eastern Aegean Sea; holds 126 pots and bottles for various drugs, some containing the original contents; the painting on the lid was added at a later date. | Courtesy of Science Museum of London |
| Unit 2<br>Page 158 | 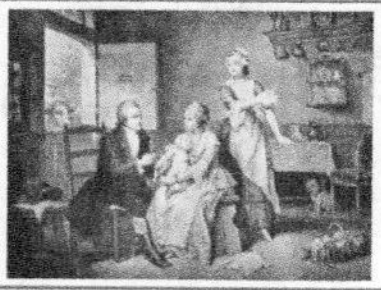 | *Vaccinating the Baby* by Ed Hamman; published in New York in 1890, the scene depicts a traveling doctor giving a baby a smallpox preventative inoculation. | Courtesy of the National Library of Medicine |
| Unit 2<br>Page 158 | 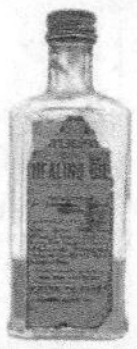 | Old bottle of cure-all healing oil, commonly called snake oil; snake oil is now a generic term to describe any medicine or treatment that claims marvelous but highly dubious medical benefits. | Shutterstock |
| Unit 2<br>Page 158 | 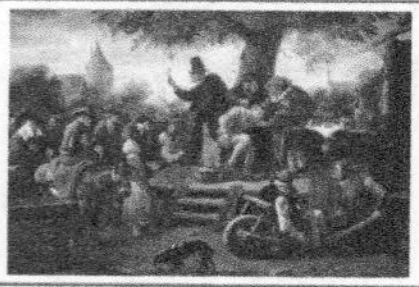 | *The Quack* by Jan Steen, a seventeenth-century Dutch genre and portrait painter; the scene depicts a seedy doctor pitching sales of different medical compounds and remedies to various townspeople. | Courtesy of the National Library of Medicine |

| Location | Image | Description | Source |
|---|---|---|---|
| Unit 2 Page 159 | 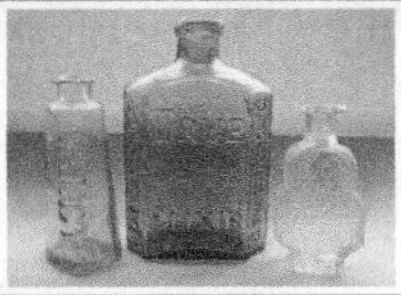 | Three antique patent medicine bottles (Daffy's Elixir, Dalby's Carminative, and Turlington's Balsam of Life) distributed by early quack medicine proprietors. | Public Domain |
| Unit 2 Page 159 | 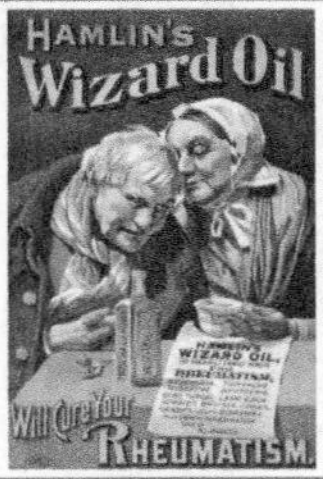  | An 1890 advertisement for Hamlin's Wizard Oil, a popular patent medicine sold under the slogan "There is No Sore It Will Not Heal, No Pain It Will Not Subdue" and used primarily as a liniment for rheumatic pain and sore muscles; it was also advertised as a treatment for pneumonia, cancer, diphtheria, earache, toothache, headache, and hydrophobia; made of 50–70% alcohol and contained camphor, ammonia, chloroform, sassafras, cloves, and turpentine. | Public Domain |
| Unit 2 Page 160 | 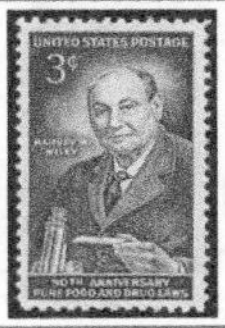 | Commemorative stamp produced in 1956 in honor of the 1906 Pure Food and Drug Act and Harvey Wiley, a chemist who led the passage of the act and the first commissioner of the Food and Drug Administration. | Public Domain |
| Unit 2 Page 160 | 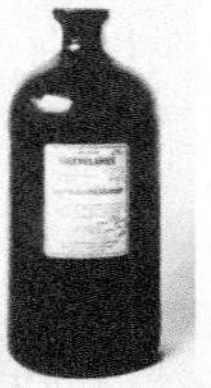 | Bottle of Elixir Sulfanilamide, the cause of 100 deaths in 1937 due to presence of unregulated poisonous compound diethylene glycol; the solvent, while useful in certain manufacturing processes, is still used in counterfeit (or unregulated) medicines and toothpastes and has led to hundreds of deaths and thousands of cases of severe illness, especially in poorer areas. | Public Domain |
| Unit 2 Page 160 | 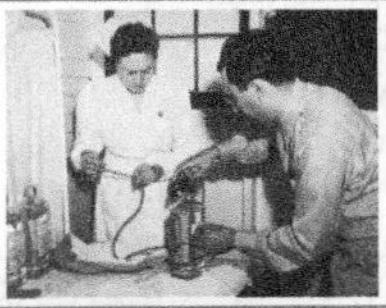 | Undated twentieth-century photograph showing a doctor and nurse preparing an IV formula for a patient; note the lack of aseptic technique due to the absence of regulation. | Courtesy of the National Library of Medicine |
| Unit 2 Page 161 | 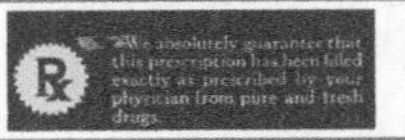 | Vintage medication label guaranteeing the quality and accuracy of the given prescription. | Courtesy of Vintage Image Madness |
| Unit 2 Page 161 | 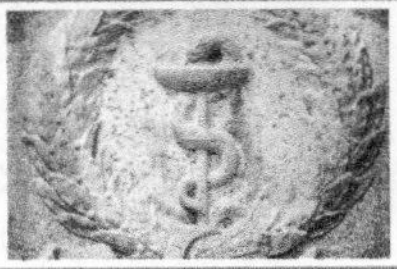 | Stylized Rod of Asclepius, a popular traditional symbol for medicine and doctors; Asclepius is the Greek god of medicine and healing, and the snake symbolism has a long and complex ancient history. | istockphoto.com |
| Chapter 6 Page 164 | 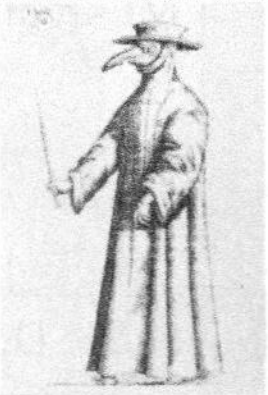 | Plague doctor wearing his distinct protective uniform: a leather hat and a mask surrounding his head and gathered at the neck; a beak that held herbs, perfumes, or spices to purify the air; a full-length gown made of heavy material and covered with wax; and leather pants and gloves; the doctor carried a wooden stick to drive away any people who got too close to him. | Courtesy of the National Library of Medicine |
| Chapter 6 Page 165 | 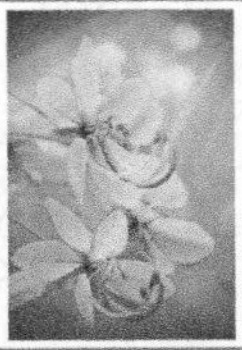 | The oils of cassia flowers were used in ancient soap recipes to produce a pleasing aroma; the plant is cultivated today mainly for its bark, which is similar to cinnamon and is used as a spice worldwide; cassia is often called "Chinese Cinnamon." | Shutterstock |
| Chapter 6 Page 166 | 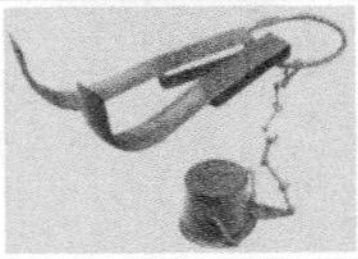 | Roman strigiles from the first century BCE; used in some ancient societies to scrape dirt and sweat from the body before the invention of effective soaps. | Public Domain |

| Location | Image | Description | Source |
|---|---|---|---|
| Chapter 6<br>Page 166 | 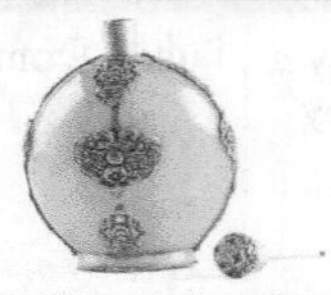 | Vintage perfume bottle; before antibacterial soaps and the widespread practice of regular bathing, perfumes were often used to mask bodily and environmental odors. | Shutterstock |
| Chapter 6<br>Page 166 | 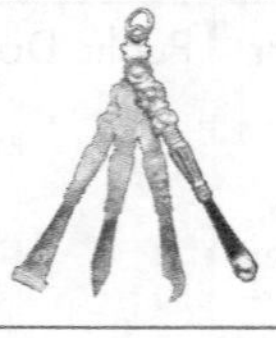 | Made in England in the 1670s, this silver manicure set is marked with the initials M. E., after a young girl named Martha Edlin; its four implements (though not clear in their purpose) were possibly an earspoon for removing ear wax, a tongue scraper, a tool for cleaning dirt from under fingernails, and a toothpick or cuticle pusher. | © Victoria and Albert Museum |
| Chapter 6<br>Page 167 | 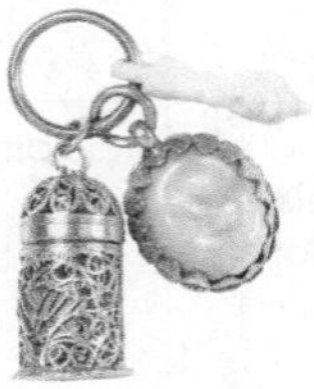 | German-made amulets from 1750–1800: the bone fist dates back to the ancient Romans and protects against evils; the operculum shell in a silver setting is a generic amulet worn to promote fertility; the small filigree case is a symbol of Walburgis oil. (St. Walburga was a British missionary to Germany in the eighth century; after her death, a liquid [Walburgis oil] was collected from her bones; Walburgis oil was considered highly effective against all kinds of infection and wounds.) | © Victoria and Albert Museum |
| Chapter 6<br>Page 167 | 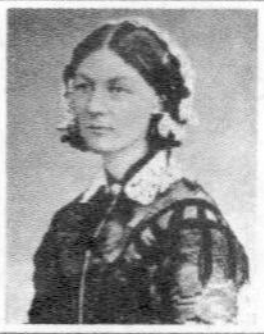 | Rare portrait of Florence Nightingale, the famous English nurse who inspired nineteenth-century England to embrace hygiene and sanitary standards after her experiences with infection and disease during the Crimean War. | Public Domain |
| Chapter 6<br>Page 168 | 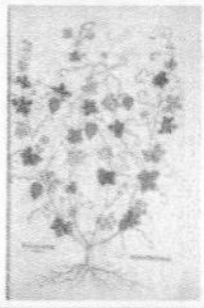 | Colored print of a 1542 woodcut of the balsam plant by Veit Rudolph Specklin; the various balsam plants produce pleasantly scented oils that have been popular for many centuries as ingredients for soap and botanical medicines. | Courtesy of the National Library of Medicine |
| Chapter 6<br>Page 168 | 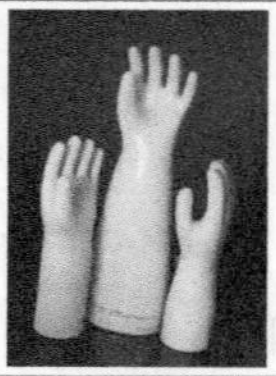 | Glove molds used to knit and sew various-length gloves for children. | Courtesy of Tara Grosse |
| Chapter 6<br>Page 169 | 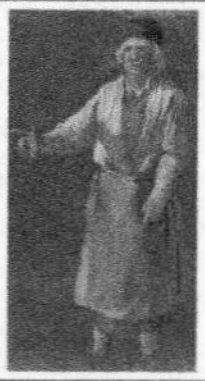 | *A Man Wearing an Apron* by Luca Carlevarijs, circa 1700–1710; this oil painting possibly depicts either a doctor/surgeon or apothecary from the time period. | © Victoria and Albert Museum |
| Chapter 6<br>Page 169 | 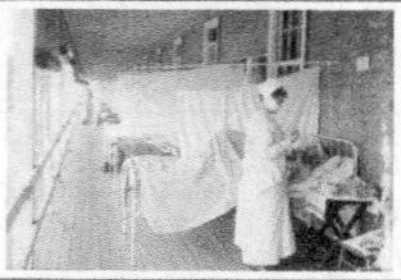 | Nurses tending to patients at Walter Reed Army Hospital during the Spanish flu pandemic of 1918–1919, which killed 50 to100 million people and spread quickly across the world. | Public Domain |
| Chapter 7<br>Page 188 | 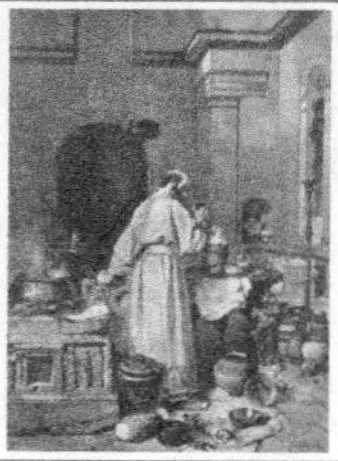 | *The Alchemist* by A. Adams, published by the *American Druggist* magazine in 1887; this engraving depicts an alchemist in the midst of his experiments, surrounded by various storage vessels and organic compounds. | Courtesy of the National Library of Medicine |

| Location | Image | Description | Source |
|---|---|---|---|
| Chapter 7<br>Page 189 | 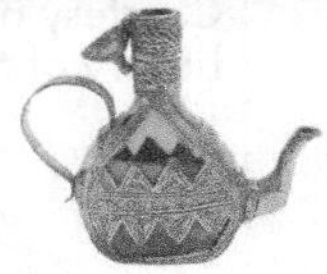 | Antique oil lamp used to hold essential oils such as cedarwood, myrrh, and eucalyptus; these oils were prized for their pleasing aromas and cleansing properties (both physical and spiritual). | Shutterstock |
| Chapter 7<br>Page 190 | 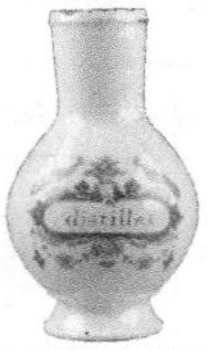 | Eighteenth-century drug vase made of tin-glazed earthenware painted with cartouche with two peacocks and inscribed "A Distillat" (Distilled Water), possibly from Delft, Netherlands. | © Victoria and Albert Museum |
| Chapter 7<br>Page 190 | 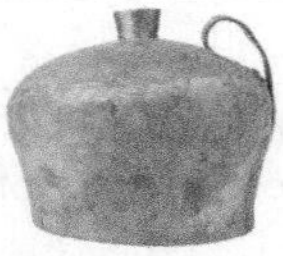 | Aged water pitcher made from copper, a popular and easily manipulated metal that also possesses antiseptic properties. | Shutterstock |
| Chapter 7<br>Page 191 | 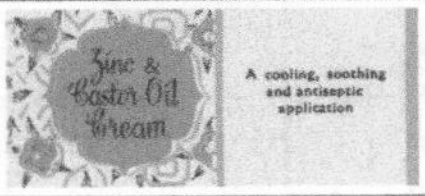 | Label from a package of Zinc & Castor Oil Cream; used as a moisturizer and rash treatment and advertised as a germ-killing medication. | Courtesy of Vintage Image Madness |
| Chapter 7<br>Page 191 | 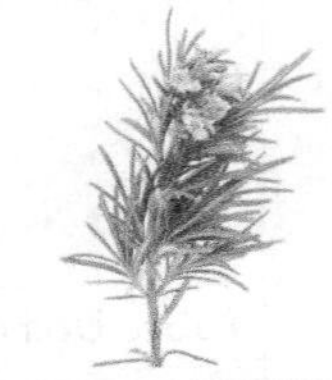 | Blooming rosemary, a fragrant herb used as an aromatic for thousands of years and once thought to ward off infection when burned indoors. | Shutterstock |
| Chapter 7<br>Page 192 | 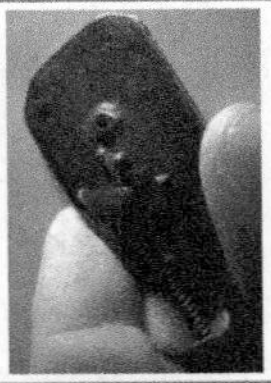 | Replica of Anton Van Leeuwenhoek's handmade microscope; Van Leeuwenhoek jealously guarded the microscope's production secret, which was not rediscovered until more than 100 years after his death. | Courtesy of Professor Brian J. Ford |
| Chapter 7<br>Page 192 | 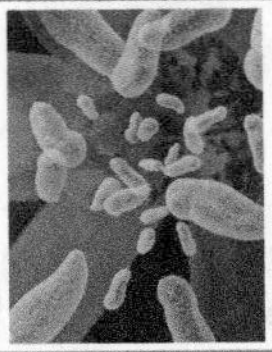 | Computerized representation of microscopic bacteria. | Shutterstock |
| Chapter 7<br>Page 192 | 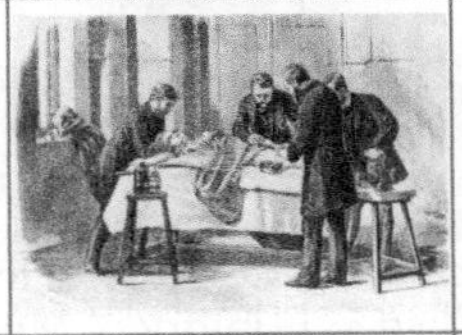 | Engraving from *History of Medicine: Operating and Surgery* showing a surgery utilizing Lister's carbolic acid spray pump; carbolic acid (often called phenol) was an irritating but effective disinfectant that gained popularity in the nineteenth century but was replaced with antiseptic practices due to the damage it inflicted on living tissue. | Courtesy of the National Library of Medicine |
| Chapter 7<br>Page 193 | 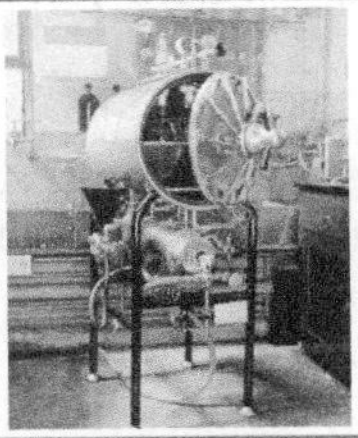 | Autoclave sterilizer from 1942; invented in 1879 by Charles Chamberland, the autoclave utilized high-pressure steam to sanitize instruments and dressings; sterilizer was a much safer and more practical alternative to destructive germ-killing chemicals such as phenol. | Courtesy of the National Library of Medicine |
| Chapter 7<br>Page 193 | 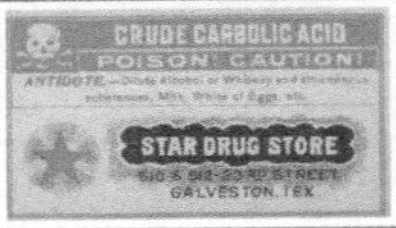 | Vintage American warning label from a package of carbolic acid, a highly irritating substance that is an effective germ-killer but can be destructive to living tissue. | Vintage Image Madness |

| Location | Image | Description | Source |
|---|---|---|---|
| Chapter 8 Page 210 | 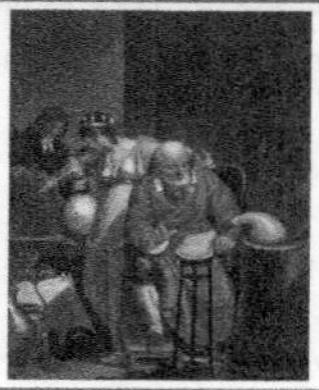 | *The Alchemist's Laboratory* by Richard Corbould; an eighteenth-century painting showing an alchemist and his assistants at work. | Courtesy of the National Library of Medicine |
| Chapter 8 Page 211 | 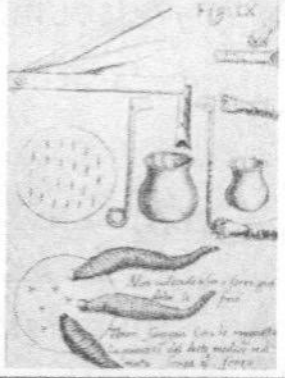 | Drawing from a 1671 Italian medical publication *Napoli: Appresso Geronimo Fasuloof*, depicting the primary methods of bloodletting: fleam, thumb lancet, cups, and leeches; image also shows a scarification pattern and incision patterns on veins. | Courtesy of the National Library of Medicine |
| Chapter 8 Page 212 | 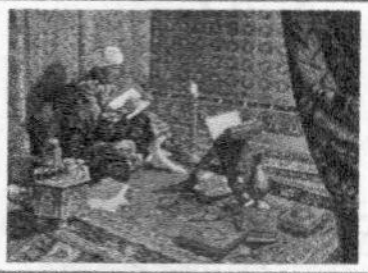 | Modern representation of Avicenna (or Ibn Sīnā), the most famous thinker of the Islamic Golden Age, from *A History of Pharmacy in Pictures* published in 1953; drawn by Robert Thom. | Courtesy of the National Library of Medicine |
| Chapter 8 Page 212 | 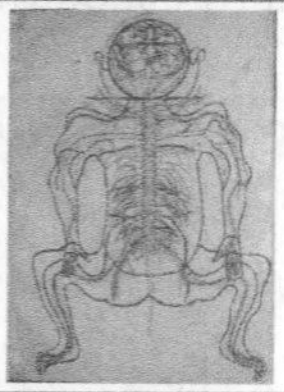 | Drawing of human circulatory system from book *Tashrih al-Badan* (Anatomy of the Body) by Mansur Ibn Ilyas, a fourteenth-century Persian physician. | Public Domain |
| Chapter 8 Page 213 | 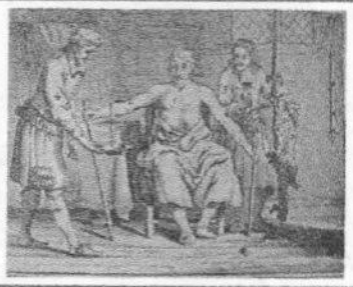 | A 1693 drawing by Ioannis Sculteti called *Armamentium Chirugiae*; it depicts the (inevitably doomed) attempted transfusion of sheep's blood to a human recipient. | Public Domain |
| Chapter 8 Page 213 | 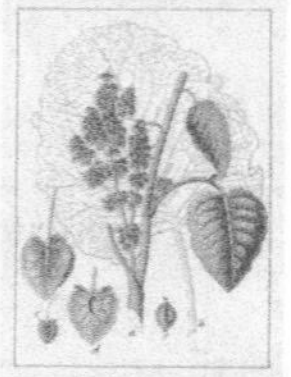 | Illustration of munk's rhubarb; engraving by Jacob Sturm from the book *Deutschlands Flora in Abbildungen nach der Natur mit Beschreibungen* (Native German Plants with Illustrations and Descriptions) published in 1862; rhubarb is often used as a purgative and was a failed treatment against the Indian blue cholera epidemic. | istockphoto.com |
| Chapter 8 Page 214 | 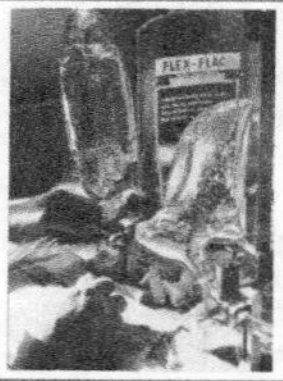 | A "Flex-Flac" being filled with a rehydration solution and a full package about to be sealed; these containers are early examples of the modern IV bag. | Courtesy of the National Library of Medicine |
| Chapter 8 Page 214 | 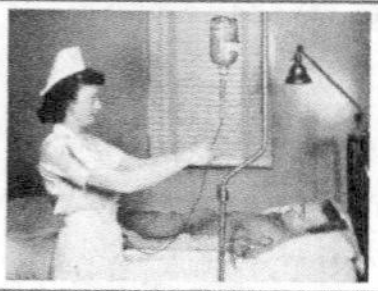 | Nurse checking a patient's IV bottle at Bolling Air Force Base, Washington, D.C., in the 1950s; at this time, IV fluid therapy was nearly universally accepted and utilized. | Courtesy of the National Library of Medicine |
| Chapter 9 Page 250 | 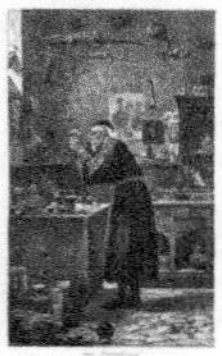 | An 1876 wood engraving called *The Apothecary*, which is a copy of the drawing by Henry Stacy Marks. | istockphoto.com |

| Location | Image | Description | Source |
|---|---|---|---|
| Chapter 9 Page 251 | 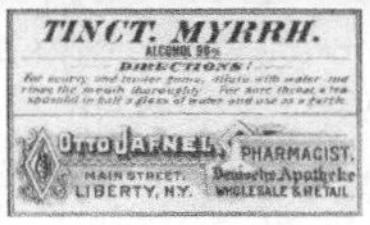 | American pharmacy label for a tincture of myrrh, a substance utilized for its antiseptic properties and success in dealing with gum conditions, as well as an ancient wound dressing and aromatic. | Courtesy of Vintage Image Madness |
| Chapter 9 Page 252 | 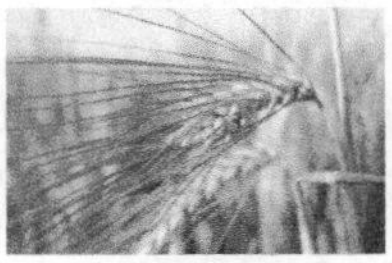 | Field of barley, a staple grain present through all of human history; many ancient civilizations used moldy and fermented grains to wrap wounds and fight infections, though the scientific understanding of mold's antibacterial properties is more recent. | Shutterstock |
| Chapter 9 Page 252 | 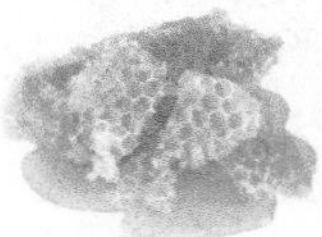 | Honeycomb, one of the oldest antibacterial substances in human history; though only recently proven to have antibacterial and antifungal properties, honey was used by ancient Egyptians, Greeks, Romans, and other civilizations to combat infection. | Shutterstock |
| Chapter 9 Page 252 | 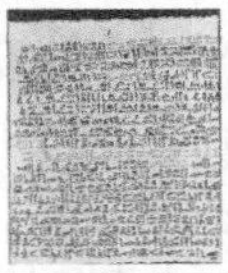 | Ebers Papyrus, the ancient Egyptian medical document from 1535 BCE; over 20 meters of parchment list about 700 remedies and formulas combining magic, prayer, and a highly advanced understanding of natural medicines and health techniques. | Courtesy of the National Library of Medicine |
| Chapter 9 Page 253 | 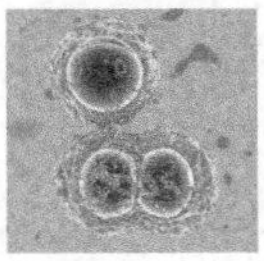 | The bacteria known as *Staphylococcus aureus*, a common cause of staph infections and nosocomial infections, as well as serious illnesses such as pneumonia and meningitis; copper has proven effective in killing this highly resistant bacteria. | Shutterstock |
| Chapter 9 Page 253 | 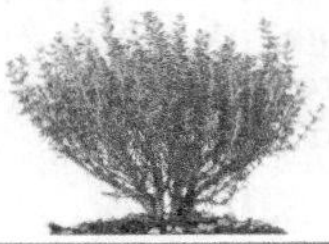 | Bush of thyme, an herb and natural antibiotic of early civilizations. | istockphoto.com |
| Chapter 9 Page 253 | 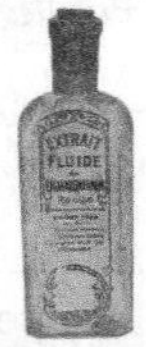 | A 1908 French medicine bottle for Quinquina, containing quinine (also known as cinchona or Peruvian bark); quinine, an effective malaria-fighting antibiotic, was so bitter in taste that French chemists mixed it with herbs and spices to create a wine-based liquor that also proved popular as a digestive aid before large meals. | Shutterstock |
| Chapter 9 Page 254 | 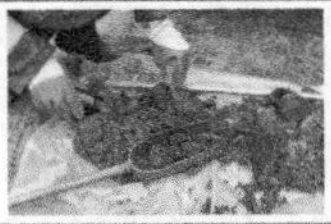 | Scientist collecting soil samples for lab testing; bacteria and other organisms discovered in soil have led to the development of important medicines, such as erythromycin. | istockphoto.com |
| Chapter 9 Page 254 | 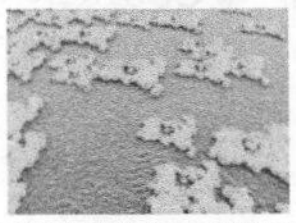 | A 3-D image of a generic streptococcal infection, a spherical gram-positive bacterium that is a common cause of meningitis and bacterial pneumonia and can be killed by sulfonamides such as the synthetic Prontosil developed by Gerhard Domagk. | Shutterstock |
| Chapter 9 Page 255 | 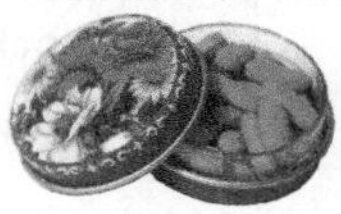 | Antique decorative pillbox from an unspecified time period; used to hold a patient's daily medications such as painkillers or digestive aids. | istockphoto.com |
| Chapter 9 Page 255 | 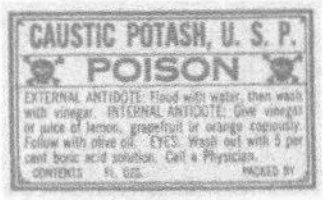 | A vintage label for potash, a potassium compound used in soaps and antibacterial substances but irritating to the skin and organs in certain forms. | Courtesy of Vintage Image Madness |
| Chapter 10 Page 288 | 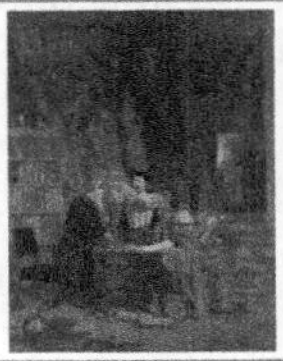 | *The Alchemist*, an 1885 oil painting by William Fettes Douglas; possibly the most famous work by the Scottish painter, who obsessed over the subjects of alchemy and the occult. | © Victoria and Albert Museum |

| Location | Image | Description | Source |
|---|---|---|---|
| Chapter 10<br>Page 289 | 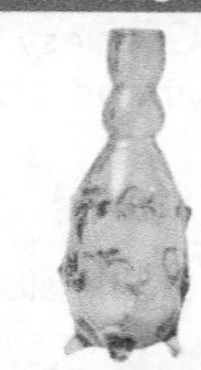 | Elongated glass flask from Syria, dated between the fifth and eighth centuries; based on earlier tear bottles, this flask was likely decorative and used for ceremonial purposes. | © Victoria and Albert Museum |
| Chapter 10<br>Page 290 | 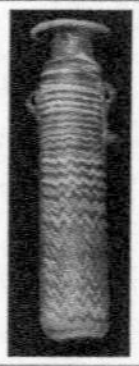 | Kohl flask from the Eastern Mediterranean region, circa 1200 BCE; kohl is an ancient eye cosmetic (usually black or green) created by grinding galena (lead sulfide) and other natural ingredients; this flask is a possible precursor to modern-day ampules. | John Noltner/Carleton College Art Collection |
| Chapter 10<br>Page 290 | 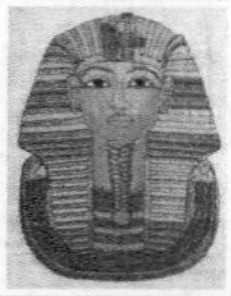 | Modernized image of a pharaoh on papyrus; the ancient Egyptians viewed magic and the supernatural as essential aspects of their advanced knowledge of science and medicine. | Shutterstock |
| Chapter 10<br>Page 290 | 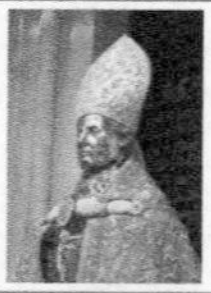 | Bust of San Gennaro at the Naples Cathedral in Italy; every year, thousands of Catholics gather around this bust to view his blood miracle. | Public Domain |
| Chapter 10<br>Page 291 | 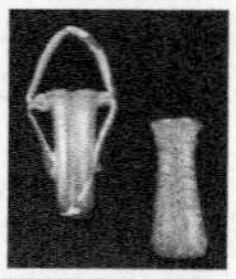 | Unguentaria used to hold oils, salves, or other liquids; the vessel with the handles was hung in order to fill a room with perfumes and pleasant aromas; from the Eastern Mediterranean region, these unguentaria date to the second or third century CE. | John Noltner/Carleton College Art Collection |
| Chapter 10<br>Page 291 | 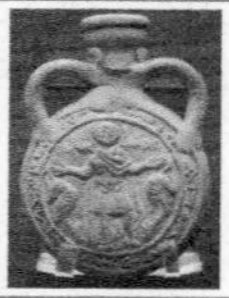 | Ampule or flask from the pilgrimage site of Abu Mena (near Alexandria, Egypt), made from terracotta in the sixth or seventh century; ampules like these were mass-produced and sold to pilgrims, much like tourists purchasing souvenirs. | Public Domain |
| Chapter 10<br>Page 291 | 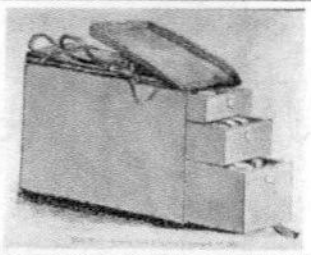 | Civil War medic's knapsack from 1862; in the fast-paced and dangerous environment of war, single-use medications like those kept in ampules were essential, as they were light enough to carry and could be quickly administered. | Courtesy of the National Library of Medicine |
| Chapter 10<br>Page 292 | 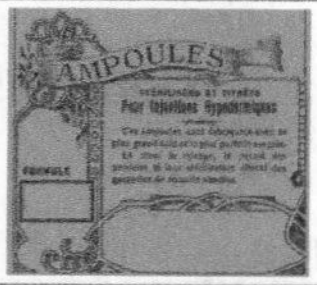 | Vintage French label for a package of ampules containing an additive for sterile injection. | Courtesy of Vintage Image Madness |
| Chapter 10<br>Page 292 | 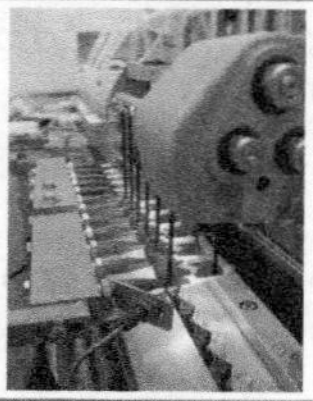 | Automated factory process of heat-sealing ampules, which ensures consistency and strength in the thin and easily broken ampule necks. | Shutterstock |
| Chapter 11<br>Page 320 | 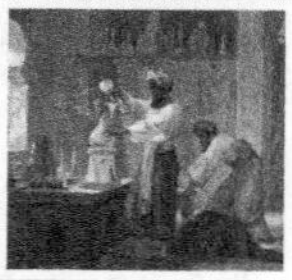 | Drawing of Abu Bakr al-Hazi Rhazes (867–925) also known as Rhazes, the Persian physician and alchemist in his laboratory in Baghdad with an assistant; from Louis Figuer's *Vies des Savants Moyen Age* (Scientists of the Middle Ages), published in Paris in 1867. | iStockphoto.com |

| Location | Image | Description | Source |
|---|---|---|---|
| Chapter 11 Page 321 | 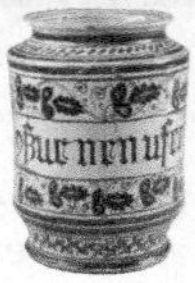 | Italian drug jar from circa 1490; the transcription translates as "water-lily juice," indicating its use as a medication storage vessel kept by an apothecary or doctor. | © Victoria and Albert Museum |
| Chapter 11 Page 322 | 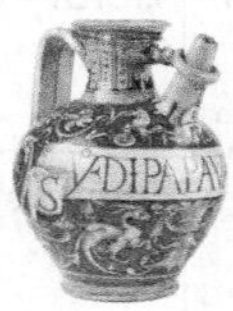 | The globular syrup jar from circa 1515 was a favorite form of drug vessel in Tuscany; the patriarchal cross above the heraldic shield indicates this jug was intended for a monastic pharmacy; the transcription indicates that this jar likely held papaver or opium alkaloids that were compounded into a liquid form. | © Victoria and Albert Museum |
| Chapter 11 Page 322 | 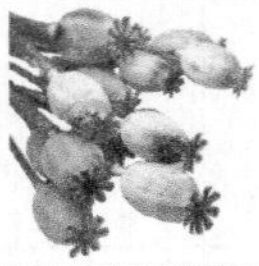 | A gathered bunch of dried poppyheads; opium and its derivatives have been utilized (and sometimes worshipped) in many cultures for thousands of years. | Shutterstock |
| Chapter 11 Page 322 | 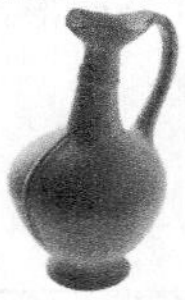 | Earthenware jug in the shape of an opium poppy exported from Cyprus; probably stored opium mixed with wine. | Courtesy of Science Museum of London |
| Chapter 11 Page 322 | 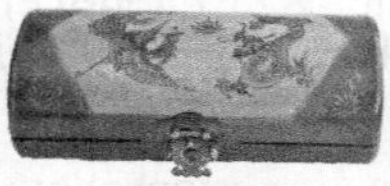 | Eastern opium box used to store paraphernalia or processed poppies; opium was a popular painkiller and recreational drug for many cultures, though is often associated with eighteenth- and nineteenth-century China. | Shutterstock |
| Chapter 11 Page 323 | 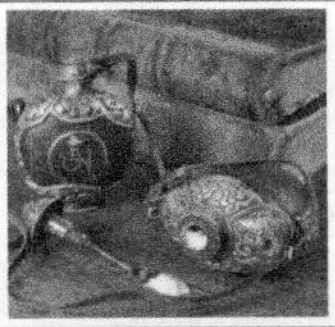 | Decorative vessel used to store powdered opium. | Shutterstock |
| Chapter 11 Page 323 | 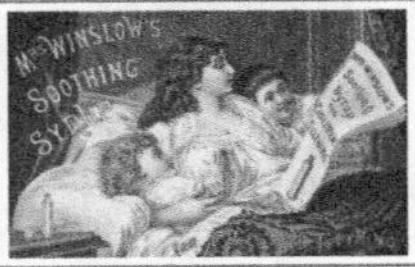 | Advertisement for Mrs. Winslow's Soothing Syrup, an opium-based preparation used to quiet fussy, teething, or colicky children. | Courtesy of the National Library of Medicine |
| Chapter 11 Page 323 | 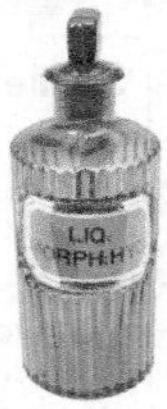 | Bottle of morphine (one of the most common and still-used products of opium), used to induce drowsiness and to alleviate pain. | Courtesy of Science Museum of London |
| Chapter 11 Page 323 | 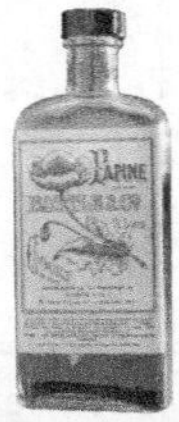 | Bottle of "Papine," an effective over-the-counter painkiller utilizing opium extracts. | Courtesy of Science Museum of London |
| Chapter 11 Page 324 | 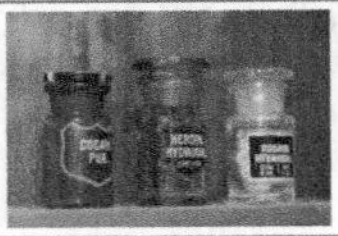 | Medicinal bottles of heroin and cocaine in an old pharmacy, dating from the late nineteenth century. | istockphoto.com |

| Location | Image | Description | Source |
|---|---|---|---|
| Chapter 11 Page 324 | 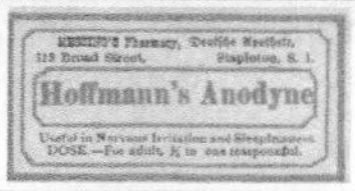  | Vintage label for Hoffman's Anodyne, a pain reliever and general soothing medication with unspecified ingredients. | Courtesy of Vintage Image Madness |
| Chapter 11 Page 324 | 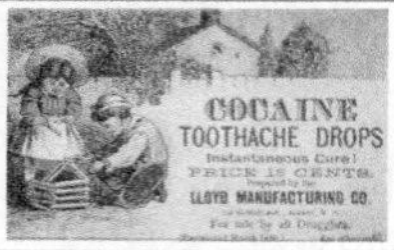  | An 1885 advertisement for toothache medication containing cocaine; the drops were produced by Lloyd Manufacturing Company. | Courtesy of the National Library of Medicine |
| Chapter 11 Page 325 | 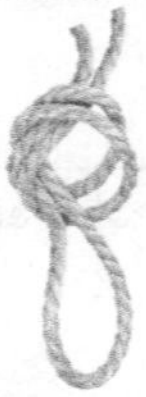 | Rope produced from hemp, the strong and popular fibrous material cultivated from the stems of the *Cannabis* plant. | Shutterstock |
| Chapter 11 Page 325 | 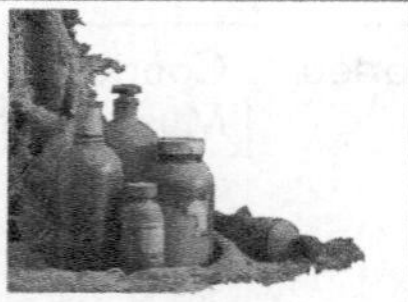 | Various dusty drug and liquid bottles resting on hemp canvas. | Shutterstock |
| Chapter 11 Page 326 | 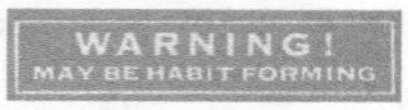  | Vintage warning label typical of those placed on certain drugs or medications in the early twentieth century, as the addictive properties of many substances were realized. | Courtesy of Vintage Image Madness |
| Chapter 11 Page 326 | 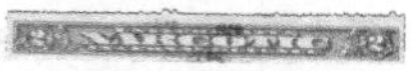 | Narcotic tax stamp issued between 1919 and 1927; the Harrison Narcotics Tax Act was implemented in 1914 to regulate and tax the production, importation, and distribution of opiates. | istockphoto.com |
| Chapter 12 Page 356 | 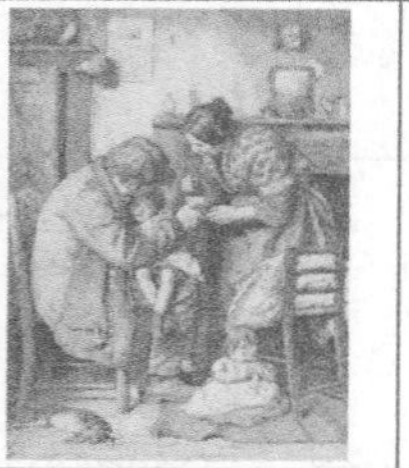 | Etched version by Joseph Clark of his own painting called *The Sick Child*, published in England circa 1858. | © Victoria and Albert Museum |
| Chapter 12 Page 357 | 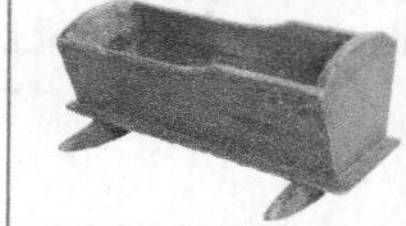 | Antique wooden infant bed, likely from the late nineteenth century; solid wooden cribs like this one were often designed to rock slowly and were passed through generations of a single family. | Shutterstock |
| Chapter 12 Page 358 | 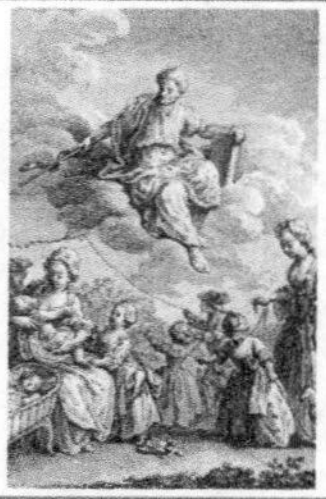 | Engraving from French artist Joseph Raulin, published in 1769 and depicting Aesculapius (Greek god of medicine), seated on a cloud holding a caduceus and book and observing the care of infants and children below. | Courtesy of the National Library of Medicine |
| Chapter 12 Page 358 | 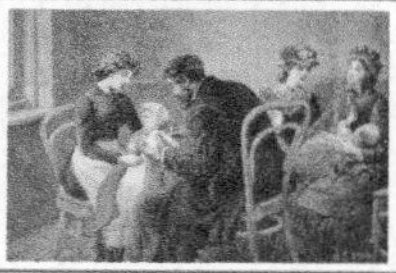 | *Vaccination from the Calf* by Charles Joseph Staniland, an engraving published in London in 1883 depicting the smallpox vaccination of two infants. | Courtesy of the National Library of Medicine |

| Location | Image | Description | Source |
|---|---|---|---|
| Chapter 12 Page 359 | 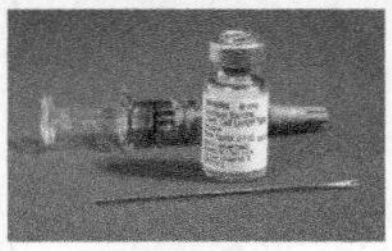 | A modern vial of a smallpox vaccine and a bifurcated needle; virtually erased from the modern world, smallpox was a deadly worldwide force prior to the pioneering work of Dr. Edward Jenner and the proliferation of the smallpox vaccine. | James Gathany/Centers for Disease Control and Prevention |
| Chapter 12 Page 359 | 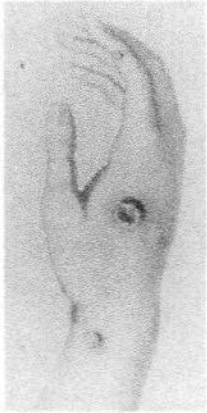 | Sketch drawn by Edward Jenner depicting the hand of the cowpox-infected dairymaid Jenner studied in his development of a smallpox vaccination. | Courtesy of the National Library of Medicine |
| Chapter 12 Page 359 | 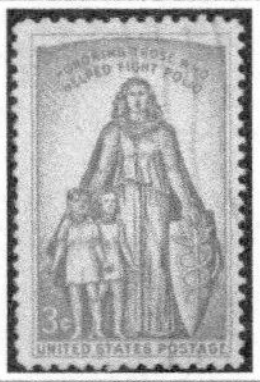 | A 1956 U.S. postage stamp dedicated to the doctors and caregivers working toward the eradication of polio. | istockphoto.com |
| Chapter 12 Page 360 | 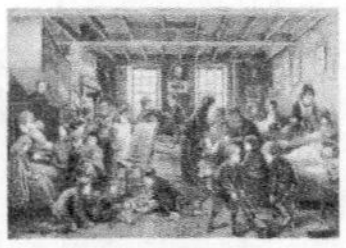 | An 1872 engraving of the East London Hospital for Children, an early pediatric hospital; prior to these dedicated facilities, sick and disabled children were often left in orphanages or churches in the hope that someone would care for them, but with little success. | Courtesy of the National Library of Medicine |
| Chapter 12 Page 360 | 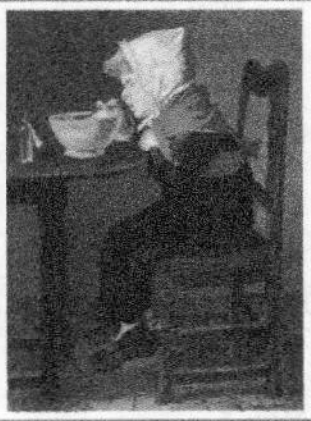 | Painting by W. Hunt titled *Rather Queer* depicting a sick and ill-tempered young boy forced to take his medicine; date unknown. | Courtesy of the National Library of Medicine |
| Chapter 12 Page 360 | 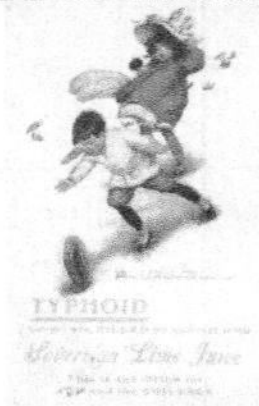 | A 1909 advertising poster for Sovereign Lime Juice, a remedy for typhoid, a historically destructive and painful disease linked to poor hygiene and public sanitation issues; contraction of the disease was greatly reduced by the development of vaccines and antibacterial medicines. | Courtesy of the National Library of Medicine |
| Chapter 12 Page 361 | 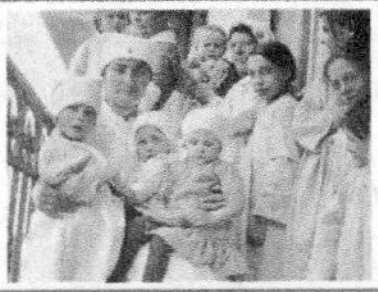 | Nurses and their young patients from the U.S. American National Red Cross Hospital in Evian, France, circa 1920. | Courtesy of the National Library of Medicine |
| Chapter 12 Page 361 | 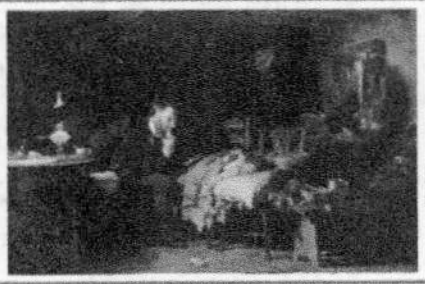 | Early twentieth-century oil painting by Sir Luke Fildes called *The Doctor*, depicting a worried doctor sitting at the bed of an ill child. | Courtesy of the National Library of Medicine |
| Chapter 12 Page 362 | 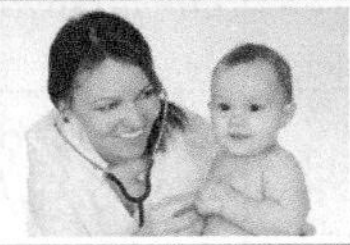 | Modern pediatrician and young patient; the existence of doctors dedicated to the health of infants and children has dramatically improved pediatric care. | Shutterstock |

| Location | Image | Description | Source |
|---|---|---|---|
| Chapter 12 Page 362 | 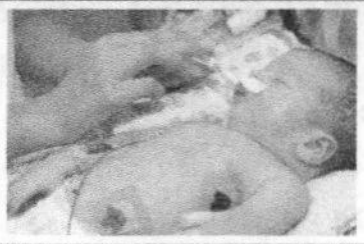 | Infant hospitalized in a neonatal intensive care unit and being supported by various IV and feeding tubes. | Shutterstock |
| Chapter 12 Page 362 | 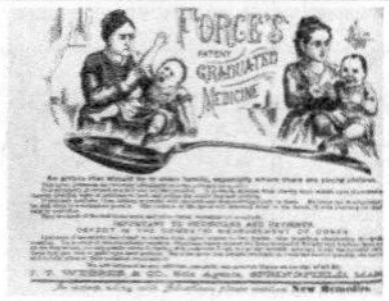 | An 1879 advertisement for Force's Patent Graduated Medicine Spoon, designed to make accurate dosing and effective administration much easier. | Courtesy of the National Library of Medicine |
| Chapter 12 Page 363 | 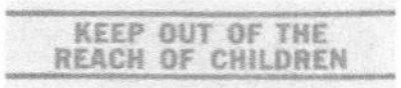 | Vintage medicine label from an unknown date, typical of warnings on strong or potentially poisonous medication, as the effects of most ingredients were not widely known. | Vintage Image Madness |
| Chapter 12 Page 363 | 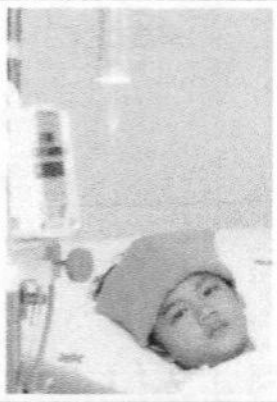 | Recovering child resting in a bed at a pediatric intensive care unit and assisted by IV fluid therapy. | Shutterstock |
| Chapter 13 Page 392 | 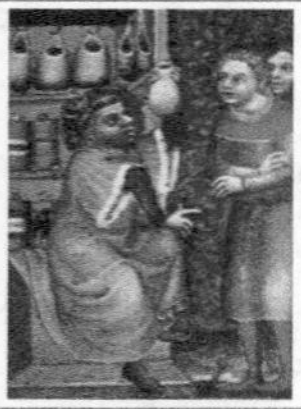 | Undated and untitled painting from the Middle Ages depicting an apothecary offering advice and medicine to an ailing customer. | Courtesy of the National Library of Medicine |
| Chapter 13 Page 393 | 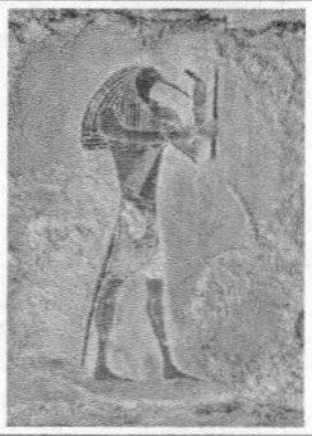 | Painted stone relief of Thoth, the powerful Egyptian god associated with the system of writing, development of science, and judgment of the dead; Thoth was considered to be the heart (which housed intelligence) and tongue of the sun god Ra; Thoth is occasionally pictured with the head of a baboon. | istockphoto.com |
| Chapter 13 Page 394 | 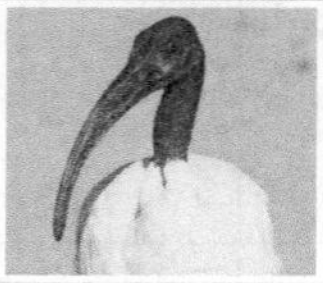 | African Sacred Ibis, the inspiration for the god Thoth and a revered creature in ancient Egypt; a common animal in Egyptian mythology, the ibis is also a potential inspiration for the first human use of enemas. | Shutterstock |
| Chapter 13 Page 394 | 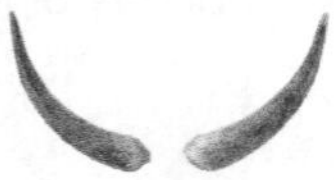 | Pair of bull horns; genuine horns grow around a bone core, creating a hollow cavity when the horn is removed and cleaned; horns have been used for thousands of years for drinking vessels, hand tools, musical instruments, and funnels, among other things. | istockphoto.com |
| Chapter 13 Page 394 | 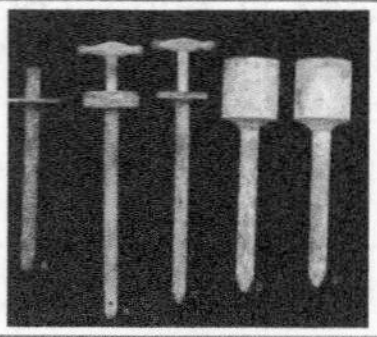 | Ancient Greek and Roman clyster syringes of the type available during the times of Hippocrates and Galen; these clysters are precursors to bulb syringes and other enema-delivery devices. | Courtesy of Historical Collections & Services, Claude Moore Health Sciences Library, University of Virginia |
| Chapter 13 Page 394 | 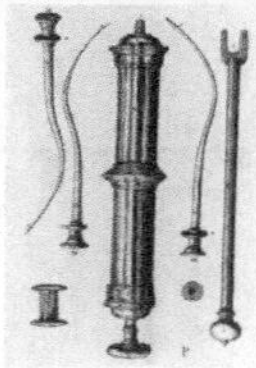 | Clyster syringe and various attachments detailed in an Italian medical text from 1648; it's possible that the attachments were used for administering different levels of liquid, or for self-administration. | Courtesy of the National Library of Medicine |

| Location | Image | Description | Source |
|---|---|---|---|
| Chapter 13 Page 395 | 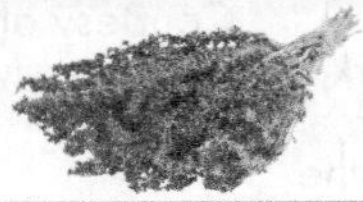 | Dried bunch of flowering sage; the many types of ornamental sage plants have had medical, cooking, and aromatic uses for thousands of years. | Shutterstock |
| Chapter 13 Page 395 | 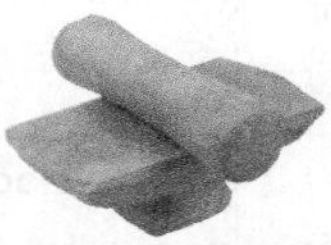 | Ancient mortar and pestle carved from local stone; unknown date and origin, though its simplicity hints at its use by a small village healer or apothecary. | Shutterstock |
| Chapter 13 Page 395 | 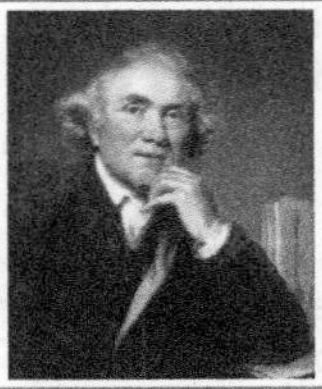 | Painted engraving of John Hunter, a famous scientist and medical thinker who, in 1790, became the first person to successfully administer a nasogastric feeding. | Courtesy of the National Library of Medicine |
| Chapter 13 Page 395 | 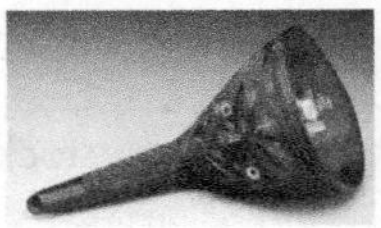 | Feeding funnel from the Maori culture of New Zealand, dating between 1890 and 1925; this carved wood funnel is inset with abalone shells and is known as a "Korere"; this funnel is designed to feed and medicate high-status individuals (such as a chief) when they have limited ability to consume food as a result of a facial tattooing ceremony. | Courtesy of the Science Museum of London |
| Chapter 13 Page 396 | 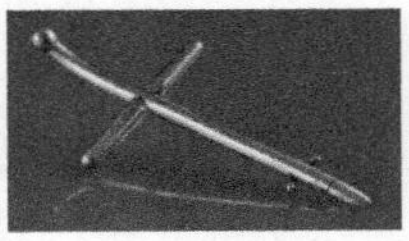 | Forcible feeding tube invented by English doctor Henry Blandford, dating from 1920; this feeding tube was used for the severely physically disabled or mentally ill people who refused food; the tube was inserted into the mouth and twisted so the cross bars held the mouth open while the food was poured down the throat. | Courtesy of the Science Museum of London |
| Chapter 13 Page 396 | 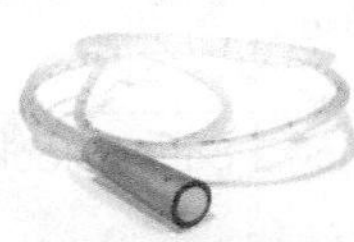 | Modern nasogastric or Levin tube; though now made from lightweight polyurethane, these tubes mimic the first Levin tubes made in the 1920s, allowing for nasogastric feeding and stomach content removal. | istockphoto.com |
| Chapter 13 Page 396 | 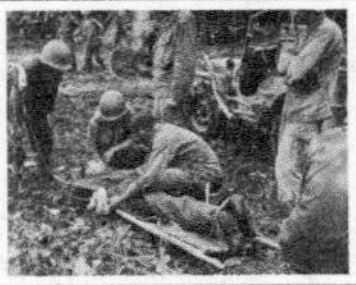 | An American soldier receiving TPN therapy after being wounded in World War II; though in the field in the Philippines, this soldier is assisted by lightweight and pre-packaged sterile supplies, allowing him to immediately receive essential nutrients. | Courtesy of the National Library of Medicine |
| Chapter 13 Page 397 | 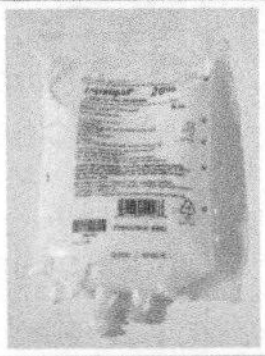 | A 500-mL bag of Intralipid 20% IV Fat Emulsion; utilizing the formula pioneered 50 years ago by Arvid Wretlind, this TPN ingredient is essential for providing balanced nutrient therapy. | © Paradigm Publishing |
| Chapter 13 Page 397 | 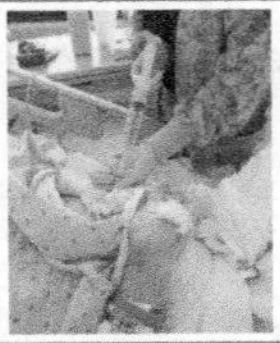 | Nurse giving a bolus (large dose of medication) feeding through a patient's gastrostomy tube; this type of modern G tube allows for TPN therapy in cases where enteral feeding is required over more than a few days; use of a G tube avoids extended patient discomfort with NG tubes. | © B. Slaven, MD / Custom Medical Stock Photo |
| Chapter 13 Page 398 | 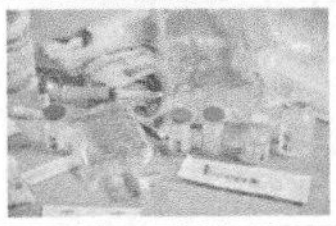 | Assorted supplies common to TPN therapy; though the processes of nutrient consumption and enteral feeding are well-understood, compounding TPN still requires intensive training and concentration. | George Brainard |

| Location | Image | Description | Source |
|---|---|---|---|
| Chapter 14 Page 444 | 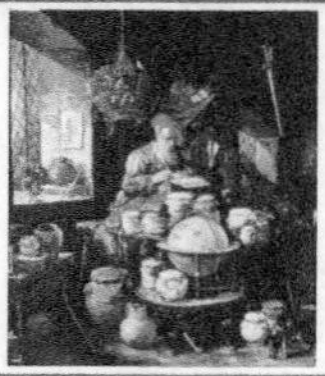 | Late seventeenth or early eighteenth century oil painting titled *An Alchemist in His Study*, by Egbert Van Heemskerk, a Dutch artist; the name belonged to a father and his son, both painters; their work is nearly indistinguishable from the other, leading to consistent confusion over the true creator of "his" many works. | Courtesy of the National Library of Medicine |
| Chapter 14 Page 445 | 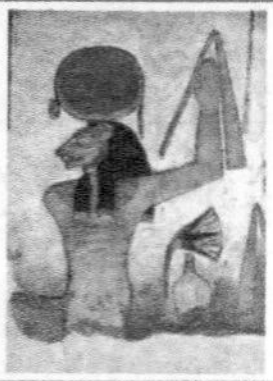 | Painted relief of Sekhmet, an important Egyptian deity depicted as a lioness and symbol of warriors and disease; it was said that the hot desert wind was her breath and that her wrath and pleasure brought deadly diseases and their cures (respectively) to those who worshipped her. | Shutterstock |
| Chapter 14 Page 446 | 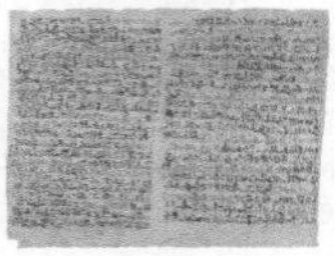 | Section of the Edwin Smith Papyrus, circa 1600 BCE; traded between collectors and museums for several hundred years, the papyrus was finally translated in 1930 and revealed medical knowledge that was largely free of the spiritual and magic content of similar known documents. | Public Domain |
| Chapter 14 Page 446 | 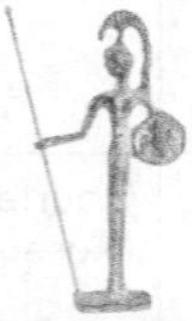 | Aged bronze sculpture of the Greek goddess Athena, the patron deity of Athens; Athena was a highly important figure, representing wisdom, strategic warfare, justice, and skill and was occasionally a source of prayers for medical knowledge and healing. | Shutterstock |
| Chapter 14 Page 446 | 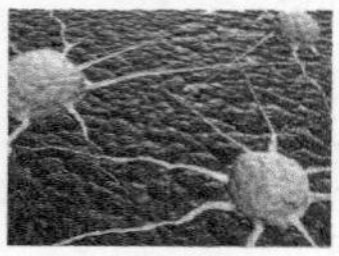 | Computer-illustrated cancer cells; although he only observed the appearance of tumors after they broke through the skin, Hippocrates made note of cancer's spreading, crab-like appendages, coining the name we use today for the disease. | Shutterstock |
| Chapter 14 Page 446 | 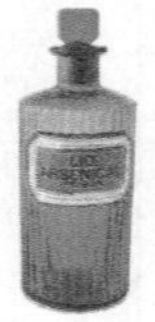 | Bottle of arsenic; called the "poison of kings" for its potency and difficulty in postmortem detection, arsenic has been used for thousands of years for medicine, cosmetics, rituals, ceremonies, and (in literature and dramatic history) stealthy murder in the halls and bedrooms of royalty. | Shutterstock |
| Chapter 14 Page 447 | 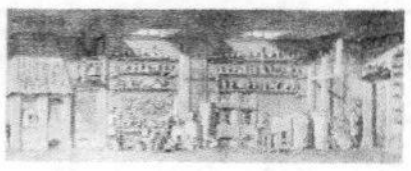 | Drawing of the early eighteenth-century London laboratory owned and operated by Ambrose Godfrey and Charles Cook; the successful businessmen operated the lab and adjoining pharmacy as town apothecaries and research scientists. | Courtesy of Fisher Scientific Co., Pittsburgh, and the National Library of Medicine |
| Chapter 14 Page 447 | 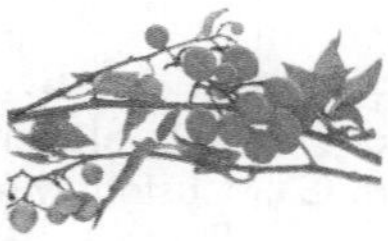 | Leaves and berries of belladonna or deadly nightshade, a popular medicine, cosmetic, and poison for thousands of years; deadly nightshade is one of the most toxic plants in the Western hemisphere; the consumption of 2 to 5 berries by children and 10 to 20 berries by adults can be lethal, and a single leaf is also fatal. | Shutterstock |
| Chapter 14 Page 447 | 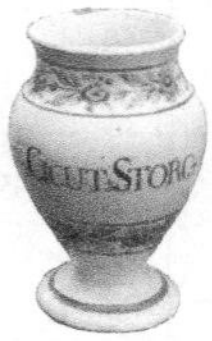 | Dispensing pot for hemlock extract, made in Italy between 1771 and 1830; this jar was used by apothecaries to store Störck's Extract of Hemlock, invented by Viennese medical professor Anton von Störck. | Courtesy of the Science Museum of London |

| Location | Image | Description | Source |
|---|---|---|---|
| Chapter 14 Page 447 | 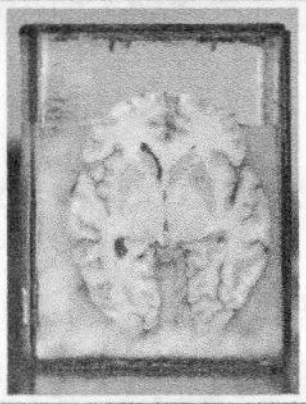 | Aged bisected section of a brain preserved in formaldehyde and glass; this object was recently discovered in an abandoned American mental hospital. | Shutterstock |
| Chapter 14 Page 448 | 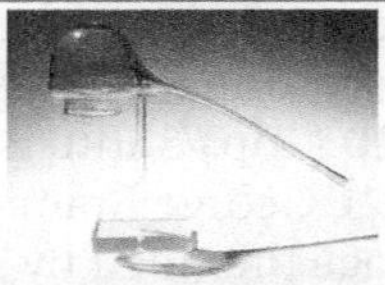 | German alembic cap from the nineteenth century; used by alchemists and scientists for thousands of years, the alembic cap is placed over a flask of heated material, so that rising steam enters the cap and then, as liquid, travels down the tube into another container. | © Victoria and Albert Museum |
| Chapter 14 Page 448 | 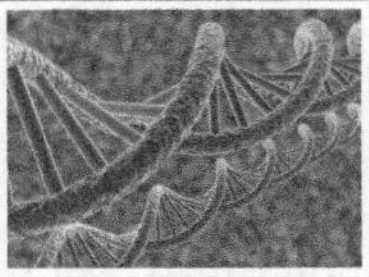 | Computerized representation of a DNA strand; the discovery of DNA and its properties was an essential landmark in medical science, allowing doctors and researchers to begin isolating genetic disease to their very origins. | Shutterstock |
| Chapter 14 Page 449 | 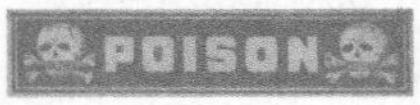 | Vintage poison label used by doctors and apothecaries on the many caustic substances used sparingly as medicine, such as arsenic, mercury, and hemlock. | Vintage Image Madness |
| Chapter 14 Page 449 | 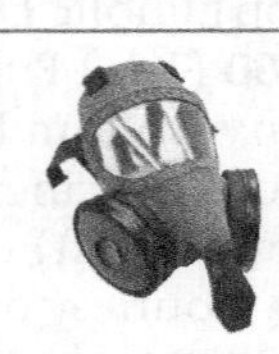 | Gas mask from the decades following World War II, most likely issued for civilian use; designed to protect the wearer from dangerous airborne substances such as nitrogen mustard; interestingly, such substances have potential medical benefits when used in small quantities and precise targeting, such as reducing the size and strength of a tumor. | istockphoto.com |
| Chapter 14 Page 449 | 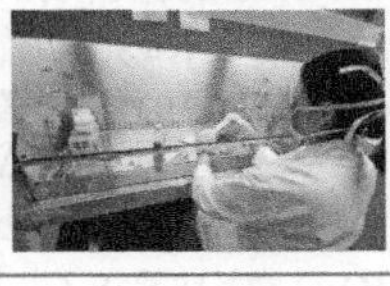 | Modern cancer research lab; research in highly controlled areas like state-of-the-art clean rooms have allowed scientists to study the effects of potentially dangerous caustic drugs on cancer cells, while being protected from the toxic chemicals. | Shutterstock |

# Photo Credits

**Photo Credits:** **1** (Right) Courtesy of the National Library of Medicine; (Left) Shutterstock; **2** (Top Left) Shutterstock; (Top Right) Shutterstock; (Middle) istockphoto.com; (Bottom) Courtesy of the National Library of Medicine; **3** (Top) istockphoto.com; (Middle) Shutterstock; (Bottom) istockphoto.com; **4** Courtesy of the National Library of Medicine; **5** Shutterstock; **6** (Top) Shutterstock; (Bottom Left) Shutterstock; (Bottom Right) Shutterstock; **7** (Top) George Brainard; (Bottom) George Brainard; **8** George Brainard; **9** George Brainard; **10** © United States Pharmacopeia; **14** George Brainard; **15** (Top) George Brainard; (Bottom) Courtesy of Vintage Image Madness; **16** George Brainard; **18** George Brainard; **25** istockphoto.com; **26** Courtesy of the National Library of Medicine; **27** Shutterstock; **28** (Top) Courtesy of the National Library of Medicine; (Bottom) istockphoto.com; **29** (Top) Courtesy of the National Library of Medicine; (Bottom) Oregon State University and the Oregon Nanoscience and Microtechnologies Institute; **30** George Brainard; **33** George Brainard; **34** George Brainard; **35** George Brainard; **39** George Brainard; **44** © United States Pharmacopeia; **46** George Brainard; **47** George Brainard; **51** istockphoto.com; **52** Courtesy of the National Library of Medicine; **53** Public Domain; **54** (Top) Courtesy of the National Library of Medicine; (Bottom) Courtesy of the National Library of Medicine; **55** (Top) Courtesy of the National Library of Medicine; (Middle) istockphoto.com; (Bottom) Shutterstock; **56** *Journal of the American Medical Association*, p. 68, 1926; **57** George Brainard; **59** (All) George Brainard; **60** (All) George Brainard; **61** George Brainard; **62** George Brainard; **63** (All) George Brainard; **64** George Brainard; **72** George Brainard; **74** © Paradigm Publishing; **75** © Paradigm Publishing; **76** George Brainard; **77** (All) George Brainard; **83** istockphoto.com; **84** Courtesy of the National Library of Medicine; **85** istockphoto.com; **86** (Left) Shutterstock; (Right) istockphoto.com; (Bottom Middle) Shutterstock; **87** (Top Left) © Paradigm Publishing; (Top Right) Courtesy of the National Library of Medicine; (Bottom Middle) Courtesy of Vintage Image Madness; **88** (Top) Courtesy of the National Library of Medicine; (Bottom Left) Shutterstock; (Bottom Middle) istockphoto.com; (Bottom Right) Shutterstock; **89** (Top) Courtesy of the National Library of Medicine; (Bottom) Courtesy of Science Museum London; **94** George Brainard; **103** © Paradigm Publishing; **105** George Brainard; **113** istockphoto.com; **114** Courtesy of the National Library of Medicine; **115** Shutterstock; **116** (Top Left) Shutterstock; (Middle) istockphoto.com; (Top Right) Image courtesy of Phisick Medical Antiques (www.phisick.com); (Bottom Right) Courtesy of Vintage Image Madness; **117** (Top Left) Courtesy of Science Museum London; (Middle Right) Shutterstock; (Bottom Left) Shutterstock; **118** (Top) Shutterstock; (Bottom) Courtesy of the National Library of Medicine; **119** Shutterstock; **120** (Top) Shutterstock; (Bottom) Shutterstock; **121** George Brainard; **122** George Brainard; **127** Image provided by APP Pharmaceuticals, LLC. Used with permission; **138** (All) © Paradigm Publishing; **144** George Brainard; **145** istockphoto.com; **155** istockphoto.com; **156** Courtesy of Science Museum London; **157** Courtesy of the National Library of Medicine; **158** (Top Left) Courtesy of the National Library of Medicine; (Top Right) Shutterstock; (Bottom) Courtesy of the National Library of Medicine; **159** (Top) Public Domain; (Bottom) Public Domain; **160** (Top) Public Domain; (Middle Left) Public Domain; (Bottom Right) Courtesy of the National Library of Medicine; **161** (Top Right) istockphoto.com; (Bottom Left) Courtesy of Vintage Image Madness; **164** Courtesy of the National Library of Medicine; **165** Shutterstock; **166** (Left) Public Domain; (Top Right) Shutterstock; (Bottom Right) © Victoria and Albert Museum; **167** (Top) Public Domain; (Middle) © Victoria and Albert Museum; **168** (Top) Courtesy of the National Library of Medicine; (Bottom) Photo courtesy of Tara Grosse; **169** (Left) © Victoria and Albert Museum; (Right) Public Domain; **171** (Top) istockphoto.com; (Bottom) George Brainard; **172** (Top) George Brainard; (Bottom) istockphoto.com; **174** (Top) Shutterstock; (Bottom) Shutterstock; **175** Shutterstock; **176** (Top) Shutterstock; (Bottom) George Brainard; **177** George Brainard; **178** George Brainard; **179** istockphoto.com; **180** George Brainard; **182** (All) George Brainard; **183** George Brainard; **187** istockphoto.com; **188** Courtesy of the National Library of Medicine; **189** Shutterstock; **190** (Top) © Victoria and Albert Museum; (Bottom) Shutterstock; **191** (Top) Courtesy of Vintage Image Madness; (Middle) Shutterstock; **192** (Top Left) Courtesy of Professor Brian J. Ford; (Top Right) Shutterstock; (Bottom) Courtesy of the National Library of Medicine; **193** (Top) Courtesy of the National Library of Medicine; (Bottom) Courtesy of Vintage Image Madness; **194** George Brainard; **195** George Brainard; **198** George Brainard; **199** George Brainard; **201** George Brainard; **205** (All) George Brainard; **209** istockphoto.com; **210** Courtesy of the National Library of Medicine; **211** Courtesy of the National Library of Medicine; **212** (Top) Public Domain; (Bottom)

Courtesy of the National Library of Medicine; **213** (Top) Public Domain; (Bottom) istockphoto.com; **214** (All) Courtesy of the National Library of Medicine; **219** George Brainard; **220** George Brainard; **224** George Brainard; **226** George Brainard; **227** (All) George Brainard; **230** George Brainard; **231** George Brainard; **232** George Brainard; **234** (All) George Brainard; **236** George Brainard; **237** George Brainard; **238** (All) George Brainard; **239** (All) George Brainard; **240** (All) George Brainard; **241** (All) George Brainard; **242** George Brainard; **249** istockphoto.com; **250** istockphoto.com; **251** Courtesy of Vintage Image Madness; (Top Right and Middle) Shutterstock; (Bottom) Courtesy of the National Library of Medicine; **253** (Top) Shutterstock; (Bottom Left) istockphoto.com; (Bottom Right) Shutterstock; **254** (Top) istockphoto.com; (Bottom) Shutterstock; **255** (Top) istockphoto.com; (Bottom) Courtesy of Vintage Image Madness; **256** (Top) Shutterstock; (Middle and Bottom) George Brainard; **259** © Allen W. Mathies, MD; **263** George Brainard; **265** George Brainard; **267** (All) George Brainard; **268** (All) George Brainard; **269** (All) George Brainard; **270** (Top) George Brainard; (Bottom Left) George Brainard; (Bottom Right) © Paradigm Publishing; **275** George Brainard; **276** (All) George Brainard; **278** (All) George Brainard; **280** (All) George Brainard; **281** (All) George Brainard; **287** istockphoto.com; **288** © Victoria and Albert Museum; **289** © Victoria and Albert Museum; **290** (Top) Photo credit: John Noltner/Carleton College Art Collection; (Bottom Left) Shutterstock; (Bottom Right) Photo by Julia Janssen; **291** (Top) Photo Credit: John Noltner/Carleton College Art Collection; (Bottom Left) Photo by Marie-Lan Nguyen; (Bottom Right) Courtesy of the National Library of Medicine; **292** (Middle Right) Shutterstock; (Bottom Left) Courtesy of Vintage Image Madness; **293** (All) Shutterstock; **294** (Top) Shutterstock; (Bottom) © Paradigm Publishing; **295** © Paradigm Publishing; **298** (All) © Paradigm Publishing; **299** © Paradigm Publishing; **300** © Paradigm Publishing; **302** George Brainard; **303** George Brainard; **304** (Top) Shutterstock; (Middle) George Brainard; **305** (All) George Brainard; **306** (All) © Paradigm Publishing; **308** George Brainard; **310** George Brainard; **311** George Brainard; **312** George Brainard; **313** (All) George Brainard; **314** (All) George Brainard; **319** istockphoto.com; **320** istockphoto.com; **321** © Victoria and Albert Museum; **322**(Top Left) © Victoria and Albert Museum; (Top Right) Courtesy of Science Museum London; (Bottom Left) Shutterstock; (Bottom Right) Shutterstock; **323** (Top) Shutterstock; (Bottom Left) Courtesy of the National Library of Medicine; (Bottom Middle) Courtesy of Science Museum London; (Bottom Right) Courtesy of Science Museum London; **324** (Top) istockphoto.com; (Middle) Courtesy of Vintage Image Madness; (Bottom) Courtesy of the National Library of Medicine; **325** (All) Shutterstock; **326** (Top) Courtesy of Vintage Image Madness; (Bottom) istockphoto.com; **327** (Top) istockphoto.com; (Bottom) Shutterstock; **328**; Public Domain; **329** (All) Shutterstock; **330** George Brainard; **331** (All) © Paradigm Publishing; **333** Public Domain; **336** (All) © Paradigm Publishing; **338** (Top) George Brainard; (Bottom) istockphoto.com; **339** © Paradigm Publishing; **340** (Top) istockphoto.com; (Bottom) George Brainard; **345** George Brainard; **349** © Paradigm Publishing; **355** istockphoto.com; **356** © Victoria and Albert Museum; **357** Shutterstock; **358** (All) Courtesy of the National Library of Medicine; **359** (Top) James Gathany/Centers for Disease Control and Prevention; (Bottom Left) Courtesy of the National Library of Medicine; (Bottom Right) istockphoto.com; **360** (All) Courtesy of the National Library of Medicine; **361** (All) Courtesy of the National Library of Medicine; **362** (Top Left) Shutterstock; (Top Right) Shutterstock; (Bottom) Courtesy of the National Library of Medicine; **363** (Top) Courtesy of Vintage Image Madness; (Bottom) Shutterstock; **364** (Top) Shutterstock; (Bottom) istockphoto.com; **365** istockphoto.com; **366** (Middle Left) istockphoto.com; (Bottom Left) Shutterstock; **367** (Top) © Paradigm Publishing; (Bottom) alwardoc/photobucket; **368** Shutterstock; **369** Shutterstock; **371** George Brainard; **372** Image Courtesy of Teva Pharmaceuticals. Used with permission; **372** © Paradigm Publishing; **375** George Brainard; **376** George Brainard; **377** © Paradigm Publishing; **379** Image Courtesy of Teva Pharmaceuticals. Used with permission; **382** (All) George Brainard; **383** (All) George Brainard; **384** George Brainard; **385** (All) George Brainard; **386** © Paradigm Publishing; **391** istockphoto.com; **392** Courtesy of the National Library of Medicine; **393** istockphoto.com; **394** (Top) Shutterstock; (Middle) Courtesy of Historical Collections & Services, Claude Moore Health Sciences Library, University of Virginia; (Bottom Left) istockphoto.com; (Bottom Right) Courtesy of the National Library of Medicine; **395** (Middle Right) Courtesy of the National Library of Medicine; (Middle Left) Shutterstock; (Bottom Left) Shutterstock; (Bottom Right) Courtesy of Science Museum of London; **396** (Top Right) istockphoto.com; (Middle Left) Courtesy of Science Museum of London; (Bottom Right) Courtesy of the National Library of Medicine; **397** (Middle) © Paradigm Publishing; (Bottom Right) © B. Slaven, MD/Custom Medical Stock Photo; **398** George Brainard; **400** Shutterstock; **401** istockphoto.com; **403** © Paradigm Publishing; **404** © Paradigm Publishing; **405** (Top) © Tova Wiegand Green; (Bottom) George Brainard; **406** Public Domain; **409** istockphoto.com; **412** (Top) © Paradigm Publishing; (Bottom) George

Brainard; **416** (All) © Paradigm Publishing; **417** © Paradigm Publishing; **418** © Paradigm Publishing; **420** © Paradigm Publishing; **421** (All) © Paradigm Publishing; **422** © Paradigm Publishing; **423** (Top Middle and Top Right) © Paradigm Publishing; (Bottom) George Brainard; **424** © Paradigm Publishing; **428** George Brainard; **430** © Paradigm Publishing; **431** © Paradigm Publishing; **432** istockphoto.com; **433** George Brainard; **434** George Brainard; **443** istockphoto.com; **444** Courtesy of the National Library of Medicine; **445** Shutterstock; **446** (Top Left) Public Domain; (Top Middle) Shutterstock; (Middle) Shutterstock; (Bottom Right) Shutterstock; **447** (Top) Courtesy of the National Library of Medicine; (Middle Left) Shutterstock; (Middle) Courtesy of Science Museum of London; (Bottom Right) Shutterstock; **448** (Middle Right) Shutterstock; (Bottom Left) © Victoria and Albert Museum; **449** (Top Right) Courtesy of Vintage Image Madness; (Bottom Left) istockphoto.com; (Bottom Right) Shutterstock; **451** istockphoto.com; **454** istockphoto.com; **456** (All) George Brainard; **457** (Top Right) istockphoto.com; (Bottom Right) George Brainard; **459** (Top Right and Middle Right) © Paradigm Publishing; (Bottom) Shutterstock; **460** Shutterstock; **461** Shutterstock; **465** (All) © Paradigm Publishing; **466** (All) © Paradigm Publishing; **467** (Top) George Brainard; (Bottom) © Paradigm Publishing; **468** (Top) © Paradigm Publishing; (Bottom) Shutterstock; **474** (All) © Paradigm Publishing; **475** George Brainard; **476** © Paradigm Publishing; **477** © Paradigm Publishing; **480** George Brainard; **481** George Brainard; **483** Shutterstock; **484** © Paradigm Publishing; **486** George Brainard; **487** © Paradigm Publishing; **496** istockphoto.com;

# Index

Page numbers with *f* indicate figures and page numbers with t indicate tables

## A

## B

## D



## E

## F



## G



## H

## I

## M

## N



## O

## P

## Q



## R

## S

## T

## U



## V



## W



## X



## Y



## Z